Postoperative Pain
Management

Postoperative Pain Management

Edited by

F. Michael Ferrante, M.D.

Assistant Professor, Department of Anaesthesia
Harvard Medical School
Director, Pain Management Center
Department of Anesthesia
Brigham and Women's Hospital
Boston, Massachusetts

Timothy R. VadeBoncouer, M.D.

Instructor, Department of Anaesthesia
Harvard Medical School
Staff Anesthesiologist, Pain Management Center
Brigham and Women's Hospital
Boston, Massachusetts
Currently:
Assistant Professor, Department of Anesthesiology
University of Illinois College of Medicine
Staff Anesthesiologist
West Side Veterans Administration Medical Center
Chicago, Illinois

Churchill Livingstone
New York, Edinburgh, London, Melbourne, Tokyo

Library of Congress Cataloging-in-Publication Data

Postoperative Pain Management / edited by F. Michael Ferrante, Timothy
  R. VadeBoncouer.
     p.   cm.
  Includes bibliographical references and index.
  ISBN 0-443-08766-0
  1. Postoperative pain. 2. Postoperative pain—Treatment.
  3. Postoperative pain—Chemotherapy. 4. Analgesia I. Ferrante,
  F. Michael. II. VadeBoncouer, Timothy R.
  [DNLM: 1. Pain, Postoperative—therapy. WO 184 P8577]
  RD98.4.P67 1993
  617'.919—dc20
  DNLM/DLC
  for Library of Congress   92-49446
                                           CIP

© **Churchill Livingstone Inc. 1993**

Distributed in the United Kingdom by Churchill Livingstone, Robert Stevenson House, 1–3 Baxter's Place, Leith Walk, Edinburgh EH1 3AF, and by associated companies, branches, and representatives throughout the world.

Accurate indications, adverse reactions, and dosage schedules for drugs are provided in this book, but it is possible that they may change. The reader is urged to review the package information data of the manufacturers of the medications mentioned.

The Publishers have made every effort to trace the copyright holders for borrowed material. If they have inadvertently overlooked any, they will be pleased to make the necessary arrangements at the first opportunity.

Acquisitions Editor: *Nancy Mullins*
Copy Editor: *Barbara L. B. Storey*
Production Designer: *Maryann King*
Production Supervisor: *Sharon Tuder*
Cover Design: *Paul Moran*

Printed in the United States of America

First published in 1993   7 6 5 4 3 2 1

To Susan:

Two roads diverged in a Southern woods,
And sorry we could not travel both
And be one partner, as it may,
So you traveled with the young academic
Throughout the lands of the Yankee,
And that has made all the difference.
I sometimes think you do not realize
How none of this is possible without you.

Michael

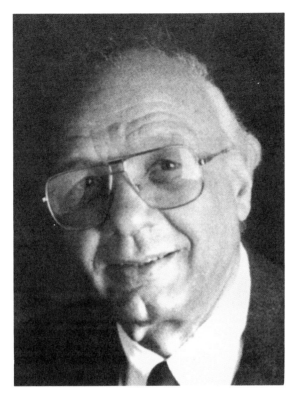

To the memory of
Benjamin G. Covino, Ph.D., M.D.
Teacher, Scholar, Administrator, Friend,
who had the wisdom to realize
that the place for the anesthesiologist
was also outside the operating room.

The editors would like to express their appreciation to Ken Bates, Amy Boches, and Diane Raeke for their artistic talents in the preparation of this book and to Heather Santosuosso for her typing skills.

Contributors

Simon C. Body, M.B. Ch.B., F.F.A.R.A.C.S.
Instructor, Department of Anaesthesia, Harvard Medical School; Associate Director
of Thoracic Anesthesia, Co-Director, Lung Transplant Anesthesia, Department of
Anesthesia, Brigham and Women's Hospital, Boston, Massachusetts

Daniel B. Carr, M.D.
Associate Professor, Departments of Anaesthesia and Medicine (Endocrinology),
Harvard Medical School; Director, Division of Pain Management, Department of
Anesthesia, Massachusetts General Hospital, Boston, Massachusetts

M. Soledad Cepeda, M.D.
Assistant Professor, Department of Anesthesia, Javeriana University School of
Medicine; Chief, Pain Unit, Department of Anesthesia, San Ignacio Hospital, Santa
Fe de Bogota, Colombia

Vincent W.S. Chan, M.D., F.R.C.P.C.
Assistant Professor, Department of Anesthesiology, University of Toronto Faculty of
Medicine, Toronto, Ontario, Canada

Mercedes Concepcion, M.D.
Assistant Professor, Department of Anaesthesia, Harvard Medical School; Director of
Orthopaedic Anesthesia, Department of Anesthesia, Brigham and Women's Hospital,
Boston, Massachusetts

Benjamin G. Covino, Ph.D., M.D.*
Professor, Department of Anaesthesia, Harvard Medical School; Chairman,
Department of Anesthesia, Brigham and Women's Hospital, Boston, Massachusetts

Gilbert J. Fanciullo, M.D.
Instructor, Department of Anaesthesia, Harvard Medical School; Staff
Anesthesiologist, Pain Management Center, Department of Anesthesia, Brigham
and Women's Hospital, Boston, Massachusetts

* Deceased

F. Michael Ferrante, M.D.
Assistant Professor, Department of Anaesthesia, Harvard Medical School; Director, Pain Management Center, Department of Anesthesia, Brigham and Women's Hospital, Boston, Massachusetts

John A. Fox, M.D.
Instructor, Department of Anaesthesia, Harvard Medical School; Staff Anesthesiologist, Department of Anesthesia, Brigham and Women's Hospital, Boston, Massachusetts

Phyllis Hoopman, M.S.N., R.N.
Director of Surgical Nursing, Department of Nursing, Brigham and Women's Hospital, Boston, Massachusetts

Niall Hughes, M.B., F.F.A.R.C.S.I.
Instructor, Department of Anaesthesia, Harvard Medical School; Staff Anesthesiologist, Department of Anesthesia, Brigham and Women's Hospital, Boston, Massachusetts

Robert N. Jamison, Ph.D.
Instructor, Departments of Anaesthesia and Psychiatry, Harvard Medical School; Staff Psychologist, Pain Management Service, Brigham and Women's Hospital, Boston, Massachusetts

Nathaniel Katz, M.D.
Instructor, Department of Anesthesia, Harvard Medical School; Staff Neurologist, Pain Management Center, Department of Anesthesia, Brigham and Women's Hospital, Boston, Massachusetts

Elisabeth Kay, M.S.W., B.C.D.
Senior Clinical Social Worker, Pain Management Center, Department of Anesthesia, Brigham and Women's Hospital, Boston, Massachusetts

Phillip Kistler, M.D.
Instructor, Department of Anaesthesia, Harvard Medical School; Staff Anesthesiologist, Pain Management Center, Department of Anesthesia, Brigham and Women's Hospital, Boston, Massachusetts

Edward M. Le Sage
Account Executive, SJ Professional Associates, Inc., Brookline, Massachusetts

Leonard J. Lind, M.D., F.C.C.M.
Assistant Professor, Department of Anaesthesia, Harvard Medical School; Anesthesiologist and Director, P.A.C.U. (Post Anesthesia Care Unit), Department of Anesthesia, Brigham and Women's Hospital, Boston, Massachusetts

Beth Minzter, M.D., M.S.

Instructor, Department of Anaesthesia, Harvard Medical School; Staff Anesthesiologist, Pain Management Center, Department of Anesthesia, Brigham and Women's Hospital, Boston, Massachusetts

P. Prithvi Raj, M.D., M.B.B.S., F.F.A.

Clinical Professor, Department of Anesthesiology, Medical College of Georgia School of Medicine, Augusta, Georgia; Executive Medical Director, Southeastern Pain Institute, Georgia Baptist Medical Center, Atlanta, Georgia

Navil F. Sethna, M.D.

Assistant Clinical Professor, Department of Anaesthesia, Harvard Medical School; Associate in Anesthesia, Associate Director of Pain Treatment Service, Department of Anesthesia and Pain Treatment Service, Children's Hospital, Boston, Massachusetts

Timothy R. VadeBoncouer, M.D.

Instructor, Department of Anaesthesia, Harvard Medical School; Staff Anesthesiologist, Pain Management Center, Brigham and Women's Hospital, Boston, Massachusetts; *Currently:* Assistant Professor, Department of Anesthesiology, University of Illinois College of Medicine; Staff Anesthesiologist, West Side Veterans Administration Medical Center, Chicago, Illinois

Preface

I am an analgesiologist. It sounds a bit awkward at first, but the name does grow on you, in time. How can I call myself an anesthesiologist when the majority of my practice is spent outside the operating room? It is good to know who and what you are, for the day-to-day practice of acute pain management is radically different from life within the operating room setting. While having its foundations in anesthesiology, acute pain management has little to do with the practice of anesthesia, but it has much to do with the practice of regional analgesia and applied analgesic pharmacology.

This important distinction is made uniformly throughout this book. Regional techniques are referred to as "anesthestics" only in the context of their administration for operative anesthesia. When administered for postoperative pain management, these techniques are referred to as "analgesics." When used in the generic sense, or when the distinction becomes blurred (e.g., thoracic epidural administration of local anesthetic and opioid with a segmental anesthetic level to pinprick), the appellation "anesthesia/analgesia" has been used.

As I am an analgesiologist, I believe in balanced analgesia. Balanced analgesia is the use of pharmacologic agents and regional analgesic techniques to discretely affect the individual physiologic processes involved in nociception: transduction, transmission, and modulation. Thus, unimodal techniques used in isolation (intravenous patient-controlled analgesia with opioids, or epidural opioids, or continuous epidural infusions of local anesthestics) may provide pain relief, but there is little data to suggest any beneficial effects upon outcome. The use of analgesics should be likened to a symphony, not a solo performance. All agents act in concert to produce analgesia, but also, perhaps, facilitation of mobilization and shortened convalescence.

Such a philosophic conceptualization of postoperative analgesic care may not always be apparent in this book. Some topics are discussed in complete isolation. This is mainly derived from ease of presentation rather than any assertion that a particular modality should not be used in concert with other analgesics. The primacy of balanced analgesia as a framework for analgesic care must always be remembered.

As an analgesiologist, I believe that regional analgesia forms the cornerstone of any effective treatment plan. It is only through the use of regional anesthetic/analgesic techniques that the neuroendocrine response to surgery may be affected (Chapter 4) and central hypersensitization and other neuroplastic changes within the spinal cord (Chapter 12) can be prevented or ameliorated. While the concept of preemptive analgesia (Chapter 12) is enticing, it is hard to imagine how the single administration of any agent could prevent both the morphologic and physiologic changes within the spinal cord induced by the afferent nociceptive barrage attendant on surgery. However, the combination of effective regional anesthesia with potent, continuous, postoperative regional analgesia and adjunctive noninvasive analgesics holds the promise of truly affecting outcome and shortening time of convalescence.

As an analgesiologist, I believe in changing the world. Too many practitioners are still looking for something akin to Ehrlich's "silver bullet," the one analgesic that will make all patients totally comfortable with a single injection. To look for such a modality is human. The realization must be reached, however, that the gate control theory of pain and all that we have learned regarding nociception points to a multimodal approach for effective pain management.

The concept of the analgesiologist does not in any way denigrate anesthesiology or anesthesiologists. On the contrary, the organized management of postoperative pain expands the role of the anesthesiologist. I was recently asked by a national group of rheumatologists to consult with them on a number of issues regarding pain. As I was introduced to each member of the panel, I was repeatedly introduced as "the analgesiologist." At first it seemed awkward, but the term was met with respect and gratitude for the presence of someone knowledgeable in pain management. All too often in the past, anesthesiology has been viewed as service-oriented and procedural in nature. Here was a group of rheumatologists who avidly sought out an anesthesiologist who was versed in pain management, not for procedural talents, but rather for thoughts and opinions. Perhaps anesthesiology has come of age.

F. Michael Ferrante, M.D.

Contents

III. Regional Anesthesia/Analgesia

IV. Nonpharmacologic Techniques

V. Surgical Subspecialties

VI. Establishment and Administration of an Acute Pain Service

VII. Analgesics in Development

1

The Problem of Postoperative Pain: An Epidemiologic Perspective

P. Prithvi Raj

Even a brief review of the pertinent literature reveals a pervasive dissatisfaction with the adequacy of postoperative pain management. The traditional technique of intramuscular administration of a fixed dose of opioid given on a fixed schedule or an as-needed basis has been rather roundly deplored. The extent of undertreatment continues to appear significant. Yet, appropriate therapeutic agents and techniques are not lacking. A variety of powerful drugs exists whose efficacy has been well established, and investigations into new routes and methods of administration have achieved some noteworthy successes.

Postoperative pain *can* be effectively managed in any individual case. The problem is that it is *not* being effectively managed in many cases. The theoretic simplicity of managing a single case belies the complexity of the problem as a whole. The general lack of clarity and consensus on such crucial areas as pain measurement, variability of response to analgesics, the incidence, causes and sequelae of uncontrolled postoperative pain, and manpower availability have combined to effectively defy a satisfactory solution.

HISTORIC BACKGROUND

A review of the historic background of current anesthetic and analgesic practice need not be extensive: a small number of significant developments have produced today's state of the art. In 1806, Friedrich Wilhelm Adam Sertürner isolated the active constituent (alkaloid) of opium. The pain-relieving properties of the opium poppy had already been recognized for centuries. Sertürner first named his new alkaloid *principium somniferum* but later changed it to *morphine*, after Morpheus, the Greek god of dreams.[1] The development of the syringe and hollow needle in the 1850s enabled physicians to dispense measured amounts of morphine. William T. G. Morton, a Boston dentist, demonstrated the effectiveness of ether as a general anesthetic in 1846, and the next year, James Simpson tried chloroform as a substitute for ether. Cocaine was recognized as a powerful local anesthetic in 1884.[2]

By enabling ever more aggressive surgical interventions, these and other related developments set the stage for existence of postoperative pain on a grand scale. Without the continuous evolution of therapeutic agents and surgical expertise, disease- and injury-related mortality would not be nearly as controllable as they are today. Yet, postoperative pain would not be so pervasive a problem either.

With the birth of effective anesthesia in the middle of the 19th century, it was not long before postoperative pain was recognized as a discipline worthy of attention in its own right. In the early 1900s, George Crile suggested that control of postoperative pain could favorably influence the results of surgery.[3]

Meperidine was introduced in 1938. By the late 1940s, postanesthesia recovery units were well established.[4] This period of the late 1940s is seen by some as the origin of modern anesthesia, and the expansion of surgical practice did not take long to produce a flurry of concern regarding postoperative pain.

With respect to present intellectual ferment, Ferrante and Covino[5] identified a group of 18 papers forming a core body of literature relating to the inadequacy of conventional intramuscular opioid regimens (Table 1-1). These papers span the time period from 1952 through 1987, with the largest number appearing during the 1980s. The continued growing perception of the inadequacy of postoperative pain management indicates that a more coordinated and effective approach is about to emerge.

Most criticisms of current practice are directed against the traditional approach to postoperative pain management: intramuscular injection of a fixed dose of opioid on a fixed or *pro re nata* (prn) schedule. It must be recognized that this approach still has a number of powerful advantages (besides the fact that it can sometimes actually work): (1) it is familiar practice for physicians and hospital staff, thus making it relatively safe in terms of avoiding excess morbidity and mortality; (2) no special support equipment is required, thus avoiding the requirements for expensive equipment along with the personnel and training required to use it, and (3) the gradual onset of analgesia attendant to intramuscular administration allows ample time to monitor the recipient for the appearance of side effects.[24] The power of these advantages must not be

TABLE 1-1. "Core" Literature Concerning the Inadequacy of Conventional Opioid Regimens

Authors	Inadequate Analgesia (%)[a]	Reference
Papper, Brodie, Rovenstine[6]	33	Surgery 32:107, 1952
Lasagna, Beecher[7]	33	JAMA 156:230, 1954
Keats[8]	26–53	J Chronic Dis 4:72, 1956
Keeri-Szanto, Heaman[9]	20	Surg Gynecol Obstet 134:647, 1972
Cronin, Redfern, Utting[10]	47	Br J Anaesth 45:879, 1973
Marks, Sachar[11]	73	Ann Intern Med 78:173, 1973
Banister[12]	12–26	Anaesthesia 29:158, 1974
Austin, Stapleton, Mather[13]		Pain 8:47, 1980
Austin, Stapleton, Mather[14]		Anesthesiology 53:460, 1980
Cohen[15]	75	Pain 9:265, 1980
Tamsen et al[16]		Clin Pharmacokinet 7:164, 1982
Tamsen et al[17]		Clin Pharmacokinet 7:252, 1982
Dahlström et al[18]		Clin Pharmacokinet 7:266, 1982
Tamsen et al[19]		Pain 13:171, 1982
Donovan[20]	31	Anaesth Intensive Care 11:125, 1983
Sriwatanakul et al[21]	41	JAMA 250:926, 1983
Weis et al[22]		Anesth Analg 62:70, 1983
Donovan, Dillon, McGuire[23]	58	Pain 30:69, 1987

[a] Percentage of proband group demonstrating inadequate analgesia.
(Data from Ferrante and Covino.[5])

underestimated, as they speak to the major areas of concern regarding postoperative pain management: safety, cost, and concern over side effects.

Despite these advantages, a litany of deficiencies has been ascribed to conventional postoperative pain management.

Smith[25] advanced the following reasons for inadequate postoperative pain control by the conventional method:

1. Postoperative patient management is often delegated to junior staff;
2. Fear of drug addiction and/or side effects (especially respiratory depression) has led nursing staff to withhold medication;
3. The task of adequately measuring pain is difficult (see Ch. 6);
4. Adjustment of dosage to achieve a measured effect is difficult.

Rawal's list[26] is a similarly broad indictment:

1. Variability of individual analgesic requirements leads to over- and undermedication;
2. Consequent fluctuation in blood levels creates similar patterns of inadequate analgesia and sedation;
3. Pain is enhanced by the delay between a patient's request and drug administration;
4. Excessive worry over side effects and the potential for addiction leads to undermedication.

In an editorial, Hug[27] also cataloged a number of factors conspiring to make the use of conventional intramuscular regimens less than optimal:

1. Excessive concerns regarding respiratory depression and the potential for addiction lead to undermedication;
2. Restrictive legislation attempting to control drug use has encouraged physicians to order fixed doses at fixed intervals;
3. Reliance on "routine" orders to save time sacrifices individualization of dosage and effective analgesia.

The consensus regarding the deficiencies of conventional postoperative pain management and the multifactorial nature of those deficiencies holds invaluable clues to the beginning of a solution to the problem. However, before analyzing some of these factors in greater detail, it seems advantageous to discuss the extent and severity of the problem of postoperative pain to provide an epidemiologic perspective.

SIZE AND SCOPE OF THE PROBLEM

A precise determination of the incidence, prevalence, and severity of postoperative pain is hampered by the innate difficulty of measuring pain. Indeed, this single factor can legitimately be seen as the foundation for the extent of inadequate pain control. Given this handicap, alternative sources of epidemiologic information on the problem of postoperative pain are (1) individual investigations documenting the incidence, prevalence, and severity of postoperative pain in selected populations, (2) more indirect yet still powerful epidemiologic data on the numbers and types of surgical procedures (and, by implication, the potential extent of the problem), (3) studies attempting to characterize the natural history of postoperative pain, and (4) comparison studies of conventional regimens with newer analgesic techniques.

Incidence from Investigations

The study by Marks and Sachar[11] in 1973 is probably the single most important investigation that has served to renew interest in the management of pain. Based on a survey of 37 patients requiring opioid analgesia, these investigators found that 32 percent continued to suffer severe distress from pain whereas 41 percent reported continuing moderate distress. The authors attributed the poor results to a general lack of sophistication regarding analgesic usage and an exaggerated apprehension of the dangers of addiction. Although these were medical inpatients, the relevance to postoperative pain management is clear.

Numerous other authors corroborate the extent of the problem of unrelieved pain (Table 1-1). The reported percentage of patients experiencing significant postoperative pain will vary from author to author. However, review of the literature as a whole shows that, on the average, one-third to one-half of surgical patients experience significant postoperative pain (Table 1-1).

Investigations involving children have generally corroborated the extent of undertreatment while highlighting the special problems that attend postoperative analgesia in that population. The report by Mather and Mackie[28] is replete with ominous implications. The investigators analyzed the incidence of postoperative pain in 170 children in two different teaching hospitals, finding 25 percent of patients to be pain-free on the day of surgery and 13 percent reporting severe pain. Fifty-three percent were pain-free on the first postoperative day and 17 percent reported severe pain. Overall, 48 percent of medicated patients reported moderate or severe pain at one time or another.

Beyer et al[29] compared the postoperative prescription and administration of analgesics after cardiac surgery in 50 children and 50 adults. In comparison with the adults, children were both prescribed and received fewer potent analgesics. Six children had no postoperative analgesics prescribed. Overall, children received 30 percent of all analgesic administrations, while adults received 70 percent. On the fifth postoperative day, only half as many children as adults had analgesics available for use. Such scenarios reflect the deficiencies inherent in the conventional management of pediatric postoperative pain.

Incidence of Surgery

In the United States, no less than 25.6 million surgical procedures were performed in 1987 (a rate of 10,616.2 per 100,000 population per year, or slightly more than 1 person in 10).[30] A considerable portion of those procedures were of sufficient magnitude to obviously be expected to produce significant postoperative pain: 655,000 hysterectomies, 536,000 cholecystectomies, and 308,000 gastrectomies with intestinal resection.[30] These figures are doubtless conservative, as they were derived from survey data from short-stay hospitals. Furthermore, the rate of surgical procedures has undoubtedly been affected more recently by various cost-control measures. Such statistics, however, demonstrate the large numbers of patients who could potentially suffer from inadequate postoperative pain management.

Investigations of the Natural History of Postoperative Pain

With wide recognition of the highly subjective nature of pain and the apparent extent of its undertreatment, it is not surprising that few papers specifically attempt to define the natural history of postoperative pain. The nature, extent, location of surgery, and psychological makeup of the patient are obviously relevant factors. Although there does not appear to be a ready formula for anticipating the extent and consequences of severe postoperative pain in any given population, a number of elements affecting its natural history have been identified.

**TABLE 1-2. Pain Associated with
Various Surgical Procedures
(decreasing order of severity)[a]**

Gastric surgery
Gall bladder
Other upper abdominal surgery
Lower abdominal surgery
Appendectomy
Inguinal and femoral herniotomy
Head/neck/limb surgery
Minor chest wall and scrotal surgery

[a] Pain estimated by amount of analgesics needed
and time to first request for analgesics.
(Data from Parkhouse et al.[31])

Rawal[26] presented a rather comprehensive list of factors thought to affect the occurrence, intensity, quality, and duration of postoperative pain. These include the physiologic and psychological makeup of the patient; the patient's preparation for surgery (both pharmacologic and psychological); the site, nature, and duration of the procedure; the occurrence of postoperative complications; the anesthetic management before, during, and after surgery; and the quality of postoperative care.

Parkhouse et al[31] investigated the incidence of postoperative pain in 1,000 general surgery patients. The interval between the return from the operating room and the administration of the first injection for pain and the total number of injections received in the first 48 postoperative hours were assessed. The authors unequivocally stated that the site of operation is the single most important factor affecting the severity of postoperative pain (Table 1–2). Operations on the upper abdomen were the most painful. (The association of upper abdominal surgery with significant postoperative pain is also corroborated by Yeager.[32])

Age did appear to have some influence on the severity of postoperative pain but only as assessed by the total number of injections. The unclear effect of age is echoed by Mather and Mackie,[28] uncovering no relationship between age and the severity of postoperative pain within a pediatric population.

Sequelae of Uncontrolled Postoperative Pain

A good overview of the potential effects of uncontrolled postoperative pain has been provided by Brown.[4] Adverse sequelae of uncontrolled postoperative pain include slow recovery from surgery, increased morbidity in the postoperative period, delayed resumption of normal pulmonary function, restriction of mobility (thus contributing to thromboembolic complications), nausea and vomiting, increased systemic vascular resistance, cardiac work, and myocardial oxygen consumption through a heightened catecholamine response. Rawal[26] echoed the concerns regarding the pulmonary complications, decreased mobility, and increased catecholamine response, also noting the possibility of cardiac arrhythmias, hypertension, and myocardial ischemia. On the subject of pulmonary complications, Yeager[32] noted that pain is generally recognized as the primary cause of pulmonary dysfunction after surgery.

Surgical Stress Response

The endocrine, metabolic, and inflammatory responses to surgical injury and infection are composed of a variety of physiologic changes called the surgical stress response[33-35] (see Ch. 4). Postoperative pain has been defined by Kehlet[33-35] as a neural stimulus and release mechanism for the surgical stress response. Kehlet argued that effective postoperative analgesia does not necessarily decrease this response (in particular for thoracic and upper abdominal procedures) because of incomplete afferent neural blockade of several fast conducting pathways.[35] Kehlet[33-35] further argued that pain relief unaccompanied by a reduction in the surgical stress response does not contribute to a reduction of postoperative morbidity.

However, Yeager[32] noted that pain affects global organ function because the stress response to surgery can be manifest in various metabolic effects. Thus, as pain is an important stimulus for neuroendocrine activation, Yeager claimed that controlling pain will produce control of the stress response.

Comparison of Analgesic Techniques (Interventional Studies)

Another way to assess the adverse effects of poor postoperative pain management is to study the results when postoperative pain *is* effectively controlled. This can be accomplished by comparing the benefits accrued from use of varying anesthetic and analgesic regimens. This approach is admittedly indirect, as it tries to assess the scope of a problem by surveying the attendant results when the cause of the problem is removed (or at least lessened). Furthermore, from a strictly scientific sense, it is possible that the beneficial impact of a specific treatment modality could result from some factor other than its efficacy in controlling pain. However, with the recent focus on analgesic agents, routes of administration, and analgesic techniques very different from the traditional intramuscular opioid regimens, a brief review of these data is appropriate.

Regional Anesthesia/Analgesia and Pulmonary Complications

Yeager noted that nearly all studies of epidural analgesia in relation to pulmonary complications have shown at least some reduction in the incidence of these complications. The author feels that this improvement probably results from the avoidance of parenteral opioids. Improved analgesia from use of a superior analgesic technique may also play a significant role.[32]

Spence and Smith[36] compared the use of conventional parenteral morphine

and continuous epidural analgesia for postoperative pain management after vagotomy with gastroenterostomy or pyloroplasty. Study groups received either
10 mg of morphine on demand or continuous epidural analgesia with 0.5 percent
bupivacaine. Forty-eight hours after surgery, seven of 10 patients receiving
parenteral morphine and two of 11 patients receiving epidural bupivacaine had
pneumonia. Furthermore, the patients receiving parenteral morphine still
showed signs of hypoxemia 5 days after surgery. The author concluded that use
of conventional opioid regimens for postoperative pain relief increased the risk
of pulmonary complications.

Similarly, Catley et al[37] encountered many more respiratory problems in
patients receiving intravenous morphine as compared with those receiving regional anesthesia. Noting episodes of oxygen desaturation in conjunction with
ventilatory disturbances during sleep, the authors emphasized the need for continuous respiratory monitoring.

Cuschieri et al[38] conducted a prospective study of patients undergoing cholecystectomy. Three different analgesic regimens were employed: intermittent
intramuscular morphine, continuous intravenous morphine, and epidural bupivacaine. Recognizing that 50–75 percent of patients experience pulmonary
problems after upper abdominal surgery, the authors found better analgesia,
significantly higher arterial oxygen tensions, and a significant decrease in pulmonary complications associated with the use of epidural bupivacaine. The
pulmonary benefits persisted, despite the fact that the epidural medication was
used for only 12 hours.

Regional Anesthesia/Analgesia and Postoperative
Morbidity

Fortunately, these comparative studies also indirectly suggest other benefits
of effective postoperative pain management. In general, Rawal[26] suggested that
adequate postoperative analgesia can beneficially affect the course of recovery
in several major areas besides that of pulmonary function: thromboembolic
complications, gastrointestinal function, and amelioration of the stress response
to surgery. Yeager[32] recounted this similarly broad range of beneficial effects.
Depending on the analgesic technique used for adequate postoperative pain
control, beneficial effects include amelioration of the neuroendocrine response
to pain, reduction of thromboembolic complications, and less conclusively,
beneficial effects on cardiovascular and gastrointestinal function, as well as
mental status.

In a randomized, controlled clinical trial, Yeager et al[39] compared 25 patients
receiving general anesthesia and postoperative intramuscular analgesics with
28 patients receiving epidural anesthesia/analgesia. Patients receiving epidural
anesthesia/analgesia displayed a reduced incidence of both cardiovascular failure and major infectious complications, an attenuated surgical stress response
(as documented by decreased urinary coritsol excretion), and a reduction in the
overall postoperative complication rate. Not surprisingly, hospital costs were
also reduced in this group. Additional rather dramatic benefits of epidural anes-

thesia/analgesia were found: a decrease in intraoperative blood loss, a decrease in postoperative catabolism, a decline in the incidence of thromboembolic events, enhanced vascular graft blood flow, and an improvement in postoperative pulmonary function.

Specifically investigating thromboembolic complications, Modig et al[40] studied 60 patients undergoing total hip replacement. Half the patients received general anesthesia with postoperative intramuscular opioids on demand, and half received epidural anesthesia with postoperative epidural bupivacaine by repeated injection every 3 hours. The authors noted that the frequency of deep venous thrombosis after this surgical procedure had been previously reported to be 20–80 percent. Patients receiving epidural anesthesia/analgesia displayed a significantly decreased incidence of this complication, as well as a decrease in blood loss and in the incidence of pulmonary embolism.

Patient-Controlled Analgesia

By means of an external drug-dispensing device, patients using patient-controlled analgesia are allowed to determine their own dosing schedule (see Ch. 10). White[41] felt that this technique provides improved analgesic response, alleviating patients' anxiety brought on by the delay in procurement of medication when requested (as well as by the time interval required before the medication begins to work). Patient-controlled analgesia also allows patients to achieve acceptable pain relief without excessive sedation and other side effects. Examining 153 post-thoracotomy patients receiving either conventional or patient-controlled analgesia, Finley et al[42] found that the latter technique enhanced early mobilization and cooperation with physiotherapy and decreased postoperative hospital stay as well.

Preoperative Medication and Anesthetic Technique

The study reported by McQuay et al[43] demonstrated the dramatic impact of different anesthetic techniques on postoperative pain. Using the time to first request for postoperative analgesia as an outcome measure, the investigators studied the use of opioid premedication and neural blockade (alone and in combination) in 929 patients undergoing a range of orthopaedic surgical procedures. The median time to first request for analgesic was less than 2 hours when neither technique was used, more than 5 hours with premedication, 8 hours with neural blockade, and greater than 9 hours when these two techniques were combined. These results imply an increase in patient comfort with use of regional anesthetic techniques and adequate premedication. Moreover, this study demonstrated a reduction in the overall amount of medication requested for pain and a reduction in the amount of nursing care required to administer analgesics.

The aforementioned investigations were primarily focused on comparison of the effects of different anesthetic and analgesic techniques. Taken together, they powerfully suggest the broad range of benefits that might be expected from superior control of postoperative pain. These include a reduction in the incidence of a variety of postoperative complications (e.g., pulmonary, thromboembolic, cardiovascular, infections, and gastrointestinal), an amelioration of the surgical stress response, and a decrease in postoperative hospital stay and cost.

FACTORS CONTRIBUTING TO INADEQUATE MANAGEMENT

The problem of uncontrolled postoperative pain can thus be looked at from a number of perspectives: the total number of surgical procedures being performed, survey of patients' postoperative hospital experiences, prescription practices of physicians, the dispensing practices of the nursing staff (and certainly, the differences between what is being prescribed and what is being administered), and the reduction of morbidity and mortality when postoperative pain is controlled. However tallied, the overwhelming consensus from the literature is that postoperative pain is not adequately managed on a grand scale.

How have we arrived at this situation? There should be no mystery: postoperative pain is a very complex multidimensional phenomenon. Its effective management seems to be hampered by a number of identifiable factors. These factors include but are surely not limited to (1) the subjective nature of pain itself, the difficulty of measuring it, and the resultant lack of routine recording, (2) the numerous and well-recognized side effects of the most widely used analgesics, (3) the variability of patients' responses to analgesics, (4) the lack of a clear understanding of the natural history of postoperative pain in all its innumerable facades, and (5) the organizational challenge of assigning specific responsibility for the management of postoperative pain. Some of these are amenable to solution by continued research. Others will require difficult organizational, administrative, and financial decisions and commitments.

Lack of Routine Quantification

Recognition of the subjective nature of pain is widespread. There are a number of eloquent testimonials to its indescribability.[44,45] There can be no doubt that the recognition of pain's subjective nature has hindered its routine measurement.

Despite the inherent difficulties in assessment, the routine quantification of postoperative pain is absolutely vital. The need to begin routine quantification in some rudimentary fashion is perhaps even more important than the accuracy or reliability of the method used. The directness and simplicity of the visual analogue scale[46] strongly suggests its ready applicability for widespread use. Regardless of any other impediments to improvement of the management of postoperative pain, routine quantification must first be addressed.

Analgesic Side Effects

There can be no doubt that the widespread knowledge of, and concern over, the side effects of analgesics (particularly the traditionally used opioids) has been a powerful factor limiting their use. Indeed, White[41] went so far as to claim that in no other part of medicine has such a concern over side effects so markedly limited treatment.

According to Brown,[4] the side effects associated with systemic opioids include respiratory depression, nausea and vomiting, constipation, hypotension, and sphincter of Oddi spasm (which may be manifest as epigastric or chest pain). A similarly broad indictment was offered by Mitchell and Smith,[24] noting that all opioids can produce respiratory depression, euphoria, decreased gut motility, nausea, suppression of cough, and urinary retention, in addition to analgesia.

Interestingly, neither of these lists includes the possibility of physiologic or psychological dependence, a concern that has greatly shaped attitudes in the past. In their landmark study, Marks and Sachar[11] found an overestimation and exaggerated apprehension of the addiction potential of opioids administered for pain relief. This was particularly evident in the nursing staff they investigated, a finding echoed by Cohen.[15] Consequently, treatment of postoperative pain was limited by this fear of addiction. Perhaps the social concerns that once served to aggravate the fear of addiction on the part of caregivers have in the longer term been responsible for the generation of data that assuage these worries. Today, it seems to be more widely recognized that physical and psychological dependence on opioids is rare in patients treated for postoperative pain if the medication is discontinued within 3 weeks.[4]

Of these side effects, the one that has undoubtedly received the most attention is respiratory depression. Brown[4] presented a good overview of the kinds of respiratory effects to be expected with the use of systemic opioids. A 20 percent increase in arterial carbon dioxide tension can be expected in patients receiving adequate analgesia. Reduction of minute volume can persist for 4–5 hours after a dose of morphine. Maximal respiratory depression occurs approximately 7 minutes after an intravenous injection of morphine. Maximal respiratory depression may occur up to 30 minutes after an intramuscular injection or up to 90 minutes if given subcutaneously.

Certainly, analgesic side effects and fear of addition have conspired to limit their effective use. Practitioners must have a greater appreciation and understanding of the actual rather than presumed risk of particular analgesic modalities. Clinicians must come to understand that surgical sequelae, immobility, pain, and pain medication all pose a potential threat to the well-being of the patient.

Individual Variability of Response to Analgesics

The variability of human response to analgesic medication has been investigated in a number of reports. Ferrante and Covino[5] subtly underscored the difficulties inherent in providing analgesia for all patients by noting two prerequisites for effective analgesia: achieving an effective plasma level by individual-izing the dosage and maintaining this level over time. Hug[27] characterized the major theoretic factors influencing individualization of dosage as pharmacody-namic variability (i.e., that exhibited by tissue when exposed to the same con-centration of an agent) and pharmacokinetic variability (i.e., the combination of metabolic influences, such as absorption, biotransformation, and excretion, that determine the concentration to which the tissue is actually exposed).

Wood[47] provided an excellent overview of the pharmacokinetic influences that produce variability in response. These include the dose; the existence of concomitant drug therapy (with the consequent potential for interactions); the age, sex, and health or disease states of the patient; genetic polymorphism; and the specific anesthetic and surgical procedures involved. In the presence of disease, the author attributes variations in drug disposition to altered blood flow to organs, to a decline in the capacity of drug-metabolizing enzymes, and to alterations in drug-protein binding.

Obviously, anesthesia and surgery will also affect drug disposition. As an example of such pharmacokinetic and pharmacodynamic variability, it is noted that 48 percent of the variability in alfentanil clearance, as well as 33 percent of the variability of distribution in the central compartment, cannot be explained after accounting for age, weight, and sex. With this large degree of interindivid-ual variability in drug response, the author emphasized the need for careful titration and monitoring.[47]

In addition to large variations in individual pharmacokinetic and pharmacody-namic processes, the particular route of administration also accounts for much of the variable response to analgesic agents. Indeed, there is broad consensus that research of more optimal routes of administration is the most productive area for investigation. Ferrante and Covino,[5] Rawal,[26] Mitchell and Smith,[24] and Austin et al[13,14] all echoed this refrain: it is not the agents but the routes of administration that need to be optimized.

TOWARD A SOLUTION

Donovan et al[23] studied the incidence and characteristics of pain in a group of medical-surgical patients. They formulated their findings in terms of a table showing "common beliefs" that were undermined by the results of their study (Table 1-3). Less than half of the patients reporting pain in the study had a caregiver inquire about pain or note it in the patient's record. Although the awareness of the problem of uncontrolled postoperative pain has been slow to gain critical mass, Yeager[32] saw the beginnings of change. Signs of change include the introduction of new analgesic techniques, the increased involvement of anesthesiologists both in postoperative care and pain management generally, and the pressures from third-party payers to reduce hospital costs.

The adequate large-scale management of postoperative pain is by no means impossible; it is merely extraordinarily complicated. Yet, it is clear that much progress is being made, particularly in the area of alternate routes and tech-

TABLE 1-3. Common Beliefs Challenged by Donovan et al[23]

Common Belief	Evidence
Patients in pain make sure caregivers know about it	For $\frac{1}{2}$ of those in pain, no evidence that caregiver knew
Pain generally well controlled in hospital	58% reported excruciating or horrible pain at some time (7% at time of interview)
Patients take too many analgesics	Average daily dose equivalent to 12.4 mg morphine
Interventions other than narcotics only effective for mild pain	Nonpharmacologic interventions effective in $\frac{1}{3}-\frac{1}{2}$ of patients; more likely to be effective for moderate than mild or severe pain
Patients who sleep do not experience pain	Some patients with mild pain had sleep interrupted; some with moderate to severe pain did not have sleep interrupted; 61% of all patients had been awakened by pain

Data from Donovan et al.[23]

niques of analgesic administration. The clinical and organizational problems are more vexing, still. However, with a better quantitative understanding of the magnitude of the problem (both on an individual and population basis) and with the continuing evolution of medical, administrative, and reimbursement practices, there is perhaps cause for optimism.

References

1. Macht DI: The history of opium and some of its preparations and alkaloids. JAMA 64:477, 1915
2. Madigan SR, Raj PP: History and current status of pain management. p. 3. In Raj PP (ed): Practical Management of Pain. 2nd Ed. Mosby-Year Book, Malvern, PA, 1992
3. Crile GW, Lower WE: Anoci-Association. WB Saunders, Philadelphia, 1914
4. Brown JG: Systemic opioid analgesia for postoperative pain management. Anesth Clin North Am 7:51, 1989
5. Ferrante FM, Covino BG: Patient-controlled analgesia: a historical perspective. p. 3. In Ferrante FM, Ostheimer GW, Covino BG (eds): Patient-Controlled Analgesia. Blackwell Scientific Publications, Boston, 1990
6. Papper EM, Brodie BB, Rovenstine EA: Postoperative pain: its use in comparative evaluation of analgesics. Surgery 32:107, 1952
7. Lasagna L, Beecher HK: The optimal dose of morphine. JAMA 156:230, 1954
8. Keats AS: Postoperative pain: research and treatment. J Chronic Dis 4:72, 1956
9. Keeri-Szanto M, Heaman S: Postoperative demand analgesia. Surg Gynecol Obstet 134:647, 1972
10. Cronin M, Redfern PA, Utting JE: Psychometry and postoperative complaints in surgical patients. Br J Anaesth 45:879, 1973
11. Marks RM, Sachar EJ: Undertreatment of medical inpatients with narcotic analgesics. Ann Intern Med 78:173, 1973
12. Banister EHD'A: Six potent analgesic drugs: a double-blind study in post-operative pain. Anaesthesia 29:158, 1974
13. Austin KL, Stapleton JV, Mather LE: Multiple intramuscular injections: a major source of variability in analagesic response to meperidine. Pain 8:47, 1980
14. Austin KL, Stapleton JV, Mather LE: Relationship between blood meperidine con-

centrations and analgesic response: a preliminary report. Anesthesiology 53:460, 1980

15. Cohen FL: Postsurgical pain relief: patients' status and nurses' medication choices. Pain 9:265, 1980
16. Tamsen A, Hartvig B, Fagerlund C, Dahlström B: Patient-controlled analgesic therapy, Part II: individual analgesic demand and analgesic plasma concentrations of pethidine in postoperative pain. Clin Pharmacokinet 7:164, 1982
17. Tamsen A, Bondesson U, Dahlström B, Hartvig P: Patient-controlled analgesic therapy, Part III: pharmacokinetics and analgesic concentrations of ketobemidone. Clin Pharmacokinet 7:252, 1982
18. Dahlström B, Tamsen A, Paalzow L, Hartvig P: Patient-controlled analgesic therapy, Part IV: pharmacokinetics and analgesic plasma concentrations of morphine. Clin Pharmacokinet 7:266, 1982
19. Tamsen A, Sakurada T, Wahlström A et al: Postoperative demand for analgesics in relation to individual levels of endorphins and substance P in cerebrospinal fluid. Pain 13:171, 1982
20. Donovan BD: Patient attitudes to postoperative pain relief. Anaesth Intensive Care 11:125, 1983
21. Sriwatanakul K, Weis OF, Alloza JL et al: Analysis of narcotic analgesic usage in the treatment of postoperative pain. JAMA 250:926, 1983
22. Weis OF, Sriwatanakul K, Alloza JL: Attitudes of patients, housestaff and nurses toward postoperative analgesic care. Anesth Analg 62:70, 1983
23. Donovan M, Dillon P, McGuire L: Incidence and characteristics of pain in a sample of medical-surgical inpatients. Pain 30:69, 1987
24. Mitchell RWD, Smith G: The control of acute postoperative pain. Br J Anaesth 63:147, 1989
25. Smith G: Management of post-operative pain. Can J Anaesth, suppl. 36:S1, 1989
26. Rawal N: Postoperative pain and its management. p. 367. In Raj PP (ed): Practical Management of Pain. 2nd Ed. Mosby-Year Book, Malvern, PA, 1992
27. Hug CC: Improving analgesic therapy. Anesthesiology 53:441, 1980
28. Mather L, Mackie J: The incidence of postoperative pain in children. Pain 15:271, 1983
29. Beyer JE, DeGood DE, Ashley LC, Russell GA: Patterns of postoperative analgesic use with adults and children following cardiac surgery. Pain 17:71, 1983
30. Graves EJ: Utilization of short-stay hospitals. Vital Health Stat 96:1, 1988
31. Parkhouse J, Lambrechts W, Simpson BRJ: The incidence of postoperative pain. Br J Anaesth 33:345, 1961
32. Yeager MP: Outcome of pain management. Anesth Clin North Am 7:241, 1989
33. Kehlet H: The stress response to anaethesia and surgery: release mechanisms and modifying factors. Clin Anaesth 2:315, 1984
34. Kehlet H: The stress response to surgery: release mechanism and the role of pain relief. Acta Chir Scand, suppl. 550:22, 1988
35. Kehlet H: Surgical stress: the role of pain and analgesia. Br J Anaesth 63:189, 1989
36. Spence AA, Smith G: Postoperative analgesia and lung function: a comparison of morphine with extradural block. Br J Anaesth 43:144, 1971
37. Catley DM, Thorton C, Jordan C et al: Pronounced, episodic oxygen desaturation in the postoperative period: its association with ventilatory pattern and analgesic regimen. Anesthesiology 63:20, 1985
38. Cuschieri RJ, Morran CG, Howie JC, McArdle CS: Postoperative pain and pulmonary complications: comparison of three analgesic regimens. Br J Surg 72:495, 1985

39. Yeager MP, Glass DD, Neff RK, Brinck-Johnsen T: Epidural anesthesia and analgesia in high-risk surgical patients. Anesthesiology 66:729, 1987

40. Modig J, Borg T, Karlström G et al: Thromboembolism after total hip replacement: role of epidural and general anesthesia. Anesth Analg 62:174, 1983

41. White PF: Patient-controlled analgesia: an update on its use in the treatment of postoperative pain. Anesth Clin North Am 7:63, 1989

42. Finley RJ, Keeri-Szanto M, Boyd D: New analgesic agents shorten postoperative hospital stay, abstracted. Pain 2:S397, 1984

43. McQuay HJ, Carroll D, Moore RA: Postoperative orthopaedic pain—the effect of opiate premedication and local anaesthetic blocks. Pain 33:291, 1988

44. Donald I: At the receiving end: a doctor's personal recollections of second-time cardiac valve replacement. Scott Med J 21:49, 1976

45. Freed DL: Inadequate analgesia at night, letter. Lancet i:519, 1975

46. Aitken RCB: Measurement of feelings using visual analogue scales. Proc R Soc Med 62:989, 1969

47. Wood M: Variability of human drug response, editorial. Anesthesiology 71:631, 1989

2

Nociception

Nathaniel Katz
F. Michael Ferrante

Pain is defined as "an unpleasant sensory and emotional experience associated with actual or potential tissue damage or described in terms of such damage."[1] Between a site of active tissue damage and the perception of pain lies a complex series of electrochemical events, collectively called *nociception*. Nociception involves four physiologic processes[2] (Fig. 2-1):

1. *Transduction* denotes the process whereby noxious stimuli are translated into electric activity at the sensory endings of nerves.
2. *Transmission* refers to the propagation of impulses throughout the sensory nervous system. The neural pathways subserving transmission are composed of three components: (1) primary sensory afferent neurons that project to the spinal cord, (2) ascending relay neurons projecting from the spinal cord to the brain stem and thalamus, and (3) thalamocortical projections.
3. *Modulation* is the process whereby nociceptive transmission is modified through a number of neural influences.
   The aforementioned events are mechanistically similar to those processes underlying any other sensation and are intrinsic to the *sensory/discriminative* aspects of pain.
4. *Perception* is the final process whereby transduction, transmission, and modulation interact with the unique psychology of the individual to create the final, subjective, emotional experience we perceive as pain.

The experience we call pain always carries with it a distinct unpleasantness and a desire to escape. These qualities are integral to the experience of pain and are referred to as the *affective/motivational* aspects of pain.

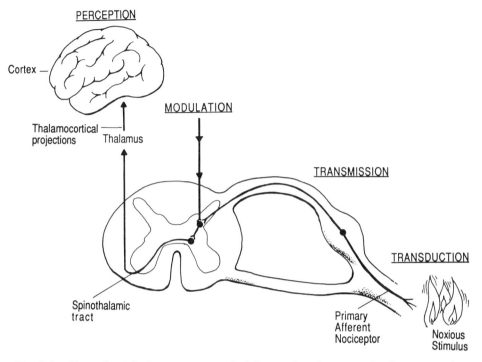

Fig. 2-1. Four physiologic processes underlying nociception: transduction, transmission, modulation, and perception.

THE PERIPHERAL NERVOUS SYSTEM

Gross Anatomy

The nervous system is composed of two parts: the central nervous system (CNS) and the peripheral nervous system (PNS). The CNS consists of the brain and spinal cord. The PNS consists of the cranial and spinal nerves and their subsequent ramifications. The autonomic nervous system (ANS) is a separate functional entity and consists of both central and peripheral components. (The ANS is extensively discussed in Ch. 3.)

The cranial nerves consist of 12 numbered nerves that leave the caudal brain and brain stem at various levels, exit the skull, and innervate structures of the head and neck, as well as the thoracoabdominal viscera.

The spinal nerves are anatomically derived from the union of the corresponding ventral and dorsal roots of the spinal cord (Fig. 2-2). Spinal nerves exit the spinal canal through the intervertebral foraminae and immediately split into dorsal and ventral rami. The dorsal rami pass posteriorly to innervate the paraspinal muscles and skin. The ventral rami combine to form plexuses at cervical and lumbosacral levels (the brachial plexus, the lumbosacral plexus). The major nerves to the limbs are derived from these plexuses. The thoracic spinal nerves form the intercostal nerves (Fig. 2-2).

The cell bodies of somatic motor nerves lie in the anterior horn of the spinal cord or in the motor nuclei of cranial nerves. Their axons pass into the ventral spinal roots or the motor rootlets of cranial nerves. Cell bodies of somatic sensory neurons reside in dorsal root ganglia that are located in the interverte-bral foraminae (Figs. 2-2 and 2-3). These ganglion cells have a peripheral axon that passes out through the dorsal root to join the spinal nerve. The central axon passes into the spinal cord via the proximal portion of the dorsal root (Fig. 2-3). Sensory nerves subserving visceral sensation also have their cell bodies in dorsal root ganglia, even though their axonal processes may travel with autonomic nerves to the periphery; they should not be viewed as autonomic nerves.

The sensory innervation of the head is analogous: cell bodies of sensory neurons are located in the trigeminal (Gasserian) ganglion. Central processes

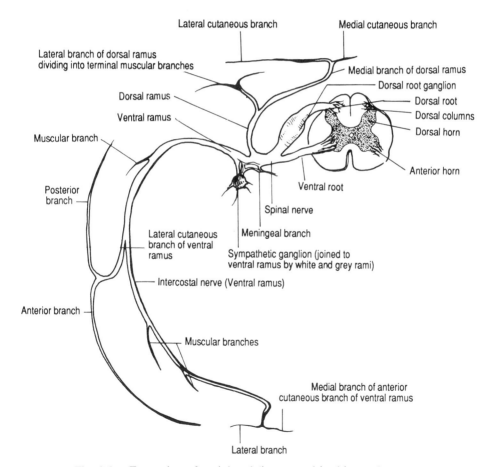

Fig. 2-2. Formation of peripheral (intercostal in this case) nerves.

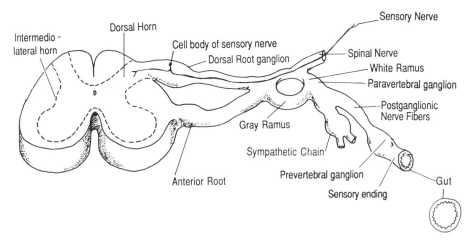

Fig. 2-3. Formation of peripheral nerves. Sensory neurons have cell bodies in the dorsal root ganglia. They send central processes into the dorsal horn via the dorsal roots and peripheral processes into the spinal nerves.

enter the brain stem via the sensory root of the trigeminal nerve. Peripheral processes exit the skull as the trigeminal nerve to innervate the anterior two-thirds of the head.

Microscopic Anatomy

A peripheral nerve is composed of both myelinated and unmyelinated nerve fibers (Fig. 2-4 and Table 2-1). A myelinated nerve fiber is surrounded by the concentric, compressed layers of a Schwann cell plasma membrane, giving rise to the myelin sheath. Unmyelinated fibers are surrounded only by Schwann cell cytoplasm.

Individual nerve fibers are invested with connective tissue called endoneurium. These nerve fibers are grouped in bundles called fascicles, which are surrounded by perineurium (Fig. 2-5).

Peripheral nerves contain axons with a variety of functions, diameters, myelination, and conduction velocities (Fig. 2-6 and Table 2-1). Electric stimulation of a nerve with recording of the voltage response at a discrete distance from the point of stimulation yields a compound action potential. The compound action potential is composed of several distinct peaks, each representing a group of nerve fibers with a different conduction velocity (Fig. 2-6).

Peripheral nerve fibers can be classified by conduction velocity, diameter, and degree of myelination (which is proportional to conduction velocity) or by function (which is again related to diameter, degree of myelination, and conduction velocity). Table 2-1 summarizes the two most commonly used systems for classification of peripheral nerve fibers.[3-6] The Lloyd-Hunt system applies only to muscle afferents. The Gasser and Erlanger system applies to all

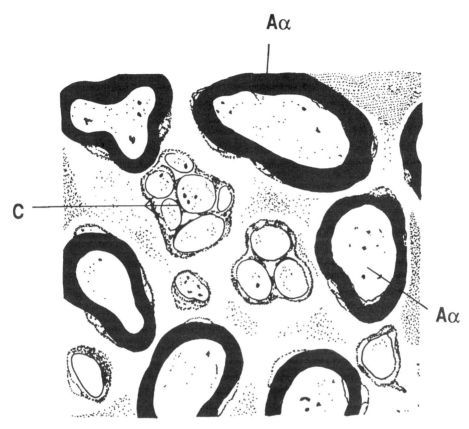

Fig. 2-4. Transverse section of a peripheral nerve as viewed by electron microscopy. Note large diameters and thick myelination of Aα fibers in contrast to smaller diameters and lack of myelination of C fibers. (Aδ fibers are not shown.)

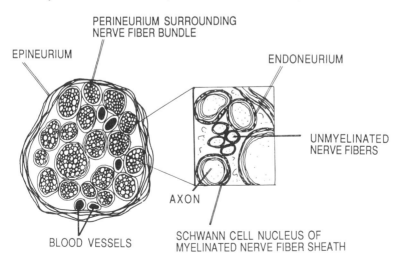

Fig. 2-5. Cross section of peripheral nerve, showing fascicles and connective tissue layers.

TABLE 2-1. Classification of Fibers in Peripheral Nerves

Fiber Group	Innervation	Mean Diameter (Range) (μm)		Mean Conduction Velocity (Range) (m/sec)	
	**Gasser and Erlanger Classification (Afferents and Efferents)**				
Aα	Primary muscle spindle motor to skeletal muscles (myelinated)	15	(12–20)	100	(70–120)
β	Cutaneous touch and pressure afferents (myelinated)	8	(5–15)	50	(30–70)
γ	Motor to muscle spindle (myelinated)	6	(6–8)	20	(15–30)
δ	Mechanoreceptors, nociceptors (myelinated)	<3	(1–4)	15	(12–30)
B	Sympathetic preganglionic (myelinated)	3	(1–3)	7	(3–15)
C	Mechanoreceptors, nociceptors, sympathetic postganglionic (unmyelinated)	1	(0.5–1.5)	1	(0.5–2)
	Lloyd/Hunt Classification (Muscle Afferents Only)				
Ia	Annulo spiral ending of muscle-spindle	13	(11–20)	75	(70–120)
b	Neurotendinous spindle				
II	Flower spray ending of neuromuscular spindle	9	(4–12)	55	(25–70)
III	Pressure sensor in muscle nociceptors	3	(1–4)	11	(10–25)
IV	Unmyelinated C fibers, mechanical nociceptors	1	(0.5–1.5)	1	(0.5–2)

peripheral nerve fibers. As is discussed below, nociceptive afferents generally fall into the Aδ and C classes of nerve fibers.

As nerve fibers approach the organs they subserve, they ramify profusely and may end in specialized structures capable of transducing stimuli. For example, group Ia and II fibers end in muscle spindles, and group II fibers end in Golgi tendon organs (Table 2-1). Most Aδ and C fibers do not terminate in specialized structures but end as free nerve endings. With respect to innervation

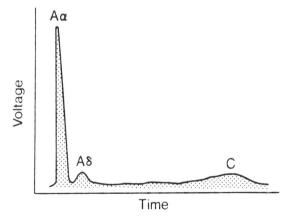

Fig. 2-6. Compound action potential recorded from stimulation of a whole nerve. The nerve is stimulated electrically, and the voltage is recorded at a discrete distance from the point of stimulation. Speed of conduction is shown to be proportional to both the diameter and the degree of myelination of individual fiber types.

of the integument, Aδ fibers lose their myelin sheath, leaving the axon surrounded by its basal lamina and a Schwann cell to terminate in the epidermis.[7] Unmyelinated C fibers may end in the superficial dermis as free penicillate nerve endings surrounded by Schwann cell cytoplasm (in hairy skin)[7] or as vertically oriented axons ending in a punctate manner in the superficial dermis (in hairless, or glabrous skin).[8] Thus, despite careful searches for a specific structure for a nociceptive receptor, it appears that transduction of noxious stimulation occurs in the free nerve ending.

TRANSDUCTION

Characterization of Nociceptors

The primary sensory afferent fiber concerned with nociception is termed the *nociceptor*. Since the actual receptor of this afferent fiber is often not well-defined, the term nociceptor is used interchangeably for the fiber and its putative receptor. (In this chapter, the term nociceptor will be used instead of ''pain fiber'' to signify fibers concerned with transduction and transmission of noxious stimuli.)

Evidence concerning the identity of nociceptive axons comes mainly from studies of cutaneous nerves. A number of factors allow the innervation of the integument to be more easily studied than the innervation of deep structures: (1) the skin is densely innervated; (2) the nerves are easily isolated and stimulated; (3) the area of skin supplied by an individual nerve (i.e., the receptive field) is easily located[2]; and (4) graded stimuli can be applied to the receptive field and the responses of the axon can be recorded. Axons most responsive to noxious stimuli can thereby be identified.

Using such models, it has been determined that large diameter myelinated afferents do not increase their firing in response to noxious stimuli and therefore cannot be involved in nociception.[6] Further confirmation has been obtained in humans where stimulation of these fibers does not produce painful sensations.[9] In contrast, many small myelinated and unmyelinated afferents respond maximally to noxious stimulation (Fig. 2-7). A categorization of the classes of nociceptors is found in the following discussion and in Table 2-2.

Myelinated Nociceptors

Myelinated fibers activated by noxious stimuli generally conduct in the Aδ range, about 20 m/sec.[10] They respond to mechanical stimulation (e.g., pressure). Although not as sensitive as large myelinated Aα fibers (so-called low threshold mechanoreceptors [LTMs]), Aδ fibers dramatically increase their firing rate as the stimulus intensity becomes greater (noxious). Thus, Aδ fibers are called high-threshold mechanoreceptors (HTMs). This illustrates a general (but not immutable) principle: nociceptive afferents generally have a higher threshold to stimulation than nonnociceptive afferents.

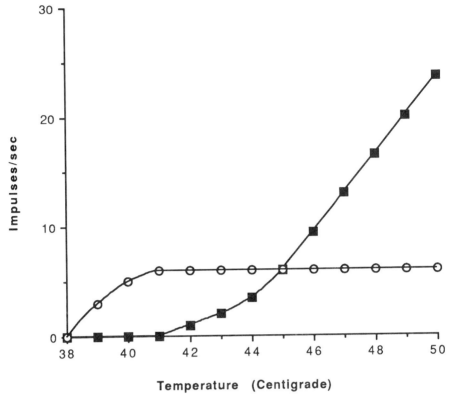

Fig. 2-7. Comparison of the response properties of a thermal nociceptor (■) and a nonnociceptive thermoreceptor (○). Both neurons may discharge at nonnoxious temperatures. As the temperature is raised so that it becomes a noxious stimulus, only the nociceptor increases its frequency of discharge.

TABLE 2-2. Categorization of Nociceptors

Myelin Type	Gasser-Erlanger Classification	Stimulus Threshold	Sensitization	Receptive Field
Myelinated				
High-threshold mechanoceptor	Aδ	High (noxious) intensity	Yes	Small
Mechanothermal	Aδ	High (noxious) intensity	Yes	Small
Unmyelinated				
C-Polymodal nociceptor	C	High (noxious) intensity	Yes	Large
Nonnociceptor, Myelinated[a]				
Low-threshold mechanoreceptor	Aα	Low intensity	No	—

[a] The low-threshold mechanoreceptor is *not* a nociceptor, but is placed here for comparison.

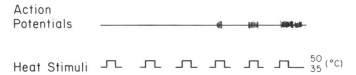

Fig. 2-8. Sensitization of an Aδ HTM using thermal stimuli. The receptor is initially insensitive to noxious thermal stimuli but responds with repeated stimulation.

HTMs do not fire in response to thermal stimulation unless stimuli are applied repeatedly. After repeated thermal stimulation, HTMs will become more sensitive (achieve a lower threshold to thermal stimulation) and will increase their frequency of discharge. This process is known as *sensitization* (Fig. 2-8). The threshold for mechanical stimulation is unchanged by this process.

Approximately 20–50 percent of Aδ nociceptors normally respond to heat, as well as mechanical stimuli, without sensitization.[10] These are called Aδ mechanothermal nociceptors and are also subject to sensitization. Some respond to cold stimulation as well.[11]

Unmyelinated Nociceptors

A large proportion of the fibers in a peripheral nerve are C fibers. Most, if not all, of these fibers are nociceptive.[2,12] Most C fibers respond to noxious mechanical, thermal, and chemical stimuli and are called C-polymodal nociceptors (C-PMNs). The receptive field for a C-PMN may be quite large (up to 17 mm²). This is in contrast to the Aδ nociceptors, whose receptive fields tend to be small clusters of spots.[11] C-PMNs do sensitize after repeated noxious stimulation and may develop an ongoing discharge. Irritant chemicals may produce discharges lasting several minutes.[13] Reports of pain correlate with C-fiber discharge during application of thermal, chemical, or mechanical noxious stimulation in humans.[11,14,15]

Role of Nociceptors in Pain Perception

Thus, there are three major classes of nociceptors: HTMs, Aδ mechanothermal nociceptors, and C-PMNs. The role played by these fibers in pain perception can be analyzed by electric stimulation of nerves. Low-intensity stimulation will preferentially activate the largest fibers.[6,9] As currents are reached that activate Aδ fibers, single stimuli evoke a sensation of intense tingling; repetitive stimuli evoke pain. When C fibers are stimulated, intense prolonged pain is experienced.[16]

Different fiber types can be preferentially blocked as well (within limits).[6] At very low concentrations, local anesthetics preferentially block small unmyelinated fibers, whereas application of pressure more easily blocks myelinated fibers. Pain perception will survive application of pressure. The remaining degree of pain perception after pressure application correlates with C-fiber activity.[17,18]

In the early part of this century, Lewis and Pechin[19] observed that application of a brief noxious stimulus will initially be experienced as a brief, sharp pain (first pain). A more prolonged, dull sensation (second pain) follows after a short lull. Application of pressure will block first pain; application of local anesthetics will block second pain.[20] Measurement of the latency between application of a noxious stimulus and detection of first pain correlates with a minimum conduction velocity in the Aδ range.[21] As first pain can occur in response to a thermal stimulus and is preferentially blocked by pressure, first pain must be mediated by the Aδ mechanothermal nociceptor.

Sensitization and Hyperalgesia

The actual mechanism whereby noxious stimuli are transduced into electric signals within the peripheral nerve fiber is uncertain. Different stimuli are probably transduced by different mechanisms, as response thresholds are different for mechanical and thermal stimuli within the same nociceptor.[22]

Lewis[23] noted a characteristic sequence of events following a skin injury known as the triple response: (1) intense vasodilation, (2) local edema (wheal), and (3) secondary vasodilation spreading to adjacent regions (flare). The subject will note a decreased threshold for nonnoxious stimuli (hyperesthesia), a decreased threshold to noxious stimuli, and increased pain in response to noxious stimulation (primary hyperalgesia) in the injured area. These changes soon spread to adjacent, noninjured areas (secondary hyperalgesia). It is important to remember that hyperalgesia, which refers to the responses of a subject, must be distinguished from sensitization, which refers to the responses of a nociceptive afferent fiber.

With respect to specific mechanisms of primary hyperalgesia, sensitization of C-PMNs is known to occur in an area of injury and may contribute to the phenomenon of thermal hyperalgesia.[23] The mechanism of thermal hyperalgesia varies with the particular tissue under study, however. In glabrous hand skin, primary hyperalgesia is mediated by sensitization of HTMs.[24]

Mechanical hyperalgesia, however, cannot be explained on the basis of sensitization of nociceptors. The threshold for mechanical stimulation of nociceptors is unchanged in the setting of mechanical hyperalgesia.[25] Other potential mechanisms for mechanical hyperalgesia include spatial summation (more peripheral nociceptors are activated for a given stimulus), existence of a novel receptor, central changes, and decreased inhibition of nociception caused by decreased responsiveness of LTMs.[26]

Secondary hyperalgesia depends on activity in unmyelinated primary afferents with sensitization of C-PMNs. After injury just outside their receptive fields, C-PMNs become sensitized and develop spontaneous depolarization.[27] This activity of C-PMNs in areas of undamaged tissue causes spreading vasodilation, edema, and further sensitization of other C-PMNs within adjacent receptive fields. This sequence of events has been termed *neurogenic inflammation* because of its similarity to the inflammatory process.

Finally, using a thermal injury model, primary hyperalgesia is noted in response to subsequent mechanical and thermal stimuli. However, secondary hyperalgesia occurs only in response to subsequent mechanical stimuli.[28] Thus, the mechanisms of primary and secondary hyperalgesia are probably different.

In summary, a sequence of events occurs after tissue injury resulting in spreading vasodilation, edema, and hyperalgesia (neurogenic inflammation). Sensitization of C-PMNs accounts for some but not all of these events.

Biochemical Substrates

Accumulation of algogenic substances in the area of injury is an integral part of the mechanisms underlying transduction and sensitization. A number of such substances have been identified, including potassium, hydrogen ion, serotonin, histamine, bradykinin, acetylcholine, prostaglandins, leukotrienes, and substance P[29] (Table 2-3). The source of origin of these substances is varied: injured cells, nociceptors, enhanced capillary permeability, and generation by local enzymatic activity. The process of transduction may be initiated and augmented through several mechanisms: (1) direct activation of nociceptors, (2) sensitization of nociceptors with consequent increased nociceptor activity, or (3) extravasasation of algogenic substances from the plasma.[30]

A number of cellular constituents are released after tissue injury. Among these, potassium and adenosine diphosphate have been shown to excite C-PMNs. Pain is produced on injection of these substances into humans.[2]

Bradykinin is a 9-amino acid peptide produced at sites of tissue injury by enzymatic action. Exposure of factor XII to injured tissue results in its conversion to the activated form. Activated factor XII converts prekallikrein to kallikrein. Kallikrein in turn acts on a precursor protein, kininogen, converting it to bradykinin. Bradykinin produces pain in humans at concentrations equivalent to those found in injured tissue.[31] Binding sites for bradykinin are found on sensory fibers and in the dorsal horn.[32] Bradykinin also increases vascular permeability, enhances leukocyte chemotaxis, and sensitizes nociceptors.[32]

Other classes of compounds that appear in areas of tissue damage are the prostanoids (the arachidonic acid metabolites of the cyclooxygenase pathway that comprise the thromboxanes, the prostacyclins, and the prostaglandins) and the eicosanoids (arachidonic acid metabolites of the lipoxygenase pathway

TABLE 2-3. Algogenic Substances Involved in Transduction

Substance	Source	Enzyme	Effect on Primary Afferent
Potassium	Damaged cells	—	Activate
Serotonin	Platelets		Activate
Bradykinin	Plasma kininogen	Kallikrein	Activate
Histamine	Mast cells	—	Activate
Prostaglandins	Arachidnoic acid-damaged cells	Cyclooxygenase	Sensitize
Leukotrienes	Arachidonic acid-damaged cells	Lipoxygenase	Sensitize
Substance P	Primary afferent	—	Sensitize

including 5-HETE, and the leukotrienes) (Fig. 2-9) (see Ch. 7). Arachidonic acid is normally esterified to cell membrane phospholipids. After cell injury, arachidonic acid is liberated from the cell membrane by an activated enzyme, phospholipase A. A number of stimuli and substances can activate phospholipase A, including norepinephrine and dopamine. Prostaglandins are then produced from arachidonic acid by action of the enzyme cyclooxygenase. Prostaglandins enhance transduction by sensitizing nociceptors to the action of other algogenic substances,[29,33] a process that underlies their role in inflammatory pain.[34]

Leukotrienes are produced from arachidonic acid by the enzyme lipoxygenase (Fig. 2-9). The leukotrienes produce hyperalgesia on injection in humans,[35] the process seemingly dependent on polymorphonuclear leukocytes.[36] Their role in the natural process of transduction is uncertain.

When unmyelinated afferents are electrically stimulated, they release a substance into the extracellular space that activates C fibers and causes pain on injection.[37,38] Substance P is a likely constituent of this effluent. Substance P is an 11-amino acid peptide that was first identified in 1931[39] and later found to be associated with sensory transmission and vasodilation. Substance P is synthesized in neuronal cell bodies in the dorsal root ganglia and transported to peripheral and central terminals where it is stored in vesicles.[40] It is released on stimulation of primary afferent nociceptors and causes vasodilation and edema.[41] Substance P also causes release of histamine from mast cells, resulting in further vasodilation and edema.

Several pieces of evidence suggest that substance P mediates neurogenic inflammation. Administration of substance P provokes plasma extravasation; other peptides do not produce extravasation.[42] Capsaicin depletes substance P and also prevents plasma extravasation evoked by nerve stimulation.[43] Despite its role in the initiation and augmentation of neurogenic inflammation, substance P does not produce pain on local injection, nor does it activate nociceptors.

Histamine is released from injured cells and from mast cells stimulated by substance P. Histamine causes activation of nociceptors, vasodilation, and edema. It has been suggested that the flare and secondary hyperalgesia of tissue injury are due to release of substance P, with consequent release of histamine and sensitization of nociceptors.[44] Controversy has arisen, however, from the demonstration that injection of histamine produces only pruritis at neutral pH.[26]

Serotonin has also been implicated as an algogenic substance. Serotonin is released by platelets in response to platelet-activating factor, a substance released by degranulating mast cells. Serotonin causes pain directly[45] and by potentiation of the nociceptive effect of bradykinin.[46] Serotonin receptors are found on peripheral nerves, and antagonists will block the nociceptive effects of serotonin.[47]

Evidence also exists for the role of catecholamines in transduction. After tissue injury, sympathetic efferent activity will stimulate Aδ mechanothermal afferents through α-receptors.[48] Epinephrine also activates C fibers in experimental neuromas, a phenomenon likewise mediated by α-receptors.[49]

Thus far we have looked at the process of transduction and nociception with

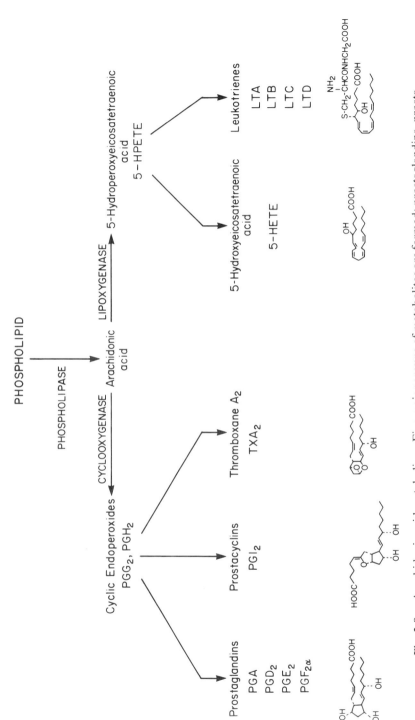

Fig. 2-9. Arachidonic acid metabolism. Five major groups of metabolites are formed: prostaglandins, prostacyclins, thromboxanes, 5-HETE, and leukotrienes.

respect to cutaneous noxious stimuli. The rest of this section reviews the process of transduction in deep somatic and visceral tissue.

Transduction in Deep Somatic Tissue

Pain from joints, muscles, and other deep somatic structures is universal, yet little studied. From the few animal studies that have been performed, transduction in deep somatic tissue is mechanistically analogous to cutaneous transduction.

Muscle

Muscle is innervated by free nerve endings of Aδ and C nociceptors.[50] The Aδ fibers respond to noxious and nonnoxious pressure, chemical irritants, or heat. The C fibers react to chemical irritants, noxious heat, and intense pressure.[51–53] There are three types of C fibers: (1) nociceptive fibers unresponsive to muscle activity, (2) nonnociceptive fibers responsive to muscle activity, and (3) fibers responsive to both.

Skeletal muscle pain is described as diffuse, poorly localized, and most intense during contraction or under ischemic conditions. In fact, a group of skeletal muscle afferents discharges maximally under the aforementioned conditions.[51] These fibers also undergo sensitization in response to algogenic agents[54] and are found in cardiac muscle as well.[55]

Joint

Joints[56–58] are innervated by Aδ and C nociceptors ending as free nerve endings in widespread plexuses in the joint. Approximately half the Aδ and all the C fibers respond only to extreme joint movement or pressure. These nociceptors become sensitized under conditions of inflammation and become activated by normally nonnoxious joint movement or pressure. They may also develop a continuous background discharge.

Bone

Bone[59] is innervated by Aδ and C fibers forming a plexus around the periosteum and investing the cancellous bone. The cortex and marrow do not receive nociceptive fibers. Bone is said to have the lowest pain threshold of the deep somatic structures.[60]

Transduction in Visceral Tissue

Observations during surgery have disclosed that viscera are relatively insensitive to stimuli that are noxious to the integument (e.g., cutting, heating, or pinching). Viscera are sensitive, however, to movements such as twisting and distension.[60,61] The viscera are, in general, supplied by Aδ and C afferents.

Visceral afferents generally travel with sympathetic fibers, which has led to their erroneous designation as "sympathetic afferent" fibers. This nomenclature is inappropriate and confusing, as visceral afferents are not autonomic fibers. Visceral afferents generally have large confluent receptive fields and can sensitize in response to certain conditions (e.g., inflammation).

Summary of Transduction

Information about noxious stimulation is carried into the CNS by nerve fibers called primary afferent nociceptors. Primary afferent nociceptors are of several types: (1) Aδ mechanoreceptors (HTMs) responding to mechanical stimulation, (2) Aδ mechanothermal nociceptors responding to mechanical and thermal stimuli, and (3) C-PMNs responding to chemical, mechanical, and thermal stimuli. First pain is carried by Aδ fibers and second pain by C fibers. After local injury, nociceptors become hypersensitive to noxious stimuli, a process called sensitization. This response is probably mediated by the release of algogenic substances in the periphery. A sequence of events is noted after local tissue injury: local vasodilation, edema (wheal), spreading vasodilation (flare), hyperalgesia in the injured area (primary hyperalgesia), and spreading (secondary) hyperalgesia. Stimulation of nociceptors can produce a similar picture called neurogenic inflammation. Sensitization may account for primary hyperalgesia, but central mechanisms need to be invoked for secondary hyperalgesia.

THE CENTRAL NERVOUS SYSTEM

Before any discussion of the physiologic processes of transmission and modulation, it is important for the reader to understand the gross and ultrastructural anatomy of the CNS.

The CNS consists of the brain and spinal cord. The brain is further subdivided into the cerebral cortex, diencephalon (thalamus and hypothalamus), basal ganglia, cerebellum, and brain stem (Fig. 2-10). These neural structures are surrounded by connective tissue layers called the meninges and are encased in the bony skull and spine.

Chapter 5 deals extensively with the bony anatomy of the vertebral column and the gross anatomy of the spinal cord. Thus, this section looks at the ultrastructural anatomy of the spinal cord and the gross anatomy of the brain.

Ultrastructural Anatomy of the Spinal Cord

As in the PNS, the functional unit of the CNS is the neuron. A chain of communicating neurons is called a pathway. A bundle of axons within a pathway is referred to as a tract, fasciculus, peduncle, or lemniscus. In the PNS, a bundle of axons is called a nerve.[62]

A transverse section of the spinal cord discloses a butterfly-shaped region

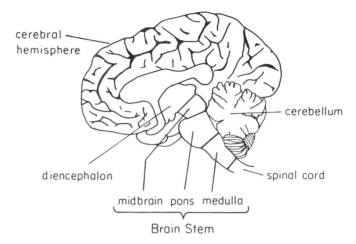

Fig. 2-10. Sagittal section of the brain.

of central gray matter composed of neuronal cell bodies (Fig. 2-11). This is surrounded by axonal tracts, making up the white matter. The gray matter is divided into a dorsal (posterior) horn, ventral (anterior) horn, and central gray commissure. The anterior and posterior roots emerge from the respective horns. The emerging roots divide the white matter into three segments: the dorsal, lateral, and ventral funiculi (Fig. 2-11).

The major tracts of the spinal cord are illustrated in Figure 2-12. The spinothalamic tract (Figs. 2-12 and 2-13) subserves the sensations of pain and temperature. Primary afferent nociceptors synapse in the dorsal horn. The tracts of the second-order neurons cross to the opposite anterior aspect of the lateral funiculus.

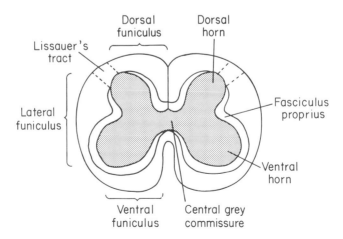

Fig. 2-11. Transverse section of the spinal cord showing gray and white matter.

ASCENDING   DESCENDING

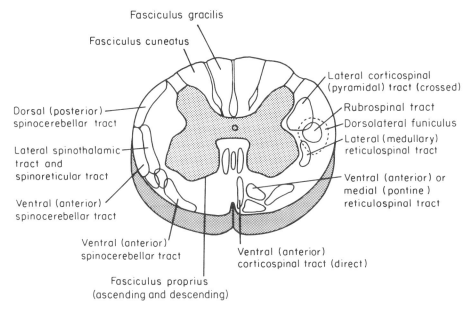

Fasciculus gracilis

Fasciculus cuneatus

Lateral corticospinal
(pyramidal) tract (crossed)

Dorsal (posterior)
spinocerebellar tract

Rubrospinal tract

Dorsolateral funiculus

Lateral (medullary)
reticulospinal tract

Lateral spinothalamic
tract and
spinoreticular tract

Ventral (anterior) or
medial (pontine)
reticulospinal tract

Ventral (anterior)
spinocerebellar tract

Ventral (anterior)
spinocerebellar tract

Ventral (anterior)
corticospinal tract (direct)

Fasciculus proprius
(ascending and descending)

Fig. 2-12. Transverse section of the spinal cord. Major ascending tracts are illustrated on the left: the dorsal columns (the fasciculus gracilis and the fasciculus cuneatus), the spinocerebellar tracts, the spinoreticular tract, and the spinothalamic tract. The major descending tracts are illustrated on the right: the lateral and ventral corticospinal tracts, the rubrospinal tract, and the reticulospinal tracts. The dorsolateral funiculus (*broken lines in diagram*) is extremely important with respect to descending antinociceptive pathways. The gray matter is surrounded by the fasciculus proprius, which consists of short ascending and descending fibers.

lus (the *anterolateral quadrant*). The spinothalamic tract then ascends through the brain stem to the thalamus (Fig. 2-13).

Fibers associated with proprioception and crude touch enter the dorsal horn and ascend ipsilaterally in the dorsal (posterior) columns (fasciculus gracilis and fasciculus cuneatus) (Figs. 2-12 and 2-14). These fibers cross in the medulla, ascend to the thalamus as the medial lemniscus, and are distributed to the cortex.

Unconscious sensation is mediated by the spinocerebellar tract (Figs. 2-12 and 2-15). Fibers ascend ipsilaterally in the lateral funiculus, exit from the pons, and terminate in the ipsilateral cerebellum.

The major descending tract is the corticospinal tract, which is responsible for motor activity. The corticospinal tract descends from the cerebral cortex into the brain stem, crosses in the medulla, and descends in the lateral funiculus to synapse in the ventral horn at multiple levels (Fig. 2-16).

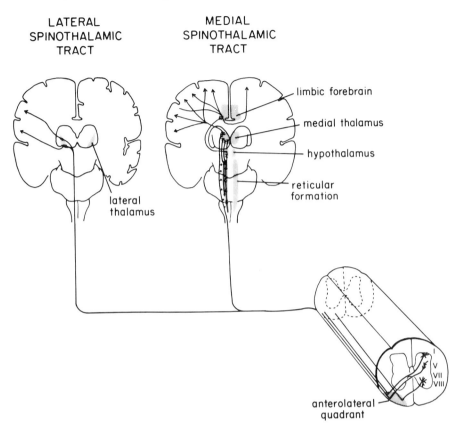

LATERAL SPINOTHALAMIC TRACT

MEDIAL SPINOTHALAMIC TRACT

limbic forebrain

medial thalamus

hypothalamus

reticular formation

lateral thalamus

anterolateral quadrant

Fig. 2-13. Spinothalamic tract. The cell bodies of the spinothalamic tract are located in laminae I, V, VII, and VIII. Their axons cross to the contralateral side of the spinal cord and ascend in the anterolateral quadrant. As the spinothalamic tract approaches the thalamus, it segregates into medial and lateral divisions. The medial spinothalamic tract projects to the brain stem reticular formation, the hypothalamus, the periaqueductal gray matter and the medial thalamic nuclei, the central lateral nucleus of the intralaminar complex, and the nucleus submedius. Subsequent ramifications are to widespread areas of the cortex and limbic system. The medial spinothalamic tract is thought to subserve the affective/motivational aspects of pain perception. The lateral division of the spinothalamic tract terminates in the lateral, ventral basal, and posterior thalamic nuclei. The lateral spinothalamic tract is thought to be involved in the sensory/discriminative aspects of the perception of pain.

Ultrastructural Anatomy of the Brain

The Brain Stem

The brain stem is the most caudal portion of the brain and consists of the medulla (myelencephalon), pons (metencephalon), and midbrain (mesencephalon). The rhombencephalon refers to the pons and medulla. The brain stem is bounded rostrally by the thalamus, caudally by the spinal cord, ventrally by a

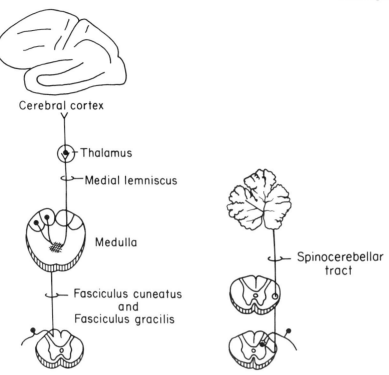

Fig. 2-14. Posterior (dorsal) columns (conscious proprioception and stereognosis). (Modified from Goldberg, [62] with permission.)

Fig. 2-15. Spinocerebellar tract. (Modified from Goldberg, [62] with permission.)

flat bone called the clivus, and dorsally is roofed by the fourth ventricle and cerebellum (Fig. 2-10). The brain stem consists of ascending and descending tracts and numerous nuclei, including those that give rise to the cranial nerves and the diffuse constellation of nuclei called the reticular formation.

The medulla is the most caudal portion of the brain stem (Fig. 2-10). Its major features are the fourth ventricle forming its roof, the pyramids, and the olives (Figs. 2-17 and 2-18 and Table 2-4). The ascending spinothalamic tract, medial lemniscus, the medullary reticular formation, and the nuclei and exiting axons of the trigeminal, vestibulocochlear, glossopharyngeal, vagus, and hypoglossal nerves comprise the important structures (Figs. 2-17 to 2-21).

The major features of the pons (Table 2-4) are the fourth ventricle forming its roof, flanked by the cerebellar peduncles, which attach the pons to the cerebellum (Fig. 2-19). The prominent base of the pons contains the corticospinal tracts (Figs. 2-18 and 2-22). Other important structures include the nuclei and exiting axons of the trigeminal, abducens, facial and vestibulocochlear nerves, the ascending spinothalamic tract, central tegmental tracts, medial lemniscus, and pontine reticular formation (Figs. 2-17 to 2-19 and 2-22).

At the level of the midbrain, the fourth ventricle has tapered into the narrow cerebral aqueduct surrounded by the periaqueductal gray matter. The roof of

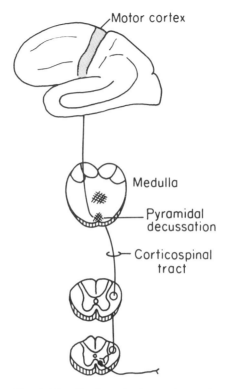

Fig. 2-16. Corticospinal tract (motor).
(Modified from Goldberg,[62] with permission.)

TABLE 2-4. Important Structures of the Brain Stem

Brain Stem Portion	Gross Structures	Nuclei and Tracts
Medulla	Fourth ventricle (roof) Pyramids (contain CSTs)[a] Olives	Nuclei: V, VIII, IX, X, XII Spinothalamic tract Medial lemniscus Medullary reticular formation
Pons	Fourth ventricle (roof) Cerebellar peduncles Base (contains CSTs)[a]	Nuclei: V, VI, VII, VIII Spinothalamic tract Central tegmental tract Medial lemniscus Pontine reticular formation
Midbrain	Cerebral aqueduct Periaqueductal gray Colliculi Cerebral peduncles (contain CSTs)[a]	Nuclei: III, IV, red, locus ceruleus, substantia nigra Medial lemniscus Spinothalamic tract

[a] CSTs, corticospinal tracts

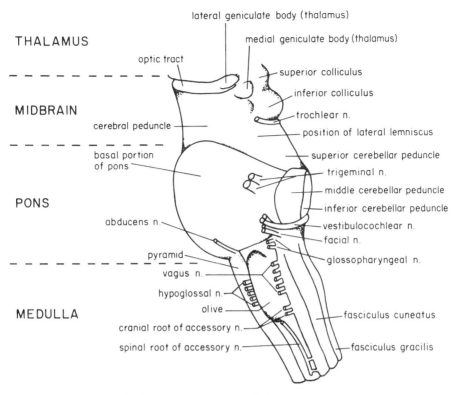

THALAMUS

lateral geniculate body (thalamus)

medial geniculate body (thalamus)

optic tract

superior colliculus

inferior colliculus

MIDBRAIN

trochlear n.

cerebral peduncle

position of lateral lemniscus

basal portion of pons

superior cerebellar peduncle

trigeminal n.

middle cerebellar peduncle

PONS

inferior cerebellar peduncle

abducens n.

vestibulocochlear n.

facial n.

pyramid

glossopharyngeal n.

vagus n.

hypoglossal n.

olive

MEDULLA

cranial root of accessory n.

fasciculus cuneatus

spinal root of accessory n.

fasciculus gracilis

Fig. 2-17. Lateral view of the brain stem.

the midbrain consists of the four paired colliculi (Figs. 2-17 and 2-19 and Table 2-4). Its ventral aspect is composed of the cerebral peduncles, which contain the corticospinal tracts (Fig. 2-18). Other important structures include the nuclei and exiting axons of the oculomotor and trochlear nerves, the red nucleus, the locus ceruleus, and the substantia nigra (Fig. 2-23).

The Thalamus

The thalamus and basal ganglia are paired subcortical nuclear structures with multiple interconnections. The basal ganglia consist of the caudate, putamen, and globus pallidus, and are concerned with motor activity. The basal ganglia will not be discussed further, as they have little role in nociception. The thalamus, however, is extremely important.

The thalamus (Figs. 2-24 and 2-25) is divided into medial and lateral nuclear groups by a band of fibers called the internal medullary lamina. The medial group contains the dorsomedial nucleus. The medial nuclei are often grouped with the nuclei located within the lamina itself (the intralaminar nuclei). The internal medullary lamina also contains the centromedial and centrolateral nuclei.

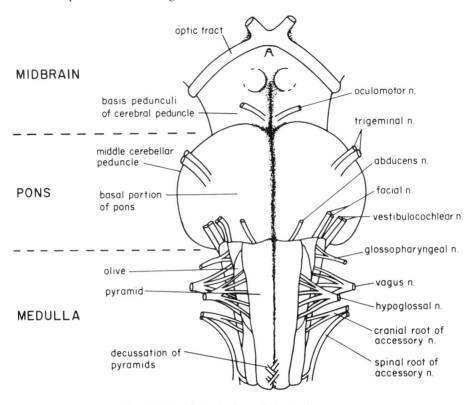

Fig. 2-18. Ventral view of the brain stem.

The lateral nuclear group is divided into dorsal and ventral tiers (Fig. 2-25). The dorsal tier contains the pulvinar, lateral dorsal, and lateral posterior nuclei. The ventral tier contains the ventral anterior, ventral lateral, ventral posterior lateral, and ventral posterior medial nuclei. As will be seen, the ventral posterior lateral and ventral posterior medial nuclei (Figs. 2-24 and 2-25) are particularly concerned with the perception of pain and the neuroendocrine response to surgical stress (see Ch. 4).

TRANSMISSION

The Fate of Primary Afferents—
The Dorsal Root

As previously noted, primary afferent neurons have their cell bodies in the dorsal root ganglia. A peripheral process is sent out through the dorsal root, and a central process is sent to the spinal cord through the proximal portion of the dorsal root (Fig. 2-3). Some experiments indicate that dorsal root ganglion cells may send central processes into the cord through the ventral root[63] (Fig.

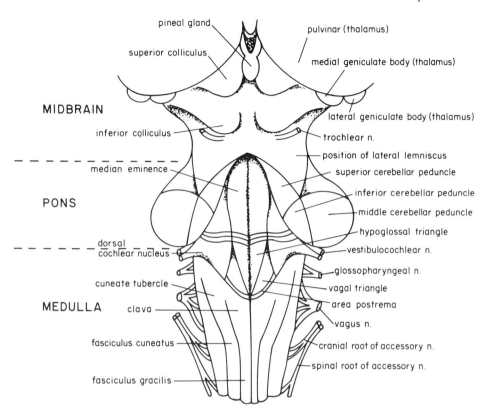

Fig. 2-19. Dorsal view of the brain stem.

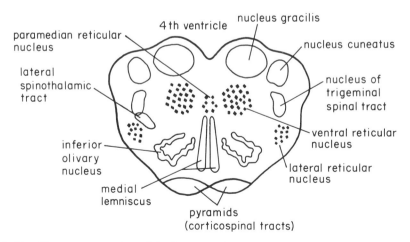

Fig. 2-20. Transverse section of the lower medulla at the level of the caudal portion of the inferior olivary nucleus.

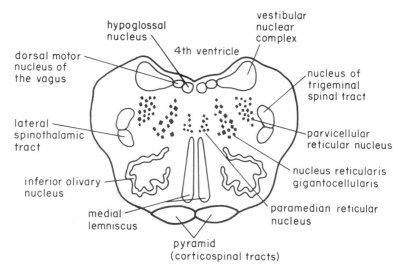

Fig. 2-21. Transverse section of the upper medulla at the level of the rostral portion of the inferior olivary nucleus.

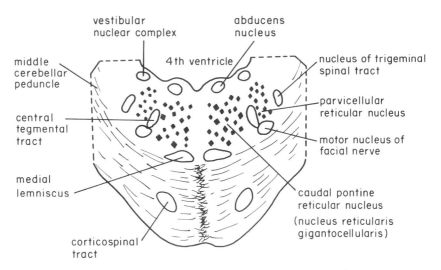

Fig. 2-22. Transverse section of the caudal portion of the pontine tegmentum.

2-26). Dorsal root ganglion cells receive no synaptic connections and thus play little, if any, role in information processing. Most of the axons in the dorsal root are unmyelinated, implying a role in nociception.

As the dorsal root approaches the cord it splits into 12–15 rootlets. Unmyelinated and small myelinated fibers migrate ventrolaterally and large myelinated

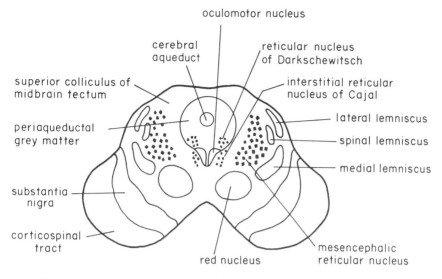

Fig. 2-23. Transverse section of the rostral region of the midbrain.

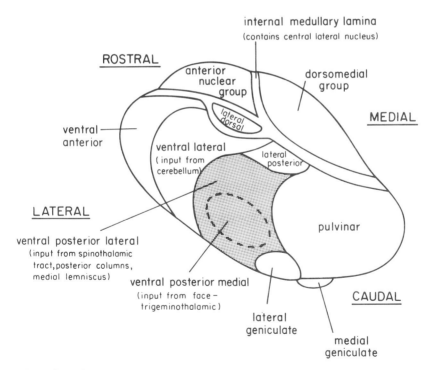

Fig. 2-24. Superior oblique (longitudinal) view of the thalamus. The internal medullary lamina divides the thalamus into medial and lateral nuclear groups. The ventral posterior lateral and ventral posterior medial nuclei are particularly concerned with the perception of pain and the neuroendocrine response to surgical stress.

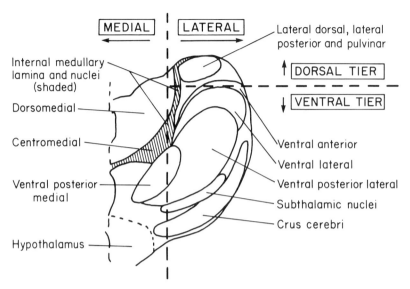

Fig. 2-25. Coronal section through half the thalamus. The lateral nuclear group is divided into dorsal and ventral tiers. The ventral tier includes the ventral anterior, ventral lateral, and ventral posterior (lateral and medial) nuclei.

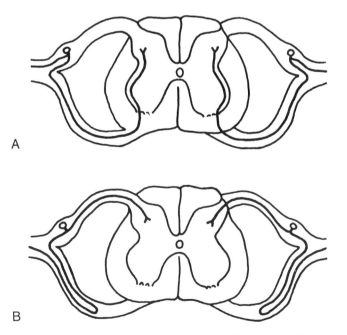

Fig. 2-26. Possible arrangements for ventral sensory afferents. (A) The central process of the dorsal root ganglion cell reaches the dorsal horn via the ventral root. (B) The central process enters the ventral root but loops back on itself.

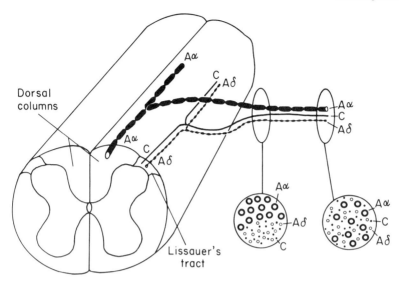

Fig. 2-27. Entry of primary afferents into the spinal cord. At a distance from the cord, the axons of different fiber types are intermingled. Near the dorsal root entry zone, the axons segregate into two groups. The Aα axons come to lie in the dorsomedial zone of the dorsal root and enter the dorsal columns. The small diameter Aδ and C axons (which include all nociceptors) assume a ventrolateral position in the dorsal root and enter Lissauer's tract. (Modified from Fields,[2] with permission.)

fibers migrate dorsomedially (Fig. 2-27). The large fibers enter medially and bifurcate into ascending and descending branches in the dorsal columns; collaterals from these fibers enter the dorsal horn.

The small fibers enter laterally and bifurcate into ascending and descending branches extending one or two segments from the entry point. Most of these fibers join Lissauer's tract, a band of fibers that caps the dorsal horn (Fig. 2-27). After ascending or descending one or two segments, these small afferents enter the spinal gray matter and give rise to numerous branches.

The Fate of Primary Afferents— The Spinal Cord

The gray matter of the spinal cord is organized into rostrocaudal layers, or laminae, first described by Rexed in cats[64] (Fig. 2-28). The laminae are given Roman numerals from dorsal to ventral. The dorsal horn is capped by Lissauer's tract, which consists mainly of ascending and descending Aδ and C fibers.[65,66] Lesions of Lissauer's tract cause degeneration in laminae I and II, implying that Aδ and C primary afferent nociceptors terminate in these laminae.[67]

Lamina I is the most superficial layer of the dorsal horn and is called the marginal layer. It contains large, flat "marginal cells" and intermediate-sized neurons. Lamina II is called the substantial gelatinosa because of its gelatinous

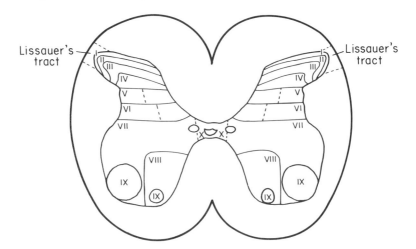

Fig. 2-28. Rexed's laminae.

appearance in freshly cut cord sections. It consists of small, densely packed cells. Lamina III contains larger, loosely packed cells. Lamina IV is the thickest layer in the dorsal horn and consists of large neurons with dendrites that spread into other layers. Laminae III and IV constitute the nucleus proprius. Lamina V consists of small neurons. Lamina VI is located at the base of the dorsal horn and is found only at the cervical and lumbar enlargements. Laminae I–VI constitute the dorsal horn (Fig. 2-28).

Lamina VII is an irregular area in the center of the spinal gray matter. Lamina VIII occupies the medial half of the ventral horn in the cervical and lumbar enlargements. Lamina IX corresponds to the motor neuron pools in the ventral horn, and lamina X surrounds the central canal. Lamina VII–IX constitute the ventral horn.

Terminals of Primary Afferents

Small-diameter myelinated and unmyelinated afferents terminate in laminae I, II, and V of the dorsal horn. C fibers terminate mainly in laminae I and II.[66] Aδ nociceptors end largely in laminae I and V and, to some extent, in lamina X.[68] Visceral afferents end mainly in laminae I and V.[69] Large myelinated afferents (entering via the dorsomedial division of the dorsal root) terminate in lamina III or deeper. Most afferent fibers end in the ipsilateral dorsal horn, although some cross just dorsal to the central canal and end in the contralateral dorsal horn.

Neurotransmitters of Primary Afferents

Criteria for proving that a substance is a neurotransmitter for a primary afferent nociceptor are (1) presence of the substance in the dorsal horn synapse of the primary afferent, (2) release of the substance on noxious stimulation, (3) release of the substance has the same effect as stimulation of the primary afferent, and (4) administration of an antagonist blocks the effect of both the substance and the primary afferent.[2] A number of peptides have been proposed to be neurotransmitters of primary afferent nociceptors. These include substance P, somatostatin, and vasoactive intestinal polypeptide. Thus far, no putative neurotransmitter has satisfied all the aforementioned criteria.

Substance P stains densely in laminae I and II, somatostatin in lamina II, and vasoactive intestinal polypeptide in lamina I. Concentrations of all these peptides in the dorsal horn decrease rapidly after sectioning the dorsal root.[2] Substance P produces depolarization of second-order neurons in the dorsal horn in a fashion similar to stimulation of primary afferent fibers.[70] Substance P cannot be the only primary afferent neurotransmitter, as it is present in less than 25 percent of dorsal root ganglion cells. Furthermore, nociception can take place despite depletion of substance P.[71] Other peptides including cholecystokinin, gastrin-releasing peptide, dynorphin, enkephalin, angiotensin II, and bombesin have also been found in primary afferents and may play a role in nociception.

There is growing evidence that excitatory neurotransmitters function as primary afferent neurotransmitters.[72] It has been shown that there are slow and fast components to the stimulation of dorsal horn neurons by primary afferents. Substance P mimics the slow component; excitatory amino acids, such as glutamate and aspartate, may mediate the fast component.[73]

Transmission Cells in the Spinal Cord

Anatomy

Three classes of cells are found in the dorsal horn: (1) projection cells relay information to rostral centers; (2) excitatory interneurons relay nociceptive transmission to projection cells, to other interneurons, or to motor cells concerned with reflexes; and (3) inhibitory interneurons modulate nociceptive transmission.[74] Features identifying a neuron as a projection neuron include maximal discharge on noxious stimulation, decreased perception of pain with decreased firing of the cell, increased perception of pain with stimulation of the neuron, and projection of the neuron to a site known to be involved in nociception. Neurons meeting these criteria are concentrated in laminae I, II, and V.

Most neurons in lamina I respond to noxious stimulation. Several primary afferents usually converge onto one lamina I neuron. Thus, the receptive fields of these neurons are several times larger than the receptive fields of individual primary afferents. Lamina I cells may receive input from myelinated or unmyelinated fibers. Some cells are excited only by nociceptors (nociceptive-specific [NS] or high-threshold neurons); most lamina I cells are NS. Other cells receive additional input from nonnociceptive afferents. These cells are called wide dynamic range (WDR) neurons and respond to a wide range of stimuli, from low

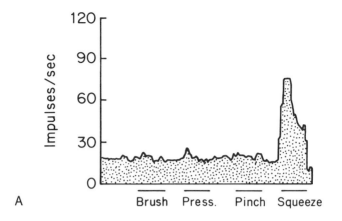

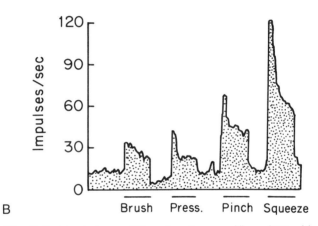

Fig. 2-29. The distinction between **(A)** nociceptive-specific and **(B)** wide dynamic range neurons in the dorsal horn. **(A)** The nociceptive-specific neuron responds little if at all to innocuous stimuli (brush, pressure, pinch) but responds vigorously to noxious stimulation (squeeze). **(B)** The wide dynamic range neuron responds to innocuous stimuli. As stimulus intensity increases into the noxious range, the neuron responds with increasing frequency of discharge. (Modified from Fields,[2] with permission.)

to high intensity (Fig. 2-29). Most lamina I cells are projection cells relaying afferent input to the thalamus.

Lamina II also contains many nociceptive cells. Most are interneurons connecting within one or two segments to other lamina II cells. Many cells in other laminae have dendrites that penetrate into lamina II, thereby implying that lamina II cells may influence other parts of the spinal gray matter. One type of cell, the stalk cell, sends excitatory input into lamina I.[75,76] Another type of cell, the islet cell, is thought to be inhibitory. Some of these islet cells are thought to be GABAergic and some enkephalinergic.[77,78,79]

Most laminae III and IV neurons respond maximally to nonnoxious stimuli and synapse mainly with large myelinated afferents. Some of these cells project to other laminae and modulate nociception. Many lamina IV cells project to the thalamus.

Like lamina I, lamina V is concerned mainly with nociception. Lamina V cells have large receptive fields, due to the convergence of afferent input from many sources. Dendrites of lamina V cells extend to laminae I and II. Afferent input from laminae I through IV are transmitted through interneurons to lamina V. Most lamina V cells are of the WDR type. The largest proportion of the cell bodies of the spinothalamic tract are found in lamina V. Most lamina V cells project to the thalamus.

Several points of evidence indicate that laminae I, II, and V are crucial in rostral nociceptive transmission: (1) cells from these areas project to the thalamus;[67] (2) cutting this projection abolishes cutaneous pain;[79] (3) stimulating the projections of laminae I and II produces pain;[79] (4) discharge of these cells increases with increasing noxious stimulation;[80] and (5) in response to a brief noxious stimulus, laminae I and V neurons have early and late discharges, analogous to first and second pain.[20,81]

Lamina VI receives mainly proprioceptive input and projects to the cerebellum.

Laminae VII and VIII contain many nociceptive neurons with complicated inputs and large receptive fields.[82] These neurons project to the thalamus and the reticular formation.

Lamina X cells have predominantly nociceptive afferent input and small receptive fields (similar to laminae I and II cells).[83]

In summary, laminae I, II, and V are the major areas for convergence of nociceptive transmission at the spinal cord. Laminae I, V, VII, and VIII contain most of the rostrally projecting neurons. Lamina II is composed mostly of interneurons; lamina I contains mainly NS cells, and lamina V contains mainly WDR cells. Laminae VII and VIII neurons possess complex afferent inputs and large receptive fields.

Central Hypersensitization or Wind-Up

If a neuron mediating nociception in the dorsal horn is repetitively stimulated by a stimulus of sufficient intensity to activate C fibers, the frequency of discharge of that neuron will dramatically increase over time (Fig. 2-30).[84–86] The perception of pain will increase concomitantly.[87] This process is called central hypersensitization or wind-up.[84–90] Wind-up will occur in the absence of sensitization of peripheral nociceptors, and is thought to represent a central mechanism for long-term enhancement of nociception.[90] The characteristics of central hypersensitization are similar to responses induced by excitatory amino acids that act at the N-methyl-D-aspartate (NMDA) receptor.[88] In fact, NMDA receptor antagonists, such as ketamine and MK801, will abolish central hypersensitization without altering the usual response of dorsal horn cells to noxious stimulation.[88]

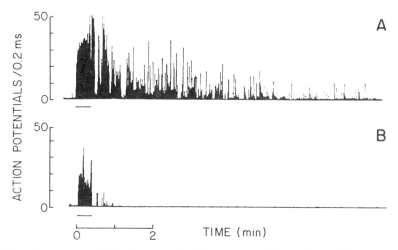

Fig. 2-30. Frequency of discharge evoked in posterior biceps femoris/semitendinous α-motor neurons of the rat by stimulation of a chronically sectioned sciatic nerve for 20 sec at 10 Hz at C-fiber strength. The period of stimulation is denoted by horizontal lines under each recording. (**A**) Stimulation of sectioned nerve produces a very long after-discharge ("wind-up"). (**B**) Stimulation of intact sciatic nerve results in a smaller number of action potentials for a shorter time period. (From Wall and Woolf,[84] with permission.)

The possible role of central hypersensitization in the production of acute[91,92] and chronic[93] pain is of more than passing significance. Its potential clinical impact is discussed in Chapter 12.

Ascending Nociceptive Pathways

More than a century ago, the anterolateral quadrant (ALQ) of the spinal cord was determined to be essential for transmission of nociception in animals. This has been confirmed many times over in humans.[60] The major ascending nociceptive tract in the ALQ is the spinothalamic tract (STT) (Fig. 2-13). Other tracts of the ALQ that are thought to be involved in pain perception are (1) the ventral STT, (2) the spinoreticular tract (SRT), (3) the spinomesencephalic tract (SMT), (4) the dorsal column postsynaptic spinomedullary system, and (5) the propriospinal multisynaptic ascending system.

The Spinothalamic Tract

The cell bodies of the STT are located in laminae I, V, VII, and VIII.[67] Their axons cross to the contralateral side of the spinal cord within a few segments of entry into the STT, ascend in the ALQ, and project to multiple nuclei in the brain stem and the thalamus. As the STT approaches the thalamus, it segregates into a medial and lateral division[94] (Fig. 2-13). The medial division terminates in the medial thalamic nuclei, the central lateral nucleus of the intralaminar complex, and the nucleus submedius (Figs. 2-24 and 2-25). The lateral division terminates in the lateral, the ventral basal, and posterior thalamic nuclei (Figs. 2-24 and 2-25).

Most axons of the lateral STT arise from laminae I and V (Fig. 2-13). These cells are either NS (lamina I) or WDR (lamina V) neurons. Their receptive fields are small discreet areas on a limb. They synapse in the lateral thalamus and project to the somatosensory cortex in a somatotopically organized manner. The lateral STT is sometimes referred to as the neospinothalamic tract, as it does not exist in lower animals.[95,96] Its function is thought to be localization and characterization of a nociceptive stimulus: the sensory/discriminative aspects of pain perception.

Most axons of the medial STT arise in laminae VII and VIII (Fig. 2-13). These neurons have large, complex receptive fields that may be bilateral. Their axons project to the medial thalamus but also to the brain stem reticular formation, periaqueductal gray matter, and hypothalamus (Fig. 2-13). Projections from these structures have been shown to terminate in widespread regions of the cortex and limbic system (Fig. 2-13). The medial STT does occur in lower animals, and is called the paleospinothalamic tract.[95,96] The medial STT is believed to mediate the general arousal and autonomic responses to pain: the affective/motivational aspects of pain perception.

The Ventral Spinothalamic Tract

The STT has a ventral component, the ventral STT, whose cell bodies are found in laminae I and IV–VII. The ventral STT ascends in the ventral funiculus of the spinal cord and terminates in multiple brain stem and thalamic nuclei. Evidence for its role in nociception is indirect.[97]

The Spinoreticular Tract

Cells of origin of the SRT are found in laminae I and V–VII.[98] The axons of the SRT ascend intermixed with the STT and terminate bilaterally in the brain stem reticular formation. The SRT is believed to participate in the affective/motivational aspects of the perception of pain.

The Spinomesencephalic Tract

Cells of origin of the SMT are located mainly in laminae I and V. Most project contralaterally and ascend in the ALQ and other areas of the cord.[60] The SMT is also believed to participate in the affective/motivational aspects of pain perception.

The SRT, SMT, and the medial forebrain bundle are sometimes grouped as

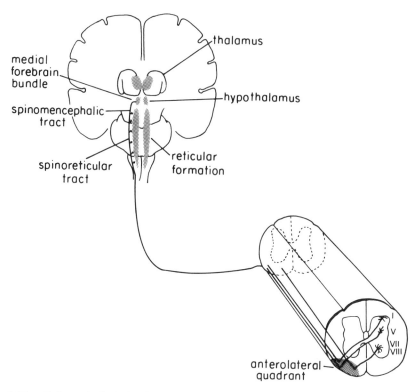

Fig. 2-31. Spinoreticulothalamic tract. The spinoreticular tract, the spinomesencephalic tract, and the medial forebrain bundle are sometimes grouped as a functional unit called the spinoreticulothalamic tract. They form a pathway of multiple synapses among the spinal cord, brain stem reticular formation, thalamus, and hypothalamus. As the pathway ends in the paraventricular nucleus of the hypothalamus via the medial forebrain bundle, the spinoreticulothalamic tract is believed to be involved in the neuroendocrine response to pain.

a functional unit called the spinoreticulothalamic tract[99] (Fig. 2-31). They form a pathway of multiple synaptic connections among the spinal cord, brain stem reticular formation, thalamus, and hypothalamus (via the medial forebrain bundle). In particular, fibers reach the paraventricular nucleus of the hypothalamus, a major integrating center for global hormonal and autonomic responses.[100] Thus, the spinoreticulothalamic tract is believed to be implicated in the neuroendocrine response to pain and the genesis of the surgical stress response (see Ch. 4).

The Dorsal Column Postsynaptic Spinomedullary System

Although the dorsal columns have traditionally been conceptualized as consisting of first-order neurons subserving proprioception and crude tactile sensations, they also contain postsynaptic neurons that respond to noxious stimuli.[101]

These fibers originate in laminae III and IV and ascend in the dorsal columns. They terminate in the dorsal column nuclei of the medulla, which subsequently give rise to projections that ascend in the medial lemniscus to the lateral thalamus.[102] The role of the dorsal column polysynaptic system in human sensation is uncertain. It may modulate information transmitted via the STT.

The Propriospinal Multisynaptic Ascending System

The spinal gray matter is immediately surrounded by white matter tracts consisting of short ascending and descending fibers (the fasciculus proprius) (Fig. 2-11). Several observations suggest a role in nociception for the fasciculus proprius: (1) certain visceral pains persist even after bilateral cordotomy,[103] and (2) reaction time to painful stimulation in animal models may not be decreased after simultaneous bilateral hemitransection of the cord at different levels.[104] The role of this tract in pain perception in humans is uncertain.

Rostral Centers

The Reticular Formation

The reticular formation consists of a number of vaguely defined nuclei situated in the core of the brain stem and extending throughout its rostrocaudal aspect (Figs. 2-20–2-23). Axons arising from the reticular formation are long and have extensive connections throughout the neuraxis. The reticular formation participates in the regulation of motor, sensory, and autonomic functions.

Many reticular neurons respond to noxious stimulation,[105] and many respond exclusively to specific noxious modalities.[106] Stimulation of Aδ and C fibers has been shown to excite cells in a reticular nucleus in the cat.[107] Stimulation of peripheral Aδ and C fibers correlated with escape behavior. Direct stimulation of the nucleus itself reproduced the behavior.[107] The reticular formation is thought to participate in the affective/motivational component of pain and in the integration of pain with autonomic and motor behavior.

The Thalamus

Within the thalamus (Figs. 2-24 and 2-25), the ventrobasal complex, the posterior nuclear group of the lateral nuclei, and the central lateral nucleus and nucleus submedius of the medial nuclei are involved in nociception.

Ventrobasal Complex

The ventrobasal complex is composed of two nuclei: the ventral posterior lateral nucleus and the ventral posterior medial nucleus (Fig. 2-24). The ventral posterior lateral nucleus receives nociceptive transmission from the lateral STT, nonnociceptive input from the dorsal columns, and input from the periaqueductal gray matter. The ventral posterior medial nucleus receives similar information from the face through the lateral trigeminothalamic tract (Fig. 2-24).

Most ventrobasal neurons respond to noxious as well as nonnoxious stimuli. The ventrobasal complex projects in a highly organized manner to the somatosensory cortex. The ventral posterior medial nucleus projects, in particular, to the cortical region concerned with facial sensation.

POSTERIOR NUCLEAR GROUP

This region receives nociceptive transmission from the STT and dorsal columns and projects without somatotopic organization to the retroinsular cortex, an additional somatosensory area. The receptive fields of these neurons are large and complex.

CENTRAL LATERAL NUCLEUS

The central lateral nucleus of the internal medullary lamina receives bilateral transmission from the deep laminae of the spinal cord through the medial STT and the reticular formation. Input from deep somatic structures is extensive.[60] Excitation results from stimulation of the medullary reticular formation as well as peripheral Aδ and C fibers.[108] Projections are not topographic and are diffuse to widespread areas of the brain.[109] The central lateral nucleus is believed to mediate general arousal and motor responses to pain.

NUCLEUS SUBMEDIUS

Although located in the medial thalamus, this nucleus receives topographically organized projections from lamina I.[110] This nucleus is organized like the ventrobasal complex but projects to the orbitofrontal cortex,[111] an area not known to play a role in pain sensation.

The Hypothalamus and the Limbic System

The limbic system consists of a ring of cortex on the medial aspect of each hemisphere (the cingulate, subcallosal, and parahippocampal gyri), subcortical nuclei, parts of the thalamus and midbrain, and the hypothalamus. The limbic system is phylogenetically very old. It is concerned with regulation of the ANS, visceral activity, emotion, motivation, arousal, and complex behaviors. Limbic structures are interconnected through numerous pathways, including the mamillothalamic tract, medial forebrain bundle, and dorsal longitudinal fasciculus.

As the regulator of the ANS, the hypothalamus governs autonomic and neuroendocrine responses to stimuli of all types including pain. Hypothalamic cells respond to noxious and nonnoxious stimuli and are not organized to provide discriminative information. Stimulation of parts of the limbic system may evoke escape behavior or an "approach" response.[60] Lesions of the cingulum (as formerly performed in "prefrontal lobotomies" for intractable pain) produce loss of the affective component of pain perception, leaving the sensory/discriminative component intact.[112]

Thus, the limbic system is thought to subserve the affective/motivational aspects of the perception of pain.

The Cerebral Cortex

Early observations on the role of the cortex in pain perception were contradictory. Removal of large areas of cortex left pain perception intact,[113] and electric stimulation of cortical areas did not produce pain.[114] However, some later reports on the production of pain by electric stimulation did appear.[67] Epileptic discharges are known to cause pain on occasion.[115] Some cortical lesions do decrease pain sensation contralaterally.[116] Although the reasons for these early discrepancies are not clear, evidence of a role for the cortex in pain perception has emerged.

THE SOMATOSENSORY CORTEX

The primary somatosensory area (Brodmann areas 3, 1, 2) (Fig. 2-32) receives direct, topographically organized projections from the lateral thalamus. A population of cells responds largely to noxious stimulation.[117] Some cells are NS and some are WDR neurons. The NS neurons are of two types, possessing either small contralateral receptive fields (e.g., neurons of the lateral STT) or large, complex receptive fields (e.g., those of the medial STT). The primary somatosensory cortex is thought to mediate the sensory/discriminative aspects of pain perception.

THE FRONTAL LOBE

Frontal lobotomies were once used for intractable pain.[113] Patients continued to report their pain if questioned, but they seldom asked for medications and no longer seemed to care about their pain. The frontal lobotomies had removed the motivational/affective component of their pain perception. A similar picture is seen in bilateral thalamic lesions.[2] The frontal lobe receives diffuse projections from the medial thalamic nuclei, which are thought to subserve the affective/motivational aspects of pain perception through their frontal–limbic connections.

Summary of Transmission

The spinal cord is organized into discrete layers called laminae. Within the laminae are found both excitatory and inhibitory interneurons, as well as projection cells relaying afferent input to rostral centers. Certain cells within the laminae respond only to nociceptive transmission (NS neurons). Other second-order neurons respond to a wide range of stimuli (WDR neurons).

Large myelinated afferents (Aα and Aβ fibers) enter the dorsal root in a

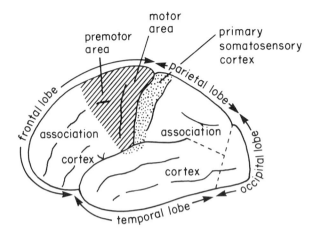

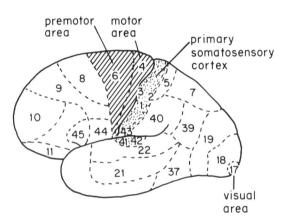

Fig. 2-32. The cerebral cortex is divided into frontal, parietal, temporal, and occipital lobes. Brodmann numbers are assigned to numerous discrete, functional areas. The primary somatosensory cortex corresponds to areas 3, 1, 2. The motor cortex corresponds to areas 4 and 6.

dorsomedial orientation and bifurcate into ascending and descending branches within the dorsal columns. Collaterals of these fibers synapse in laminae III and IV. Aδ and C fibers enter the dorsal root in a ventrolateral orientation and subsequently enter Lissauer's tract to ultimately synapse in laminae I, II and V.

The major ascending tract is the STT, whose cell bodies are located in laminae I, V (mainly), VII, and VIII. The rostrally projecting axons of these neurons enter the ALQ. The ALQ in turn gives rise to two distinct pathways as the STT approaches the thalamus. The lateral STT or neospinothalamic tract synapses in the lateral thalamus and subsequently projects to the somatosensory cortex. The lateral STT subserves the sensory/discriminative aspects of pain perception. The medial STT or paleospinothalamic tract has multiple synapses in the brain stem reticular formation, the medial thalamus, periaqueductal gray matter, and hypothalamus. Subsequent projections are to diffuse areas of the cortex and limbic system. Thus, the medial STT subserves the affective/motivational aspects of pain perception.

MODULATION

It has long been observed that injuries of similar severity can give rise to dramatically different degrees of pain perception in different individuals, depending on psychological, situational, cultural, or other factors. For example, battlefield injuries may be associated with little or no pain compared with civilian injuries of similar severity.[118] Furthermore, administration of an inert substance or placebo can produce significant analgesia.[119] Thus, the ability of the CNS to modulate pain has long been recognized. The mechanisms by which it does so have only recently come to light.

Stimulus-Produced Analgesia

Reynolds[120] first observed profound analgesia in rats during electric stimulation of the periaqueductal gray matter surrounding the cerebral aqueduct (Fig. 2-23). The duration of this stimulation-produced analgesia[121,122] outlasted the application of the stimulus and inhibited withdrawal reflexes, irrespective of the intensity of subsequent noxious stimuli.[123] Such withdrawal reflexes in the rat are spinally mediated. Stimulation-produced analgesia inhibits these withdrawal reflexes through activation of descending antinociceptive pathways. The lack of alteration of other sensory or motor behaviors indicates a specific effect on the pain modulating system. Stimulation-produced analgesia has also been noted in humans.[124]

Opioid-Mediated Analgesia

Several regions of the brain have been found to evoke stimulation-produced analgesia in both animals and humans.[125] Such regions have been found to contain or to overlap areas with a high concentration of endogenous opioid neurotransmitters.[126] Extensive evidence indicates a common anatomy, physiology, and pharmacology between stimulation-produced analgesia and opioid-mediated analgesia. Injection of minute quantities of morphine into sites known to produce stimulation-produced analgesia will result in intense analgesia.[127] Patients or experimental animals can become tolerant to stimulation-produced analgesia, and cross-tolerance exists between morphine and stimulation-produced analgesia.[128] Furthermore, stimulation-produced analgesia can be attenuated by opioid antagonists.[124,129] However, the stimulation-produced and opioid-mediated analgesic systems are not identical, as there are other forms of stimulation-produced analgesia that are not mediated by the endogenous opioid system.

Anatomy of the Descending Modulating System[130]

Midbrain

Stimulation-produced analgesia can be most consistently induced in humans by stimulation of the periaqueductal gray matter (midbrain) (Figs. 2-23 and 2-33) or the periventricular gray matter lateral to the hypothalamus[131] (Fig. 2-33). These two areas are connected anatomically to each other and to a medullary region with similar properties called the rostroventral medulla[132,133] (Fig. 2-33). The rostroventral medulla receives input from the periventricular and periaqueductal gray matter and widespread regions of the brain and spinal cord.[134] The rostroventral medulla projects through the reticulospinal tracts (Fig. 2-12) and the dorsolateral funiculus (Figs. 2-12 and 2-33) to laminae I, II, and V of the dorsal horn.[135] As noted, these laminae receive the densest nociceptive afferent transmission.

The Pons

Stimulation of the lateral and dorsolateral pontine tegmentum produces analgesia in animals[136] (Fig. 2-33). This region contains noradrenergic neurons that project to the periaqueductal gray matter, rostroventral medulla, and the spinal cord.

The Medulla

Stimulation of the rostroventral medulla reliably generates stimulation-produced analgesia.[137] As discussed, the periaqueductal gray matter sends a major projection to the rostroventral medulla. The rostroventral medulla in turn projects to the dorsal horn via the reticulospinal tracts and the dorsolateral funiculus, terminating in laminae I, II, and V (Figs. 2-12 and 2-33). Indeed, the periaqueductal gray matter appears to produce its inhibitory effect on the dorsal horn through this projection pathway.[138] The rostroventral medulla includes the midline serotonin-containing nucleus raphe magnus. Thus, serotonin is implicated as the neurotransmitter of this pathway.

The Cortex and Diencephalon

Stimulation of the primary somatosensory cortex in animals can inhibit the responses of WDR neurons in the spinal cord to C-fiber input.[131] Such inhibition appears to be mediated by the corticospinal tract. Stimulation of various subcor-

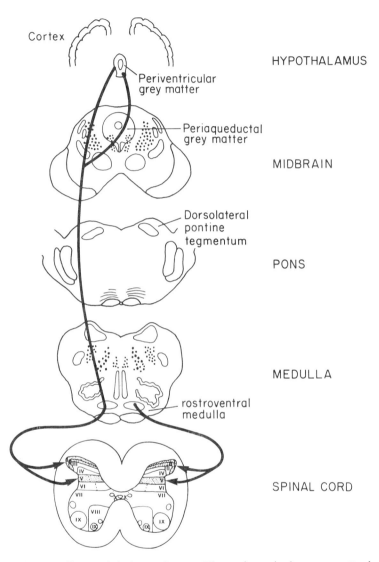

Fig. 2-33. Descending modulating pathways. The periventricular gray matter lateral to the hypothalamus and the periaqueductal gray matter of the midbrain are anatomically interconnected. They give rise to a descending projection that passes through the rostroventral medulla and descends in the dorsolateral funiculus of the spinal cord to synapse with nociceptive neurons in laminae I, II, and V. As there is only a minor direct projection from the periaqueductal gray matter to the spinal cord, the rostroventral medulla acts as a relay to the spinal cord for more rostral centers. Separate from this projection pathway, noradrenergic neurons in the dorsolateral pontine tegmentum and serotonergic neurons of the rostroventral medulla also discretely project to the dorsolateral funiculus and then to laminae I, II, and V.

tical structures, including the thalamus, can also produce analgesia,[139] although the exact mechanism underlying this process is unknown.[60]

Neurotransmitters of the Descending Pathways[130,140]

Norepinephrine

Much evidence implicates an α-receptor-mediated descending inhibitory influence on nociception. The dorsolateral pons (which is conducive to stimulation-produced analgesia) contains noradrenergic neurons.[141] There is a high concentration of α$_2$-receptors in the dorsal horn.[142] Application of norepinephrine to the spinal cord inhibits discharge of dorsal horn nociceptive neurons[143] and decreases the response of animals to noxious stimulation.[144] Such effects appear to be mediated by an α$_2$-receptor.

Clonidine (an α$_2$-agonist) inhibits discharge of nociceptive neurons in the dorsal horn[145] and produces analgesia when applied to the spinal cord in animals[146] and humans.[147] Yohimbine, an α$_2$-antagonist, reduces the antinociceptive effect of brain stem stimulation.[148] Norepinephrine may be an important element of opioid-mediated analgesia as well. Administration of α-antagonists has been shown to reduce the analgesia produced by systemic administration of opioids, as well as that produced by microinjection of morphine into neural tissue.[149]

Serotonin

Evidence analogous to that for norepinephrine implicates serotonin as a neurotransmitter in descending antinociceptive pathways.[150] The rostroventral medulla is rich in serotonergic neurons that project to the spinal cord.[151] Stimulation of neurons in the rostroventral medulla with serotonergic terminals in the dorsal horn inhibits nociceptive neurons in laminae I and II.[72] Serotonin antagonists can attenuate analgesia produced by stimulation of the rostroventral medulla.[152] Finally, application of serotonin to the spinal cord inhibits discharge of STT neurons[153] and relieves pain.[154]

Endogenous Opioids

SITES OF ACTION

Opioids are the most powerful systemic analgesics known and have been used for millennia. Many observations indicate that exogenously administered opioids exert their analgesic effects by acting directly on the CNS.[2,155] In particular, injection of minute amounts of morphine into multiple discrete areas of the brain and spinal cord can produce profound analgesia at doses well below those required systemically.[2,155] The major anatomic areas involved in opioid-mediated analgesia include the periventricular and periaqueductal gray matter and the rostroventral medulla (all also involved in stimulation-produced analgesia). Injection of naloxone into these regions attenuates analgesia from systemic opioids, implying that exogenously administered opioids act at these sites to produce analgesia. Rats with bilateral lesions of the dorsolateral funiculus of the spinal cord require significantly greater amounts of morphine to achieve analgesia, implying that opioids act by activating descending antinociceptive pathways.[2,155]

Administration of exogenous opioids may also activate descending monoaminergic antinociceptive pathways.[155] Supraspinal administration of opioids results in increased release of serotonin and norepinephrine at the spinal cord. The antinociceptive effects of morphine administered to the periaqueductal gray matter are mimicked by application of serotonin or norepinephrine to the spinal cord and antagonized by spinal adrenergic and serotonergic antagonists.[155]

Activation of descending brain stem pathways does not entirely account for opioid-mediated analgesia, however. Systemic administration does not produce the local tissue concentrations attained by microinjection into the periaqueductal gray matter or rostroventral medulla. Application of opioid directly to the spinal cord produces profound analgesia without affecting other sensory or motor systems in both animals and in humans.[73,156] Concomitant administration of morphine to the brain stem and spinal cord demonstrates synergistic action.[157] Thus, systemic opioids produce analgesia by acting synergistically at multiple CNS sites and by activation of descending monoaminergic antinociceptive pathways.

The biochemistry of the endogenous opioids as well as a discussion of the opioid receptor and receptor classes is extensively discussed in Chapter 8. The reader is referred to that source for a discussion of this very important topic.

Summary of Modulation

There are descending antinociceptive pathways within the CNS. Important centers of this descending modulating system include the periventricular and periaqueductal gray matter, the dorsolateral pons, the nucleus raphe magnus, and the rostroventral medulla. Biogenic amines (serotonin and norepinephrine), as well as endogenous opioids, are implicated as neurotransmitters. The ultimate projection of these descending pathways is to laminae I, II, and V through the dorsolateral funiculus of the spinal cord. These descending antinociceptive pathways can be activated by electric stimulation, systemic or neuraxial injection of opioids, and neuraxial injection of α_2-agonists, as well as by stress, suggestion, and pain.

THE SYNTHESIS: THE GATE CONTROL THEORY OF PAIN

Knowledge of the neuroanatomy and neurophysiology of nociception is of more than academic interest. Such knowledge is of practical importance, as it forms the basis for a rational approach to the treatment of postoperative pain by

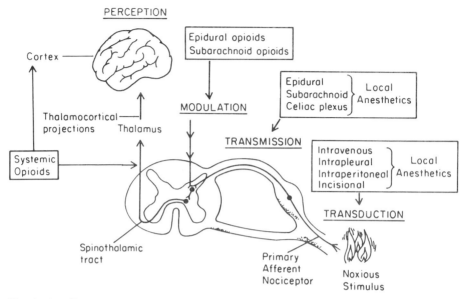

Fig. 2-34. Gate control theory of pain. The physiologic process underlying nociception (transduction, transmission, and modulation) all converge on and impact on the discharge of nociceptive neurons in laminae I, II, and V of the dorsal horn. Thus, the dorsal horn is the focal point or *gate* for the integration and modulation of nociception. The pharmacologic manipulation of the processes of transduction, transmission, and modulation with highly specific agents can effectively "close the gate." This key concept forms the philosophic underpinning of the effective management of postoperative pain.

manipulation of the physiologic processes involved: transduction, transmission, and modulation. All three physiologic processes converge on and impact on the discharge of nociceptive neurons in laminae I, II, and V of the dorsal horn. Therefore, the dorsal horn is the focal point or *gate* for the integration and modulation of nociception (Fig. 2-34). Thus, the neural pathways for pain sensation are not "labeled lines" or mere cables in the complex circuitry of the PNS and CNS. Nociception is a dynamic and fluid process, capable of modification and modulation at discrete levels with particular highly specific agents. Thus, the concept of the dorsal horn as a "gate" that can be "closed" by the pharmacologic manipulation of transduction, transmission, and modulation forms the underlying philosophic tenet for effective management of postoperative pain (Fig. 2-34).

References
1. Mersky H: Classification of chronic pain: description of chronic pain syndromes and definition of pain terms. Pain, suppl. 3:S1, 1986
2. Fields HL: Pain. McGraw-Hill, New York, 1987
3. Gasser HS: Pain-producing impulses in peripheral nerves. Proc A Res Nerv Ment Dis 23:44, 1943
4. Hursh JB: Conduction velocity and diameter of nerve fibers. Am J Physiol 127: 131, 1939

5. Lloyd DPC: Neuron patterns controlling transmission of ipsilateral hind limb reflexes in cat. J Neurophysiol 6:293, 1943
6. Bishop GH: Neural mechanisms of cutaneous sense. Physiol Rev 26:77, 1946
7. Cauna N: The free pencillate nerve endings of human hairy skin. J Anat 115:277, 1973
8. Cauna N: Fine morphological characteristics and microtopography of the free nerve endings of the human digital skin. Anat Rec 198:643, 1980
9. Collins WF Jr, Nulsen FE, Randt CT: Relation of peripheral nerve fiber size and sensation in man. Arch Neurol 3:381, 1960
10. Adriaensen H, Gybels J, Handwerker H, Van Hees J: Response properties of thin myelinated (Aδ) fibers in human skin nerves. J Neurophysiol 49:111, 1983
11. Besson P, Perl ER: Response of cutaneous sensory units with unmyelinated fibers to noxious stimuli. J Neurophysiol 32:1025, 1969
12. Torebjork HE: Afferent C units responding to mechanical, thermal and chemical stimuli in human nonglabrous skin. Acta Physiol Scand 92:374, 1974
13. Van Hees J, Gybels JM: Pain related to single afferent C fibers from human skin. Brain Res 48:397, 1972
14. Gybels J, Handwerker HO, Van Hees J: A comparison between the discharges of human nociceptive nerve fibres and the subject's ratings of his sensations. J Physiol 292:193, 1979
15. LaMotte RH, Campbell JN: Comparison of responses of warm and nociceptive C-fiber afferents in monkey with human judgements of thermal pain. J Neurophysiol 41:509, 1978
16. Price DD, Dubner R: Neurons that subserve the sensory-discriminative aspects of pain. Pain 3:307, 1977
17. Torebjork HE, Hallin RG: Perceptual changes accompanying controlled preferential blocking of A and C-fibre responses in intact human skin nerves. Exp Brain Res 16:321, 1973
18. Torebjork HE, Hallin RG: Identification of afferent C units in intact human skin nerves. Brain Res 67:387, 1974
19. Lewis T, Pechin EE: The double pain response of the human skin to a single stimulus. Clin Sci 3:67, 1937
20. Price DD, Hu JW, Dubner R, Gracely RH: Peripheral suppression of first pain and central summation of second pain evoked by noxious heat pulses. Pain 3:57, 1977
21. Campbell JN, LaMotte RH: Latency to detection of first pain. Brain Res 266:203, 1983
22. Georgopoulos AP: Functional properties of primary afferent units probably related to pain mechanisms in primate glabrous skin. J Neurophysiol 39:71, 1976
23. Lewis T: Pain. Macmillan, New York, 1942
24. Meyer RA, Campbell JN: Myelinated nociceptive afferents account for the hyperalgesia that follows a burn to the hand. Science 213:1527, 1981
25. Campbell JN, Meyer RA, LaMotte RH: Sensitization of myelinated nociceptive afferents that innervate monkey hand. J Neurophysiol 42:1669, 1979
26. Campbell JN, Raja SN, Cohen RH et al: Peripheral neural mechanisms of nociception. p. 22. In Wall PD, Melzack R (eds): Textbook of Pain. 2nd Ed. Churchill Livingstone, Edinburgh, 1989
27. Fitzgerald M: The spread of sensitization of polymodal nociceptors in the rabbit from nearby injury and by antidromic nerve stimulation. J Physiol 297:207, 1979
28. Raja SN, Campbell JN, Meyer PA: Evidence for different mechanisms of primary and secondary hyperalgesia following heat injury to the glabrous skin. Brain 107:1179, 1984

29. Juan H, Lembeck F: Action of peptides and other algesic agents on paravascular pain receptors of the isolated perfused rabbit ear. Naunyn Schmiedebergs Arch Pharmacol 283:151, 1974

30. Yaksh TL, Hammond DL: Peripheral and central substrates in the rostral transmission of nociceptive information. Pain 13:1, 1982

31. Armstrong D: Bradykinin, kallidin and kallikrein. p. 434. In Erdos EG (ed): Handbook of Experimental Pharmacology. Vol. 25. Springer-Verlag, Berlin, 1970

32. Beck PW, Handwerker HO: Bradykinin and serotonin effects on various types of cutaneous nerve fibres. Pflugers Arch 347:209, 1974

33. Ferreira SH: Prostaglandins, aspirin-like drugs, and analgesia. Nature New Biol 240:200, 1972

34. Fock S, Mense S: Excitatory effects of 5-hydroxytryptamine, histamine and postassium ions on muscular group IV afferent units: a comparison with bradykinin. Brain Res 105:459, 1976

35. Bisgaard H, Kristensen JK: Leukotriene B4 produces hyperalgesia in humans. Prostaglandins 30:791, 1985

36. Levine JD, Lau W, Kwiat G, Goetzl EJ: Leukotriene B4 produces hyperalgesia that is dependent upon polymorphonuclear leukocytes. Science 225:743, 1984

37. Chahl LA, Ladd RJ: Local oedema and general excitation of cutaneous sensory receptors produced by electrical stimulation of the saphenous nerve in the rat. Pain 2:25, 1976

38. Chapman LF, Ramos AO, Goodell H, Wolff HG: Neurohumoral features of afferent fibers in man. Arch Neurol 4:617, 1961

39. von Enler US, Gaddum JH: An unidentified depressive substance in certain tissue extracts. J Physiol 72:74, 1931

40. Brimijoin S, Lundberg JM, Brodin E et al: Axonal transport of substance P in the vagus and sciatic nerves of the guinea pig. Brain Res 191:443, 1980

41. Otsuka M, Konishi S, Yanagisawa M et al: Role of substance P as a sensory transmitter in the spinal cord and sympathetic ganglia. Ciba Found Symp 91:13, 1982

42. Gamse R, Petsche U, Lembeck F, Jancso G: Capsaicin applied to peripheral nerve inhibits axoplasmic transport of substance P and somatostatin. Brain Res 239:447, 1982

43. Jansco N, Jansco-Gabor A, Szolcsanyi J: Direct evidence for neurogenic inflammation and its prevention by denervation and by pretreatment with capsaicin. Br J Pharmacol 31:138, 1967

44. Lambeck F: Sir Thomas Lewis's nocifensor system, histamine and substance-P-containing primary afferent nerves. Trends Neurosci 6:106, 1983

45. Richardson BP, Engel G, Donatsch P, Stadler PA: Identification of serotonin M-receptor subtypes and their specific blockade by a new class of drugs. Nature 316:126, 1985

46. Sicuteri F, Fanciullacci M, Franchi G, Del Bianco PL: Serotonin-bradykinin potentiation of the pain receptors in man. Life Sci 4:309, 1965

47. Richardson BP, Engel G: The pharmacology and function of 5-HT3 receptors. Trends Neurosci 9:424, 1986

48. Roberts WJ, Elardo SM: Sympathetic activation of Aδ nociceptors. Somatosensory Res 3:33, 1985

49. Korenman EMD, Devor M: Ectopic adrenergic sensitivity in damaged peripheral nerve axons in the rat. Exp Neurol 72:63, 1981

50. Mense S, Meyer H: Different types of slowly conducting afferent units in cat skeletal muscle tendon. J Physiol 363:403, 1985

51. Mense S, Stahnke M: Responses in muscle afferent fibres of slow conduction velocity to contractions and ischaemia in the cat. J Physiol 342:383, 1983
52. Kumazawa T, Mizumura K: Thin-fibre receptors responding to mechanical, chemical, and thermal stimulation in the skeletal muscle of the dog. J Physiol 273:179, 1977
53. Mense S: Nerve outflow from skeletal muscle following chemical noxious stimulation. J Physiol 267:75, 1977
54. Mense S: Sensitization of group IV muscle receptors to bradykinin by 5-hydroxytryptamine and prostaglandin E2. Brain Res 225:95, 1981
55. Brown AM: Excitation of afferent cardiac sympathetic nerve fibres during myocardial ischaemia. J Physiol 190:35, 1967
56. Schaible HG, Schmidt RF: Activation of groups III and IV sensory units in medial articular nerve by local mechanical stimulation of knee joint. J Neurophysiol 49:35, 1983
57. Schaible HG, Schmidt RF: Responses of fine medial articular nerve afferents to passive movements of knee joints. J Neurophysiol 49:1118, 1983
58. Coggeshall RE, Hong KA, Langford LA et al: Discharge characteristics of fine medial articular afferents at rest and during passive movements of inflamed knee joints. Brain Res 272:185, 1983
59. Hurrell DJ: The nerve supply of bone. J Anat 72:54, 1937
60. Bonica JJ: The Management of Pain. 2nd Ed. Lea & Febiger, Philadelphia, 1990
61. Cervero F, Morrison JFB: Visceral Sensation. Elsevier, Amsterdam, 1986
62. Goldberg SG: Clinical Neuroanatomy Made Ridiculously Simple. Medmaster, Miami, 1990
63. Coggeshall RE: Afferent fibers in the ventral root. Neurosurgery 4:443, 1979
64. Rexed B: A cytoarchitectonic atlas of the spinal cord in the cat. J Comp Neurol 96:415, 1952
65. Coggeshall RE, Chung K, Chung JM, Langford LA: Primary afferent axons in the tract of Lissauer in the monkey. J Comp Neurol 196:431, 1981
66. LaMotte C: Distribution of the tract of Lissauer and the dorsal root fibers in the primate spinal cord. J Comp Neurol 172:529, 1977
67. Willis WD: The Pain System. S Karger, Basel, 1985
68. Light AR, Perl ER: Spinal termination of functionally identified primary afferent neurons with slowly conducting myelinated fibers. J Comp Neurol 186:133, 1979
69. Willis WD Jr: Visceral inputs to sensory pathways in the spinal cord. Prog Brain Res 67:207, 1986
70. Urban L, Randic M: Slow excitatory transmission in rat dorsal horn: possible mediation by peptides. Brain Res 290:336, 1984
71. Bittner MA, Lahann TR: Biphasic time-course of capsaicin-induced substance P depletion: failure to correlate with thermal analgesia in the rat. Brain Res 322:305, 1984
72. Ruda MA, Bennet GJ, Dubner R: Neurochemistry and neurocircuitry in the dorsal horn. Prog Brain Res 66:219, 1986
73. Yaksh TL, Noueihed R: The physiology and pharmacology of spinal opiates. Annu Rev Pharmacol Toxicol 25:433, 1985
74. Dubner R, Bennet GJ: Spinal and trigeminal mechanisms of nociception. Annu Rev Neurosci 6:381, 1983
75. Price DD, Hayashi H, Dubner R, Ruda MA: Functional relationship between neurons of marginal and substantia gelatinosa layers of primate dorsal horn. J Neurophysiol 42:1590, 1979

76. Gobel S: Golgi studies of the neurons in layer II of the dorsal horn of the medulla (trigeminal nucleus caudalis). J Comp Neurol 180:395, 1978
77. Cervero F, Iggo A: The substantia gelatinosa of the spinal cord: a critical review. Brain 103:717, 1980
78. Gobel S: Neural circuitry in the substantia gelatinosa of Rolando: anatomical insights, p. 175. In Bonica JJ, Liebeskind J, Albe-Fessard D (eds): Advances in Pain Research and Therapy. Vol. 3. Raven Press, New York, 1979
79. Mayer DJ, Price DD, Becker DP: Neurophysiological characterization of the anterolateral spinal cord neurons contributing to pain perception in man. Pain 1:51, 1975
80. Kenshalo DR Jr, Leonard RB, Chung JM, Willis WD: Responses of primate spinothalamic neurons to graded and repeated noxious heat stimuli. J Neurophysiol 42: 1370, 1979
81. Chung JM, Kenshalo DR Jr, Gerhart KD, Willis WD: Excitation of primate spinothalamic neurons by cutaneous C-fiber volleys. J Neurophysiol 42:1354, 1979
82. Fields HL, Clanton CH, Anderson SD: Somatosensory properties of spinoreticular neurons in the cat. Brain Res 120:49, 1977
83. Nahin RL, Madsen AM, Giesler GJ Jr: Anatomical and physiological studies of the grey matter surrounding the spinal cord central canal. J Comp Neurol 220:321, 1983
84. Wall PD, Woolf CJ: The brief and the prolonged facilitatory effects of unmyelinated afferent input on the rat spinal cord are independently influenced by peripheral nerve section. Neuroscience 17:1199, 1986
85. Wall PD, Coderre TJ, Stern Y, Wiesenfeld-Hallin Z: Slow changes in the flexion reflex of the rat following arthritis or tenotomy. Brain Res 447:215, 1988
86. Woolf CJ: Evidence for a central component of post-injury pain hypersensitivity. Nature 306:686, 1983
87. Price DD, Hayes RL, Ruda M, Dubner R: Spatial and temporal transformations of input to spinothalamic tract neurons and their relation to somatic sensations. J Neurophysiol 41:933, 1978
88. Dickenson AH: A cure for wind-up: NMDA receptor antagonists as potential analgesics. Trends Pharmacol Sci 11:307, 1990
89. Cook AJ, Woolf CJ, Wall PD, McMahon SB: Dynamic receptive field plasticity in rat spinal cord dorsal horn following C-primary afferent input. Nature 325:151, 1987
90. Coderre TJ, Melzack R: Cutaneous hyperalgesia: contributions of the peripheral and central nervous systems to the increase in pain sensitivity after injury. Brain Res 404:95, 1987
91. Tverskoy M, Cozacov C, Ayache M et al: Postoperative pain after inguinal herniorrhaphy with different types of anesthesia. Anesth Analg 70:29, 1990
92. Wall PD: The prevention of postoperative pain (editorial). Pain 33:289, 1988
93. Bach S, Noreng MF, Tjéllden NU: Phantom limb pain in amputees during the first 12 months following limb amputation, after preoperative lumbar epidural blockade. Pain 33:297, 1988
94. Mehler WR: The anatomy of the so-called "pain tract" in man: an analysis of the course and distribution of the ascending fibers of the fasciculus anterolateralis, p. 26. In French JD, Portor RW (eds): Basic Research in Paraplegia. Charles C Thomas, Springfield, 1962
95. Mehler WR: Some neurological species differences—a posteriori. Ann NY Acad Sci 167:424, 1969
96. Kevetter GA, Willis WD: Collateralization in the spinothalamic tract: new methodology to support or deny phylogenetic theories. Brain Res 319:1, 1984

97. Kerr FWL: The ventral spinothalamic tract and other ascending systems of the ventral funiculus of the spinal cord. J Comp Neurol 159:335, 1975
98. Kevetter GA, Haber LH, Yezierski RP et al: Cells of origin of the spinoreticular tract in the monkey. J Comp Neurol 207:61, 1982
99. Yaksh TL: Neurologic mechanisms of pain. p. 791. In Cousins MJ, Bridenbaugh PO (eds): Neural Blockade in Clinical Anesthesia and Management of Pain. 2nd Ed. JB Lippincott, Philadelphia, 1988
100. Swanson LW, Sawchenko PE: Hypothalamic integration: organization of the paraventricular and supraoptic nuclei. Annu Rev Neurosci 6:269, 1983
101. Bennett GJ, Nishikawa N, Lu GW et al: The morphology of dorsal column postsynaptic spinomedullary neurons in the cat. J Comp Neurol 224:568, 1984
102. Dennis SG, Melzack R: Pain-signalling systems in the dorsal and ventral spinal cord. Pain 4:97, 1977
103. White JC, Sweet WH: Pain and the Neurosurgeon. Charles C Thomas, Springfield, IL 1969
104. Basbaum AI: Conduction of the effects of noxious stimulation by short-fiber multisynaptic systems of the spinal cord in rat. Exp Neurol 40:699, 1973
105. Bowsher D: Role of the reticular formation in responses to noxious stimulation. Pain 2:361, 1976
106. Casey KL: Reticular formation and pain: toward a unifying concept. p. 93. In Bonica JJ (ed): Pain. Raven Press, New York, 1980
107. Casey KL: Somatosensory responses of bulboreticular units in awake cat: relation to escape-producing stimuli. Science 173:77, 1971
108. Dong WK, Ryu H, Wagman IH: Nociceptive responses of neurons in medial thalamus and their relationship to spinothalamic pathways. J Neurophysiol 41:1592, 1978
109. Kaufman EF, Rosenquist AC: Efferent projections of the thalamic intralaminar nuclei in the cat. Brain Res 335:257, 1985
110. Craig AD Jr, Burton H: Spinal and medullary lamina I projection to nucleus submedius in medial thalamus: a possible pain center. J Neurophysiol 45:443, 1981
111. Albe-Fessard D, Berkley KJ, Kruger L et al: Diencephalic mechanisms of pain sensation. Brain Res 9:217, 1985
112. Foltz EL, White LE: Pain "relief" by frontal cingulotomy. J Neurosurg 19:89, 1962
113. Barber TX: Toward a theory of pain: relief of chronic pain by prefrontal cencotomy, opiates, placebos, and hypnosis. Psychol Bull 56:430, 1959
114. Penfield W, Boldrey E: Somatic motor and sensory representation in cerebral cortex of man as studied by electrical stimulation. Brain 60:389, 1937
115. Young GB, Blume WT: Painful epileptic seizures. Brain 106:537, 1983
116. Lewin W, Phillips CG: Observations on partial removal of the postcentral gyrus for pain. J Neurol Neurosurg Psychiatry 15:143, 1952
117. Kenshalo DR Jr, Isensee O: Responses of primate SI cortical neurons to noxious stimuli. J Neurophysiol 50:1479, 1983
118. Beecher HK: The Measurement of Subjective Responses. Oxford University Press, New York, 1959
119. Fields HL, Levine JD: Placebo analgesia—a role for endorphins? Trends Neurosci 7:271, 1984
120. Reynolds DV: Surgery in the rat during electrical analgesia induced by local brain stimulation. Science 164:444, 1969
121. Mayer DJ, Price DD: Central nervous system mechanisms of analgesia. Pain 2: 379, 1976

122. Fields HL, Basbaum AI: Brain stem control of spinal pain-transmission neurons. Annu Rev Physiol 40:217, 1978
123. Mayer DJ, Wolfle TL, Akil H et al: Analgesia from electrical stimulation in the brainstem of the rat. Science 174:1351, 1971
124. Hosobuchi Y, Adams JE, Linchitz R: Pain relief by electrical stimulation of the central gray matter in humans and its reversal by naloxone. Science 197:183, 1977
125. Baskin DS, Mehler WR, Hosobuchi Y et al: Autopsy analysis of the safety, efficacy and cartography of electrical stimulation of the central gray in humans. Brain Res 371:231, 1986
126. Snyder SH: Brain peptides as neurotransmitters. Science 209:976, 1980
127. Yaksh TL, Rudy TA: Narcotic analgesics: CNS sites and mechanisms of action as revealed by intracerebral injection techniques. Pain 4:299, 1978
128. Mayer DJ, Hayes RL: Stimulation-produced analgesia: development of tolerance and cross-tolerance to morphine. Science 188:941, 1975
129. Akil H, Mayer DJ, Liebeskind JC: Antagonism of stimulus-produced analgesia by naloxone, a narcotic antagonist. Science 191:961, 1976
130. Basbaum AI, Fields HL: Endogenous pain control systems: brainstem spinal pathways and endorphin circuitry. Annu Rev Neurosci 7:309, 1984
131. Hammond DL: Control systems for nociceptive afferent processing: the descending inhibitory pathways. p. 363. In Yaksh TL (ed): Spinal Afferent Processing. Plenum Press, New York, 1986
132. Abels IA, Basbaum AI: Afferent connections of the rostral medulla of the cat: a neural substrate for midbrain-medullary interactions in the modulation of pain. J Comp Neurol 201:285, 1981
133. Mantyh PW: The ascending input to the midbrain periaqueductal grey in the primate. J Comp Neurol 211:50, 1982
134. Mantyh PW: Connections of midbrain periaqueductal gray in monkey. II. Descending efferent projections. J Neurophysiol 49:582, 1983
135. Basbaum AI, Marley NJ, O'Reefe J, Clanton CH: Reversal of morphine and stimulus-produced analgesia by subtotal spinal cord lesions. Pain 3:43, 1977
136. Hodge CJ Jr, Apkarian AV, Stevens RT et al: Dorsolateral pontine inhibition of dorsal horn cell responses to cutaneous stimulation: lack of dependence of catecholaminergic system in the cat. J Neurophysiol 50:1220, 1983
137. Zorman G, Hentall ID, Adams JE, Fields HL: Naloxone-reversible analgesia produced by microstimulation in the rat medulla. Brain Res 219:137, 1981
138. Fields HL, Heinricher MM: Anatomy and physiology of a nociceptive modulatory system. Philos Trans R Soc Lond [Biol] 308:361, 1985
139. Sedan R, Lazorthes Y, Verdie JC et al: La neurostimulation electrique thérapeutique. Neurochirurgie, suppl. 24:S1, 1978
140. Duggan AW: Pharmacology of descending control systems. Philos Trans R Soc Lond [Biol] 308:375, 1985
141. Westlund KN, Bowker RM, Ziegler MG, Coulter JD: Origins and terminations of descending noradrenergic projections to the spinal cord of the monkey. Brain Res 292:1, 1984
142. Unnerstall JR, Kopajtic TA, Kuhar MJ: Distribution of α_2 agonist binding sites in the rat and human central nervous system: analysis of some functional, anatomic correlates of the pharmacologic effects of clonidine and related adrenergic agents. Brain Res 319:69, 1984
143. Belcher G, Ryall RW, Schaffner R: The differential effects of 5-hydroxytryptamine, noradrenaline, and raphe stimulation on nociceptive and non-nociceptive dorsal horn interneurons in the cat. Brain Res 151:307, 1978

144. Reddy SV, Yaksh TL: Spinal noradrenergic terminal system mediates antinociception. Brain Res 189:391, 1980
145. Fleetwood-Walker SM, Mitchell R, Hope PJ et al: An α_2 receptor mediates the selective inhibition by noradrenaline of nociceptive responses of identified dorsal horn neurones. Brain Res 334:243, 1985
146. Yaksh TL, Reddy SV: Studies in the primate on the analgetic effects associated with intrathecal actions of opiates, α-adrenergic agonists and baclofen. Anesthesiology 54:451, 1981
147. Sosnowski M, Yaksh TL: Spinal administration of receptor-selective drugs and analgesics: new horizons. J Pain Symptom Manag 5:204, 1990
148. Barbaro NM, Hammond DL, Fields HL: Effects of intrathecally administered methysergide and yohimbine on microstimulation-produced antinociception in the rat. Brain Res 343:223, 1985
149. Hammond DL: Pharmacology of central pain-modulating networks (biogenic amines and non-opioid analgesics). p. 499. In Fields HL, Dubner R, Cervero F (eds): Advances in Pain Research and Therapy. Vol. 9. Raven Press, New York, 1985
150. Roberts MH: 5-Hydroxytryptamine and antinociception. Neuropharmacology 23: 1529, 1984
151. Bowker R, Westlund KN, Coulter JD: Origins of serotonergic projections of the spinal cord in rat: an immunocytochemical-retrograde transport study. Brain Res 226:187, 1981
152. Yezierski RP, Wilcox TK, Willis WD: The effects of serotonin antagonists on the inhibition of primate spinothalamic tract cells produced by stimulation in nucleus raphe magnus or periaqueductal gray. J Pharmacol Exp Ther 220:266, 1982
153. Jordan LM, Kenshalo DR Jr, Martin RF et al: Depression of primate spinothalamic tract neurons by iontophoretic application of 5-hydroxytryptamine. Pain 5:135, 1978
154. Yaksh TL, Wilson PR: Spinal serotonin terminal system mediates antinociception. J Pharmacol Exp Ther 208:446, 1979
155. Yaksh TL, Al-Rodhan NR, Jensen TS: Sites of action of opiates in production of analgesia. Prog Brain Res 77:371, 1988
156. Cousins MJ, Mather LE: Intrathecal and epidural administration of opioids. Anesthesiology 61:276, 1984
157. Yeung JC, Rudy TA: Sites of antinociceptive action of systemically injected morphine: involvement of supraspinal loci as revealed by intracerebroventricular injections of naloxone. J Pharmacol Exp Ther 215:626, 1980

3

The Autonomic Nervous System

F. Michael Ferrante

The sympathetic nervous system together with the parasympathetic nervous system constitute the autonomic nervous system (ANS) and regulate circulatory, respiratory, alimentary, and genitourinary functions. Many of the pharmacologic manipulations and invasive techniques used to treat postoperative pain will in some way affect autonomic function. Thus, to intelligently and safely use these techniques, the practitioner must have a working knowledge of the anatomy, pharmacology, and physiology of the autonomic nervous system.

GENERAL CONSIDERATIONS

The ANS is composed of both central and peripheral parts (Fig. 3-1). Central elements are located within multiple areas of the central nervous system (CNS) including the cortex, hypothalamus, midbrain, medulla, and spinal cord. The peripheral portion is divided into sympathetic and parasympathetic divisions consisting of afferent and efferent neurons whose axons are located outside of the CNS.[1,2]

Aggregates of neurons within the aforementioned areas of the CNS are functionally connected with the ANS by extensive neural ramifications. In the hypothalamus, however, autonomic centers are most clearly anatomically delineated. Sixteen distinct nuclei are found, some of which subserve either sympathetic or parasympathetic function. Autonomic centers within the brain stem and spinal cord are connected to the various hypothalamic nuclei by the axons of the dorsal longitudinal fasciculus. The axons of the dorsal longitudinal

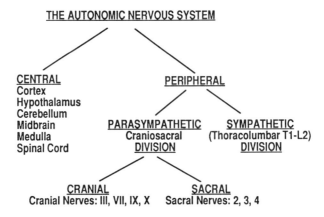

Fig. 3-1. Divisions of the autonomic nervous system.

fasciculus pass caudally from the hypothalamus through the mesencephalon and pons to terminate in the reticular formation, cranial nerve nuclei of the brain stem (parasympathetic division), and intermediolateral gray of the spinal cord (sympathetic thoracolumbar outflow; parasympathetic sacral outflow) (Fig. 3-2).[1]

THE PERIPHERAL AUTONOMIC NERVOUS SYSTEM

The peripheral ANS consists of preganglionic and postganglionic efferent and afferent axons. The cell bodies of preganglionic neurons are located in the intermediolateral gray of the spinal cord or in visceral efferent nuclei in the brain stem. The axons of these cell bodies reach outlying peripheral ganglia through the anterior roots of spinal nerves or through cranial nerves. Cell bodies of postganglionic neurons are found within the peripheral ganglia (Table 3-1). Their axons pass to their final destinations within viscera, blood vessels, sweat glands, etc.[3]

On the basis of anatomic, physiologic, and pharmacologic considerations, the peripheral ANS is divided into the parasympathetic and sympathetic nervous systems.

TABLE 3-1. Autonomic Ganglia

Sympathetic	Parasympathetic
Paravertebral	Cephalic
Prevertebral	Terminal (intrinsic)

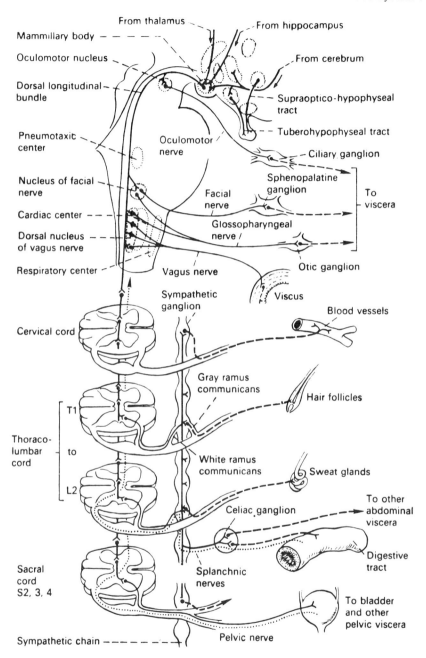

Fig. 3-2. Central and efferent peripheral autonomic pathways. Autonomic nuclei in the hypothalamus are connected to autonomic centers in the brain stem and spinal cord by the dorsal longitudinal fasciculus. The caudal termination of the dorsal longitudinal fasciculus is the intermediolateral gray cell column of the spinal cord. Cell bodies of preganglionic sympathetic neurons are located in the intermediolateral gray in spinal cord segments T1–L2. Cell bodies of parasympathetic neurons are found in cranial nerve nuclei of the oculomotor, facial, glossopharyngeal, and vagus nerves. (From Bonica,[1] with permission.)

Parasympathetic Nervous System

The parasympathetic nervous system consists of cranial and sacral portions (Figs. 3-1 and 3-2). The cell bodies of preganglionic parasympathetic fibers are located in cranial nerve nuclei of the brain stem. Their axons pass to peripheral ganglia as part of the oculomotor, facial, glossopharyngeal, and vagus nerves. The long preganglionic fibers of the oculomotor, facial, and glossopharyngeal nerves synapse with short postganglionic fibers of the ciliary, sphenopalatine, and otic ganglia (Fig. 3-2). The very long preganglionic fibers of the vagus synapse in intramural ganglia of the heart, lungs, and gastrointestinal tract.

Preganglionic neurons of the sacral portion of the parasympathetic nervous system have cell bodies located in the intermediolateral gray of the second, third, and fourth sacral cord segments. Leaving through anterior spinal nerve roots, their axons travel as the pelvic splanchnic nerves to the pelvic plexuses. The axons finally terminate in the terminal ganglia of the pelvic or vesical plexuses, or the intramural ganglia of the urinary bladder, the descending and sigmoid colon, rectum, and genitalia.

Sympathetic Nervous System

Cell bodies of preganglionic sympathetic neurons lie within the intermediolateral gray of spinal cord segments T1–L2 (Fig. 3-2). There is some evidence that cell bodies of preganglionic neurons can also be found at spinal cord segments C7, C8, L3, and L4.[4,5]

Axons from these preganglionic neurons pass by way of anterior spinal roots and rami communicantes to reach paravertebral ganglia of the sympathetic chain (Figs. 3-2 and 3-3). On reaching the paravertebral ganglia of the sympathetic chain, preganglionic sympathetic axons may (1) synapse, (2) pass cephalad or caudad for variable distances within the sympathetic chain before synapsing, or (3) pass without interruption to prevertebral ganglia/plexuses (celiac, superior mesenteric, etc.).

Paravertebral ganglia are segmentally arrayed in bilateral vertical rows extending from the second cervical vertebra to the coccyx. Longitudinal ascending and descending nerve fibers connect adjacent ganglia thereby forming the chain or trunk. Cervical ganglia lie anterior to the base of the respective transverse processes. Lumbar ganglia lie on the anterolateral surface of the respective vertebrae. The anatomic locations are important for the approach of the needle during sympathetic neural blockade.

Prevertebral ganglia lie distal to the sympathetic chain in close proximity to their end organs.

GANGLIA AND PLEXUSES OF THE PERIPHERAL AUTONOMIC NERVOUS SYSTEM

Although the term *plexus* and *ganglion* are casually interchangeable and informally refer to prevertebral ganglia, the term *plexus* is more inclusive. More correctly, *ganglion* refers to a site of synaptic connections specific to the sympa-

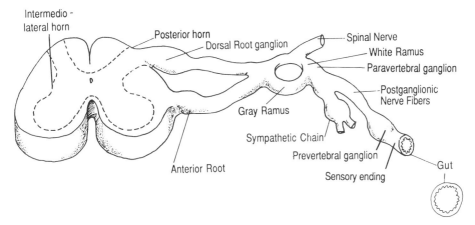

Fig. 3-3. Course of preganglionic and postganglionic sympathetic neurons. Cell bodies of preganglionic sympathetic neurons are located in the intermediolateral gray cell column of spinal cord segments T1–L2. Axons of these preganglionic neurons travel by way of anterior spinal roots and the white rami communicantes to reach the paravertebral ganglia of the sympathetic chain. On reaching the paravertebral ganglia, preganglionic sympathetic axons may (1) synapse, (2) pass cephalad or caudad for variable distances within the sympathetic chain before synapsing, or (3) pass without interruption to prevertebral ganglia.

thetic or parasympathetic systems. *Plexus* refers to a number of ganglia and axons (sympathetic and parasympathetic, as well as visceral afferent) converging in a well-defined anatomic location. The following is a short listing of important ganglia and plexuses.

Cephalic Ganglia (Plexuses)

Autonomic ganglia include the ciliary, sphenopalatine, otic, and submaxillary ganglia, which are situated in relation to the respective cranial nerves (III, VII, and IX). Each ganglion receives sympathetic postganglionic fibers, parasympathetic preganglionic fibers, and sensory fibers. (Thus, they should be more correctly termed *plexuses*.)

Stellate Ganglion

The superior, middle, intermediate, and inferior ganglia comprise the sympathetic chain within the cervical region. In approximately 80 percent of individuals, the inferior cervical ganglion and first thoracic ganglion are fused to form the stellate ganglion. Cell bodies of preganglionic sympathetic neurons supplying the head, neck, and upper extremity are found in the intermediolateral gray from T1 through T6.

Autonomic Plexuses of the Chest

The cardiac, pulmonary, and esophageal plexuses consist of prevertebral sympathetic ganglia and interconnecting sympathetic, parasympathetic, and visceral afferent fibers. A full discussion of their physiology is beyond the scope of this book. A more definitive discussion may be found in the work of Bonica.[6]

Abdominal Autonomic Plexuses

Similar to the thorax, the abdomen contains three large plexuses composed of prevertebral sympathetic ganglia, parasympathetic fibers from the vagus or sacral parasympathetics, and visceral afferent fibers. The celiac plexus (sometimes also called the splanchnic plexus, the abdominal brain of Bichat, or the solar plexus) (Fig. 3-4) innervates the abdominal viscera (above the pelvis). Preganglionic fibers to the celiac plexus arise from the greater, lesser, and least splanchnic nerves. The greater splanchnic nerve (arising from spinal segments T5 or T6 to T9 or T10), the lesser splanchnic nerve (arising from T10 and T11), and the least splanchnic nerve (arising from T11 and T12) pass through the crux of the diaphragm to synapse in the celiac ganglia. Postganglionic fibers radiate to celiac, aortorenal, superior and inferior mesenteric, and other subsidiary plexuses supplying innervation to the abdominal viscera above the pelvis. The other two great abdominal plexuses include the superior and inferior hypogastric plexuses supplying the pelvic viscera (Fig. 3-4).

PHARMACOLOGY OF THE AUTONOMIC NERVOUS SYSTEM

Certainly, an all-inclusive discussion of the pharmacology of the ANS is beyond the scope of this book. This section is included to discuss a few basic pharmacologic principles pertaining to the ANS.

Acetylcholine is released at all preganglionic nerve endings (both sympathetic and parasympathetic) and postganglionic parasympathetic nerve endings (Fig. 3-5). Sympathetic postganglionic innervation to sweat glands is also cholinergic.

Acetylcholine activates two different receptor types: muscarinic and nicotrinic receptors.[7] The muscarinic receptors are located in all effector cells stimulated by postganglionic parasympathetic neurons as well as postganglionic cholinergic sympathetic neurons. Nicotinic receptors are located in the ganglionic synapses between pre- and postganglionic neurons of the sympathetic and parasympathetic nervous systems. Nicotinic receptors are also found in the membranes of skeletal muscle fibers at the neuromuscular junction. The nicotinic action of acetylcholine can be blocked by ganglionic blocking agents such as the quaternary ammonium bases. The muscarinic action of acetylcholine can be blocked by atropine.

Norepinephrine is the neurotransmitter found in postganglionic sympathetic (adrenergic) nerve endings. The cells of the adrenal medulla are homologous to

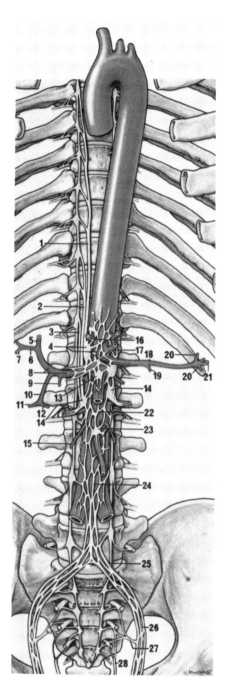

Fig. 3-4. Splanchnic nerves, celiac ganglia and plexus, and secondary ganglia and plexuses.
1. Greater splanchnic nerve
2. Lesser splanchnic nerve
3. Least splanchnic nerve
4. Celiac ganglion and plexus
5. Left branch of hepatic artery
6. Right branch of hepatic artery
7. Cystic artery
8. Common hepatic artery
9. Right gastric artery
10. Gastroduodenal artery
11. Superior pancreatico-duodenal artery
12. Right gastroepiploic artery
13. Superior mesenteric ganglion and plexus
14. Aorticorenal ganglion and renal artery with plexus
15. Ovarian/testicular artery and plexus
16. Phrenic plexus
17. Left gastric artery and plexus
18. Splenic artery and plexus
19. Pancreatic branch
20. Gastric arteries
21. Splenic branch
22. Abdominal aortic plexus
23. Inferior mesenteric ganglion and plexus
24. Superior hypogastric plexus
25. Inferior hypogastric plexus
26. Pelvic plexus
27. Pelvic splanchnic nerve
28. Pudendal nerve
(From Katz and Renck,[14] with permission.)

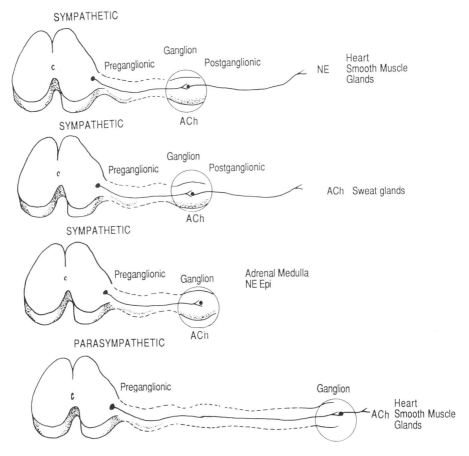

Fig. 3-5. Neurotransmitters of the autonomic nervous system. ACh = acetylcholine, NE = norepinephrine, Epi = epinephrine.

postganglionic sympathetic neurons and contain both epinephrine (80 percent) and norepinephrine (20 percent) (Fig. 3–5).

The end organ response to catecholamines is mediated by two types of receptors: α-adrenergic and β-adrenergic. Two classes of α-receptors have been demonstrated: α_1 and α_2. The α_1-adrenergic receptors[8] are located in smooth muscle of the coronary arteries, skin, uterus, intestinal mucosa, and splanchnic beds. Activation of α_1-adrenergic receptors results in either decreased or increased tone, depending on the individual end organ.

The α_2-receptors are found in both presynaptic and postsynaptic locations. Stimulation of presynaptic α_2-receptors inhibits norepinephrine release, serving as a negative feedback mechanism.[9–10] Norepinephrine acts at both α_1- and α_2-receptors, serving to activate smooth muscle contraction (α_1) while at the same time inhibiting its own release by presynaptic α_2-receptors. Postsynaptic α_2-receptors, like the α_1-receptor, affect vasoconstriction. Differentiation of the two receptor types is based on differences in the potency of varying agonists and antagonists.[11]

The β-adrenergic receptors have also been divided into two groups.[11,12] The β_1-adrenergic receptors are located in the myocardium, the sinoatrial node, the ventricular conduction system, and adipose tissue. The β_1-receptor is equally sensitive to norepinephrine and epinephrine, which distinguishes it from the β_2-adrenergic receptor. Effects of β_1-receptor stimulation include increased cardiac rate, contractility and conduction velocity, coronary vasodilation, and lipolysis.[13]

The β_2-adrenergic receptors are found in bronchial smooth muscle and vascular smooth muscle in the skin, muscle, and mesentery. β_2-receptors are more sensitive to stimulation by epinephrine than norepinephrine.[8] Stimulation produces bronchodilation and vasodilation.[13]

CONCLUSION

The physiologic importance of the ANS cannot be overstated. This chapter was not meant to be an exhaustive review but to provide the practitioner with a working fund of knowledge. Please refer to the excellent texts listed in the references for more detailed information.

References

1. Bonica JJ: Applied anatomy relevant to pain: B. The autonomic nervous system. p. 146. In Bonica JJ (ed): The Management of Pain. Vol 1. 2nd Ed. Lea & Febiger, Philadelphia, 1990
2. Pick J: The Autonomic Nervous System: Morphological, Comparative, Clinical and Surgical Aspects. JB Lippincott, Philadelphia, 1970
3. Bonica JJ: Autonomic innervation of the viscera in relation to nerve block. Anesthesiology 29:793, 1968
4. Laruelle LL: Les bases anatomiques du système autonome cortical et bulbospinal. Rev Neurol 72:349, 1940
5. Neuwirth E: Current concepts of the cervical portion of the sympathetic nervous system. Lancet ii 80:337, 1960
6. Bonica JJ: General considerations of pain in the chest. p. 959. In Bonica JJ (ed): The Management of Pain. Vol 2. 2nd Ed. Lea & Febiger, Philadelphia, 1990
7. Flacke WE, Flacke JW: Cholinergic and anticholinergic agents. p. 160. In Smith NT, Corbascio AN (eds): Drug Interaction in Anesthesia. Lea & Febiger, Philadelphia, 1986
8. Osswald W, Guimaraes S: Adrenergic mechanisms in blood vessels: morphological and pharmacological aspects. Rev Physiol Biochem Pharmacol 96:54, 1983
9. Langer SZ: Presynaptic regulation of catecholamine release. Biochem Pharmacol 23:1973, 1974
10. Hoffman BB, Lefkowitz RJ: Alpha-adrenergic receptor subtypes. N Engl J Med 302:1390, 1980
11. Ariens EJ, Simonis AM: Physiological and pharmacological aspects of adrenergic receptor classification. Biochem Pharmacol 32:1539, 1983

12. Lands AM, Arnold A, McAnliff JP et al: Differentiation of receptor systems activated by sympathomimetic amines. Nature 214:597, 1967
13. Durrett LR, Lawson NW: Autonomic nervous system physiology and pharmacology. p. 165. In Barash PG, Cullen BF, Stoelting RK (eds): Clinical Anesthesia. JB Lippincott, Philadelphia, 1989
14. Katz J, Renck H: Handbook of Thoraco-abdominal Nerve Block. Grune & Stratton, Orlando, FL, 1987

4

The Neuroendocrine Response to Postoperative Pain

M. Soledad Cepeda
Daniel B. Carr

THE STRESS RESPONSE: DEFINITION AND BACKGROUND

The collection of global, linked, endocrinologic, immunologic, and inflammatory effects that occur in response to surgery or to the pain that is perceived afterward is commonly considered to exemplify "the stress response." Selye[1] defined "stress" as "the nonspecific response of the organism to any demand made upon it." The broadness of Selye's definition might in theory encompass any physiologic response and any external stimulus. Because surgery and pain evoke responses within numerous, linked, physiologic systems, formulation of a more precise and restrictive definition of the stress response has been an elusive goal.

During the past two decades, an operational definition of the stress response has come to include neuroendocrine phenomena through the introduction of sensitive hormone assays that quantitate physiologic responses. The hormones

TABLE 4-1. Site of Secretion and Action of Hormones of the Stress Response to Surgery

Site of Secretion Hormone	Action
Hypothalamus	
Corticotropin-releasing hormone (CRH)	Stimulates ACTH and β-endorphin secretion by adenohypophysis Analgesic Anti-inflammatory
Vasopressin (ADH)	Free water retention Synergistic effect with CRH on adenohypophyseal secretion
Pituitary	
Adrenocorticotropic hormone (ACTH)	Stimulates zonae fasciculata and reticularis of adrenal cortex to secrete cortisol
β-Endorphin	Endogenous opioid (analgesic) Anti-inflammatory
Growth hormone (GH) and prolactin	Carbohydrate intolerance Lipid mobilization Immunostimulation
Adrenal cortex	
Cortisol (glucocorticoids)	Stimulates glycogenolysis, protein, and fat catabolism Immunosuppression Anti-inflammatory Negative feedback inhibition of ACTH and β-endorphin secretion Long-term facilitation of adrenomedullary catecholamine synthetic enzymes
Adrenal medulla	
Catecholamines	Stimulate glycogenoylsis and gluconeogenesis, protein, and fat catabolism Reduce pancreatic insulin secretion Immunosuppression
Leu- and met-enkephalin	Endogenous opioids (analgesics) Anti-inflammatory Inhibit gonadotropin, GH, and prolactin secretion Feedback inhibition of ACTH secretion
Pancreas	
Insulin	Anabolic regulation of carbohydrate metabolism
Inflammatory response	
Interleukin-1 (IL-1)	Synthesized by macrophages Stimulates adenohypophysis to secrete ACTH and β-endorphin Pyrogen Stimulation of acute-phase protein synthesis Stimulates protein catabolism Activation of T and B lymphocytes
Substance P	Neurotransmitter of primary nociceptive afferents Stimulation of IL-1 release from white blood cells Stimulation of GH and prolactin release from adenohypophysis Inhibition of glucose-induced insulin secretion
Tumor necrosis factor	Secretion by lymphocytes and monocytes/macrophages Stimulates carbohydrate, protein, and fat catabolism Pyrogen

TABLE 4-2. Neuroendocrine Response to Surgery

Endocrine
Increased catabolism
Secondary to *increased*: adrenocorticotropic hormone, cortisol, vasopressin, growth hormone, catecholamines, interleukin-1
Decreased anabolism
Secondary to *decreased*: insulin

Metabolic
Carbohydrate
Hyperglycemia
Glucose intolerance
Insulin resistance
Increased glycogenolysis
Increased gluconeogenesis
Secondary to *decreased*: insulin secretion and decreased intrinsic effect
Secondary to *increased*: epinephrine, glucagon (increased glycogenolysis)
Secondary to *increased*: cortisol, glucagon, growth hormone, epinephrine, free fatty acids (increased gluconeogenesis)
Protein
Enhanced catabolism
Enhanced synthesis of acute phase reactants
Secondary to *increased*: cortisol, epinephrine, glucagon, interleukin-1
Fat
Enhanced oxidation
Enhanced lipolysis
Secondary to *increased*: cortisol, glucagon, growth hormone, catecholamines

of the pituitary-adrenal axis, the catecholamines of the adrenal medulla, and the multiple circulating hormones regulating carbohydrate, protein, and lipid metabolism are particularly implicated in the neuroendocrine response to surgery (Tables 4-1 and 4-2).[2] To this "classical" (i.e., humoral) concept of stress responses have been added perioperative cardiovascular and immune adaptations.[3] Although stress inhibits the release of certain pituitary hormones such as gonadotropins and thyroid-stimulating hormone, these inhibitory responses do not figure prominently in the literature on pain and hormone secretion.

This chapter presents evidence that normal physiologic responses to surgery, trauma, or pain contribute to the deleterious effects produced by such stimuli. Undesirable effects include marked catabolism, increased cardiac work and arrhythmogenesis, hypercoagulability, and immunosuppression. Happily, the analgesic techniques described throughout this book reduce or even nullify the stress response.[4] It still remains uncertain as to whether the improvements in postoperative morbidity and mortality associated with the use of such techniques are the direct result of reductions in the stress responses.

STIMULATORY MECHANISMS

Much clinical and experimental evidence points to the prime importance of *afferent neurogenic stimuli* in classic stress responses. The activation of afferent neural pathways during surgical injury is of primary importance in evoking cardiovascular[5] and hypothalamic-pituitary responses.[6] However, the local release of mediators from damaged tissue (e.g., interleukin-1 [IL-1], prostaglandins, bradykinin, substance P) stimulates global inflammatory responses.[7] Mediators released from injured tissue directly contribute to the stress response by traveling through the circulation to evoke hormonal responses at distant target organs (e.g., pituitary). Mediators also indirectly contribute to the stress response by augmenting afferent nociceptive transmission, thereby evoking and potentiating the secretion of hypothalamic releasing hormones.

Thus, the nature of the responses triggered by surgical injury is heterogeneous (both humoral and inflammatory).[8] It is not possible to outline a single set of mechanisms that apply in fixed proportions to each component of the complex linked set of responses.[9,10]

Neurologic Mechanisms

The nociceptive signal is transmitted from the surgical site to the central nervous system primarily through small myelinated Aδ and unmyelinated C fibers. Recent evidence indicates that fast conducting fibers may also participate in the hypothalamic activation characteristic of the initial endocrine response to surgery.[11,12]

On entering the spinal cord, primarily through the dorsal root, nociceptive fibers ascend and descend one or two segments in Lissauer's tract and synapse within the six anatomically distinct layers of the dorsal horn. Cutaneous nociceptive afferents project to laminae I, II, and V, whereas visceral and muscle nociceptive afferents project to laminae I and V but not lamina II.[6,12] After decussation, pain fibers ascend in the anterolateral quadrant of the spinal cord, principally in the spinothalamic and the spinoreticulothalamic tracts. The spinothalamic tract divides into medial and lateral components (Fig. 4-1) as it approaches the thalamus (Fig. 4-2). The lateral division terminates in the ventrobasal nuclei (which have the clearest role in pain transmission)[6] and in the posterior nuclear complex. (For an explanation of thalamic nuclear anatomy, please see Ch. 2.) Lateral and medial divisions ultimately project to the somatosensory cortex.

Of greater importance for the autonomic, hormonal, and affective reaction to pain is the spinoreticulothalamic system (Fig. 4-3).[13] Spinorecticular fibers terminate bilaterally in the medulla, principally within or near the nucleus reticularis gigantocellularis. They then ascend in the ventral tegmental tract and enter the hypothalamus, where they join the medial forebrain bundle. Through the medial forebrain bundle, fibers reach the hypothalamic paraventricular nucleus (PVN), a major integrating center for global hormonal and autonomic responses.[14]

Neurons containing vasopressin (antidiuretic hormone [ADH]) and corticotropin-releasing hormone (CRH) are located within the PVN[15,16] (Fig. 4-4). CRH is the principal hypothalamic releasing hormone for stimulation of anterior pituitary secretion of adrenocorticotropic hormone (ACTH) and β-endorphin

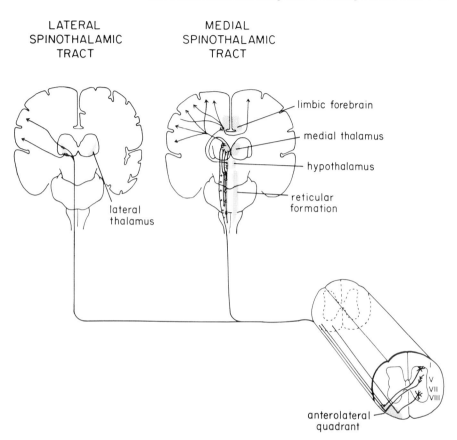

LATERAL
SPINOTHALAMIC
TRACT

MEDIAL
SPINOTHALAMIC
TRACT

limbic forebrain

medial thalamus

hypothalamus

reticular
formation

lateral
thalamus

anterolateral
quadrant

Fig. 4-1. Axons from cell bodies in Rexed's laminae I, V, VII, and VIII mainly project to the contralateral anterolateral quadrant of the spinal cord (with a smaller ipsilateral contribution). Ascending fibers form spinothalamic and spinoreticulothalamic tracts. As fibers of the spinothalamic tract approach the thalamus, they segregate into medial and lateral components. The **medial spinothalamic tract** projects to the medial thalamus, hypothalamus, and limbic forebrain. Fibers of the **lateral spinothalamic tract** synapse in ventrobasal and posterior nuclei and project to the cerebral cortex.

(an endogenous opioid—see Ch. 8). Vasopressin is transported from the PVN and stored in the posterior pituitary (Fig. 4-4) from which it is secreted into the blood. Plasma levels of vasopressin are considered to be indices of stress. Prolonged elevation of these levels is seen after major surgery, particularly after thoracic procedures.[17] Vasopressin stimulates free water retention and also exerts a synergistic effect with CRH on ACTH and β-endorphin secretion from the pituitary.[16,18]

Recently, direct nociceptive projections from the spinal cord to the hypothalamus, septal nuclei, and nucleus accumbens have been identified as the spinohypothalamic tract.[19] Cells contributing to this pathway originate not only from

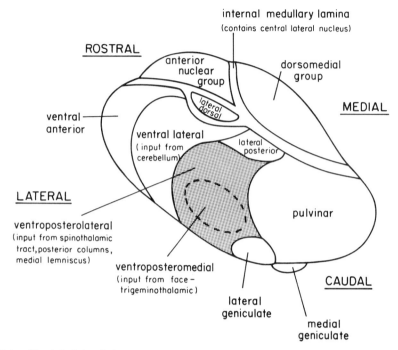

Fig. 4-2. Nuclei of the thalamus (longitudinal view). Thalamic nuclei that receive direct input from the spinal cord include (1) the **ventrobasal complex** (ventroposterolateral and ventroposteromedial nuclei), (2) the **posterior nuclear complex** (not shown), (3) the **central lateral nucleus** (part of the intralaminar complex), and (4) the **nucleus submedius** (not shown).

the lateral reticulated area of the spinal cord (which also contributes to the spinothalamic tract) but also from the lateral spinal nucleus and areas adjacent to the central canal (which do not contribute to the spinothalamic tract).[20] A further distinction between spinohypothalamic and spinothalamic tracts is the degree of bilaterality of their projections. Forty percent of neurons in the former tract project ipsilaterally, compared with fewer than 10 percent in the latter.[21] Spinohypothalamic neurons are a potentially important route by which segmental nociceptive stimuli may trigger hypothalamic-pituitary responses. However, their quantitative contribution to stress hormone secretion has not yet been defined.

The correlation between the site and extent of surgery and the magnitude of the resultant hormonal stress response presumably reflects the graded actions of neural pathways. Several studies have provided good evidence that such a correlation is clinically evident.[22] Diagnostic biopsies of superficial tissue, ocular surgery, and aural procedures elicit modest metabolic and hormonal responses. Thoracic procedures or those involving bone or deep tissue in the abdomen evoke quantitatively greater responses.

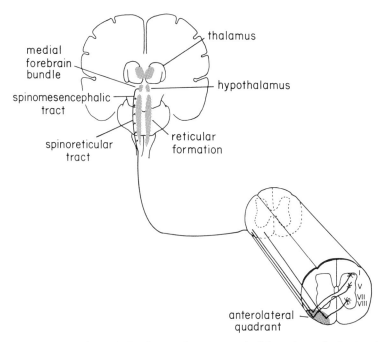

Fig. 4-3. The spinoreticulothalamic tract is composed of the **spinoreticular tract** (SRT), the **spinomesencephalic tract** (SMT), and the **medial forebrain bundle** (MFB). Cells of origin of the SRT are found in Rexed's laminae I and V–VIII and ascend intermixed with the spinothalamic tract. Axons of the SRT terminate in the brain stem reticular formation, principally within or near the nucleus gigantocellularis. Cells of origin of the SMT are mainly located in Rexed's laminae I and V. Axons ascend in the anterolateral quadrant and enter the hypothalamus where they join the MFB to eventually synapse in the paraventricular nucleus of the hypothalamus.

Inflammatory Mediators

Tissue injury releases inflammatory mediators such as substance P, cytokines, eicosanoids, and bradykinin that contribute to the initiation and maintenance of the stress response.[23–25] The neural stimulus is the principal release mechanism for the surgical stress response. However, the observation that tissue injury in animals without brain-pituitary connections still elicits a pituitary-adrenal response indicates the importance of extraneural factors in this process.[7]

Substance P[26] acts as a neurotransmitter in nociceptive afferents in the periphery and within the spinal cord. In addition, it has broad actions as an immunomodulator, including stimulation of IL-1 release from white blood cells.[27] Substance P stimulates the release of growth hormone (GH) and prolactin from anterior pituitary cells[28] and modulates exocrine and endocrine pancreatic function (e.g., inhibits glucose-induced insulin release). The diverse systemic effects of substance P illustrate how a locally generated mediator can augment or maintain global stress responses.

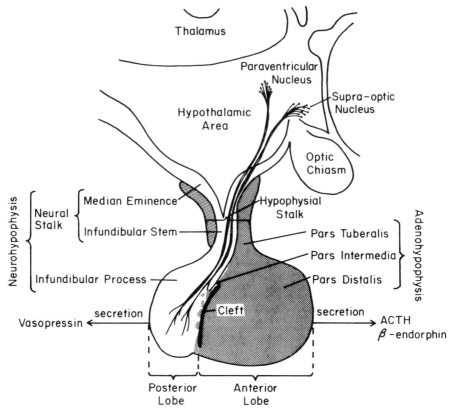

Fig. 4-4. The hypothalamus and pituitary gland (neurohypophysis and adenohypophysis).

IL-1 is a protein produced by macrophages and other marrow-derived cells (apart from erythrocytes). Two distinct genes give rise to two forms of IL-1, termed α and β. Each form of IL-1 is variably glycosylated. Originally termed *lymphocyte activating factor*, other synonyms for IL-1 include (among other terms) *endogenous pyrogen* and *B-cell activating factor*. Some postoperative cellular responses or clinical signs mimicked by IL-1 administration include fever, slow-wave sleep, anorexia, acute-phase protein synthesis, amino acid release from skeletal muscle, and activation of T and B lymphocytes and natural killer cells. Apart from its function as an inflammatory mediator and immunostimulant, IL-1 directly stimulates the release of ACTH and β-endorphin from the anterior pituitary.[29] This is another example of a peripherally derived humoral factor that augments, perhaps synergistically, the magnitude of the postsurgical stress response evoked by afferent nociceptive transmission.[23,25,30,31]

Tumor necrosis factors (TNFs) are also important mediators of the injury response. TNF-α (previously termed *cachectin*) and TNF-β are closely related polypeptides that are secreted by lymphocytes and monocyte/macrophage cell lines and act through the same receptor. Experimental studies have demonstrated that TNF-α induces fever, anorexia, acute-phase protein synthesis, release of amino acids from skeletal muscle, increased lactate production, hyperglycemia, lipolysis, and decreased vascular resistance when given in vivo.[30–33] TNF-α is at present considered to be the key physiologic trigger for numerous manifestations of sepsis, inflammation, and multiple organ failure.[25]

Significant increases in circulating levels of platelet release products have also been observed during and after surgical trauma. Increases in thromboxane B_2 and 5-hydroxytryptamine (serotonin) are found to be closely related to the more traditional indices of the surgical stress response. Peak concentrations of thromboxane B_2 and serotonin occur 1–2 hours after skin incision. A preoperative increase in platelet release products has also been observed and interpreted to reflect adrenomedullary activation caused by psychological stress.[34]

The aforementioned substances are but a few examples of the multiple mediators recognized within injured tissue. Other examples include bradykinin and eicosanoids (see Ch. 2). Mediators released from injured tissue directly contribute to the stress response by traveling through the circulation to influence distant target organs.[35] Mediators indirectly contribute to the stress response by augmenting afferent nociceptive transmission, thereby evoking and potentiating the secretion of hypothalamic releasing hormones.[36] Prophetically, Selye's original letter describing the stress response (which he termed the *general adaptation syndrome*) considered that this response may be initiated by substances released from injured tissue.

THE STRESS HORMONES

There are two major hormonal secretory systems (axes) for the neuroendocrine response to surgical stress: the hypothalamic-pituitary-adrenal axis (HPA) (Fig. 4-5) and the sympathoadrenomedullary system. The sympathoadrenomedullary system stores and releases catecholamines (norepinephrine from peripheral nerves and epinephrine from the adrenal medulla). Adrenomedullary opioids are also released, particularly the leu- and met-enkephalins derived from proenkephalin A (see Ch. 8).[37,38] With respect to the HPA, trophic hormones released from the hypothalamus (not only CRH—see below) stimulate pituitary release of ACTH, β-endorphin, GH, and prolactin. Circulating ACTH stimulates the adrenal gland to secrete cortisol and aldosterone.

After a 40-year search for the major active principle that elicits the secretion of ACTH from the pituitary,[39] CRH was isolated and characterized as a 41-amino acid peptide by Vale and colleagues in 1981.[40] Neurons of the PVN of the hypothalamus synthesize CRH and project to the median eminence region of the pituitary stalk (Fig. 4-4). CRH is then secreted directly into the portal blood. Transported in the portal blood vessels to the anterior pituitary, CRH stimulates the release of ACTH and β-endorphin into the systemic circulation[41,42] (Fig. 4-5). Circulating ACTH acts on cell membrane receptors in the zona fasciculata and zona reticularis of the adrenal cortex to activate adenylate

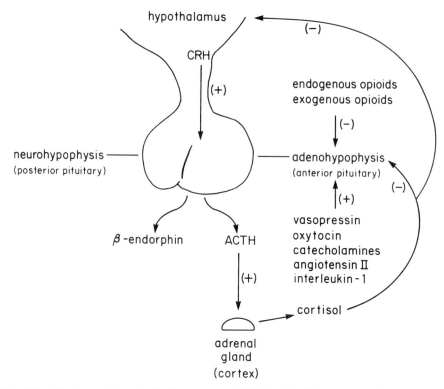

Fig. 4-5. The hypothalamic-pituitary-adrenal (HPA) axis. The negative sign (−) refers to negative feedback inhibition by various substances. The positive sign (+) signifies a stimulatory effect on secretion.

cyclase. Elevated intracellular levels of cyclic AMP elicit the immediate synthesis and secretion of cortisol and aldosterone.[43] Glucocorticoids such as cortisol exert immediate negative feedback on the synthesis and release of both CRH and ACTH.[43–45] They also exert a longer-term facilitatory action on catecholamine synthetic enzymes within the adrenal medulla.[9]

Recent evidence suggests that CRH is widely distributed throughout the brain, spinal cord, and adrenal gland.[46] Thus, it is plausible that CRH acts as a neurotransmitter in addition to its governing role within the HPA axis (Fig. 4-5).

Intracerebral administration of CRH stimulates sympathetic nervous system and adrenomedullary activity, causing behavioral activation similar to that observed during stress. These autonomic changes include elevation of arterial pressure and pulse rate[47] and increases in the plasma concentrations of norepinephrine and epinephrine. CRH-induced elevations of arterial pressure and heart rate are demonstrable in hypophysectomized animals and hence are not secondary to the pituitary actions of this peptide. Thus, CRH-induced autonomic changes are manifestations of its central effects.[41]

CRH also possesses intrinsic analgesic and anti-inflammatory activity. CRH binding sites have been identified on peripheral nerves and on lymphocytes. When CRH is injected locally into an inflamed paw, it inhibits hyperalgesia by a peripheral mechanism.[48] Systemic injections of CRH can also produce analgesia and reduce plasma extravasation caused by antidromic nerve stimulation.[49]

Despite the paramount importance of CRH, it is important to remember that the secretion of ACTH is multihormonally regulated[42] (Fig. 4-5). Catecholamines and several peptides such as vasopressin, oxytocin, and angiotensin II have a stimulatory effect on the release of ACTH.[2,17,35,42,44] Vasopressin, in particular, stimulates ACTH release by both a direct action on anterior pituitary cells and by potentiating the activity of CRH.[17,20,44,50]

Just as CRH does not act by itself to regulate ACTH secretion, ACTH is neither synthesized nor secreted in isolation. ACTH and β-endorphin[51-53] are derived from the same precursor molecule, pro-opiomelanocortin (POMC).[54] POMC undergoes a series of ordered proteolytic cleavages and modifications in the corticotrophs of the anterior pituitary to yield ACTH and β-lipotropin (β-LPH).[55] β-LPH in turn gives rise to daughter molecules, including β-endorphin. Endogenous opioid peptides, as well as exogenous opioids, inhibit gonadotropin secretion and exert biphasic actions on the secretion of other pituitary hormones such as vasopressin,[37] GH, and prolactin. Besides their central analgesic effects, endogenous opioids that are secreted into the systemic circulation have analgesic and anti-inflammatory actions in the periphery at the site of tissue injury.[56,57] These actions overlap with immune aspects of the stress response (see below). As secretion of opioid peptides is a component of HPA activation, it is not surprising that HPA activation is under inhibitory opioid control.[42,43,58] Therefore, the reduction of HPA responses during opioid therapy does *not* necessarily imply that adequate analgesia has been provided.

Increases in circulating levels of GH and prolactin have also been described during and after surgery.[9,59] GH secretion is affected by numerous hormones, including ACTH, vasopressin, cortisol, and catecholamines.[59] Mediators such as PGE_2 stimulate GH release by activating the receptor for GH releasing hormone. GH and prolactin have strong sequence homology and have similar immune and metabolic effects (lipid mobilization and carbohydrate intolerance).[60] Specific binding sites for prolactin have been demonstrated on lymphocytes, and leukocytes synthesize GH.[61] As a rule, the marked perioperative elevations of GH and prolactin are inhibited by opioids, although opioids given under basal nonstressed conditions do provoke transient increases in plasma levels of these hormones.

Limited and somewhat conflicting data suggest that thyroid hormone dynamics are altered during stress. Pituitary secretion of thyroid-stimulating hormone is reduced; plasma levels of active forms of thyroid hormones such as triiodothyronine and thyroxine are reduced, and levels of inactive forms such as "reverse T_3" are increased.[59] Normalization of thyroid hormone alterations is seen by 1 week after acute trauma or surgery.[24,52]

In summary, the general pattern of the neuroendocrine response involves the release of trophic hormones from the hypothalamus that stimulate the pituitary release of ACTH, β-endorphin, GH, and prolactin.[9,10,62] Secretion of other pituitary hormones such as thyroid-stimulating hormone and gonadotropins is inhibited by stress. Vasopressin is released from the posterior pituitary as the result of hypothalamic neural control. Blood levels of catabolic hormones such as catecholamines, cortisol, or glucagon increase, while levels of anabolic hormones such as insulin decline.[63,64]

METABOLIC RESPONSES TO SURGERY OR TRAUMA

More than 50 years ago, Cuthbertson recognized the presence of a "disturbance of metabolism produced by bony and nonbony injury" and divided this disturbance into "ebb" and "flow" phases[24,65,66] (Table 4-3). The ebb phase is a hypometabolic state. The metabolic rate does not rise to the extent expected from the degree of fuel availability. The ebb phase is characterized by relatively low oxygen consumption and diminished capacity for heat production. Depending on many factors, such as the severity of the injury and the treatment applied, the ebb phase typically lasts no more than a day.[24,25] Plasma concentrations of catecholamines, cortisol, glucagon, and GH are generally high during this phase, whereas plasma insulin concentrations are depressed in relation to plasma glucose.[24]

The ebb phase evolves into a more prolonged flow phase in which catabolism occurs. Metabolic rate, core temperature, pulse rate, oxygen consumption, urinary excretion of nitrogen, and other indices of protein breakdown (e.g., 3-methylhistidine, zinc, creatinine)[67] are all increased during the flow phase. The duration and intensity of these catabolic changes vary according to the severity and nature of the injury.

Glucose Metabolism

After severe injury, several mechanisms disrupt the normal regulation of both the release and uptake of glucose. Hyperglycemia after surgery reflects a failure of the dual negative feedback processes by which an elevated plasma glucose

TABLE 4-3. "Ebb" and "Flow" Phases of the Stress Response

Ebb Phase (shock-like)	Flow Phase
Early (first 24 h)	Late (2–5 days)
Increased or decreased cardiac output	Increased cardiac output
Decreased oxygen consumption	Increased oxygen consumption
Vasoconstriction (mainly α effects)	Increased regional blood flow (mainly β effects)
Decreased urine flow	Hypermetabolic state
Hypometabolic state	Increased temperature
Decreased temperature	Increased protein catabolism
Decreased insulin levels	Increased fatty acid oxidation
	Glucose intolerance
	Increased gluconeogenesis
	Increased glycogenolysis

concentration inhibits hepatic gluconeogenesis and increases peripheral glucose use.[66,68] Stimulation of hepatic gluconeogenesis reflects an increased substrate supply, particularly amino acids such as alanine from skeletal muscle,[68] glycerol released from adipose tissue lipolysis, and lactate derived from ischemic tissues and areas of inflammation.[67,69]

In uninjured individuals, a rise in plasma glucose concentration stimulates pancreatic insulin secretion. Insulin acts to increase peripheral glucose clearance by muscle and adipose tissue.[59] Yet, immediately after injury, high circulating levels of catecholamines reduce pancreatic insulin secretion. Later, plasma insulin concentrations consistently rise, even to levels that are inappropriately high for the plasma glucose concentration.[63] The delayed elevation in insulin levels reflects, in part, the subsiding of adrenergic restraint on secretion and the stimulation of insulin release by amino acids, particularly arginine (a potent insulin secretagogue).[24,70] Despite the elevation of insulin concentrations, however, insulin fails to exert its expected anabolic effects ("insulin resistance"). Thus, postoperative glucose production is enhanced, glucose storage is reduced, fat mobilization and oxidation are increased, and protein turnover is also resistant to the normal anabolic effect of insulin. Studies evaluating individual or concurrent infusions of epinephrine, cortisol, and glucagon suggest that these three hormones act synergistically to promote and sustain hepatic glucose production, increase metabolic rate, and lower glucose clearance.[24] During the initial phase of such infusions, as shortly after trauma, the increase in insulin is appropriately low for the level of hyperglycemia.[24,66,70]

Lipid Metabolism

A rise in free fatty acids (FFA) and glycerol is observed as early as 2 hours after trauma or surgery. Increased fat oxidation regularly accompanies the flow phase, as the major part of any energy requirement is provided by fat. The number of calories derived from this process correlates positively with the severity of the injury.[66,71] Adipose tissue lipolysis is stimulated by epinephrine and potentiated by cortisol, GH, and glucagon. As described above, elevated circulating levels of these catabolic hormones impair the ability of insulin to inhibit lipolysis effectively, leading to increased FFA turnover.[71] Indeed, fat continues to be mobilized after trauma or surgery, even during administration of sufficient glucose to meet energy requirements.

Protein Metabolism

Protein synthesis and degradation both increase after injury.[69,72] Catabolism of protein stores (particularly skeletal muscle), loose connective tissue, and intestinal viscera predominate.[64] The extent of catabolism varies with the severity of the stress and is often assessed using the urinary excretion of 3-methylhistidine.[69] There is a marked increase in the peripheral oxidation of the branched chain amino acids to provide substrates for gluconeogenesis. These amino acids are thus rendered unavailable for reincorporation into body protein.[25] Hence, nitrogen is excreted as urinary urea, and body protein stores are progressively depleted.[68,72] The major source for the protein-derived energy mobilization after surgery or trauma is skeletal muscle, in which protein synthesis decreases and catabolism increases. In the liver, however, stress-induced increases in the synthesis of "acute-phase" proteins and decreases in the synthesis of other proteins (albumin and transferrin) are well described.[67,69,72]

THE IMMUNOLOGIC RESPONSE

Ample clinical and experimental evidence points to globally impaired humoral and cellular immune mechanisms after surgery and trauma. Decreases in responsiveness to mitogens and antigens, lymphocyte-mediated cytotoxicity, delayed hypersensitivity, skin graft rejection, antibody response, and natural killer cell activity have all been observed after stress. Stress has also been shown to enhance experimental tumor growth.[61,73,74]

Because of the well-known immunosuppressive effects of corticosteroids, many aspects of stress-induced immune deficiency have tentatively been related to the enhanced release of glucocorticoids. Glucocorticoids are not only lympholytic, but also inhibit secretion of T-cell growth factor (TCGF), which is essential for the proliferation of antigen-activated T cells. Both mitogenesis and IL-1 production are thereby inhibited.[44]

Apart from glucocorticoids, other stress hormones function as immune modulators: catecholamines, GH, prolactin, and endogenous opioids. Surface α_1- and α_2-adrenoreceptors are present on macrophages, and both epinephrine and norepinephrine have adverse effects on immune function. These catecholamines depress chemotactic and phagocytic activities, block the activation of macrophages to a tumoricidal and antiviral state and inhibit the production of reactive oxygen intermediates.[60,75,76]

Not all stress-released substances are immunosuppressive. GH and prolactin may act as endogenous restorative agents that counteract stress-induced immune dysfunction.[77] GH and prolactin stimulate macrophage tumoricidal activity and synthesis of interferon-γ.[61] Administration of exogenous GH and prolactin can reverse the immune impairment produced by glucocorticoids or correct immunologic deficiencies present in hypophysectomized rats.[60]

The role of endogenous opioids in stress-induced alterations of the immune system is supported by extensive evidence.[78–82] Frankly conflicting effects have been ascribed to opioids (immunoenhancement versus immunosuppression).[75,79] Disparate results have been reported after in vivo and in vitro studies, after acute and chronic opioid administration, and with use of opioids of differing chemical class (e.g., peptides versus alkaloids). The intensity of analgesia can also confound experimental findings, given the experimental observation that the opioid form of stress-induced analgesia (i.e., naloxone-reversible) reduces natural killer cell activity. The latter form of immunosuppression appears to be centrally mediated in that it is mimicked by central[80] or peripheral[81,82] morphine administration and blocked by opioid antagonists.[80]

Under appropriate conditions, cells of the immune system synthesize POMC-like molecules and release β-endorphin and ACTH indistinguishable from that produced by pituitary corticotrophs.[80,83] ACTH released by lymphocytes stimulates glucocorticoid release from the adrenal cortex,[60,83,84] giving rise to the term *lymphoadrenal axis*.[85] As described earlier for the CRH-like effects of IL-1, cytokines produced by immune cells act not only in paracrine fashion to stimulate the immune response, but also in an endocrine manner on distant targets to stimulate stress hormonal secretion.[61] Conversely, CRH has lymphocyte modulatory properties.[47–49] Thus, the sensitivity of the immune system to stress is due to a network of reciprocal regulatory influences that exist between the immune system and the central nervous system. Bidirectional communication occurs through shared neuroendocrine and cytokine hormones and hormone receptors, as well as the autonomic nervous system. By these means, the immune system transmits and receives signals from the brain as part of the integrated behavioral and physiologic response to stress.[60,61,86]

NEURAL EFFECTS: CARDIOVASCULAR

For the cardiovascular system, paracrine factors such as endothelin and nitric oxide are crucial to the local regulation of vascular tone. Neural outflow also figures prominently in the perioperative redistribution of blood flow among and within organs. Broadly speaking, unrelieved pain produces a state of heightened sympathetic tone and a resetting of the baroreceptor reflex. Thus, heart rate and blood pressure are both elevated.[87] Cardiac work and myocardial oxygen consumption increase, predisposing to myocardial ischemia if coronary artery disease is present. Decreased cardiac perfusion may induce arrhythmias in ischemic tissue. Yet even in the absence of myocardial ischemia, stress appears to be arrhythmogenic.[5] Because cardiac dysfunction (including arrhythmia) contributes to perioperative morbidity and mortality, the cardiovascular effects of pain are of special interest.

Randich and Maixner[88] convincingly argued that ''systems controlling cardiovascular function are closely coupled to systems modulating the perception of pain,'' as these systems share neurochemical and neuroanatomic substrates. Activation of C-fiber afferents leads to an increase in neural activity in the paraventricular nucleus of the hypothalamus,[14] the locus ceruleus of the brain stem,[89] and segmental sympathetic neurons within the intermediolateral columns of the spinal cord.[90] Activation of each can increase sympathetic outflow. Within the hypothalamus, pain- or stress-induced CRH release is likely to be an important mechanism to elicit enhanced global sympathetic tone.[41]

Besides increasing circulating catecholamines and sympathetic neural outflow, pain also produces a reflex reduction in parasympathetic outflow. The distorted balance of sympathetic and parasympathetic tone that accompanies pain alters the normal relation between heart rate and arterial blood pressure (baroreceptor reflex). This "resetting" of the baroreceptor reflex yields an abnormally high heart rate for a given blood pressure.[91] Intriguingly, hypertension and/or baroreceptor stimulation inhibit pain transmission at spinal and supraspinal levels during experimental pressor-induced hypertension or essential hypertension.[92] In other words, the reflex rise in blood pressure evoked by pain is itself a "gate" that inhibits pain perception. This gate phenomenon is mediated at least in part by endogenous opioids, because naloxone abolishes hypertension-induced analgesia.[93] Enhanced secretion of endogenous opioids into the peripheral circulation also occurs during hemodynamic states in which blood pressure is dependent on sympathetic outflow, such as in cardiac failure.[94,95] Giving exogenous opioids during varied stressors (e.g., hemorrhage, physical restraint) protects against the heightened ventricular vulnerability to fibrillation inherent in such settings. This protection results from antagonism of catecholamine-induced inotropy and chronotropy[96,97] and normalization of the baroreceptor-directed balance of sympathetic and parasympathetic neural outflow to the myocardium.[5,90]

ANALGESIA, STRESS REDUCTION, AND OUTCOME

Kehlet,[23,98–100] Wilmore,[64] and others recently reviewed evidence that the neurohumoral response to surgery is largely undesirable, resulting in erosion of body mass and tissue reserve, immunosuppression, and an increase in postoperative morbidity and mortality. Pain-induced reflexes can increase cardiac oxygen demand and/or vulnerability to fibrillation, impair respiratory function, and increase the risk of postoperative thromboembolism. Thus, the "homeostatic value" of the surgical stress response is questionable.[30,99] In the following sections we review how different analgesic modalities[101–104] (Fig. 4-6) may perhaps beneficially influence the stress response and thereby improve patient outcome.

Epidural Local Anesthetics

Numerous clinical trials document that pain control by epidural administration of local anesthetics inhibits the stress response (Fig. 4-6), particularly if the operative site is on the lower part of the body.[4,105] The clearest inhibitory effects have been observed for operations such as hysterectomy, vaginal surgery, inguinal herniotomy, prostatectomy, and orthopaedic procedures of the lower extremities. In contrast, use of epidural local anesthetics for procedures of the upper abdomen and thorax has failed to show a pronounced inhibitory effect on the surgical stress response (despite excellent analgesia).[101,106–108]

Thus, satisfactory analgesia per se is not sufficient to reduce the stress response to surgery of the upper abdomen and thorax (incomplete somatosensory blockade). Residual afferent nociceptive activity below the threshold where conscious perception of pain would be elicited may still evoke the surgical stress response. Evidence for the latter explanation is provided by clinical observa-

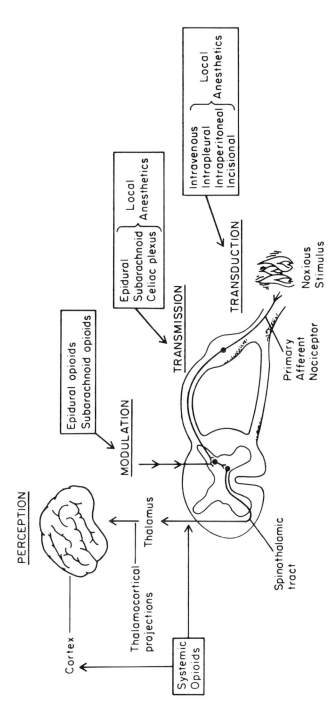

Fig. 4-6. Postoperative analgesic modalities that may affect the neuroendocrine response to surgery and pain.

tions of persistent evoked potential responses to somatic stimulation during thoracic epidural anesthesia/analgesia.[109] Incomplete sympathetic afferent blockade may also contribute to persistent stress responses, as addition of intraoperative splanchnic nerve block has been found to further decrease the stress response during epidural anesthesia.[100] Other nociceptive pathways not blocked by epidural local anesthetics include vagal and phrenic afferents. The importance of these pathways for the stress response appears minor.[106]

A correlation has been demonstrated between the level of sensory blockade and reduction of the cortisol and glucose response to surgery.[110] Suppression of adrenocortical and hyperglycemic responses to lower abdominal surgery requires maintenance of afferent blockade to about the fourth thoracic segment.[17,105,110,111] The duration of neural blockade is also an important variable, as brief blockade (i.e., <4 hours) has only a transient inhibitory effect on the adrenocortical and hyperglycemic response to surgery.

The hormonal and metabolic correlates of epidural local anesthesia/analgesia for surgery of the lower abdomen or lower extremities are well studied. Intra- and postoperative plasma catecholamine and cortisol concentrations are reduced. Elevations of plasma prolactin, GH, vasopressin, ACTH, and β-endorphin levels are prevented.[4,59] Such elevations are otherwise seen with general anesthesia and postoperative systemic analgesia.[4,59] The usual hyperglycemic response to surgery is reduced or blocked by epidural anesthesia/analgesia[110] because of these and other hormonal effects and through suppression of efferent sympathetic neural activity to the liver. Intraoperative lipolysis is inhibited as assessed by reduced levels of plasma FFAs and glycerol.[4]

Postoperative protein catabolism, a potentially life-threatening consequence of the surgical stress response, can be improved by epidural anesthesia/analgesia with local anesthetics. Brandt and colleagues[112] found that patients receiving continuous epidural anesthesia/analgesia for 24 hours after surgery were in neutral nitrogen balance from the second postoperative day onward. Patients receiving general anesthesia and parenteral postoperative analgesia were in negative nitrogen balance throughout the 5 days of study.[112] Similar studies that provided continuous epidural analgesia for 24 hours after surgery have supported these findings, demonstrating a beneficial metabolic effect in the late postoperative period.[17] Cumulative nitrogen balance improved, and plasma creatinine phosphokinase levels remained below those of controls.[17] In suppressing endocrine and metabolic responses to surgery, epidural anesthesia/analgesia with local anesthetics also inhibits the usual increase in postoperative oxygen consumption. Thus, demands on the cardiovascular system are reduced.[112]

Peripheral Neural Blockade

Neural afferent activity is a necessary step in eliciting the stress response. Thus, it is logical to suppose that interruption of peripheral neural pathways by infiltration anesthesia or peripheral neural blockade might decrease the stress response by reducing afferent neurogenic stimuli (Fig. 4-6). Unfortunately, this idea has not been borne out in practice.

Application of local anesthetics at the site of the surgical incision provides pain relief but does not produce any consistent or important modification of the stress response after abdominal or major thoracic surgery.[4,98] Specifically, bilateral intercostal nerve blocks were found to have no effect on perioperative plasma cortisol and only a modest inhibitory effect on hyperglycemia,[98] despite significant pain relief.[101] Intraoperative paravertebral blocks provided pain relief for 1–6 hours after abdominal surgery but minimally attenuated the stress response.[102] Innovative techniques such as interpleural administration of bupivacaine[103] or continuous intraperitoneal infusion of the same agent[104] likewise did not reduce the stress response despite achieving a satisfactory degree of analgesia.

Before drawing the conclusion that peripheral neural blockade is ineffective in suppressing the surgical stress response, it is important to remember that the aforementioned studies involved upper abdominal and thoracic surgery. Once again, analgesia per se is not sufficient to reduce the stress response. Reduction of the stress response is highly dependent on the location of the surgical site and the analgesic modalities used. Thus, further research is needed regarding the effects of peripheral neural blockade on the neuroendocrine response to lower abdominal and lower extremity surgery before any definitive conclusions can be drawn.

Systemic Opioids

Pro re nata (prn) intramuscular opioids are typically offered as "rescue" doses to the control (i.e., conventionally treated) patient groups in studies evaluating the effects of new postoperative analgesic modalities on the stress response. Given the design of such analgesic trials,[5] the magnitudes of stress responses observed with this traditional approach are by definition the standard against which novel techniques are measured. In other words, systemic as-needed opioids do not *influence* a response so much as *define* it!

Because conventional as-needed intramuscular opioid therapy dictates that a patient experience the reemergence of pain before each new request for an injection, conventional systemic opioids are relatively ineffective either for assuring continuous analgesia or for inhibiting stress responses. During such conventional treatment, the hormonal and metabolic responses outlined above are regularly observed in rough proportion to the magnitude of the operation performed.[17,108]

Even when systemic postoperative opioid analgesia is provided through a patient-controlled analgesia (PCA) paradigm, there is little effect on stress responses despite improvements in patient satisfaction and analgesia.[113] (There is a possible modest reduction in cortisol levels, however.[114]) Even though pain control is often superior using PCA as compared with as-needed injections, the persistent need for the patient to titrate analgesia to the reemergence of pain results in the persistence of stress responses.

In contrast to the minimal effects of small postoperative doses of opioids on stress responses, high (anesthetic) doses of intraoperative opioids are recognized to suppress pituitary-adrenal and sympathetic responses to intubation and surgery.[37,58,115,116] The suppressive effect does not extend beyond approximately the eighth postoperative hour unless a continuous opioid infusion is provided.[98,111] Consistent with our earlier discussion, the administration of high doses of intraoperative opioids does produce clinical benefits such as cardiovascular stability during the same time interval that stress responses are blunted.

Spinal (Epidural and Subarachroid) Opioids

Despite provision of good analgesia and improvement in certain measures of outcome such as pulmonary function, spinal opioids have no major effect on the surgical stress response. Trends toward reduced levels of cortisol, vasopressin, catecholamines, or glucose have been reported during epidural opioid analgesia. However, reductions in the correlates of the surgical stress response fall far short of the magnitude and extent observed during continuous epidural infusion of local anesthetics.[17,98,101,108,117] In particular, negative urinary nitrogen balance was found by Scott and colleagues[107] to be unaltered during a regimen of epidural morphine (4 mg every 12 hours) given for 3 days postoperatively. Furthermore, epidural morphine did not appear to augment the effectiveness of epidural bupivacaine in suppressing postoperative elevations of glucose and cortisol.[107] The experience with spinal opioids extends the concept (described above for systemic opioid administration) that analgesia and certain of its benefits may be dissociated from suppression of stress hormones.

Stress Hormones Are Not Outcomes: Some Caveats

From the above discussions it is clear that analgesia and its physiologic impact are related but not equivalent. As controversies exist concerning the best means to assess postoperative pain and standardization of assessment tools is lacking, investigators have sought other means to quickly quantitate the clinical response to analgesia. Since sensitive hormone assays became available about 20 years ago, measurements of circulating hormones have been widely used as "outcome surrogates" to assess the effectiveness of analgesic interventions. Indeed, most of the clinical studies described above were conducted with the implicit assumption that stress hormone suppression is in itself a desirable goal. Yet, particularly in the case of opioid analgesia, we must be cautious in interpreting stress hormone suppression to be as desirable an outcome or of equal significance to the suppression seen in the context of afferent neural blockade.[118]

The basis for such caution is that exogenous opioids act as surrogates for endogenous opioids. β-Endorphin is cosecreted from the pituitary along with ACTH.[54] This secretory process, as many other endocrine pathways, is subject to negative feedback control (Fig. 4–5).[59] Hence, administration of an exogenous opioid exerts negative feedback inhibition of ACTH and β-endorphin secretion in the same way that administration of thyroid hormone or estrogen inhibits the pituitary secretion of their respective trophic hormones. Thus, lowering of ACTH, β-endorphin, or cortisol levels in the plasma in response to opioid analgesia is not proof of adequate analgesia. Conversely, the persistence of elevated levels of ACTH, β-endorphin, or cortisol need not be equated with inadequate analgesia, as cells of the immune system are capable of producing and secreting ACTH and opioids.[85] Immunocytes also secrete IL-1, whose multiple effects include stimulation of pituitary secretion of ACTH and β-endorphin.[86]

Thus, administration of exogenous opioids may cause levels of stress hormones to fall, simply because of feedback inhibition of pituitary secretion of ACTH and β-endorphin. Similarly, the inflammatory response itself may cause plasma levels of stress hormones to rise by immunocyte secretion of stress hormones and stimulation of pituitary secretion. However, neither process may have any direct relation to the attendant degree of pain or analgesia.

Suppression of the Surgical Stress Response and Outcome

As previously outlined, numerous studies have looked at hormonal responses to surgery and analgesia. Few, however, have addressed the effects of reduction of the stress response on postoperative morbidity, mortality, and cost of medical care. Available data do point to the physiologic benefits of aggressive provision of analgesia. However, nearly no data exist comparing the fiscal savings afforded by reductions in postoperative length of stay and morbidity (e.g., pneumonia) and the monetary expenses or risks (e.g., epidural abscess) associated with doing so.

One important but often overlooked outcome is patient satisfaction.[119,120] Patients are more satisfied with their pain relief when PCA is used as compared with conventional as-needed opioid injections.[119,120] Furthermore, although the data are preliminary and controversial, intravenous PCA may allow quicker recovery of minute ventilation, earlier normalization of oral temperature, more rapid ambulation, and earlier discharge.[121] Nonetheless, the hormonal and metabolic effects of PCA compared with conventional treatment are limited at best. Thus, enhanced patient satisfaction and reduction in morbidity and cost of care can occur without a corresponding reduction of stress hormones.

It is clear that epidural neural blockade using local anesthetics inhibits several aspects of hypermetabolism and catabolism, particularly for procedures involving the lower abdomen and extremities.[99] Concurrent with these endocrinologic effects, postoperative epidural neural blockade has been associated with less sedation, earlier ambulation, higher pulmonary flow rates, improved oxygenation, and a decreased likelihood of deep venous thrombosis.[23]

Studies of clinical outcomes during epidural analgesia (local anesthetics and opioids) have focused on high-risk patient populations. In a randomized double-blind study of 30 grossly obese patients undergoing gastroplasty for weight reduction, Rawal et al[122] compared clinical outcomes after intramuscular and epidural morphine. They found a markedly earlier onset of postoperative mobilization in the epidural group, who also were more alert and had more rapid recovery of bowel movements.[122]

Yeager and colleagues[123] performed a provocative pilot study with ASA III patients undergoing vascular surgery with or without epidural anesthesia and postoperative analgesia. Postoperatively, patients receiving epidural anesthesia/analgesia had a reduction in urinary cortisol excretion for the initial 24 hours, a reduced morbidity from cardiovascular and infectious complications, a decreased duration of endotracheal intubation, and earlier discharge from the intensive care unit and the hospital as compared with controls. Associated with the more rapid convalescence and fewer clinical complications was a decrease in physician charges and overall hospital costs for the treatment group. Wide acceptance of this study's conclusions was impeded, however, by the relatively small number of patients studied and the unusually high incidence of morbidity and mortality (four of 25 patients) in the conventionally treated group.

Thus, despite the presence of the aforementioned studies, research regarding the relation among analgesia, stress hormone reduction, and clinical outcome remains a pressing need.

CONCLUSION

The multiple hormonal "stress" responses evident after surgery are not in themselves outcomes. In certain respects, hormone secretion itself directly mediates or contributes to undesirable postoperative metabolic sequelae such as catabolism or hyperglycemia. In such situations, suppression of hormonal responses is beneficial for outcome. In other respects, stress hormone levels in the blood may not be correlated with the return of homeostatic function (restoration of pulmonary or intestinal function, time to ambulation, or even analgesia itself). In these situations, little evidence exists that the hormone levels determine outcome.

Further, the significance of a blunted postoperative cortisol response during epidural afferent blockade using local anesthetic is quite distinct from that of a blunted cortisol response during opioid administration. The latter blunting may simply be a demonstration of a well-known endocrine feedback loop.

From an endocrinologic viewpoint, the aim of postoperative analgesia is to dissociate tissue injury and mediator release from their usual hormonal sequelae. As described above, the dissociation evident during epidural anesthesia results mainly from blockade of afferent neural impulses from the site of injury. The concomitant blockade of efferent sympathetic pathways (e.g., to the liver and adrenal medulla) may possibly be important as well.[112] Even when the stress response is not completely blocked, as in the use of epidural opioids or epidural local anesthesia for upper abdominal and thoracic surgery, there are suggestions that improved outcome occurs with provision of good analgesia. If these suggestions are borne out in large-scale, prospective outcome studies during the 1990s, the next clinical challenge will be to assure the widespread application of these analgesic techniques as an integral part of quality care.

References
1. Selye H: A syndrome produced by diverse nocuous agents. Nature 138:32, 1936
2. Axelrod J: The relationship between the stress hormones, catecholamines, ACTH and glucocorticoids. p. 3. In Usdin E, Kvetnansky R, Axelrod J (eds): Stress. The Role of Catecholamines and Other Neurotransmitters. Gordon and Breach Science Publishers, New York, 1983
3. Carr DB, Murphy MT: Operation, anesthesia, and endorphin system. Int Anesthesiol Clin 26:199, 1988
4. Kehlet H: Modification of responses to surgery by neural blockade: clinical implications. p. 145. In Cousins MJ, Bridenbaugh PO (eds): Neural Blockade in Clinical Anesthesia and Management of Pain. 2nd Ed. JB Lippincott, Philadelphia, 1988
5. Verrier RL, Carr DB: Stress-specific influences of opioids on cardiac electrical stability, abstracted. J Cardivoasc Electrophysiol, suppl. 2:S124, 1991
6. Bonica JJ: Anatomic and physiologic basis of nociception and pain. p. 28. In Bonica JJ, (ed): The Management of Pain. 2nd Ed. Lea & Febiger, Philadelphia, 1990
7. Carr DB, Ballantyne JC, Osgood PF et al: Pituitary-adrenal stress response in the absence of brain-pituitary connections. Anesth Analg 69:197, 1989
8. Hargreaves KM, Dionne RA: Evaluating endogenous mediators of pain and analagesia in clinical studies. p. 579. In Max MB, Portenoy RK, Laska EM (eds): The Design of Analgesic Clinical Trials. Advances in Pain Research and Therapy. Vol. 18. Raven Press, New York, 1991
9. Smelik PG: Factors determining the pattern of stress responses. p. 17. In Usdin E, Kvetnansky R, Axelrod J (eds): Stress. The Role of Catecholamines and Other Neurotransmitters. Gordon and Breach Science Publishers, New York, 1983
10. Smelik PG: Summary of panel discussions on stress. p. 69. In Usdin E, Kvetnansky R, Axelrod J (eds): Stress. The Role of Catecholamines and Other Neurotransmitters. Gordon and Breach Science Publishers, New York, 1983
11. Lund C, Hansen OB, Mogensen T, Kehlet H: Effect of thoracic epidural bupivacaine on somatosensory evoked potentials after dermatomal stimulation. Anesth Analg 66:731, 1987
12. Fields HL: Introduction. Pain pathways. p. 1. In Fields HL (ed): Pain Syndromes in Neurology. Butterworth, London, 1990
13. Yaksh TL: Neurologic mechanisms of pain. p. 791. In Cousins MJ, Brinenbaugh PO (eds): Neural Blockade in Clinical Anesthesia and Management of Pain. 2nd Ed. JB Lippincott, Philadelphia, 1988
14. Swanson LW, Sawchenko PE: Hypothalamic integration: organization of the paraventricular and supraoptic nuclei. Annu Rev Neurosci 6:269, 1983
15. Swanson LW, Sawchenko PE, Lind RW, Rho JH: The CRH motoneuron: differential peptide regulation in neurons with possible synaptic, paracrine, and endocrine outputs. Ann N Y Acad Sci 512:12, 1987
16. Antoni FA: Receptors mediating the CRH effects of vasopressin and oxytocin. Ann N Y Acad Sci 152:195, 1987
17. Bormann B, Weidler B, Dennhardt R et al: Influence of epidural fentanyl on stress-induced elevation of plasma vasopressin (ADH) after surgery. Anesth Analg 62:727, 1983
18. Bilezikjian LM, Vale WW: Regulation of ACTH secretion from corticotrophs: the interaction of vasopressin and CRF. Ann N Y Acad Sci 512:85, 1987
19. Burstein R, Cliffer KD, Giesler GJ Jr: Direct somatosensory projections from the spinal cord to the hypothalamus and telencephalon. J Neurosci 7:4159, 1987
20. Burstein R, Cliffer KD, Giesler GJ Jr: The spinohypothalamic and spinotelecepha-

lic tracts: direct nociceptive projections from the spinal cord to the hypothalamus and telencephalon. p. 548. In Dubner R, Gebhart GF, Bond MR (ed): Proceedings of the Vth World Congress on Pain. Elsevier Science Publishing, New York, 1988

21. Burstein R, Cliffer KD, Giesler GJ Jr: Cells of origin of the spinohypothalamic tract in the rat. J Comp Neurol 291:329, 1990

22. Chernow B, Alexander HR, Smallridge RC et al: Hormonal responses to graded surgical stress. Arch Intern Med 147:1273, 1987

23. Kehlet H: The stress response to surgery: release mechanisms and the modifying of pain relief. Acta Chir Scand Suppl 550:22, 1989

24. Frayn KN: Hormonal control of metabolism in trauma and sepsis. Clin Endocrinol (Oxf) 24:577, 1986

25. Brown JM, Grosso MA, Harken AH: Cytokines, sepsis and the surgeon. Surg Gynecol Obstet 169:568, 1989

26. Aimone LD, Yaksh TL: Opioid modulation of capsaicin-evoked release of substance P from rat spinal cord in vivo. Peptides 10:1127, 1989

27. Payan DG: Neuropeptides and inflammation: the role of substance P. Annu Rev Med 40:341, 1989

28. Payan D, Goetzl EJ: Dual roles of substance P: modulator of immune and neuroendocrine functions. Ann N Y Acad Sci 512:465, 1987

29. Matta SG, Singh J, Newton R, Sharp BM: The adrenocorticotropin response to interleukin-1 beta instilled into the rat median eminence depends on the local release of catecholamines. Endocrinology 127:2175, 1990

30. Kehlet H: Stress free anaesthesia and surgery. Acta Anaesthesiol Scand 23:503, 1979

31. Billingham MEJ: Cytokines as inflammatory mediators. Br Med Bull 43:350, 1987

32. Beutler B: Cachectin in tissue injury, shock, and related states. Crit Care Clin 5: 353, 1989

33. Simpson SQ, Casey LC: Role of tumor necrosis factor in sepsis and acute lung injury. Crit Care Clin 5:27, 1989

34. Naesh O, Friis JT, Hindberg I, Winther K: Platelet function in surgical stress. Thromb Haemost 54:849, 1985

35. Mezey E, Reisine T, Brownstein MJ et al: Peripheral catecholamines regulate in vivo ACTH release through adrenergic receptors in the rat anterior pituitary. p. 225. In Usdin E, Kvetnansky R, Axelrod J (eds): Stress. The Role of Catecholamines and Other Neurotransmitters. Gordon and Breach Science Publishers, New York, 1983

36. Palkovits M: Anatomy of neural pathways affecting CRH secretion. Ann N Y Acad Sci 512:139, 1987

37. Grossman A: Opioids and stress in man. J Endocrinol 119:377, 1988

38. Zaloga GP: Catecholamines in anesthetic and surgical stress. Int Anesthesiol Clin 26:187, 1988

39. Yasuda N, Greer MA, Aizawa T: Corticotropin-releasing factor. Endocr Rev 3: 123, 1982

40. Vale W, Speiss J, Rivier C, Rivier J: Characterization of a 41-residue ovine hypothalamic peptide that stimulates secretion of corticotropin and β-endorphin. Science 213:1934, 1981

41. Fisher LA: Corticotropin-releasing factor: endocrine and autonomic integration of responses to stress. Trends Pharmacol Sci 10:189, 1989

42. Plotsky PM: Regulation of hypophysiotropic factors mediating ACTH secretion. Ann N Y Acad Sci 512:205, 1987

43. Negro-Vilar A, Johnston C, Spinedi E et al: Physiological role of peptides and amines on the regulation of ACTH secretion. Ann N Y Acad Sci 512:218, 1987
44. Munck A, Guyre PM Holbrook NJ: Physiological functions of glucocorticoids in stress and their relation to pharmacological actions. Endocr Rev 5:25, 1984
45. Keller-Wood ME, Dallman MF: Corticosteroid inhibition of ACTH secretion. Endocr Rev 5:1, 1984
46. Bruhn TO, Engeland WC, Anthony EL et al: Corticotropin-releasing factor in the adrenal medulla. Ann N Y Acad Sci 512:115, 1987
47. Dunn AJ, Berridge CW: Is corticotropin-releasing factor a mediator of stress responses? Ann N Y Acad Sci 579:183, 1990
48. Hargreaves KM, Dubner R, Costello AH: Corticotropin releasing factor (CRF) has a peripheral site of action for antinociception. Eur J Pharmacol 170:275, 1989
49. Wei T, Kiang JG, Buchan P, Smith TW: Corticotropin-releasing factor inhibits neurogenic plasma extravasation in the rat paw. J Pharamcol Exp Ther 238:783, 1986
50. Gillies G, Lowry PJ: Corticotropin-releasing hormone and its vasopressin component. p. 45. In Ganong WF, Martini I (eds): Frontiers in Neuroendocrinology. Raven Press, New York, 1982
51. Morley JE: The endocrinology of the opiates and opioid peptides. Metabolism 30: 195, 1981
52. Oyama T, Wakayama S: The endocrine responses to general anesthesia. Int Anesthesiol Clin 26:176, 1988
53. Carr DB: Opioids. Int Anesthesiol Clin 26:273, 1988
54. Eipper BA, Mains RE: Structure and biosynthesis of proadrenocroticotropin/endorphin and related peptides. Endocr Rev 1:1, 1980
55. Carr DB, Lipkowski AW, Silbert BS: Biochemistry of the opioid peptides. p. 3. In Estafanous FG (ed): Opioids in Anesthesia II. Butterworth-Heinemann, Stoneham, MA, 1991
56. Joris J, Dubner R, Hargreaves KM: Opioid analgesia at peripheral sites: a target for opioids released during stress and inflammation? Anesth Analg 66:1277, 1987
57. Stein C: Peripheral analgesic actions of opioids. J Pain Symptom Management 6: 199, 1991
58. Dubois M, Pickar D, Cohen M et al: Effects of fentanyl on the response of plasma beta-endorphin immunocreativity to surgery. Anesthesiology 57:468, 1982
59. Frohman LA, Krieger DT: Neuroendocrine physiology and disease. p. 185. In Felig P, Baxter JD, Broadus AE, Frohman LA (eds): Endocrinology and Metabolism. 2nd Ed. McGraw-Hill, New York, 1986
60. Cavagnaro J, Waterhouse GA, Lewis RM: Neuroendocrine-immune interactions: immunoregulatory signals mediated by neurohumoral agents. Year Immunol 3:228, 1988
61. Dantzer R, Kelley KW: Stress and immunity: an integrated view of relationships between the brain and the immune system. Life Sci 44:1995, 1989
62. Anand KJ, Carr DB: The neuroanatomy, neurophysiology, and neurochemistry of pain, stress, and analgesia in newborns and children. Pediatr Clin North Am 36: 795, 1989
63. Douglas RG, Shaw JH: Metabolic response to sepsis and trauma. Br J Surg 76:155, 1989
64. Wilmore DW: Catabolic illness. Strategies for enhancing recovery. N Engl J Med 325:695, 1991
65. Cuthbertson DP: Observations on the disturbance of metabolism produced by injury to the limbs. Q J Med 25:233, 1932

66. Hensle TW, Askanazi J: Metabolism and nutrition in the perioperative period. J Urol 139:229, 1988
67. Cerra FB: Hypermetabolism-organ failure syndrome: a metabolic response to injury. Crit Care Clin 5:289, 1989
68. Wolfe RR: Carbohydrate metabolism in the critically ill patient. Implications for nutritional support. Crit Care Clin 3:11, 1987
69. Cerra FB: Metabolic manifestations of multiple systems organ failure. Crit Care Clin 5:119, 1989
70. Lange MP, Dahn MS, Jacobs LA: The significance of hyperglycemia after injury. Heart Lung 14:470, 1985
71. Wiener M, Rothkopf MM, Rothkopf G, Askanazi J: Fat metabolism in injury and stress. Crit Care Clin 3:25, 1987
72. Elwyn DH: Protein metabolism and requirements in the critically ill patient. Crit Care Clin 3:57, 1987
73. Liebeskind JC: Pain can kill (editorial). Pain 44:3, 1991
74. Saba TM, Scovill WA: Effect of surgical trauma on host defense. Surg Annu 7:71, 1975
75. Tecoma ES, Huey LY: Psychic distress and the immune response. Life Sci 36:1799, 1985
76. Felten DL, Felten SY, Bellinger DL et al: Noradrenergic sympathetic neural interctions with the immune system: structure and function. Immunol Rev 100:225, 1987
77. Clevenger CV, Altmann SW, Prystowsky MB: Requirement of nuclear prolactin for interleukin-2-simulated proliferation of T lymphocytes. Science 253:77, 1991
78. Stein C, Hassan AH, Przewlocki R et al: Opioids from immunocytes interact with receptors on sensory nerves to inhibit nociception in inflammation. Proc Natl Acad Sci USA 87:5935, 1990
79. Morley JE, Kay NE, Solomon GF, Plotnikoff NP: Neuropeptides: conductors of the immune orchestra. Life Sci 41:527, 1987
80. Shavit Y, Lewis JW, Terman GW et al: Opioid peptides mediate the suppressive effect of stress on natural killer cytotoxicity. Science 223:188, 1984
81. Bryant HU, Bernton EW, Holaday JW: Immunomodulatory effects of chronic morphine treatment: pharmacologic and mechanistic studies. NIDA Res Monogr 6:131, 1990
82. Bryant HU, Roudebush RE: Suppressive effects of morphine pellet implants on in vivo parameters of immune function. J Pharmacol Exp Ther 255:410, 1990
83. Harbour-McMenamin D, Smith EM, Blalock JE: Bacterial lipopolysaccharide induction of leukocyte-derived corticotropin and endorphins. Infect Immun 48:813, 1985
84. Kavelaars A, Ballieux RE, Heijnen CJ: In vitro beta-adrenergic stimulation of lymphocytes induces the release of immunoreactive beta-endorphin. Endocrinology 126:3028, 1990
85. Smith EM, Meyer WJ, Blalock JE: Virus-induced corticosterone in hypophysectomized mice: a possible lymphoid adrenal axis. Science 218:1311, 1982
86. Weigent DA, Carr DJ, Blalock JE: Bidirectional communication between the neuroendocrine and immune systems. Common hormones and hormone receptors. Ann N Y Acad Sci 579:17, 1990
87. Carr DB, Saini V, Verrier RL: Opioids and cardiovascular function: neuromodulation of ventricular ectopy. p. 223. In Kulbertus HE, Franck G (eds): Neurocardiology. Futura Publishing, Mount Kisco, NY, 1988

88. Randich A, Maixner W: Interactions between cardiovascular and pain regulatory systems. Neurosci Biobehav Rev 8:343, 1984
89. Aghajanian G: Tolerance of locus coeruleus neurones to morphine and suppression of withdrawal responses to clonidine. Nature 276:186, 1978
90. Franz DN, Hare BD, McCloskey KL: Spinal sympathetic neurons: possible sites of opiate-withdrawal suppression by clonidine. Science 215:1643, 1982
91. Randall DC: Plasticity of the unconditional response: evidence linking pain and cardiovascular regulation? J Cardiovasc Electrophysiol, suppl. 2:S76, 1991
92. Schramm LP, Poree LR: Medullo-spinal modulation of sympathetic output and spinal afferent input. J Cardiovasc Electrophysiol, suppl. 2:S18, 1991
93. Maixner W: Interactions between cardiovascular and pain modulatory systems: physiological and pathophysiological implications. J Cardiovasc Electrophysiol, suppl. 2:S3, 1991
94. Liang CS, Imai N, Stone CK et al: The role of endogenous opioids in congestive heart failure: effects of nalmephene on systemic and regional hemodynamics in dogs. Circulation 75:443, 1987
95. Carr DB, Athanasiadis CG, Skourtis CT et al: Quantitative relationships between plasma beta-endorphin immunoactivity and hemodynamic performance in preoperative cardiac surgical patients. Anesth Analg 68:77, 1989
96. Carr DB, Verrier RL: Opioids in pain and cardiovascular responses: overview of common features. J Cardiovasc Electrophysiol Suppl 2:S34, 1991
97. Saini V, Carr DB, Verrier RL: Comparative effects of the opioids fentanyl and buprenorphine on ventricular vulnerability during acute coronary artery occlusion. Cardiovasc Res 23:1001, 1989
98. Kehlet H: Surgical stress: the role of pain and analgesia. Br J Anaesth 63:189, 1989
99. Scott NB, Kehlet H: Regional anaesthesia and surgical morbidity. Br J Surg 75:299, 1988
100. Kehlet H: The endocrine responses to regional anesthesia. Int Anesthesiol Clin 26:182, 1988
101. Scheinin B, Scheinin M, Asantila R et al: Sympatho-adrenal and pituitary hormone responses during and immediately after thoracic surgery—modulation by four different pain treatments. Acta Anaesthesiol Scand 31:762, 1987
102. Giesecke K, Hamberger B, Jarnberg PO, Klingstedt C: Paravertebral block during cholecystectomy: effects on circulatory and hormonal responses. Br J Anaesth 61:652, 1988
103. Scott NB, Mogensen T, Bigler D, Kehlet H: Comparison of the effects of continuous intrapleural vs epidural administration of 0.5% bupivacaine on pain, metabolic response and pulmonary function following cholecystectomy. Acta Anaesthesiol Scand 33:535, 1989
104. Scott NB, Mogensen T, Greulich A et al: No effect of continuous I.P. infusion of bupivacaine on postoperative analgesia, pulmonary function and the stress response to surgery. Br J Anaesth 61:165, 1988
105. Murat I, Walker J, Esteve C et al: Effect of lumbar epidural anaesthesia on plasma cortisol levels in children. Can J Anaesth 35:20, 1988
106. Traynor C, Paterson JL, Ward ID et al: Effects of extradural analgesia and vagal blockade on the metabolic and endocrine response to upper abdominal surgery. Br J Anaesth 54:319, 1982
107. Scott NB, Mogensen T, Bigler D et al: Continuous thoracic extradural 0.5% bupivacaine with or without morphine: effect on quality of blockade, lung function, and the surgical stress response. Br J Anaesth 62:253, 1989

108. Rutberg H, Hakanson E, Anderberg L et al: Effects of the extradural administration of morphine, or bupivacaine, on the endocrine response to upper abdominal surgery. Br J Anaesth 56:233, 1984

109. Lund C, Qvitzau S, Greulinch A et al: Comparison of the effects of extradural clonidine with those of morphine on postoperative pain, stress responses, cardiopulmonary function, and motor and sensory block. Br J Anaesth 63:516, 1989

110. Moller IW, Hjortso E, Krantz T et al: The modifying effect of spinal anaesthesia on intra- and postoperative adrenocortical and hyperglycaemic response to surgery. Acta Anaesthesiol Scand 28:266, 1984

111. Blunnie WP, McIlroy PD, Merrett JD, Dundee JW: Cardiovascular and biochemical evidence of stress during major surgery associated with different techniques of anaesthesia. Br J Anaesth 55:611, 1983

112. Brandt MR, Fernandes A, Mordhorst R, Kehlet H: Epidural analgesia improves postoperative nitrogen balance. Br Med J 1:1106, 1978

113. Moller IW, Dinesen K, Sondergard S et al: Effect of patient-controlled anaglesia on plasma catecholamine, cortisol and glucose concentrations after cholecystectomy. Br J Anaesth 61:160, 1988

114. Wasylak TJ, Abbott FV, English MJ, Jeans M: Reduction of post-operative morbidity following patient-controlled morphine. Can J Anaesth 37:726, 1990

115. Campbell BC, Parikh RK, Naismith A et al: Comparison of fentanyl and halothane supplementation to general anaesthesia on the stress response to upper abdominal surgery. Br J Anaesth 56:257, 1984

116. Anand KJ, Sippell WG, Aynsley-Green A: Randomized trial of fentanyl anasthesia in preterm babies undergoing surgery: effects on the stress response. Lancet i:62, 1987

117. Tsuji H, Shirasaka CT, Asoh T, Uchida I: Effects of epidural administration of local anaesthetics or morphine on postoperative nitrogen loss and catabolic hormones. Br J Surg 74:421, 1987

118. Carr DB: Caveats in the evaluation of stress hormone responses in analgesic trials. p. 599. In Max MB, Portenoy RK, Laska EM (eds): The Design of Analgesic Clinical Trials. Advances in Pain Research and Therapy. Vol. 18. Raven Press, New York, 1991

119. Eisenach JC, Grise SC, Dewan DM: Patient-controlled analgesia following cesarean section: a comparison with epidural and intramuscular narcotics. Anesthesiology 68:444, 1988

120. Harrison DM, Sinatra R, Morgese L, Chung JH: Epidural narcotics and patient-controlled analgesia for post-cesarean section pain relief. Anesthesiology 68:454, 1988

121. Ready LB: Patient-controlled analgesia—does it provide more than comfort? (editorial). Can J Anaesth 37:719, 1990

122. Rawal N, Sjöstrand U, Christoffersson E et al: Comparison of intramuscular and epidural morphine for postoperative analgesia in the grossly obese: influence on postoperative ambulation and pulmonary function. Anesth Analg 63:583, 1984

123. Yeager MP, Glass D, Neff RK, Brinck-Johnsen T: Epidural anesthesia and analgesia in high-risk surgical patients. Anesthesiology 66:729, 1987

5

Anatomy of the Vertebral Column

F. Michael Ferrante

Epidural anesthesia/analgesia is the most commonly used regional technique for the management of acute pain. To facilitate the use of the epidural and subarachnoid routes of administration, the practitioner must have a working knowledge of spinal anatomy. This chapter briefly reviews the anatomy of the vertebral column and its contents. Of course, the best way to learn anatomy is via specimens. In lieu of this, some of the finest anatomic diagrams can be found in the suggested reading list at the end of the chapter.

BONY STRUCTURES

The vertebral column consists of 24 vertebrae (7 cervical, 12 thoracic, 5 lumbar), the sacrum, and the coccyx. The sacrum and coccyx are the result of the fusion of five sacral vertebrae and four coccygeal segments, respectively. The spinal canal extends from the foramen magnum to the sacral hiatus. It is formed from the continuum of the vertebral arches and the posterior aspect of the vertebral bodies.

An individual vertebra consists of two parts: the body (anteriorly) and the arch (posteriorly) (Fig. 5-1). The contents of the dural sac (as the spinal cord does not extend the full length of the spinal canal) are surrounded by the posterior surface of the vertebral body, the pedicles, and the laminae. Transverse processes lie at the juncture of the pedicles and the laminae. Posteriorly, the laminae are fused to form the spinous process. Superior and inferior articular

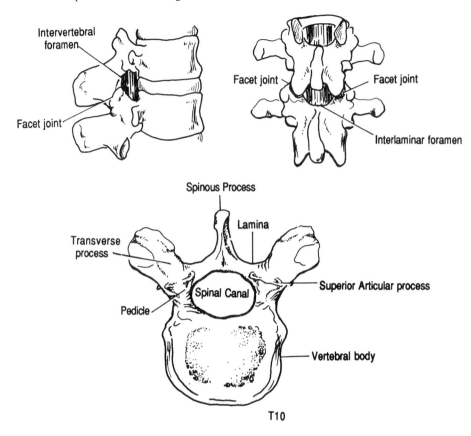

Fig. 5-1. Typical vertebra (thoracic) and articulating lumbar vertebrae.

processes form facet joints by attachment to corresponding processes on adjacent cephalad and caudad vertebrae.

A space between adjacent pedicles is formed by the articulation of two vertebrae (Fig. 5-1). Spinal nerves bilaterally exit through each of these intervertebral foraminae. The space between adjacent laminae and the respective facet joints of articulating vertebrae is called the interlaminar foramen (Fig. 5-1). Using the spinous processes as landmarks, the location of the interlaminar foraminae may be estimated in order to gain access to the spinal canal for invasive procedures.

The size and shape of vertebrae differ in the cervical, thoracic, and lumbar areas of the vertebral column (Fig. 5-2). The cervical vertebrae are the smallest and the lumbar vertebrae are the largest in size. The angulation of the spinous processes varies according to region. In the cervical, lower thoracic, and lumbar regions, spinous processes are nearly horizontal. In the midthoracic region, spinous processes have a marked caudad angulation (maximal between T3 and T7 vertebrae) (Fig. 5-2). Degree of angulation will affect the direction of the needle during a regional technique, as well as the degree of difficulty inherent in the procedure.

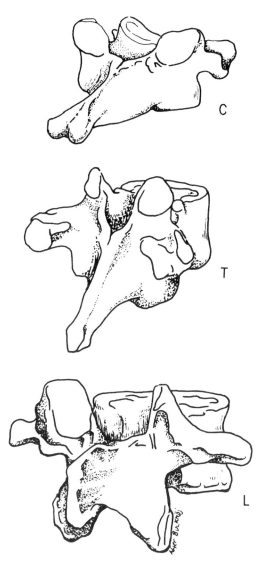

Fig. 5-2. Oblique view of typical lower cervical (C), midthoracic (T), and midlumbar (L) vertebrae. Note acute angulation of spinous processes in the midthoracic region, contributing to the difficulty of epidural technique. Angulation is maximal between T3 and T7 vertebrae. In the cervical, lower thoracic, and lumbar regions, spinous processes are nearly horizontal.

LIGAMENTS

The vertebral arches of adjacent vertebrae are joined by three ligaments (Fig. 5-3). The laminae of articulating vertebrae are connected by the ligamentum flavum. Constituting a major portion of the posterior wall of the vertebral canal, it also forms the posterior boundary of the epidural space. The spinous proc-

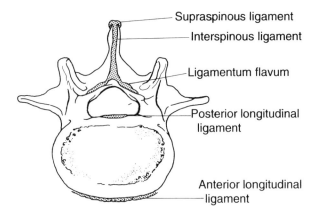

Supraspinous ligament

Interspinous ligament

Ligamentum flavum

Posterior longitudinal ligament

Anterior longitudinal ligament

Fig. 5-3. Ligaments of the vertebral column.

esses are connected by the interspinous ligament, uniting the lower border of one spinous process with the upper border of its neighbor. The supraspinous ligament runs superficial to the tips of the spinous processes and unites their apices.

The anterior and posterior longitudinal ligaments provide support for the vertebral bodies from C2 to the sacrum (Fig. 5-3). The anterior longitudinal ligament is attached to the vertebral discs and adjacent margins of the vertebral bodies. The posterior longitudinal ligament connects the posterior surface of the vertebral bodies and forms part of the anterior wall of the spinal canal.

CONTENTS OF THE SPINAL CANAL

Spinal Cord

The spinal cord extends from the foramen magnum to the level of the second lumbar vertebra. Its caudal end tapers into a conical structure (conus medularis) connected to the coccyx by the delicate filament of the filum terminale (Fig. 5-4). The lumbar, sacral, and coccygeal nerves come off in sequence from the conus medularis to form the cauda equina, bathed in cerebrospinal fluid (CSF) within the dural sac.

The spinal cord has two fusiform enlargements: the cervical and lumbar enlargements. The cervical enlargement extends from the C3 to T2 vertebrae and corresponds to nerves supplying the upper extremities. The lumbar enlargement extends from the T9 to the upper border of L1 vertebrae and corresponds to the nerves comprising the lumbar plexus.

The spinal cord is suspended at the foramen magnum, which prevents the larger medulla oblongata from moving caudad. More caudally, it is held in place by nerve roots, denticulate ligaments, and the filum terminale. The denticulate ligaments (Fig. 5-4) are lateral thickenings of the pia mater on either side of the

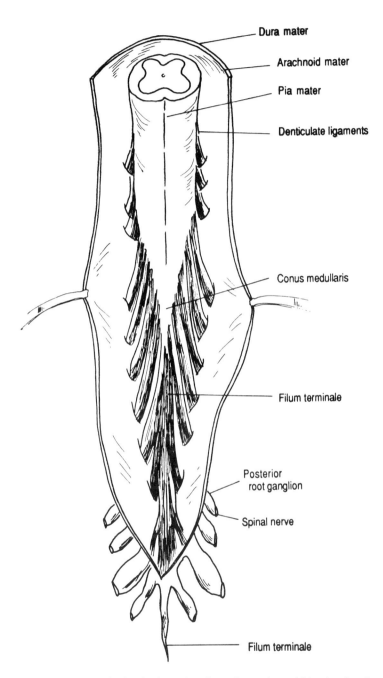

Fig. 5-4. Lower end of spinal cord and cauda equina within the dural sac.

nerve roots. The denticulate ligaments adhere to the arachnoid mater and dura mater.

As the spinal cord is shorter in adult life than the vertebral column, spinal cord segments do not lie exactly opposite the numerically corresponding vertebrae (Fig. 5-5). Because of this, it is convenient to regard the cord as being composed of segments and corresponding spinal nerves, although there is no macroscopic transverse segmentation. Thus, the eight cervical spinal cord segments lie opposite the upper six cervical vertebrae. The upper six thoracic cord segments are opposite the C7 and upper four thoracic vertebrae. The lower six thoracic spinal cord segments are opposite the T5-T9 vertebrae. The five lumbar segments are opposite the T10-T12 vertebrae. The five sacral and single coccygeal spinal cord segments lie opposite the T12 and L1 vertebrae.

Meninges

The meninges are three membranes enveloping the central nervous system. The pia mater is a delicate vascular membrane closely investing the spinal cord and each nerve root. The arachnoid mater is a nonvascular membrane closely applied to the dura mater. A small amount of fluid lubricates the lining between the arachnoid mater and the dura mater, forming a potential space called the subdural space. Thus, it is possible to make subdural extraarachnoid injections. The arachnoid mater extends to the second lumbar vertebra with the dura mater. The dura mater is the tough outermost sheath surrounding the spinal cord and invests the roots of spinal nerves, as well as mixed nerves in the intervertebral foraminae. As the spinal nerves pierce the dura, each anterior and posterior root carries a sleeve of the dura laterally. The dura eventually becomes contiguous with the epineurium of the spinal nerve. Thus, the possibility of an intradural injection always exists when performing regional techniques near the spinal canal. The dura mater is attached to the foramen magnum in its cephalad aspect and ends at the second sacral vertebra.

Subarachnoid Space

The subarachnoid space lies between the arachnoid mater and the pia mater and contains CSF. Although approximately 150 ml of CSF is contained within the spinal subarachnoid space and the ventricular system, only 30 ml bathes the cord and cauda equina.

The CSF is formed by the choroid plexuses of the lateral third and fourth ventricles. CSF is an ultrafiltrate of plasma. It bathes the spinal cord by leaving the fourth ventricle through the foraminae of Luschka and Magendie. CSF is returned to the bloodstream through the arachnoid granulations, which project into intracranial venous sinuses. Arachnoid granulations are also found in the dural cuff region of the epidural space (see below).

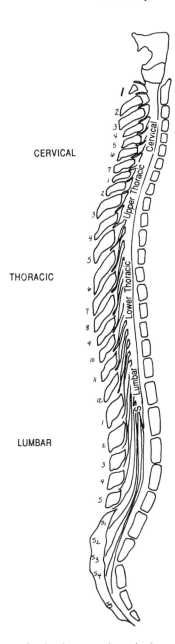

CERVICAL

THORACIC

LUMBAR

Fig. 5-5. Relation of the vertebral column to the spinal cord in the adult. Lateral view. Spinal cord segments do not lie opposite the numerically corresponding vertebrae. The eight cervical cord segments lie opposite the upper six cervical vertebrae. The upper six thoracic cord segments are opposite the C7 and upper four thoracic vertebrae. The lower six thoracic spinal cord segments are opposite the T5-T9 vertebrae. The five lumbar segments are opposite the T10-T12 vertebrae. The five sacral and single coccygeal spinal cord segments lie opposite the T12 and L1 vertebrae.

Epidural Space

The epidural space is located between the dura mater and the connective tissue covering the vertebrae and the ligamentum flavum (Fig. 5-6). The epidural space totally surrounds the dural sac. It is completely filled with connective

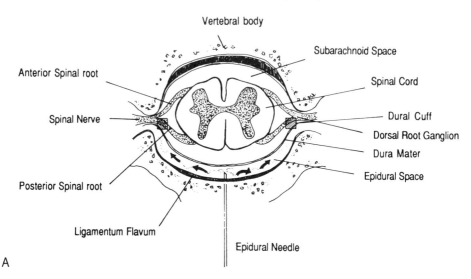

A

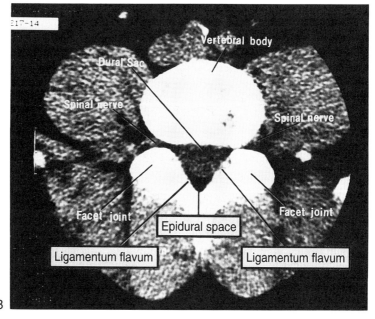

B

Fig. 5-6. (A) Cross-sectional diagram of spinal canal and (B) accompanying view by computed tomography at L3-L4. Drugs injected into the epidural space will diffuse laterally to the dural cuff. Arachnoid granulations in the region of the dural cuff allow access to the CSF.

tissue, fat, and blood vessels, particularly venous plexuses, and is therefore described as a potential space. The epidural space spans the distance of the entire spinal canal, extending from the foramen magnum to the sacral hiatus.

In actuality, the cross-sectional area between the ligamentum flavum and the dura mater varies inversely with the contents of the spinal canal (Fig. 5-7). The epidural space is narrow in the areas of the cervical and lumbar enlargements of the spinal cord. Once the spinal cord ends at L2, the epidural space widens. In the lower cervical region, the distance between the ligamentum flavum and the dura mater may be 2 mm or less. In the midthoracic region, the distance may be 3–5 mm. Below the end of the cord at L2, distances of 5–7 mm are the norm (Fig. 5-7). Thus, the amount of local anesthetic required to anesthetize a spinal segment is directly proportional to the cross-sectional area of the epidural space: approximately 0.5 ml per thoracic segment, 1.5 ml per lumbar segment, and 3 ml per sacral segment.

When injected into the epidural space, analgesics will spread laterally in the horizontal plane (Fig. 5-6). Diffusion to the region of the dural cuff will allow access to the CSF through passage across the arachnoid granulations. This mechanism is important for the eventual passage of epidural opioids to receptor sites in the cord. Further diffusion laterally through the intervertebral foramen will allow analgesics to reach the paravertebral space (Fig. 5-8). Thus, epidural anesthesia/analgesia with local anesthetics is potentially produced by two mechanisms: spinal nerve root blockade (in the dural cuff region) and paravertebral neural blockade (passage through intervertebral foraminae).

BLOOD SUPPLY OF THE SPINAL CANAL

Arterial

The blood supply to the spinal cord, nerve roots, and meninges is derived from the anterior spinal artery and two posterior spinal arteries. The anterior spinal artery descends in the anterior median sulcus on the anterior surface of the spinal cord (Fig. 5-9) to terminate as an arteriole on the filum terminale. It arises from several contributing sources. In the upper cord, the anterior spinal artery is formed by fusion of the terminal branches of the vertebral arteries and anastamotic channels from branches of the vertebral, thyrocervical, and costocervical arteries. It supplies the spinal cord to the level of T4. The anterior spinal artery of the midthoracic cord is fed by intercostal arteries (from the aorta) from T4-T9. For the rest of the cord, the anterior spinal artery is fed by a single dominant vessel, the arteria radicularis magna (the artery of Adamkiewicz). The origin of the artery is quite variable but usually arises from the aorta between T9 and L2. The anterior spinal artery supplies blood to the anterior two-thirds of the spinal cord (Fig. 5-9).

The posterior spinal arteries arise from the posterior inferior cerebellar arteries and descend on the posterior surface of the cord. The posterior spinal arteries are each located just medial to their respective posterior roots (Fig. 5-9). The posterior spinal arteries supply the posterior one-third of the spinal cord.

Variations in the anatomic patterns and continuity of the anterior spinal artery

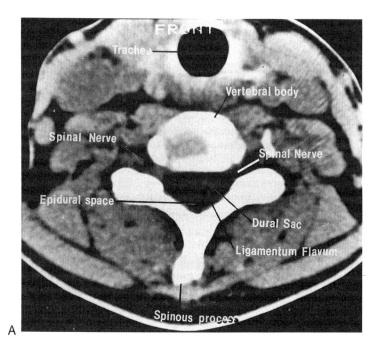

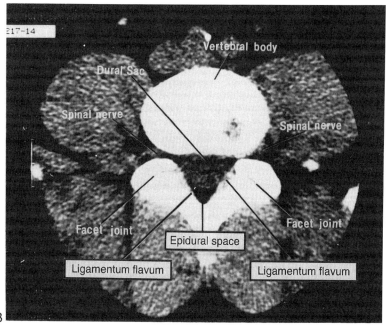

Fig. 5-7. Computed axial tomographic images at (**A**) C6-C7 and (**B**) L3-L4. Note the great increase in the cross-sectional area of the epidural space in the lumbar region. In the lower cervical region, the distance between the ligamentum flavum and the dura mater may be 2 mm or less.

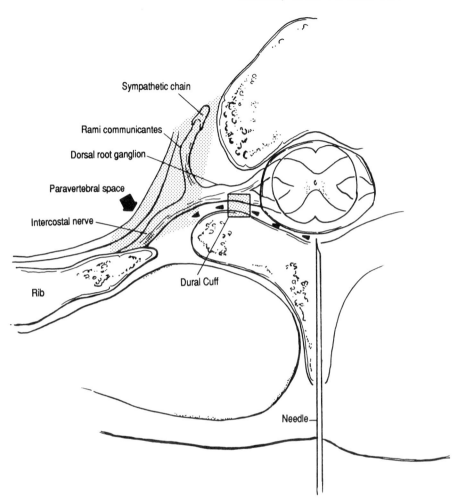

Fig. 5-8. Transverse section at level of intervertebral foramen. Local anesthetic injected into the epidural space will diffuse laterally to the dural cuff. Further diffusion laterally through the intervertebral foramen allows local anesthetic to reach the paravertebral space (triangular stippled area). Thus, epidural anesthesia can be produced by two mechanisms: spinal nerve root blockade and paravertebral neural blockade.

are clinically significant. Anastamotic blood supply often does not exist between all areas of the cord. Thus, relative areas of ischemia may exist as certain portions of the cord are limited to bloody supply from a single end artery, the artery of Adamkiewicz. Although segmental arterial supply to the cord is usually bilateral, terminal portions of the cord may be supplied by a single unilateral end artery. Interruption of flow may lead to ischemia and anterior spinal artery syndrome characterized by motor weakness with intact sensation (Fig. 5-9).

Oblique lateral entry of an epidural needle into the ligamentum flavum may cause trauma to the dural cuff region. Spinal arterial "feeder" branches enter

POSTERIOR

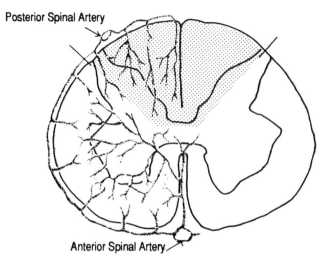

ANTERIOR

Fig. 5-9. Transverse section through the spinal cord showing the arterial blood supply. Note that the anterior spinal artery supplies the anterior two-thirds of the cord. Ischemia in the distribution of the anterior spinal artery will cause motor symptoms.

the spinal canal through the intervertebral foramen. Theoretically, it may be possible to traumatize an end artery to the anterior spinal artery during performance of epidural anesthesia/analgesia. However, the actual contribution of modern epidural techniques to the incidence of anterior spinal artery syndrome is probably minimal and remains controversial.

Venous

A complex system of epidural venous plexuses surrounds the dural sac and extends the entire length of the spinal canal. The venous plexuses drain the spinal cord, vertebral canal, and a small quantity of CSF through the arachnoid granulations. In its cephalad aspect, the epidural plexuses communicate with the cerebral venous sinuses. Blood from the cord itself drains into the azygos and hemiazygos veins. Below, the epidural plexuses drain into the inferior vena cava through the sacral and pelvic plexus veins.

Suggested Readings

Covino BG, Scott DB: Handbook of Epidural Anaesthesia and Analgesia. Grune & Stratton, Orlando, FL, 1985

Katz J, Renck H: Handbook of Thoraco-abdominal Nerve Block. Grune & Stratton, Orlando, FL, 1987

Scott DB: Techniques of Regional Anaesthesia. Appleton & Lange/Mediglobe, Norwalk, CT, 1989

6

Clinical Measurement of Pain

Robert N. Jamison

There has been a growing interest in the assessment and measurement of pain. Although pain is a subjective experience, great attention has been paid to the quantification of this experience. Initial attempts at pain measurement focused only on the fluctuation of pain intensity. It is now known that the experience of pain in humans reflects a complex system of physiologic and psychological processes resulting in endless "qualities" of pain.

Unfortunately, the measurement of pain is in its infancy, and there is no unified theoretic basis for pain measurement. In general, two main models for pain have emerged: (1) the *medical* model, in which pain represents pathology or a threat of injury, and (2) the *behavioral* model, in which pain is a perception that is influenced by cognition, behavior, and predisposing personality factors. The medical model is more traditional and relies on objective findings of pathology. The behavioral model encompasses subjective factors such as past experiences and learned behaviors. These two fundamental differences in perspective typify some of the difficulties surrounding the accurate assessment of pain.

It is important to note some of the difficulties inherent in the measurement of pain. As pain is a subjective experience, everyone has different perceptions of that experience. Idiosyncratic differences are found in how individuals quantify pain. For example, some individuals would never say that their pain was a "10" on a scale from "0 to 10," unless the pain was so severe that they would be almost unconscious from the intensity. Contrast this with other individuals reporting their pain as a constant "10," despite looking calm and relaxed. Also, all numeric scales used to measure pain have floor and ceiling effects. If patients describe their pain to be a "10" on a "0 to 10" scale, there is no way to report an increase in pain intensity.

A number of individual differences between patients make comparisons of pain measurement difficult. Patients report differences in site, duration, and pattern of pain. In addition, past experiences influence patients' present perception of pain. Demographic factors such as gender, age, and ethnic background influence the individual's perception of pain. Report of pain is influenced by medication, sleep disturbances, and affect. Also, patients who are clinically depressed and anxious tend to report increased pain intensity.

All these factors highlight the difficulties inherent in the assessment of pain in humans. Despite these limitations, a number of methods have been accepted and used to measure clinical pain. This chapter reviews some of these methods and briefly describes their benefits and limitations.

SELF-REPORT PAIN MEASURES

The most common way to quantify pain is through self-report measures. Patients may use numbers or words or mark intensity levels on a line to indicate their pain. Some scales include more than one form of measurement, although most scales are unidimensional.

The simplest way to categorize pain is to just ask patients whether they have pain (yes/no). This is certainly the easiest method, but there would be no indication of intensity. One of the first scales to categorize pain intensity was developed by Melzack and Torgerson[1] using a five-point verbal scale ranging from "mild" to "excruciating." Such scales have been criticized because they do not fully express the sensation that the individual is experiencing. Some measures have also been found to be more reliable and valid than others.

Numeric Rating Scales

Numeric rating scales are used to determine the intensity of pain. The first pain intensity ratings were developed by Budzynski et al[2] and Melzack.[3] Patients would be asked to rate their pain from "0" or "no pain" to some number representing pain as intense as it could be. Commonly, scales are "0 to 10" or "0 to 100." These scales allow for increased sensitivity of measurement. They are easy to administer and have demonstrated reliability with other measures of pain intensity.[4] Patients find these scales to be easy to use, especially if the numbers are anchored with recognizable descriptors of pain. Numeric scales can be easily given, scored, and recorded. They are readily accepted by the patient. Although different numeric scales are used, it is advisable to use an 11 point scale (0–10) or larger scale to allow for greater variability of response.

Some clinicians and investigators ask patients to rate their pain on an hourly basis during the course of their treatment. A periodic rating of pain provides information on the variability of pain over time as compared with a single global rating of pain intensity. Also, baseline ratings can be compared with subsequent ratings to determine the efficacy of treatment. Frequent pain measurement does require a level of compliance on the patient's part, which may prove to be a problem over time. Furthermore, the awareness of pain that coincides with frequent monitoring may contribute to increased anxiety, perception of lack of control, and feelings of helplessness.[5] This is especially true when pain ratings remain constant or increase in intensity.[5] Thus, frequent pain monitoring carries the potential for imprecise measurement or exaggeration of pain.[6]

Despite these criticisms, numeric pain ratings are frequently used in the clinical setting and have been shown to be valuable. They are probably the easiest method to use when treating numerous patients on a postoperative pain service.

It has been suggested that patients monitoring their pain may experience an increased sense of control over pain.[7] The act of monitoring alone may also serve as an interventional strategy to reduce pain.[8] A recent study has shown that hourly pain intensity profiles have potential clinical usefulness.[5] Patients showing no consistent trend in their pain ratings over time were found to report significantly higher levels of emotional distress. These results have been explained by suggesting that patients with particular consistency or predictability to their reports of pain also have general feelings of control. Patients demonstrating inconsistent pain patterns or a constant pain pattern that does not change over time express feelings of lack of control. It has been suggested that perception of lack of control increases anxiety. Anxiety itself can contribute to increased pain perception.

Visual Analogue Scale

The Visual Analogue Scale (VAS) uses a straight line with extremities of pain intensity on either end. The line is typically 10 cm long with one end defined as "no pain" and the other end being "excruciating, unbearable pain" (Fig. 6-1). The line can be either vertical or horizontal.[9] Patients are asked to place a mark on the line to describe the amount of pain that they are currently experiencing. The distance between the end labeled "no pain" and the mark placed by the patient is measured and rounded to the nearest centimeter.

To assist in describing the intensity of pain, words can be placed along the scale (e.g., mild, moderate, or severe). Such descriptors can help orient the patient to the degree of pain. This particular variation of the VAS has been known as a graphic rating scale.[10] Patients may tend to group their responses around the placement of the descriptors using a graphic rating scale. For this reason, graphic rating scales have become less popular.

As with other measures, careful explanation is needed by the clinician or

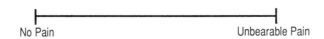

No Pain   Unbearable Pain

Fig. 6-1. Visual analogue scale used to measure pain intensity.

clinical investigator when using the VAS. Occasionally, the patient may be confused about the line, perceiving it to represent time or degree of relief rather than degree of pain intensity.

There are a number of advantages to using the VAS: (1) it has been shown to be a valid measure of pain intensity—past studies have demonstrated good correlation between the VAS and other measures of pain intensity[11]; (2) most patients find this measure easy to understand and to use—even young children (5 years old and older) are able to use this measure[12]; (3) there is an even distribution of ratings using the VAS[13]; (4) the measure is reproducible over time[9]; and (5) there is adequate sensitivity for assessment of treatment effects as compared with verbal categories of pain.[14] The VAS has been successfully used in many studies designed to determine treatment effects.

The VAS does have some disadvantages compared with other pain measures. Patients may be very random in how they place their mark. Frequently, their mark does not correspond to the mental numeric value that the patient gives to their pain. Second, the line will need to be measured to derive a value. This is time-consuming, and measurement error is possible. Third, the VAS is not easily administered to elderly patients because of problems in perceiving the line and coordinating their marks.[15] Finally, photocopying may tend to distort the line, thus affecting the measurement.[13] For these reasons, the VAS is not recommended as the best measurement for adults and the elderly but is seen as a useful measure for children.[10]

Verbal Rating Scales

Verbal rating scales are another means of assessing the varieties and intensities of pain. A verbal rating scale uses a list of words from which patients choose descriptors of their pain. Physicians have often listened for key words such as burning, stabbing, and cramping to assist in accurate diagnosis. Patients will quite commonly use multiple descriptors to convey levels of discomfort to the physician. For these reasons, verbal rating scales are readily accepted by health care professionals and patients alike.

Verbal rating scales, like numeric scales, assess pain intensity. There are a number of different verbal rating scales in the pain literature, including four-item scales,[16,17] five-item scales,[18,19] six-item scales,[3] 12-item scales,[20] and 15-item scales.[21] The words are often ranked according to severity and numbered sequentially from least intense to most intense (Fig. 6-2).

There are a number of advantages inherent in the use of verbal rating scales. They are easy to administer, simple to score, and demonstrate adequate reliability and validity. Verbal scales are highly correlated with measures of pain intensity[15] but poorly correlated with personality factors influencing pain.[22] Verbal rating scales are sensitive to change. Clinical studies have demonstrated changes in sensory and affective ratings of pain after neurosurgical procedures and/or medication regimens.[23,24]

As pain is such a personal experience, verbal ratings are better able to reflect

1. No Pain	1. None	1. No Pain
2. Mild	2. Mild	2. Mild
3. Moderate	3. Moderate	3. Discomforting
4. Severe	4. Severe	4. Distressing
	5. Very Severe	5. Horrible
		6. Excruciating

1. Not noticeable	1. None
2. Just noticeable	2. Extremely weak
3. Very weak	3. Just noticeable
4. Weak	4. Very weak
5. Mild	5. Weak
6. Moderate	6. Mild
7. Strong	7. Moderate
8. Intense	8. Uncomfortable
9. Very strong	9. Strong
10. Severe	10. Intense
11. Very intense	11. Very strong
12. Excruciating	12. Extremely intense
	13. Very intense
	14. Intolerable
	15. Excruciating

Fig. 6-2. Examples of verbal rating scales of pain intensity.

the multidimensional nature of pain. To date, verbal pain rating scales have been the most popular means of measuring pain sensation.

Unfortunately, verbal ratings also possess a number of weaknesses. Most scales are ranked according to severity. These rankings were often obtained from persons experiencing experimentally induced rather than spontaneous clinical pain. Moreover, the ranking of pain severity can be different in persons experiencing acute pain or chronic pain. To circumvent this, investigators have asked patients to rank the descriptors themselves. This is known as the *cross-modality* approach.[10] Although this helps in individualizing pain rankings, it is time-consuming. Furthermore, the cross-modality approach does not ensure equal intervals of pain intensity between descriptors (ordinal not interval data). Thus, the scale is less precise.[25]

Other problems with verbal ratings of pain include insensitivity to subtle changes in sensation and the tendency to be influenced by changes in affect. Studies have shown that sensory, affective, and evaluative pain language are correlated with anxiety.[26]

Differences in diagnosis have also been found to impact on the scoring of verbal scales. For example, patients with malignancy tend to report low levels of pain intensity and tend to endorse more affective descriptors as compared with patients with benign pain.[27] Conflicting evidence exists, however, as to how accurately verbal reports of pain correlate with medical diagnosis. Fordyce[28] and others suggested that pain language is influenced by a number of factors apart from the pathology of pain. Chronic pain patients using more than

TABLE 6-1. List of Verbal Pain Descriptors

1. Piercing	8. Stinging
2. Stabbing	9. Squeezing
3. Shooting	10. Numbing
4. Burning	11. Itching
5. Throbbing	12. Tingling
6. Cramping	13. None
7. Aching	

one word to describe their pain (e.g., burning, throbbing, aching, shooting; see Table 6-1) have been shown to experience more emotional distress and to be at greater risk for treatment failure.[29]

To date, there is no evidence to suggest that VASs are significantly more sensitive to treatment effects than verbal rating scales.[30] Both measures are acceptable for quantification of clinical pain.

The McGill Pain Questionnaire

Melzack and Torgerson[1] classified a list of words describing pain qualities into three major classes: sensory, affective, and evaluative words. From this list evolved the McGill Pain Questionnaire (MPQ). The MPQ consists of 20 subclasses of descriptors as well as a pain intensity score ranging from "0" ("no pain") to "5" ("excruciating"). The MPQ contains three types of measures: (1) pain intensity index, (2) number of words chosen, and (3) an overall pain intensity score. The MPQ has demonstrated adequate reliability and validity in measuring subjective pain.[31] A short form of the MPQ has been published.[32] The MPQ allows for measurement of different aspects of the pain experience and is sensitive to treatment effects and differential diagnosis.

There are a number of limitations in the use of the MPQ. First, the MPQ includes pain descriptors that may not be easily understood (e.g., lancinating, rasping). Thus, someone may need to be available to help define the words for the patient. Second, the three scales are highly correlated with each other. Thus, the different scores may be measuring only one dimension.[33] Finally, there has been some question about the stability and internal consistency of the subscales.[10] Despite its limitations, the MPQ has been frequently used in clinical practice over the years and has been an accepted tool in the subjective measurement of pain.

Dermatomal Pain Drawing

Pain drawings are a popular assessment tool. Patients are asked to indicate the location and distribution of their pain by shading areas of a dermatomal chart. Frequently, the chart portrays a front and back view of the human body. Other charts use oblique angles. The patient is asked to fill in areas on the chart that correspond to the location of their pain complaint. Some clinicians use colors to represent different sensations (e.g., red = pain, blue = numbness).

A number of scoring techniques have been published. Margolis and colleagues[34] divided the dermatomal chart into 45 anatomic areas (Fig. 6-3). Using a clear plastic template they were able to score each drawing by assigning a score of "1" to each area that has shading indicating the presence of pain. The areas are scored "0" if the pain shading is absent. A total score reflects the number of areas shaded. Toomey and associates[35] defined 32 regions of the body and used a similar scoring method. The use of these specific scoring systems is well documented.[34,36,37]

Other scoring techniques have been developed wherein points are assigned based on normal or abnormal distributions of the drawings. Scoring criteria include (1) unreal drawings compared with the patient's verbal description of the pain, (2) expansion or magnification of the painful area, (3) emotional overinvolvement (e.g., lengthy notes, descriptions), and (4) pain shading well removed from the primary site.

Margoles[38] found that patients with orthopaedic pain frequently drew paresthesiae that were nonanatomic. He dismissed the notion that drawings that did not follow a strict anatomic pathway represented "functional overlay." Other studies have shown a weak correlation between abnormal pain drawings and psychopathology.[39]

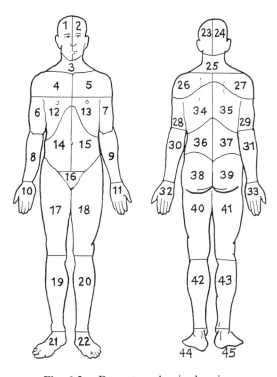

Fig. 6-3. Dermatomal pain drawing.

Pain drawings are simple, easy to use, and easy to score. They can be particularly helpful in diagnosing certain pain pathologies, as well as useful in determining the appropriateness of surgical intervention.

There are some limitations associated with the use of pain drawings: (1) patients may fabricate the drawing; (2) some patients require detailed explanations; (3) elderly patients may have difficulty in seeing and accurately drawing a description of their pain; and (4) pain drawings may be influenced by the patient's affect and the chronicity of the condition. It has been recommended that drawings should never be used to assess psychopathology but rather be incorporated as a descriptive assessment of the patient's pain.[10]

PAIN INDUCTION METHODS

Tourniquet Pain Test

The tourniquet pain test was introduced as a method to correlate clinical pain intensity with experimentally induced pain.[40] A tourniquet or pressure cuff is wrapped around the upper arm and inflated. The patient is asked to close and open the hand at a fixed rate by squeezing a hand exerciser. The patient is then instructed to indicate when the induced pain matches the clinical pain level. The patient is also asked to continue to exercise until maximum pain tolerance is reached. The measurement of clinical pain is determined by the number of seconds necessary for the patient to report that the ischemic pain and clinical pain are the same. The number of seconds that the patient takes before maximum tolerance is reached is also calculated. With these two scores, a tourniquet pain ratio can be obtained by dividing the clinical pain level by the pain tolerance score and multiplying this number by 100.

The tourniquet pain test is attractive because it gives an indication of pain intensity over time and allows for a comparison with experimentally induced pain. Some reports have attested to its adequate reliability and validity.[41] There is evidence that the tourniquet test gives a measurement of peripheral pain quite distinct from analogue measures of pain.

Some investigators have expressed reservations about the reliability, validity, and usefulness of the tourniquet test.[42] Wolff[43] reported that the technique is inferior to other methods of pain induction because of its prolonged time of administration. Furthermore, little consistency is reported among tests. Although the tourniquet pain test continues to be used, it is not considered the best choice for measurement of clinical pain intensity.

Cold Pressor Test

In this test a hand is immersed in warm water for 2 minutes and then placed in ice water. The patients are instructed to say when they initially feel "pain" and when maximum tolerance is reached. Time between the start of immersion in ice water and appreciation of pain threshold and maximum tolerance is recorded. This test has been determined to be a valid measure of pain intensity[44] but has limited use in the clinical setting.

Heat Beam Dolorimetry

This method is used for evaluation of pain tolerance. Target sites are identified, frequently on the forearm encompassing the C6–T1 dermatomes. A matte black paint is applied to the skin. When dry, a heat lamp is applied to the site, and the patient is instructed to remain still until the pain is "intolerable." Time in seconds is recorded from the onset of the beam until subject movement. Multiple measures can be taken at each site.[45,46]

This method has the advantage of being easy to administer. The use of a portable hand-held dolorimeter and timer can accurately measure response latency. Unfortunately, the test has associated affective components, such as anxiety, which influence response time. Also, some patients have developed blisters caused by prolonged burning of the tissue. For these reasons, this method is considered useful for experimental studies but has limited use in a clinical setting.

Other Pain Induction Methods

A number of other pain induction methods have been described in the literature. These include electric stimulation (electric impulses delivered to the forearm or tooth pulp[43]), chemical techniques (cutaneous and subcutaneous[47]), and pressure (pressure algometer and strain-gauge pain stimulator[48]). All these methods have the advantage of precise calibration and easy application.

It is argued that there is less interference from social, ethnic, and environmental factors with these induction methods and that they are particularly useful as part of an experimental design.[49] Unfortunately, pain induction methods have been seen as artificial and an unreliable measure of organic pain. It is difficult to determine the relationship between clinical pain, pain threshold, and tolerance as determined by induction techniques. Part of the difficulty lies in the attempt to study the process of nociception in isolation from personality and emotional/motivational factors that influence pain perception.

Furthermore, little attempt has been made to compare the sensitivity and specificity of induction methods. Quite often the technique chosen is based more on the availability of particular machinery rather than the appropriateness of technique for a particular pain problem.[50] Because of the differences in reaction thresholds and tolerances as determined by these tests, clinical trials may report disparate analgesic efficacies for a drug depending on the particular induction method. For these reasons, induction techniques should be used in conjunction with other subjective self-report measures of pain. Results should be replicated using a variety of measurement techniques.

Biochemical Analysis

Advances are being made in the correlation of endogenous opioid and other neurotransmitter levels to the perception of pain. Body fluids such as cerebrospinal fluid, blood plasma, urine, or saliva can be biochemically analyzed for the presence of specific neurotransmitters. There is evidence that external cutaneous stimulation such as acupuncture and transcutaneous electrical nerve stimulation (TENS) can increase endogenous opioid levels in the body.[51] Naloxone has been found to increase the report of pain in patients already experiencing discomfort.

This area of investigation holds much promise in the future. However, the present level of sophistication of measurement of neurotransmitters and the precision of correlation to the experience we describe as "pain" is less than perfect. This is due in part to the complexity of neuropeptide chemistry in the body.[52] One particular area of interest is substance P. It is now recognized that an important relationship exists between levels of substance P and the perception of pain.

Unfortunately, it is difficult to obtain and store body fluids for measurement in most clinical settings. Moreover, the particular methods of storage and analysis greatly influence the results. Controversy exists in the literature as to which body fluids should be obtained. Although studies in this area are relatively new, they may revolutionize the future measurement of pain.

BEHAVIORAL OBSERVATIONS

In experimental pain, a controlled stimulus is applied and a measurement is taken of the patient's reaction to that stimulus. However, as pain is such a subjective personal experience, it is difficult to measure the patient's affective response. Apart from what patients say, often the only other way to understand what they are experiencing is to watch their actions. Some patients appear stoic. Others tend to overdramatize and show negative pain behaviors such as demanding pain medication, refusing to be physically active, presenting excessive emotional distress, and avoiding work or home duties. In clinical practice, behavioral observation of pain behaviors is very important. The concept of pain behavior was first introduced by Fordyce.[28] Fordyce distinguished between behaviors that are functional during acute pain but can quickly become dysfunctional as the pain persists.

Most physicians and health professionals are taught to be aware of inconsistent or exaggerated pain behaviors during the physical examination. Typically, patients demonstrating behaviors such as excessive verbal complaints of pain, demand for opioids, and emotionality are judged to be poor risks for invasive procedures. Although physicians and other professionals freely discuss the concept of pain behavior, little attention is paid to its systematic assessment. More often than not, this assessment is determined through clinical judgment.

The daily activity diary as developed by Fordyce[28] was one of the first efforts to measure pain behavior. The daily activity diary includes hourly records of patient medication intake and time spent either sitting, reclining, or standing/walking.

The first systematic research of pain behavior patterns was conducted by Keefe and Block.[53] Using a standardized examination, patients could be rated on the following pain behaviors: guarding, bracing, rubbing, grimacing, and sighing. Patients were asked to sit, stand, walk, and recline while being video-taped. Trained raters scored each patient on the five behavioral categories during each of the observed activities. The reliability and validity of their observer rating system was very high.[54] Other investigators have examined additional behaviors including shifting of body positions, making sounds, and verbalizing physical limitations.[55]

The scoring system of Keefe and Block was developed for observation of chronic pain patients. Its applicability for acute pain is limited as patients would be expected to quite naturally demonstrate some rubbing, grimacing, and sighing behaviors. Such pain behaviors would not represent maladaptive functioning. Another limitation of this system is the time inherent in monitoring and scoring the observations.

Patient-controlled analgesia (PCA) can be a useful source of information about patient pain behavior. Patients can self-administer a preset dose of intravenous opioid by pushing a button. Most PCA infusers store information on the number of doses successfully administered and the number of attempts. The clinician can calculate a "demand ratio" for each patient by simply dividing the number of attempts by the number of successful deliveries of opioid. A low ratio (i.e., one successful delivery for each attempt) implies that the patient did not anticipate the lockout interval. A high ratio suggests that the patient made many more attempts at receiving a dose of opioid than was allotted. Although this is a crude measure, patients with high demand ratios tend to be anxious and less satisfied with their pain control. Controlled studies are needed to further investigate the usefulness of this indicator of pain behavior.

FUTURE CONSIDERATIONS

Traditionally, pain assessment consisted of self-reported pain intensity using crude and divergent methods. Until recently, little effort had been made to acknowledge a theoretic basis for pain and to use both reliable and valid instruments.

Pain measurement is complex, and determination of pain pathology is as much an art as a science. It is important to resist thinking of pain as a dichotomy between the organic and the psychogenic. An interaction clearly exists between the biologic qualities of pain and the psychosocial characteristics of the patient. The clinician needs to be sensitive to each patient's perception of their own painful experience.

Future studies are needed to acquire more sensitive self-report, biochemical, and behavioral measures for assessing clinical pain. Attempts to refine measurement instruments suitable for specific pain conditions should be encouraged. For instance, the assessment of pediatric pain has been given all too little attention. Attempts to identify ways in which psychological status influences pain should also continue. Ultimately, these continued efforts will succeed in bridging the gap between the physical and psychological measurements of the pain experience.

References

1. Melzack R, Torgerson WS: On the language of pain. Anesthesiology 34:50, 1971
2. Budzynski T, Stoyva J, Adler LS, Mullancy DJ: EMG biofeedback and tension headaches: a controlled outcome study. Psychosom Med 35:484, 1973
3. Melzack R: The McGill Pain Questionnaire: major properties and scoring methods. Pain 1:277, 1975
4. Kerns RD, Finn P, Haythornwaite J: Self-monitored pain intensity: psychometric properties and clinical utility. J Behav Med 11:71, 1988
5. Jamison RN, Brown GK: Validation of hourly pain intensity profiles with chronic pain patients. Pain 45:123, 1991
6. Blanchard EB, Andrasik F: Management of Chronic Headaches: A Psychological Approach. Pergamon Press, New York, 1985
7. Barlow OH: Anxiety and Its Disorder: The Nature and Treatment of Anxiety and Panic. Gilford Press, New York, 1988
8. Haynes SN: Principles of Behavioral Assessment. Gardner Press, New York, 1978
9. Scott J, Huskisson EC: Accuracy of subjective measurements made with or without previous scores: an important source of error in serial measurements of subjective states. Ann Rheum Dis 38:558, 1979
10. Karoly P, Jenson MP: Multimethod Assessment of Chronic Pain. Pergamon Press, New York, 1987
11. Downie WW, Leatham PA, Rhind VM et al: Studies with pain rating scales. Ann Rheum Dis 37:378, 1978
12. Scott J, Ansell BM, Huskisson EC: The measurement of pain in juvenile chronic polyarthritis. Ann Rheum Dis 36:186, 1977
13. Huskisson EC: Visual analogue scales. p. 33. In Melzack R (ed): Pain Measurement and Assessment. Raven Press, New York, 1983
14. Turner JA: Comparison of group progressive-relaxation training and cognitive-behavioral group therapy for chronic low back pain. J Consult Clin Psychol 50:757, 1982
15. Jensen MP, Karoly P, Braver S: The measurement of clinical pain intensity: a comparison of six methods. Pain 27:117, 1986
16. Seymour RA: The use of pain scales in assessing the efficacy of analysis in postoperative dental pain. Eur J Clin Pharmacol 23:441, 1982
17. Joyce CRB, Zutshi DW, Hrubes V, Mason RM: Comparison of fixed interval and visual analogue scales for rating chronic pain. Eur J Clin Phrmacol 8:415, 1975
18. Frank AJM, Moll JMH, Hort JF: A comparison of three ways for measuring pain. Rheumatol Rehabil 21:211, 1982
19. Kremer E, Atkinson JH, Ingnelzi RJ: Measurement of pain: patient preference does not confound pain measurement. Pain 10:241, 1981
20. Tursky B, Jamner LD, Friedman R: The pain perception profile: a psychological approach to the assessment of pain report. Behav Ther 13:376, 1982
21. Gracely RH, McGrath P, Dubner R: Ratio scales of sensory and effective verbal pain descriptors. Pain 5:5, 1978

22. Rybstein-Blinchik E: Effects of different cognitive strategies on chronic pain experience. J Behav Med 2:93, 1979
23. Eggebrecht DB, Bautz MT, Brenig MID et al: Psychometric evaluation. p. 71. In Comic PM, Brown FD (eds): Assessing Chronic Pain: A Multidisciplinary Clinic Handbook. Springer-Verlag, New York, 1989
24. Gracely RH, McGrath P, Dubner R: Validity and sensitivity of ratio scales of sensory and affective verbal pain descriptors: manipulation of affect by diazepam. Pain 5: 19, 1978
25. Ahles TA, Ruckdeschel JC, Blondard EB: Cancer-related pain: II. Assessment with visual analogue scales. J Psychosom Res 28:121, 1984
26. VanBaren J, Klenknecht RA: An evaluation of the McGill Pain Questionnaire for use in dental pain assessment. Pain 6:23, 1979
27. Kremer EF, Atkinson JH Jr, Ingnelzi RJ: Pain measurement: the affective dimensional measure of the McGill Pain Questionnaire with a cancer pain population. Pain 12:153, 1982
28. Fordyce W: Behavioral Methods for Chronic Pain and Illness. CV Mosby, St. Louis, 1976
29. Jamison RN, Vasterling JJ, Parris WCV: Use of sensory descriptors in assessing chronic pain patients. J Psychosom Res 31:647, 1987
30. Ohnhaus EE, Adler R: Methodological problems in the measurement of pain: a comparison between the verbal rating scale and the visual analogue scale. Pain 1: 379, 1975
31. Reading AE: The McGill Pain Questionnaire: an appraisal. p. 55. In Melzack R (ed): Pain Measurement and Assessment. Raven Press, New York, 1983
32. McCreary C: Pain description and personality disturbance. p. 137. In Melzack R (ed): Pain Measurement and Assessment. Raven Press, New York, 1983
33. Turk DC, Rudy TE, Salovey P: The McGill Pain Questionnaire reconsidered: confirming the factor structure and examining appropriate uses. Pain 21:385, 1985
34. Margolis RB, Tait RC, Krause SJ: A rating system for use with patient pain drawings. Pain 24:57, 1986
35. Toomey TC, Gover VF, Jones BN: Spatial distribution of pain: a descriptive characteristic of chronic pain. Pain 17:289, 1983
36. Feller I, Jones CA: Nursing the Burned Patient. Araum-Bromfield, Ann Arbor, MI, 1965
37. Ransford AO, Cairns DC, Mooney V: The pain drawing as an aid to the psychologic evaluation of patients with low-back pain. Spine 1:127, 1976
38. Margoles MS: The pain chart: spatial properties of pain. p. 215. In Melzack R (ed): Pain Measurement and Assessment. Raven Press, New York, 1983
39. Schwartz DP, DeGood DE: Global appropriateness of pain drawings: blind ratings predict patterns of psychological distress and litigation status. Pain 19:383, 1984
40. Smith GM, Lowenstein E, Hubbard HJ, Beecher HK: Experimental pain produced by the submaximum effort tourniquet technique: further evidence of validity. J Pharmacol Exp Ther 163:468, 1968
41. Sternbach RA: The tourniquet pain test. p. 27. In Melzack R (ed): Pain Measurement and Assessment. Raven Press, New York, 1983
42. von Graffenried B, Adler R, Abt K et al: The influence of anxiety and pain sensitivity on experimental pain in man. Pain 4:253, 1978
43. Wolff BB: Behavioral measurement of human pain. p. 121. In Sternbach RA (ed): The Psychology of Pain. 2nd Ed. Raven Press, New York, 1986
44. Wolff BB, Kontor TG, Cohen P: In Bonica JJ, Fessard DA (eds): Advances in Pain Research and Therapy. Vol 1. Raven Press, New York, 1976

45. Lipman JJ, Blumenkopf B, Parris WCV: Chronic pain assessment using heat beam dolorimetry. Pain 30:59, 1987
46. Lipman JJ, Blumenkopf B: Comparison of subjective and objective analgesic effects of intravenous and intrathecal morphine in chronic pain patients by heat beam dolorimetry. Pain 39:249, 1989
47. Keele A, Armstrong D: Substances Producing Pain and Itch. Edward Arnold, London, 1964
48. Forgione AG, Barber TX: A strain gauge pain stimulator. Psychophysiology 8:102, 1971
49. Smith GK, Covino GC: Acute Pain. Butterworth, Boston, 1985
50. Rollman GB: Measurement of experimental pain in chronic pain patients: methodological and individual factors. p. 251. In Melzack R (ed): Pain Measurement and Assessment. Raven Press, New York, 1983
51. Akil H, Richardson DE, Hughes J, Barchas JD: Enkephalin-like material elevated in ventricular cerebrospinal fluid of pain patients after analgetic focal stimulation. Science 201:463, 1978
52. Akil H, Watson SJ, Young E et al: Endogenous opioids: biology and function. Annu Rev Neurosci 7:223, 1984
53. Keefe FJ, Block AR: Development of an observation method for assessing pain behavior in chronic low back pain patients. Behav Ther 13:363, 1982
54. Keefe FJ, Crisson JE, Trainor M: Observational methods for assessing pain: a practical guide. p. 67. In Blumenthal JA, McKee DC (eds): Application in Behavioral Medicine and Health Psychology: A Clinician's Source Book. Professional Resource Exchange Inc., Sarasota, FL, 1987
55. Follick MJ, Ahern DK, Aberger EW: Development of an audiovisual taxonomy of pain behavior: reliability and discriminant validity. Health Psychol 4:555, 1985

7

Nonsteroidal Anti-inflammatory Drugs

F. Michael Ferrante

Recent pharmacologic research has focused on analgesics that decrease the sensitivity of peripheral nociceptors (desensitization).[1] Prostaglandins are generated by tissue trauma and mediate nociception by sensitization of peripheral nociceptors in synergy with other chemical mediators (e.g., histamine, bradykinin, serotonin).[1] Inhibition of cyclooxygenase (Fig. 7-1) reduces tissue levels of prostaglandins, thereby reducing or abolishing this synergy and decreasing pain.

Oral nonsteroidal anti-inflammatory drugs (NSAIDs) have long been used in medicine for their anti-inflammatory, antipyretic, and analgesic properties. Widespread use of these medications as analgesics for the treatment of postoperative pain, however, has been limited by lack of a potent parenteral preparation. Ketorolac tromethamine now provides practitioners with an adjunctive analgesic of a potency similar to opioids.

This chapter looks at the pharmacology of NSAIDs in general and the history of their use as postoperative analgesics and briefly discusses the pharmacology of ketorolac tromethamine.

MECHANISM OF ACTION

NSAIDs block the synthesis of prostaglandins by inhibition of the enzyme cyclooxygenase.[2] Cyclooxygenase (prostaglandin synthetase) catalyzes the conversion of arachidonic acid to the cyclic endoperoxide precursors of prostaglandins (Fig. 7-1).[3] Prostaglandins mediate several components of the inflam-

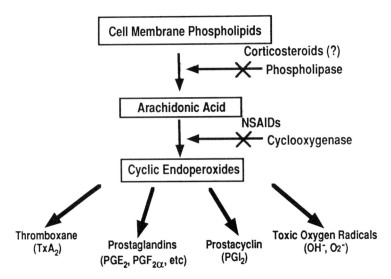

Fig. 7-1. Metabolism of arachidonic acid via the cyclooxygenase pathway. The prostanoids (thromboxanes, prostaglandins and prostacyclins) are the active metabolites of the cyclooxygenase pathway. Arachidonic acid may also be metabolized via lipoxygenase (pathway not shown) to form the eicosanoids (the leukotrienes and 5-hydroxyeicosatetraenoic acid).

matory response including fever, pain, and vasodilation.[3,4] However, NSAIDs also have prostaglandin-independent effects[5] (e.g., inhibition of neutrophil migration and lymphocyte responsiveness), which contribute to their salutary anti-inflammatory and analgesic properties.

PHARMACOLOGY

Practically all the NSAIDs in use in the United States are derivatives of carboxylic acid and can be subdivided on the basis of chemical structure into salicylic acids, acetic acids, propionic acids, and anthranilic acids (Table 7-1).[6]

The NSAIDs are rapidly absorbed from the gastrointestinal tract after ingestion.[6] Most NSAIDs are metabolized in the liver, and inactive metabolites are excreted in the urine.[6] Sulindac and salicyl salicylate, however, are inactive prodrugs that must be converted to active metabolites by the liver.[7,8] The NSAIDs are highly protein-bound after entrance into the bloodstream (>90 percent).[6]

The half-lives and recommended oral anti-inflammatory dosage ranges for NSAIDs available in the United States are listed in Table 7-1. It must be remembered that NSAIDs differ in potency with respect to their analgesic, anti-inflam-

TABLE 7-1. NSAIDs Currently Available in the United States

Drug	Dosage Range (PO) (mg/day)	T ½ Hours	Doses per Day
CARBOXYLIC ACIDS			
Salicylic acids			
Acetylsalicylic acid (aspirin)	1,000–6,000	4–15	2–4
Nonacetylated salicylates			
Choline magnesium trisalicylate (Trilisate)	1,500–4,000	4–15	2–4
Salicyl salicylate (Disalcid)	1,500–5,000	4–15	2–4
Diflunisal (Dolobid)	500–1,500	7–15	2
Acetic acids			
Indoles			
Indomethacin (Indocin)	50–200	3–11	2–4
Sulindac (Clinoril)	300–400	16	2
Pyrolle acetic acids			
Tolmetin (Tolectin)	600–2,000	1–2	3–6
Ketorolac (Toradol)	75–150 (IM or IV)	3–8	4
	40 (PO)	3–8	4
Phenyl acetic acids			
Diclofenac (Voltaren)	100–200	2	2–4
Propionic acids			
Phenylpropionic acids			
Ibuprofen (Motrin)	1,200–3,200	2	3–6
Fenoprofen (Nalfon)	1,200–3,200	2	3–4
Flurbiprofen (Ansaid)	200–300	3–4	2–3
Ketoprofen (Orudis)	100–400	2	3–4
Naphthylpropionic acids			
Naproxen (Naprosyn, Anaprox)	250–1,500	13	2
Anthranilic acids			
Fenamates			
Meclofenamate (Meclomen)	200–400	2–3	4
PYRAZOLES			
Phenylbutazone (Butazolidin)	200–800	40–80	1–4
OXICAMS			
Piroxicam (Feldene)	20	30–86	1

matory, and antipyretic properties.[9,10] For instance, ketorolac only elicits anti-inflammatory activity at doses higher than those producing analgesia.[9,10] Ketorolac is not indicated for rheumatic conditions.

Patients receiving oral NSAIDs exhibit marked variability in clinical response to a particular drug despite similar clinical conditions and uniform serum levels.[6,8] It is uncertain as to whether this phenomenon is caused by individual variations in drug handling or is specific to unrecognized differences in inflammatory responses among patients.[6] Thus, when using oral NSAIDs in general medical practice, it is important to sequentially try several agents until an adequate response is achieved.[11] No data exist as to the variability of clinical response when NSAIDs are used for postoperative analgesia.

ADVERSE EFFECTS

The three major problems associated with NSAID therapy are *gastropathy, impaired hemostasis,* and *nephrotoxicity.* All are directly related to inhibition of prostaglandin synthesis. As a group, the nonacetylated salicylates (Table 7-1) are less likely to cause these side effects than other NSAIDs.[12-17] In addition to the aforementioned side effects, NSAIDs can cause idiosyncratic central nervous system (CNS), dermatologic, hepatic, musculoskeletal, pulmonary, or systemic reactions[18-21] (Table 7-2).

Gastropathy

A variety of prostaglandins, including PGE_1, PGE_2, and prostacylcin (PGI_2), have been shown to participate in gastric mucosal cytoprotection. These autocoids (locally produced hormones) elicit a variety of protective actions: increased gastric bicarbonate secretion, blood flow, and mucus production and a reduction in gastric acid secretion.[22,23]

Suppression of prostaglandin synthesis by NSAIDs leads to decreased mucosal cytoprotection, increased gastric acid secretion, and eventually, gastric ulcerations. Symptoms of NSAID gastropathy[22,23] include dyspepsia, epigastric pain, anorexia, esophagitis, constipation, and diarrhea. A history of peptic ulcer disease and/or gastric bleeding, use of alcohol, increasing age, and high doses of NSAIDs have been identified as risk factors for the development of NSAID gastropathy.

The question of prophylaxis for NSAID-induced peptic ulceration is complex.[24,25] Histamine-H_2-antagonists reduce the incidence of gastroscopically

TABLE 7-2. Idiosyncratic Reactions to NSAID Therapy

Idiosyncratic Reaction	Manifestation	Major Implicated Agents
Bone marrow toxicity	Aplastic anemia, leukopenia, red cell aplasia	Phenylbutazone
CNS symptoms	Headaches, dizziness, mood alterations, light-headedness, blurred vision	Indomethacin
Aseptic meningitis	Headache, stiff neck, fever, photophobia	Ibuprofen, sulindac, tolmetin
Dermatologic reactions	Minor rashes to exfoliative dermatitis or toxic epidermal necrolysis	Most NSAIDs
Asymptomatic transaminasemia	No clinical signs or symptoms except elevated laboratory values	Most NSAIDs
Hepatitis	Variable mechanisms and manifestations	Sulindac, phenylbutazone, diclofenac
Bilateral pulmonary infiltrates	Dyspnea, nonproductive cough	Naproxen
Exacerbation of bronchospasm	Seen in triad of asthma, nasal polyposis, aspirin hypersensitivity	Any NSAID

verified NSAID-associated duodenal ulcers.[26] Omeprazole reduces the incidence of gastric ulcers.[27] Misoprostol (a prostaglandin analogue) inhibits both gastric and duodenal ulceration.[28–30] If prophylaxis of NSAID-associated ulceration is to be cost-effective, it should decrease the incidence of serious complications such as perforation and bleeding. At the present time, it is uncertain as to whether prophylaxis actually decreases the incidence of such complications. The optimal duration of concomitant antiulcer medication with NSAID administration is also unknown. Some studies suggest that adaptation to the antiulcer medication may occur. This would negate any benefits to be derived from long-term administration.[24,31]

Hemostatic Defects

The effects of NSAIDs on hemostasis depend on the balance between the inhibition of thromboxane A_2 (TxA_2) synthesis within platelets and inhibition of PGI_2 synthesis within endothelial cells.[2] TxA_2 is the major arachidonic acid derivative of platelets. It is a potent vasoconstrictor and stimulates the platelet-release reaction and platelet aggregation, thereby promoting clotting. PGI_2 is the major arachidonic acid derivative of the vascular endothelium. It is a potent vasodilator and inhibits platelet aggregation, thereby promoting bleeding. As NSAIDs will inhibit synthesis of both prostaglandins, the net balance determines the tendency to bleeding or clotting.[2]

With respect to NSAID therapy itself, aspirin *irreversibly* inhibits platelet cyclooxygenase.[32] Thus, the bleeding time is prolonged for 6–10 days (the lifetime of the platelet). The bleeding time will not return to normal until new platelets have been produced. In comparison, all other NSAIDs *reversibly* inhibit platelet cyclooxygenase.[33] Thus, normal hemostasis will be restored after five half-lives, the time required to clear all drugs from the body. Therefore, longer-acting NSAIDs possess a relative disadvantage in patients at risk for bleeding (Table 7-1).

All NSAIDs displace coumadin and other drugs from plasma protein binding sites, increasing the concentration of free drug in the plasma. Thus, NSAIDs must be used carefully in patients on concurrent oral anticoagulant therapy.

Nephrotoxicity

In the healthy patient, renal blood flow and glomerular filtration are not prostaglandin-dependent. This is not true, however, in patients who are volume-depleted or have congestive heart failure or hepatic cirrhosis. These conditions are associated with activation of the renin-angiotensin system and sympathetic nervous system. Besides being vasoconstrictors, both angiotensin II and norepinephrine promote local renal secretion of vasodilator prostaglandins that minimize renal ischemia. Inhibition of prostaglandin synthesis by NSAIDs in the aforementioned disease states could lead to decreased renal perfusion and glomerular filtration.[16,17]

Prostaglandins also inhibit tubular reabsorption of sodium and water, as well as renin secretion from the juxtaglomerular apparatus. In the presence of volume depletion, congestive heart failure, or hepatic cirrhosis, NSAIDs can lead to fluid retention, impaired responsiveness to diuretic therapy, and hyperkalemia.[16,17]

Idiosyncratic Reactions

The gastropathy, hemostatic defects, and nephrotoxicity induced by NSAIDs are all mediated by inhibition of prostaglandin synthesis. NSAIDs can also have idiosyncratic side effects that are not prostaglandin-mediated.[18-21] Such idiosyncratic reactions are rare but can be serious. They are reviewed in Table 7-2.

NSAIDS FOR POSTOPERATIVE PAIN MANAGEMENT

As parenteral opioid therapy for postoperative analgesia can often produce the undesirable side effects of cardiovascular, respiratory, and CNS depression, there has been much recent interest in NSAIDs as alternative or adjunctive analgesics. Until the appearance of ketorolac tromethamine, the lack of a potent parenteral preparation has limited the usefulness of NSAIDs in the United States. Until recently, most research on the use of parenteral NSAIDs as postoperative analgesics has come from the British and European literatures.[34-42]

Indomethacin rectal suppositories have been shown to provide good adjunctive analgesia after abdominal surgery and a morphine-"sparing" effect in doses higher than recommended for their oral anti-inflammatory effect.[34,35] The suppositories can be administered during the postoperative period without the need for preoperative loading.[35] A higher incidence of perioperative bleeding has been associated with use of indomethacin suppositories.[34,35]

With respect to injectable preparations, lysine acetyl salicylate has been available in Europe for some time. However, there is no consensus of opinion as to its efficacy in the treatment of severe pain.[36-40]

Intramuscular diclofenac, on the other hand, has been shown to be uniformly effective and to possess morphine-"sparing" properties.[41,42] In contrast to indomethacin, diclofenac has been shown to have no effect on perioperative blood loss (at least after transurethral prostatectomy).[43] Unfortunately, the parenteral use of diclofenac has not been sufficiently studied to advocate its widespread clinical use.

Ketorolac Tromethamine (Toradol)

Ketorolac tromethamine is a member of the pyrolle acetic acid group of NSAIDs (Fig. 7-2). Ketorolac was recently introduced into the United States as a short-term parenteral analgesic.[44] Ketorolac possesses many desirable fea-

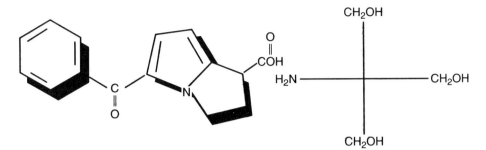

Fig. 7-2. Ketorolac tromethamine (Toradol) is a member of the pyrolle acetic acid group of NSAIDs. Ketorolac is the first NSAID available for parenteral administration in the United States.

tures as an adjunctive or alternative medication to the opioids: high analgesic potency,[45-48] suitability for parenteral administration,[45-47] rapid onset of action,[45-47] prolonged analgesic duration,[45-48] lack of irritation at injection site, paucity of side effects associated with opioids[40-50] or NSAIDs,[44,51-54] and lack of addictive potential.[55]

After intramuscular injection of ketorolac, analgesia is perceptible at about 10 minutes (similar for opioids) with a mean peak plasma concentration (C_{max}) of 2.2–3.0 µg/ml occurring within 40–60 minutes (T_{max}).[56,57] Duration of analgesia is approximately 6 hours.[45-47] Similar to other NSAIDs, ketorolac is highly bound to plasma proteins[56] and is metabolized to inactive products, which are excreted in the urine.[57] Clearance is significantly reduced in the elderly (aged 65 years or older)[58] and in patients with renal disease.[59]

Ketorolac has analgesic potency similar to opioids[45-47,60] (2 mg IM ketorolac is approximately equal to 1 mg IM morphine[45-49]; 1 mg IM ketorolac is approximately equal to 3–5 mg IM meperidine[60]). As ketorolac has a terminal plasma half-life of 5–6 hours, it should be given every 6 hours to maintain a steady-state plasma level. A loading dose of 60 mg IM should be followed by 30 mg IM every 6 hours. In patients weighing less than 60 kg or older than 65 years of age or with reduced renal function, a loading dose of 30 mg IM should be followed by 15 mg IM every 6 hours. No dosage adjustment is indicated in patients with chronic cirrhosis.[61] The pharmacokinetics of ketorolac in patients with other liver disorders is unknown.

When postoperative pain is severe, ketorolac alone may be insufficient to provide adequate analgesia.[46] Thus, ketorolac may serve an adjunctive role as an analgesic; the need for opioids may not be totally eliminated.

Unlike opioids, ketorolac does not produce respiratory depression,[48,49] reduction of gastrointestinal motility,[49] psychomotor effects,[50] or addiction.[55] However, like other NSAIDs, gastrointestinal, hematologic, and nephrotoxic side effects are possible.

Gastrointestinal Effects

In patients receiving oral doses of ketorolac of up to 120 g/day, the incidence of bleeding peptic ulceration was 0.3 percent in 6,400 patients.[44] Most incidents of bleeding occurred between 38 and 248 days of long-term oral use. With short-term use for postoperative analgesia, the incidence should be further reduced.

Hemostatic Defects

Ketorolac produces an increase in bleeding time, but this appears to have little significance in patients with normal hemostatic function.[51] There appears to be no interaction between ketorolac and the administration of low-dose heparin.[51] Ketorolac, like all NSAIDs, is highly protein-bound, and displacement of other bound agents is possible (coumadin). Despite the increase in bleeding time, ketorolac is not associated with increased perioperative bleeding.[62]

Nephrotoxicity

Ketorolac itself appears to have little nephrotoxic potential in patients with renal failure. However, in disease states in which activation of the renin-angiotensin system occurs, prostaglandins are important in the maintenance of renal blood flow. In these conditions, ketorolac, as well as all NSAIDs, should be used cautiously.

CONCLUSION

Ketorolac now adds a potent, new, nonopioid analgesic to the armamentarium of agents for the treatment of postoperative pain. With its appearance, we may expect further developments in NSAID chemistry as the search for alternative or adjunctive analgesics to the opioids continues.

References

1. Lim RKS, Guzman F, Rodgers DW et al: Site of action of narcotic and non-narcotic analgesics determined by blocking bradykinin-evoked visceral pain. Arch Int Pharmacodyn Ther 152:22, 1964
2. Vane JR: Inhibition of prostaglandin synthesis as a mechanism of action for the aspirin-like drugs. Nature New Biol 231:232, 1971
3. Moncada S, Vane JR: Arachidonic acid metabolites and the interactions between platelets and blood-vessel walls. N Engl J Med 300:1142, 1979
4. Trang LE: Prostaglandins and inflammation. Semin Arthritis Rheum 9:153, 1980
5. Abramson SB, Weissmann G: The mechanisms of action of nonsteroidal anti-inflammatory drugs. Arthritis Rheum 32:1, 1989
6. Brooks PM, Day RO: Nonsteroidal antiinflammatory drugs—differences and similarities. N Engl J Med 324:1716, 1991
7. Simon LS, Mills JA: Nonsteroidal antiinflammatory drugs (Frist of two parts). N Engl J Med 302:1179, 1980

8. Simon LS, Mills JA: Nonsteroidal antiinflammatory drugs (Second of two parts). N Engl J Med 302:1237, 1980

9. Rooks WH II, Maloney PJ, Shott LD et al: The analgesic and anti-inflammatory profile of ketorolac and its tromethamine salt. Drugs Exp Clin Res 11:479, 1985

10. Rooks WH II, Tomolonis AJ, Maloney PJ et al: The analgesic and anti-inflammatory profile of ($\pm$) -5-benzoyl-1,2-dihydro-3H pyrrolo [1,2a] pyrrole-1-carboxylic acid (RS-37619). Agents Actions 12:684, 1982

11. Champion GD: Therapeutic usage of non-steroidal anti-inflammatory drugs. Med J Aust 149:203, 1988

12. Kilander A, Dotevall G: Endoscopic evaluation of the comparative effects of acetylsalicylic acid and choline magnesium trisalicylate on human gastric and duodenal mucosa. Br J Rheumatol 22:36, 1983

13. Cohen A, Garber HE: Comparison of choline magnesium trisalicylate and acetylsalicylic acid in relation to fecal blood loss. Curr Ther Res 28:187, 1978

14. Huskisson EC: Antiinflammatory drugs. Semin Arthritis Rheum 7:1, 1977

15. Abramson S, Korchak H, Ludewig R et al: Modes of action of aspirin-like drugs. Proc Natl Acad Sci USA 82:7227, 1985

16. Clive DM, Stoff JS: Renal syndromes associated with nonsteroidal antiinflammatory drugs. N Engl J Med 310:563, 1984

17. Patrono C, Dunn MJ: The clinical significance of inhibition of renal prostaglandin synthesis. Kidney Int 32:1, 1987

18. O'Brien WM, Bagby GF: Rare adverse reactions to nonsteroidal antiinflammatory drugs. (1). J Rheumatol 12:13, 1985

19. O'Brien WM, Bagby GF: Rare adverse reactions to nonsteroidal antiinflammatory drugs. (2). J Rheumatol 12:347, 1985

20. O'Brien WM, Bagby GF: Rare adverse reactions to nonsteroidal antiinflammatory drugs. (3). J Rheumatol 12:562, 1985

21. O'Brien WM, Bagby GF: Rare adverse reactions to nonsteroidal antiinflammatory drugs. (4). J Rheumatol 12:785, 1985

22. Semble EL, Wu WC: Antiinflammatory drugs and gastric mucosal damage. Sem Arthritis Rheum 16:271, 1987

23. Roth SH, Bennett RE: Non-steroidal anti-inflammatory drug gastropathy: recognition and response. Arch Intern Med 147:2093, 1987

24. Hawkey CJ: Non-steroidal anti-inflammatory drugs and peptic ulcers. Br Med J 300:278, 1990

25. Soll AH: Pathogenesis of peptic ulcer and implications for therapy. N Engl J Med 322:909, 1990

26. Langman MJS: Treating ulcers in patients receiving anti-arthritic drugs (editorial). Q J Med 73:1089, 1989

27. Walan A, Bader JP, Classen M et al: Effect of omeprazole and ranitidine on ulcer healing and relapse rates in patients with benign gastric ulcer. N Engl J Med 320:69, 1989

28. Roth S, Agrawal N, Mahowald M et al: Misoprostol heals gastroduodenal injury in patients with rheumatoid arthritis receiving aspirin. Arch Intern Med 149:775, 1989

29. Graham DY, Agrawal N, Roth SH: Prevention of NSAID-induced gastric ulcer with misoprostol: multicentre, double-blind, placebo-controlled trial. Lancet ii:1277, 1988

30. Agrawal NM, Roth S, Graham DY et al: Misoprostol compared with sucralfate in the prevention of nonsteroidal anti-inflammatory drug-induced gastric ulcer. A randomized, controlled trial. Ann Intern Med 115:195, 1991

31. Carson JL, Strom BL, Soper KA et al: The association of nonsteroidal anti-inflammatory drugs with upper gastrointestinal tract bleeding. Arch Intern Med 147:85, 1987

32. Burch JW, Stanford N, Majerus PW: Inhibition of platelet prostaglandin synthetase by oral aspirin. J Clin Invest 61:314, 1978

33. Ali M, McDonald JWD: Reversible and irreversible inhibition of platelet cyclooxygenase and serotinin release by nonsteroidal antiinflammatory drugs. Thromb Res 13:1057, 1978

34. Reasbeck PG, Rice ML, Reasbeck JC: Double-blind controlled trial of indomethacin as an adjunct to narcotic analgesia after major abdominal surgery. Lancet ii:115, 1982

35. Engel C, Lund B, Kirstensen SS et al: Indomethacin as an analgesic after hysterectomy. Acta Anaesthesiol Scand 33:498, 1989

36. Doutre M, Périssat M, Hiriogoyen M et al: Utilisation de l'E.B.49G (acétyl salicylate de lysine) par voie intraveineuse et intramusculaire en analgésie post-operatoire. Bord Med 12:3081, 1970

37. Nicolas F, Jeanniard Du Dot X: Utilisation des propriétés analgésiques de l'acetyl-salicylate de lysine dans la période post-operatoire. L'Ouest Med 25:1191, 1972

38. Kweekel-de Vries WJ, Spierdijk J, Mattie H, Hermans JMH: A new soluble acetyl-salicylic acid derivative in the treatment of postoperative pain. Br J Anaesth 46:133, 1974

39. McAteer E, Dundee JW: Injectable aspirin as a postoperative analgesic. Br J Anaesth 53:1069, 1981

40. Cashman JN, Jones RM, Foster JMG, Adams AP: Comparison of infusions of morphine and lysine acetyl salicylate for the relief of pain after surgery. Br J Anaesth 57:255, 1985

41. Hodsman NBA, Burns J, Blyth A et al: The morphine sparing effects of diclofenac sodium following abdominal surgery. Anaesthesia 42:1005, 1987

42. Moffat AC, Kenny GNC, Prentice JW: Postoperative neofam and diclofenac. Evaluation of their morphine-sparing effect after upper abdominal surgery. Anaesthesia 45:302, 1990

43. Bricker SRW, Savage ME, Hanning CD: Peri-operative blood loss and non-steroidal anti-inflammatory drugs: an investigation using diclofenac in patients undergoing transurethral resection of the prostate. Eur J Anaesthesiol 4:429, 1987

44. Kenny GNC: Ketorolac trometamol—A new non-opioid analgesic (editorial). Br J Anaesth 65:445, 1990

45. Yee JP, Koshiver JE, Allbon C, Brown CR: Comparison of intramuscular ketorolac tromethamine and morphine sulfate for analgesia of pain after major surgery. Pharmacotherapy 6:253, 1986

46. Gillies GWA, Kenny GNC, Bullingham RES, McArdle CS: The morphine sparing effect of ketorolac tromethamine: a study of a new, parenteral non-steroidal anti-inflammatory agent after abdominal surgery. Anaesthesia 42:727, 1987

47. O'Hara DA, Fragen RJ, Kinzer M, Pemberton D: Ketorolac tromethamine as compared with morphine sulfate for treatment of postoperative pain. Clin Pharmacol Ther 41:556, 1987

48. Bravo LJC, Mattie H, Spierdijk J et al: The effects on ventilation of ketorolac in comparison with morphine. Eur J Clin Pharmacol 35:491, 1988

49. Rubin P, Yee JP, Murthy VS, Seavey W: Ketorolac tromethamine (KT) analgesia: no post-operative respiratory depression and less constipation. Clin Pharmacol Ther 41:182, 1987

50. MacDonald FC, Gough KJ, Nicoll RAG, Dow RJ: Psychomotor effects of ketorolac in comparison with buprenorphine and diclofenac. Br J Clin Pharmacol 27:453, 1989
51. Spowart K, Greer TA, McLaren M et al: Haemostatic effects of ketorolac with and without concomitant heparin in normal volunteers. Thromb Haemost 60:382, 1988
52. Conrad KA, Fagan TC, Mackie MJ, Mayshar PV: Effects of ketorlac tromethamine on hemostasis in volunteers. Clin Pharmacol Ther 43:542, 1988
53. Lanza FL, Karlin DA, Yee JP: A double-blind placebo controlled endoscopic study comparing the mucosal injury seen with an orally and parenterally administered new nonsteroidal analgesic ketorolac tromethamine at therapeutic and subtherapeutic doses, abstracted. Am J Gastroenterol 82:939, 1987
54. Orme ML: Non-steroidal anti-inflammatory drugs and the kidney (editorial). Br Med J 292:1621, 1986
55. Lopez M, Waterbury LD, Michel A et al: Lack of addictive potential of ketorolac tromethamine. Pharmacologist 29:136, 1987
56. Jung D, Mroszczak EJ, Bynum L: Pharmacokinetics of ketorolac tromethamine in humans after intravenous, intramuscular and oral administration. Eur J Clin Pharmacol 35:423, 1988
57. Jung D, Mroszczak EJ, Wu A et al: Pharmacokinetics of ketorolac and p-hydroxyketorolac following oral and intramuscular administration of ketorolac tromethamine. Pharm Res 6:62, 1989
58. Montoya-Iraheta C, Garg DC, Jallad NS et al: Pharmacokinetics of single dose oral and intramuscular ketorolac tromethamine in elderly vs young healthy subjects, abstracted. J Clin Pharmacol 26:545, 1986
59. Martinez JJ, Garg DC, Pages LJ et al: Single dose pharmacokinetics of ketorolac in healthy young and renal impaired subjects, abstracted. J Clin Pharmacol 27:722, 1987
60. Yee J, Bradley R, Stanski E et al: A comparison of analgesic efficacy of intramuscular ketorolac tromethamine and meperidine in postoperative pain, abstracted. Clin Pharmacol Ther 39:237, 1986
61. Pages LJ, Martinez JJ, Garg DC et al: Pharmacokinetics of ketorolac tromethamine in hepatically impaired vs young healthy subjects, abstracted. J Clin Pharmacol 27: 724, 1987
62. Power I, Noble DW, Douglas E, Spence AA: Comparison of IM ketorolac trometamol and morphine sulfate for pain relief after cholecystectomy. Br J Anaesth 65: 448, 1990

8

Opioids

F. Michael Ferrante

The origins of the medicinal use of the juice of the poppy plant are lost in antiquity. Although the Ebers Papyrus (circa 1552 BC) contains several ancient Egyptian prescriptions using opium,[1] the first authentic reference to the milky juice of the poppy is from Theophrastus at the beginning of the third century BC.[2] The word *opium,* in fact, is derived from the Greek word meaning "juice." Opium is the dried powdered mixture of 20 alkaloids obtained from the unripe seed capsules of the poppy plant (Fig. 8-1).

Our understanding of opioids has, of course, advanced greatly since the time of Theophrastus and Hippocrates, particularly so in the past two decades. The shifting terminologies resulting from enhanced understanding of the pharmacology of these agents has unfortunately provided an opportunity for confusion. *Opiate* refers to any agent derived from opium (i.e., an alkaloid). The term *opioid* refers to all endogenous and exogenous (natural or synthetic) substances that possess morphine-like properties. Thus, the proper "generic" term for this class of agents is *opioid.*

STRUCTURE-ACTIVITY RELATIONSHIP

The alkaloids derived from opium can be divided into two distinct chemical classes: the phenanthrenes and the benzylisoquinolones. The principal phenanthrene alkaloids derived from opium include morphine, codeine, and thebaine (Table 8-1). The principal benzylisoquinolone alkaloids in opium are papaverine (a vasodilator) and noscapine, which lack morphine-like properties.

Morphine is the prototypic opioid. Its molecular skeleton is composed of five interlocked rings. Modification of functional groups on the skeleton (giving rise to the *semisynthetic* opioids, see Fig. 8-2 and Table 8-1) changes its pharmaco-

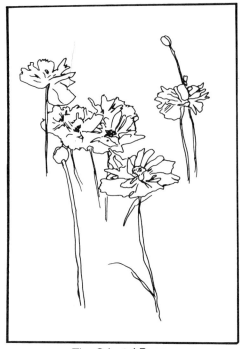

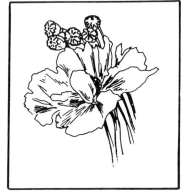

The Oriental Poppy   Poppy and Seed Pods

Fig. 8-1. Oriental poppy. Opium is dried powder obtained from unripe seed capsules of the poppy plant.

logic properties. For example, substitution of a methyl group for the hydroxyl group on carbon 3 results in codeine. Substitution of acetyl groups on carbons 3 and 6 gives rise to heroin (diacetylmorphine).

Synthetic opioids (Table 8-1) are created not by modification of functional groups on the phenanthrene moiety but by progressive reduction of the number of fused rings (Fig. 8-3). However, a "common core" is derived from the morphine molecule and envisaged as T-shaped. A piperidine ring forms the crossbar (and is believed to confer "opioid-like" properties), and a hydroxylated phenyl group forms the vertical axis (Fig. 8-3).[3]

A number of other structural characteristics are shared among the potent opioids[4]: a quaternary carbon, a phenolic hydroxyl (in morphine derivatives) or ketone group (meperidine, methadone), and a tertiary amine nitrogen. At pH = 7.4, the tertiary amine nitrogen is highly ionized, contributing to the water solubility of the opioids. While remaining basic features of many opioids, these characteristics are no longer considered essential for morphine-like activity.[5] Interestingly, stereochemical structure does influence morphine-like activity, with levorotatory isomers being most active.[6]

TABLE 8-1. Classification of Opioids on the Basis of Intrinsic Activity[a] and Synthetic Origin

Agonists	Agonist-Antagonists	Antagonists
Phenanthrene alkaloids	Semisynthetic opioids	Naloxone
Morphine	Buprenorphine	Naltrexone
Codeine	Nalbuphine	
Thebaine		
	Synthetic opioids	
Semisynthetic opioids	Benzomorphan derivatives	
Diacetylmorphine (heroin)	pentazocine	
Hydrocodone		
Hydromorphone	Morphinan derivatives	
Oxycodone	butorphanol	
Oxymorphone	dezocine	
Synthetic opioids		
Morphinan derivatives		
levorphanol		
Phenylpiperidine derivatives		
meperidine		
fentanyl		
sufentanil		
alfentanil		
Propioanilide derivatives		
methadone		
propoxyphene		

[a] Intrinsic activity refers to the intensity of the pharmacologic effect initiated by the drug-receptor complex (see below).

PHARMACODYNAMIC CONSIDERATIONS

Endogenous Opioid Peptides

The endogenous opioids[7] form one part of an endogenous analgesic system that modulates nociception (see Ch. 2). All endogenous opioids contain the amino acid sequence *tyrosine-glycine-glycine-phenylalanine* and are formed from cleavage of larger precursor molecules. Endogenous opioids can be grouped by their derivation from three precursor molecules: proenkephalin A, pro-opiomelanocortin, and prodynorphin (proenkephalin B) (Table 8-2).

Both met-enkephalin and leu-enkephalin are derived from proenkephalin A. Enkephalins are found in the gastrointestinal tract, sympathetic nervous system, and adrenal medulla. They are found in high density in areas of the central nervous system (CNS) important for antinociception: the periaqueductal gray matter, the rostroventral medulla, and Rexed's laminae I, II, V, and X (Fig. 8-4).

β-Endorphin is derived from pro-opiomelanocortin and is released with adrenocorticotropic hormone (ACTH) from the pituitary. β-Endorphin is the most potent of the endogenous opioids and is found in the hypothalamus, periaqueductal gray matter, and locus ceruleus (Fig. 8-4). In the past, the word *endorphins* has been used as a generic term for the endogenous opioids. This practice

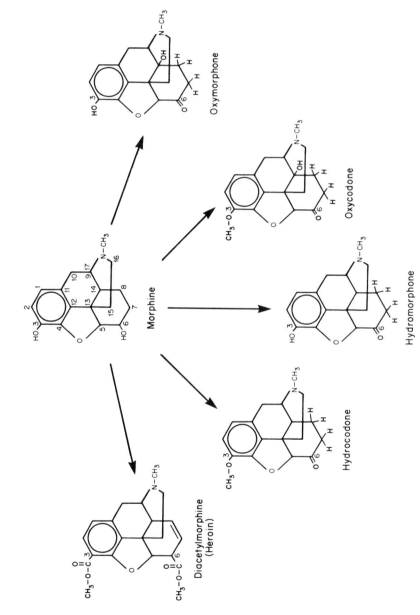

Fig. 8-2. Semisynthetic opioids are created by modification of functional groups on the morphine molecular skeleton.

148

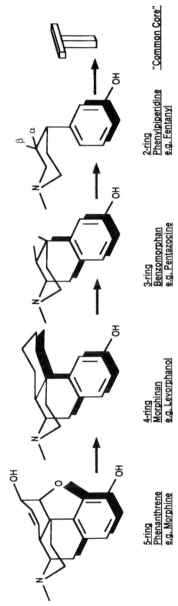

Fig. 8-3. Synthetic opioids are produced by successive removal of ring structures from the five-ring phananthrene structure of morphine. However, a common core, envisaged as a T, is shared by all opioids. A piperidine ring (which is believed to confer "opioid-like" properties to a compound) forms the crossbar and a hydroxylated phenyl group forms the vertical axis.

149

TABLE 8-2. Classification of Endogenous Opioid Peptides

Group	Precursor	Anatomic Locations
Enkephalins Leu-enkephalin Met-enkephalin	Proenkephalin A	Amygdala Hypothalamus-pituitary gland Periaqueductal gray matter Rostroventral medulla Rexed's laminae I, II, V, X Gastrointestinal tract Sympathetic nervous system Adrenal medulla
β-Endorphin	Pro-opiomelanocortin	Arcuate nucleus of basal hypothalamus Pituitary gland Nucleus of the solitary tract Periaqueductal gray matter Locus ceruleus
Dynorphins Dynorphin α-Neoendorphin	Prodynorphin	Similar distribution to the enkephalins

is declining in popularity because of the potential confusion with the specific moiety, β-endorphin.

Prodynorphin (proenkephalin B) gives rise to dynorphin and α-neoendorphin. Despite having an anatomic location similar to that of the enkephalins (Fig. 8-4), the dynorphins are not potent analgesics. Dynorphin is the prototypic ligand for the κ-receptor. Otherwise, its physiologic function remains obscure.

For a full description of the neuroanatomy and physiology of the endogenous opioid modulating system, see Chapter 2.

Opioid Receptors

Exogenously administered opioids produce analgesia by mimicking the actions of endogenous opioid peptides at specific receptors within the CNS.[7] The receptor can be envisaged as a common molecular site of action for a diverse group of analgesic compounds. The receptor subserves two distinct functions: chemical recognition and biologic action. These functions occur in different regions of the receptor complex. The recognition site is highly specific: only levorotatory isomers exhibit analgesic activity.[6] Opioids will bind to the recognition site with varying strength. The strength of attachment is termed *binding affinity* (Table 8-3).[8] Using various bioassay systems it is possible to determine the rank order of binding affinities, which correlates with the rank order of analgesic potencies.[9]

Continued exposure of the receptor to high concentrations of opioid will cause tolerance, which refers to the progressive decline in potency of an opioid with continued use, so that increasingly higher concentrations are required to achieve the same analgesic effect. The phenomenon is characteristic of opioids as a class of analgesics and is receptor-mediated. When tolerance develops to a particular opioid, cross-tolerance to other opioids concomitantly develops.

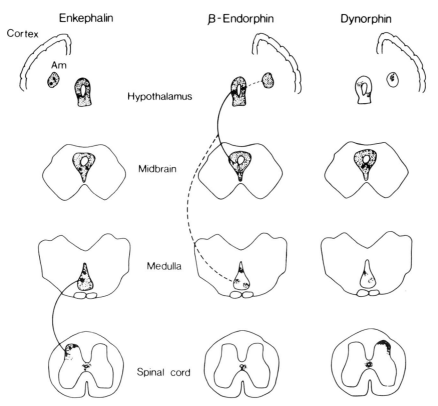

Fig. 8-4. Distribution of endogenous opioid peptides in CNS. Only structures involved in pain modulation or transmission are included. (**Left**) Proenkephalin-derived peptides have the most extensive distribution. They are present in cells and terminals in the amygdala (*Am*), the hypothalamus, the midbrain periaqueductal gray matter, the rostroventral medulla, and the dorsal horn of the spinal cord and lamina X. (**Middle**) β-Endorphin in CNS. β-Endorphin is largely derived from cells in the arcuate nucleus of the hypothalamus. There is a significant amount of β-endorphin in the periaqueductal gray matter and much less in the medulla and spinal cord. (**Right**) Dynorphin-related peptides. Dynorphin-related peptides roughly parallel the distribution of enkephalins, but there is much less dynorphin in the hypothalamus and the rostroventral medulla. (From Fields,[7] with permission.)

There are several types of opioid receptors (Table 8-4). Each receptor type mediates a spectrum of pharmacologic effects.[10–15]

Most endogenous, naturally occurring, semisynthetic and synthetic opioids bind to "morphine-preferring" or μ-receptors. The prototypic endogenous ligand is β-endorphin. The prototypic exogenous ligand is morphine. Using autoradiography, it has been shown that μ-receptors are specifically located in areas of the brain that are intimately involved with opioid-induced analgesia: the periaqueductal gray, the nucleus raphe magnus, and the medial thalamus.[16–18] (The other opioid receptors that mediate analgesia [δ- and κ-receptors] are so-

TABLE 8-3. Receptor Binding Affinities of Opioids (in order of decreasing affinity)

	Binding Affinity[a]	Specific Binding[b]
Sufentanil	0.1	92
Fentanyl	1.6	25
Morphine	5.7	60
Alfentanil	19.0	—
Meperidine	193.0	—

[a] Binding affinity is measured by the equilibrium inhibition constant (K_i) for [^{3}H]sufentanil (nM). The lower the value of K_i, the higher the affinity for the μ-receptor.

[b] Specific binding refers to the percentage of administered opioid bound to receptor sites (specific binding) as opposed to nonspecific (extraneous lipid) sites.

(Data from Leysen et al.[8])

matotopically localized to the spinal cord, though μ-receptors are also found at the cord.) Thus, activation of μ-receptors is largely responsible for supraspinal analgesia.

Two subtypes of μ-receptors have been proposed.[19–21] Activation of $μ_1$-receptors is responsible for the analgesic effects of μ-agonists. Activation of $μ_2$-receptors mediates the production of respiratory depression, cardiovascular effects such as bradycardia, and inhibition of gastrointestinal motility. Unfortunately, no presently developed opioid agonist selectively activates $μ_1$-receptors without concomitant $μ_2$-receptor activation. Similarly, naloxone antagonizes both $μ_1$- and $μ_2$-receptor effects by attaching to but not activating the receptors. However, derivatives of naloxone (naloxononazine and naloxazone) are $μ_1$-selective antagonists.[20,22] The receptor specificity of naloxonazine and naloxazone suggests the tantalizing possibility of synthesis of a $μ_1$-selective agonist.

Spinal analgesia mainly involves activation of δ- and κ-receptors.[15] Enkephalins are the prototypic ligands for the δ-receptor. In a classic series of studies, Yaksh and co-workers[23–25] demonstrated that enkephalin analogues are more potent segmental (spinal) analgesics than morphine when administered into the

TABLE 8-4. Classification Schema for Opioid Receptor Types and Proposed Actions

Receptor Type (or subtype)	Prototypic Ligand		Proposed Actions
	Endogenous	Exogenous	
$μ_1$	β-Endorphin	Morphine	Supraspinal analgesia
$μ_2$	β-Endorphin	Morphine	Respiratory depression Cardiovascular effects Gastrointestinal tract transit
δ	Enkephalin	—	Spinal analgesia
κ	Dynorphin	Ketocyclazocine	Spinal analgesia Sedation
ε	β-Endorphin	—	Hormone (?)
σ	—	N-allylnormetazocine	Psychotomimetic effects Dysphoria

subarachnoid space. In humans, the δ-ligand [D-Ala^2, D-Leu^5] enkephalin (DADL) has been reported to be up to five times more potent than morphine when administered into the subarachnoid space.[26]

μ-Agonists are presently used for spinal (epidural and subarachnoid) analgesia (see Ch. 11). If δ-receptors mediate opioid-induced analgesia at the level of the spinal cord, δ-selective agonists would appear to be better choices as agents for spinal analgesia. Furthermore, spinal analgesia mediated by δ-receptor activation is not associated with concomitant respiratory depression (μ_2-receptor effects). Unfortunately, enkephalins are rapidly degraded by peptidases on administration. Inhibition of these degradative enzymes enhances the analgesic effect of enkephalins.[27,28] Metabolically stable, potent analogues of enkephalin have also been synthesized.[29] However, the development of a δ-selective agonist clinically useful for segmental analgesia awaits further research.

Activation of κ-receptors causes spinal analgesia but also sedation. As with activation of δ-receptors, analgesia occurs without concomitant respiratory depression. Dynorphin is the protypic endogenous agonist while ketocyclazocine is the prototypic exogenous agonist. Morphine also acts as an agonist at the κ-receptor. However, the relative affinity of morphine for the μ-receptor is 200 times greater than its affinity for the κ-receptor. The analgesic properties of opioid agonist-antagonists are principally derived from κ-receptor activation.

The ϵ-receptor has been described using in vitro binding studies in the rat vas deferens. The receptor is not well characterized. The proposed endogenous agonist is β-endorphin. As β-endorphin is released in a one-to-one molar ratio with ACTH from the pituitary, ϵ-receptors may mediate a hormonal effect of β-endorphin.[15]

Another poorly characterized opioid receptor is the σ-receptor. This receptor is responsible for production of psychotomimetic effects including dysphoria and hallucinations, as well as tachycardia, tachypnea, and mydriasis. Most agonist-antagonist opioids at least partially activate the σ-receptor.

Relationship Between Receptor Binding and Response: Intrinsic Activity

The intensity of the biologic response (analgesia, sedation, etc.) that is produced by administration of an opioid can be used to define its intrinsic activity. Opioids such as morphine, which produce a maximal biologic response through receptor binding (μ_1 and μ_2 in this case), are termed *agonists*. Agents such as naloxone have low or no intrinsic activity and antagonize the effects of agonists by preventing their access to the receptor. Such drugs are called *antagonists* (Fig. 8-5).[30]

Other opioids produce a submaximal response at a particular receptor type, even at high doses (e.g., buprenorphine's action at the μ-receptor). Such drugs are termed *partial agonists*. Partial agonists exhibit certain characteristic pharmacologic properties: (1) the slope of the dose-response curve is less steep than that of a full agonist (Fig. 8-5); (2) the dose-response curve exhibits a ceiling effect (i.e., a submaximal response as compared with a full agonist) (Fig. 8-

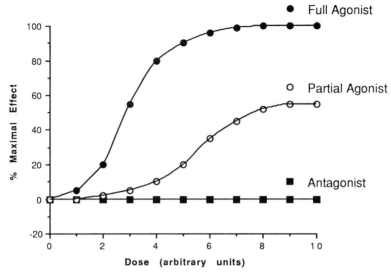

Fig. 8-5. Concept of intrinsic activity. Full agonists produce a maximal biologic response (e.g., analgesia, respiratory depression), whereas partial agonists produce a submaximal response even at high doses. Antagonists reverse the biologic response to opioids. Therefore, their effect is listed here as zero.

5); and (3) concomitant administration of a partial and full agonist can reduce (antagonize) the effect of the full agonist.

The aforementioned terms imply interaction at a single receptor type. However, opioids may have divergent activities on different receptors, acting simultaneously as an agonist at one receptor and an antagonist at another. Such agents are called *agonist-antagonists* or *mixed agonist-antagonists*.[31,32] For example, morphine acts as a full agonist at μ-receptors. Naloxone is an antagonist at μ- and κ-receptors but has greater binding affinity for the μ-receptor. Naloxone is devoid of agonist activity. Pentazocine is a weak competitive antagonist at the μ-receptor, a strong κ-agonist, and a σ-agonist. Nalbuphine reverses opioid-induced respiratory depression through μ-receptor antagonism while providing analgesia through partial κ-agonism.[33] Thus, pentazocine and nalbuphine are excellent examples of agonist-antagonist opioids. A list of the interactions of opioids at various receptor subtypes is found in Table 8-5.

Molecular Mechanisms Underlying Production of a Biologic Response

The opioid receptor site is anionic, requiring an opioid to be in the ionized state for strong binding to occur.[34] Binding of an opioid to the receptor produces inhibition of adenylate cyclase activity.[35] Furthermore, opioid-receptor binding inhibits transmembrane transport of calcium ions, presynaptically interfering with the release of other neurotransmitters.[36,37] Opioid-mediated inhibition of

TABLE 8-5. Intrinsic Activity of Opioids at Various Receptor Types

Opioid	Receptor Type			
	μ	κ	σ	δ
"Classic" agonists				
Morphine	Agonist	—	—	—
Meperidine	Agonist	—	—	—
Hydromorphone	Agonist	—	—	—
Oxymorphone	Agonist	—	—	—
Levorphanol	Agonist	—	—	—
Fentanyl	Agonist	—	—	—
Sufentanil	Agonist	—	—	—
Alfentanil	Agonist	—	—	—
Methadone	Agonist	—	—	—
Agonist-antagonists				
Buprenorphine	Partial agonist	—	—	—
Butorphanol	Antagonist	Agonist	Agonist	—
Nalbuphine	Antagonist	Partial agonist	Agonist	—
Pentazocine	Antagonist	Agonist	Agonist	—
Dezocine	Partial agonist	—	—	Agonist
Antagonists				
Naloxone	Antagonist	Antagonist	Antagonist	Antagonist

the release of acetylcholine from nerve endings may play a prominent role in the production of analgesia.

PHARMACOKINETIC CONSIDERATIONS

In order to have any pharmacologic effect, exogenous opioids must gain access to the receptor through use of drug delivery systems (Table 8-6). *Direct* systems involve application of the drug to the neuraxis and place the opioid in the region of the receptor. *Indirect* delivery systems rely on blood-borne carriage of the opioid to the receptor after (1) direct systemic absorption, (2) forma-

TABLE 8-6. Drug Delivery Systems

Direct (to neuraxis)	Indirect (via blood-borne carriage)
Epidural	Via systemic absorption
Subarachnoid	Oral
Intraventricular	Sublingual
	Rectal
	Inhalational
	Via depot formation
	Transcutaneous
	Intramuscular
	Subcutaneous
	Direct instillation
	Intravenous

tion of a depot for sustained release, or (3) direct instillation into the blood. The pharmacokinetics of direct delivery systems are only beginning to be explored.[38-40] Thus, this discussion will concentrate on the pharmacokinetics of indirect delivery and, in particular, direct intravenous administration.

After intravenous administration, opioid will be dispersed throughout the plasma volume, distributed to blood cells and other intravascular binding sites, distributed to tissues as a function of the distribution of cardiac output and tissue blood partition coefficient, and eventually to receptors (Fig. 8-6). Regions of the body containing receptors have been collectively referred to as the biophase. It is here that an opioid will bind to a receptor to produce a pharmacologic effect. Thus, what we view as the intensity of clinical effect or potency is determined by two processes: (1) access of opioid to the receptor (distribution)

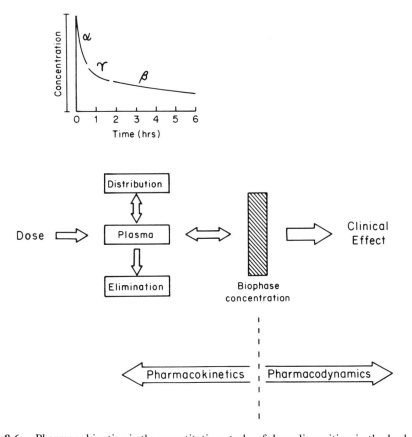

Fig. 8-6. Pharmacokinetics is the quantitative study of drug disposition in the body. It includes processes of absorption from the site of administration, distribution to body tissues and fluids, and elimination through biotransformation and excretion. Opioids bind to receptors in the biophase to produce an effect. For μ-agonists, global pharmacokinetic principles determine the concentration of opioid delivered to the biophase. Pharmacodynamics is the study of receptor responsiveness and the clinical actions of the opioids.

TABLE 8-7. Physicochemical and Pharmacokinetic Properties of Several Opioids

Opioid	Partition Coefficient at pH = 7.4[a]	pKa	% Unionized at pH = 7.4	% Unbound at pH = 7.4	V_D (L/kg)	TBCl (L/min)	Binding Affinity
Morphine	1	7.9	5	80	3.2	0.8–1.2	5.7
Meperidine	21	8.7	24	60	3.8	0.4–0.8	193.0
Methadone	115	9.3	1	10	4.1	0.1–0.2	—
Alfentanil	130	6.5	89	10	0.86	0.2–0.6	19.0
Fentanyl	950	8.4	9	20	4.1	0.8–1.3	1.6
Sufentanil	1,750	8.1	20	10	1.7	0.5–1.0	0.1

Abbreviations: V_D = Volume of distribution, TBCl = total body clearance.
[a] *n*-Octanol: pH 7.4 buffer.

and (2) the "fit" of the opioid onto the receptor (i.e., the binding affinity; see Table 8-3). The chemical structures of the opioids inevitably determine their access to and "fit" onto receptors through their physicochemical properties.[41] Table 8-7 reviews the physicochemical and pharmacokinetic properties of opioids that will be shown to be important in determination of potency in the following discussion.

Access to Receptors

Clinical pharmacokinetic data appear to relate blood or plasma concentrations of opioid to global responses (analgesia, respiratory depression). Opioid concentrations within the blood have been correlated to changes seen on electroencephalography (EEG),[42] although the relationship between these changes and analgesia remains to be determined. In so far as opioid concentrations at the receptor are in equilibrium with concentrations in the blood or plasma, any pharmacologic effect of an opioid must be affected by the global pharmacokinetic properties of the opioid (Fig. 8-6). The pharmacokinetic properties of individual opioids determine the resultant blood or plasma concentrations and their time course.

Influence of Physicochemical Properties on Potency

The physicochemical properties of lipid solubility and pKa (Table 8-7) are the primary determinants of access of an opioid to the receptor.[41,43,44] All opioid agonists are basic amines and are reasonably lipophilic (except for morphine). The innate lipophilicity of an opioid is described in terms of a partition coefficient. The partition coefficient describes how a drug "partitions" itself between aqueous and lipid phases at a particular pH after thorough mixing in an experimental setting. Lipid solubility and pKa are functionally related, as it is the unbound unionized form of an opioid that is free to diffuse across membranes and bind to receptors. The pKa value (defined as the negative logarithm of the acid dissociation constant of the protonated form of a base or conjugate acid) is functionally equal to the pH at which 50 percent of molecules are ionized. Thus, the pKa of an opioid determines the fraction of cationic (hydrophilic) versus base or unionized (lipophilic) moieties at a particular pH. Consequently, differences in pKa among opioids result in a range of unionized fractions and apparent lipid solubilities at physiologic plasma and tissue pH (Table 8-7).[41,44]

Similarly, there will be a range of binding to plasma proteins (Table 8-7) and uptake by red blood cells based on lipophilicity and pKa. With increasing unionized fraction, there is increasing plasma protein binding (implying that hydrophobic binding is involved). Although increasing unionized fraction would facilitate diffusion into red blood cells, no opioids are significantly concentrated in blood cells relative to the plasma.[41]

Thus, the apparent potency of an opioid correlates with the ease with which the lipid-soluble, unionized, unbound fraction diffuses across membranes to reach the receptor-containing biophase. This concept explains the apparent difference in potency between morphine and fentanyl or sufentanil. A much greater fraction of a dose of fentanyl or sufentanil reaches the receptor site. When this is corrected for, these agents really have the same potency.[8,45,46] Thus, all opioids, whether administered by direct or indirect delivery systems, can be made equianalgesic or equipotent by correcting for dose (see below).

Influence of Pharmacokinetic Properties on Potency

Although the lipid-soluble, unionized, unbound fraction of a dose of opioid is potentially available for receptor binding, the amount of opioid actually reaching receptors will also depend on the fraction of a dose remaining in the blood in comparison with distribution to other tissues. Thus, the apparent volume of distribution (which reflects the tissue:blood partition coefficient) becomes important in determining the clinical effects of highly lipophilic opioids. The apparent volume of distribution may be conceptualized as the volume into which a given dose of opioid must be diluted in order to achieve a particular concentration in the blood. Thus, the larger the volume of distribution, the smaller the blood concentration for a given dose of opioid. For example, the rapid onset and short duration of action of alfentanil in comparison with fentanyl may be explained by its smaller volume of distribution (i.e., smaller degree of tissue uptake) (Table 8-7).[42]

Biophase and Receptor Kinetics

Physiocochemical properties have a paradoxical effect on the central actions of opioids. As we have stated, high lipid solubility and an abundance of unbound unionized moieties facilitate opioid transfer across the blood-brain barrier to reach the biophase. However, such properties at the same time confer slow receptor kinetics on the lipophilic opioids. Not all opioid-receptor bonds are made or broken at the same rate and are proportional to the association-dissociation constants of particular drugs and receptors. Time to reach equilibrium may differ among the opioids.[8,47] This may be so because penetration of a hydrophilic barrier is necessary before the conjugate acid of the opioid can occupy an anionic site on a receptor.[34] Thus, once across the blood-brain barrier, highly lipophilic opioids with large unionized fractions are at a distinct disadvantage and would be expected to pierce the hydrophilic barrier rather slowly. This may have tremendous implications for the concept of potency with respect to the direct delivery of opioids to the receptor (i.e., epidural and subarachnoid routes of administration).[48]

Differences in receptor kinetics for partial μ-receptor agonists (e.g., buprenorphine) and the agonist-antagonist opioids are not governed by considerations of the degree of lipophilicity or ionization. For such opioids the kinetics of the analgesic response are dominated by the kinetics of dissociation from the receptor (i.e., the binding affinity of the particular opioid) (Table 8-7).[41,44] Binding affinity may be determined by competitive displacement analysis.[8,9,49]

The consequence of such receptor kinetics is that pharmacokinetic profiles and blood concentrations are not useful in designing dosage regimens for the partial agonists and the agonist-antagonists.[50,51] However, differences in receptor kinetics for the μ-agonists are small, so that their time-effect relationships are governed by the global pharmacokinetic principles that determine systemic concentrations of opioids. The pharmacokinetic behavior of μ-agonists can be characterized by their respective distribution volumes and clearances (see Table 8-7) independent of compartmental pharmacokinetic models.[51]

PHARMACOLOGIC CONSIDERATIONS

Central Nervous System Effects

Opioids can both depress and excite the CNS. Depression of the CNS is clinically expressed as analgesia, change in respiratory pattern, reduced level of consciousness, and associated electroencephalographic changes. The stimulating or excitatory effects include miosis, nausea, and vomiting.

Analgesia

All exogenously administered opioids produce their analgesic effects by mimicking the actions of endogenous opioid neurotransmitters at specific receptors in the CNS.[7] The neural pathways and the receptor mechanisms underlying the production of analgesia have been extensively discussed in Chapter 2, as well as in preceding sections of this chapter.

Concept of Equianalgesic Dosing

As discussed previously, the intensity of analgesic effect or potency of individual opioids is dependent on (1) access to the receptor, and (2) binding affinity ("fit" at the receptor site). Access to the receptor for μ-agonists is dependent

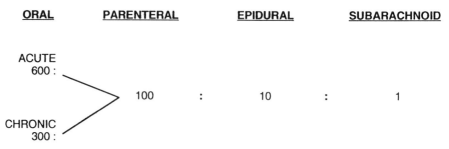

Fig. 8-7. Equianalgesic conversions among routes of administration. These conversion ratios are approximations, and practitioners should not be dogmatic in their interpretations.

on a number of physicochemical and global pharmacokinetic properties (Table 8-7): (1) liphophilicity, (2) pKa, (3) the degree of ionization, (4) the portion of a dose that is unbound, (5) the apparent volume of distribution, (6) the clearance, and (7) the route of administration. Thus, apparent differences in potency among opioids are really a function of physicochemical and pharmacokinetic differences among individual opioids rather than pharmacodynamic distinctions. This concept is extremely important in the clinical use of opioids. Thus, all opioids can be made equipotent or equianalgesic by adjusting for physicochemical and pharmacokinetic differences by correcting for dosage and route of administration (Fig. 8-7 and Table 8-8). This is known as the concept of equianalgesic dosing.[52,53]

Equianalgesic conversion schemas such as those outlined in Figure 8-7 and Table 8-8 should be used as only guidelines. As there are a number of methodologic problems inherent in the genesis of such conversion tables, practitioners should not be dogmatic in their interpretations.

STUDY DESIGN

Equianalgesic dosing schemas are traditionally based on single-dose studies in which intramuscular opioids are compared with morphine to establish potency ratios.[52] Inherent in any intramuscular dosing regimen, however, is a severalfold variability in the peak concentration achieved and/or the time to reach that concentration.[54] (For a full discussion of the vagaries inherent in absorption from an intramuscular depot, please see Ch. 10). Comparisons using intravenous administration would seem more practicable.

Furthermore, single doses of opioid are rarely administered in clinical practice to achieve prolonged analgesia. More realistic conversion guidelines could be developed from multiple dose studies. Intravenous patient-controlled analgesia (IV-PCA) has been used for such studies.[55,56] Use of IV-PCA eliminates experimenter bias by allowing patients to determine when and how much opioid they receive. IV-PCA also allows determination of mean analgesic consumption despite great interpatient variation in analgesic requirements.[55–59]

TABLE 8-8. Opioid Analgesic Equivalents[a]

Opioid	Route	Equianalgesic Dose[b]
Morphine	Parenteral[c]	10 mg
	Oral	30 mg
Codeine	Parenteral	130 mg
	Oral	200 mg
Oxycodone	Parenteral	15 mg
	Oral	30 mg
Levorphanol	Parenteral	2 mg
	Oral	4 mg
Hydromorphone	Parenteral	1.5 mg
	Oral	7.5 mg
Meperidine	Parenteral	75 mg
	Oral	300 mg
Methadone	Parenteral	10 mg
	Oral	20 mg
Fentanyl	Parenteral	100 μg
	Oral	Not available

[a] Based on single-dose studies in which an IM dose of each listed drug was compared with morphine to establish relative potency.

[b] Conversion of dosage among the different opioids does not take into account the property of incomplete cross-tolerance (see text).

[c] For acute or postoperative pain and single doses, the oral to parenteral potency ratio for morphine is 1:6. The oral to parenteral potency ratio may decrease to 1:2 or 1:3 with repetitive dosing (e.g., for the treatment of chronic pain).

(Adapted from Foley,[52] with permission.)

INCOMPLETE CROSS-TOLERANCE

Patients who become tolerant to the analgesic effect of a given opioid can have another opioid substituted to provide better analgesia because of incomplete cross-tolerance.[60,61] One-half of the equianalgesic dose of the new opioid is recommended as the initial dose.[52] This dosage is empirically derived and suggests that the relative potency of some opioids may increase with repetitive dosing.[52] Please note that the potency ratios listed in Table 8-8 do *not* take incomplete cross-tolerance into account.

ORAL TO PARENTERAL POTENCY RATIO

The bioavailability of oral morphine has been found to vary between 15 and 64 percent (mean, 38 percent).[62] Parenteral bioavailability is in the order of 100 percent as suggested by some authors (see below). Thus when converting from oral to parenteral morphine, it is important to allow for the significant first-pass metabolism seen with this opioid.[63]

For acute pain and single doses, the oral to parenteral potency ratio for morphine is 1:6.[64] For chronic pain and repetitive prolonged dosing, the oral to parenteral potency ratio for morphine is 1:2 or 1:3.[62,65,66] These ratios have been empirically adopted for oral to parenteral conversion with the other opioids.

EQUIVALENCE OF POTENCY AMONG
PARENTERAL ROUTES

Many equianalgesic conversion schemes assume equivalent potency among the intramuscular (IM), subcutaneous (SC), and intravenous (IV) routes of administration. Such an assumption presupposes equivalent bioavailability among the three routes of administration. Although little data exist, several authors have questioned this assumption.

In a study by Urquhart et al,[67] patients receiving hydromorphone via subcutaneous-PCA (SC-PCA) in comparison with IV-PCA had significantly higher dosage requirements, suggesting unequal bioavailability between the two routes of administration. According to the data of Urquhart et al,[67] the subcutaneous to intravenous potency ratio should be 1:1.5 or 1:2.

Respiration

All μ-agonists and the partial agonist buprenorphine produce a dose-dependent reduction in the responsiveness of brain stem respiratory centers to increases in carbon dioxide tension (P_{CO_2}).[68,69] The agonist-antagonist opioids do not produce a dose-related depression of sensitivity but appear to have a limited or "ceiling effect."[32] Opioid agonists also depress the pontine and medullary centers involved in regulating respiratory rhythmicity, leading to prolonged pauses between breaths, delayed exhalation, and periodic breathing.[68,69]

The reduction in the responsiveness of the respiratory center to P_{CO_2} produced by μ-agonists is characterized by an increase in resting P_{CO_2} and displacement of the CO_2 response curve to the right (Fig. 8-8).[70] When administered at equianalgesic dosages, μ-agonists will produce the same degree of respiratory depression and an equivalent shift of the CO_2 response curve.[70–72] Agonist-antagonists will also displace the CO_2 response curve to the right, but when given in increasing doses, the CO_2 response curve is characteristically "bell-shaped."[32]

Clinically, opioid-induced respiratory depression manifests as a reduction in the rate of breathing and is often accompanied by a compensatory increase in tidal volume. However, the compensation is incomplete, as evidenced by elevation of P_{CO_2}. After therapeutic doses, respiratory minute volume may be reduced for as long as 4–5 hours. High doses of μ-agonists or partial agonists result in apnea. The asleep elderly patient is more sensitive to the respiratory depressant effects of opioids. Conversely, postoperative pain counteracts the respiratory depression produced by opioids.[71]

Reduction in Level of Consciousness

Opioids are mood-altering drugs. Patients in pain can report feelings of warmth and well-being, drowsiness and euphoria. Alterations in mood and perception of surroundings is believed to be mediated through the limbic system.[73]

Opioids may eventually produce sleep although unconsciousness is not as-

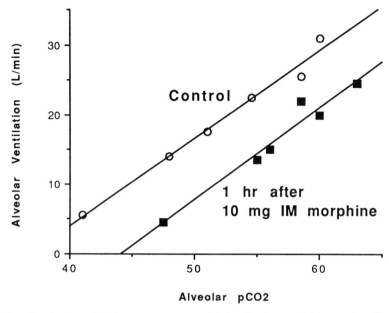

Fig. 8-8. Respiratory (CO_2) response curve obtained before and 1 hour after 10 mg IM morphine. Equianalgesic dosages of opioids produce equivalent changes in responsiveness of respiratory centers and equally displace the CO_2 response curve to the right.

sured even at high doses. Even at high or ''anesthetic'' doses, arousal may be produced by noxious stimulation.[74] The opioids differ in their intrinsic potential to produce sleep even after administration in equianalgesic dosages (Table 8-9).[75]

The effects of the opioids on EEG resemble changes associated with sleep. There is replacement of rapid α waves by slower δ waves (Fig. 8-9).[76]

Antitussive Effects

All opioids depress the cough reflex at least in part by a direct effect on the cough center in the medulla. There is no obligatory relationship between depression of respiration and depression of coughing.[72] The opioids differ in their intrinsic potential for cough suppression (Table 8-10).

TABLE 8-9. Hypnotic Effects of Opioids (Decreasing Order of Potency)

Diacetylmorphine = hydromorphone
Meperidine = nalbuphine = pentazocine
Morphine
Methadone
Codeine
Fentanyl

(Data from Freye.[75])

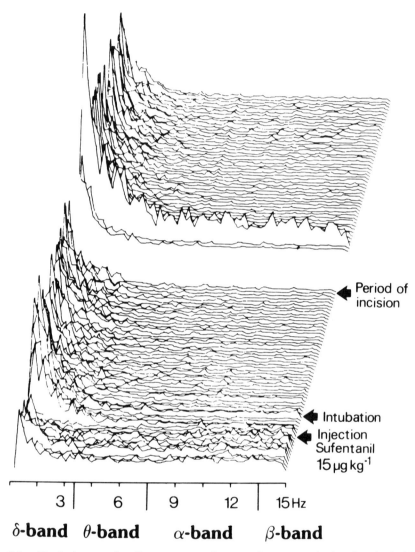

Fig. 8-9. Typical example of a compressed spectral array analysis of a single EEG derivative (T3-Co) during anesthesia with sufentanil, 15 μg/kg. Note shift to high power of activity. (From Bovill et al,[76] with permission.)

TABLE 8-10. Antitussive Effects of Opioids (Decreasing Order of Potency)

Diacetylmorphine = fentanyl = hydromorphone = hydrocodone
Methadone
Codeine
Morphine
Levorphanol
Meperidine = pentazocine

(Data from Freye.[75])

Pupillary Effects

Most μ- and κ-agonists cause constriction of the pupil in humans. Miosis is due to an excitatory action of the opioids on the autonomic segment of the Edinger-Westphal nucleus of the oculomotor nerve. After high doses of opioids, the pupils may become pinpoint. Miosis may be antagonized by atropine.

Nausea and Vomiting

Opioids produce nausea and vomiting by stimulation of the chemoreceptor trigger zone in the area postrema of the medulla.[72] This may reflect the role of opioids as partial dopamine agonists at dopamine receptors. Opioids may also cause nausea and vomiting by delaying gastrointestinal transit. When given in equianalgesic dosages, all opioids are equipotent in the production of nausea and vomiting.

Tolerance, Physical Dependence, and Addiction

With continued use of substantial amounts of opioid, the potency of the opioid declines so that progressively more and more drug is required to produce the same degree of analgesia. This phenomenon, called *tolerance,* is characteristic of the opioids as a class of drugs. All opioid analgesics produce tolerance, and when tolerance develops, there is cross-tolerance to other opioids, although incomplete.[7] Tolerance can occur without physical dependence.

Physical dependence is not synonymous with addiction. Physical dependence is a physiologic state characterized by withdrawal (abstinence) syndrome on discontinuation of the opioid. Initial manifestations of withdrawal include yawning, diaphoresis, lacrimation, coryza, and tachycardia. Abdominal cramps, nausea, and vomiting ensue and reach a peak in 72 hours. During withdrawal, tolerance to the opioid is rapidly lost.

Addiction is defined by the World Health Organization as

> *A state, psychic and sometimes also physical, resulting from the interactions between a living organism and a drug, characterized by behavioral and other responses that always include a compulsion to take the drug on a continuous or periodic basis in order to experience its psychic effects, and sometimes to avoid the discomfort of its absence. Tolerance may or may not be present.*[77]

This definition closely approximates the popular conception of addiction as a compulsion or overpowering drive to obtain a drug in order to experience its

TABLE 8-11. Addiction Potential of Opioids (Decreasing Potential)

Diacetylmorphine = oxymorphone
Fentanyl = methadone
Levorphanol = morphine
Meperidine
Codeine
Nalbuphine = pentazocine

(Data from Freye.[75])

psychologic effects. Addiction implies compulsive behavior and psychologic dependence and is conceptually and phenomenologically distinct from tolerance (a pharmacologic property of the class of drugs) and physical dependence (a physiologic effect also characteristic of this class of drugs).

It is commonly asked whether administration of opioids for medically appropriate reasons (e.g., postoperative analgesia) can induce addiction. The incidence of opioid addiction has been examined prospectively in 12,000 hospitalized patients who received at least one strong opioid.[78] There were only four reasonably well-documented cases of subsequent addiction in patients without a prior history of drug abuse. Thus, opioid addiction rarely occurs iatrogenically.[78]

The tendency of opioids to cause addiction is somewhat related to their analgesic potency (Table 8-11).[75] Only the agonist-antagonists have low abuse potential, probably due to the antagonist component of these mixed analgesics.[75] However, the overall liability for abuse of an opioid is not established on the psychic properties of the drug alone. Long-term use of opioids without addiction has been demonstrated in patients with pain of nonmalignant origin.[79,80] Drug use alone is not the major factor in the development of addiction,[79,80] but underlying personality, social environment, and the availability of money may be more important factors in its development.[81]

Effects on the Gastrointestinal Tract

Stomach and Small and Large Intestine

Opioids reduce the propulsive peristaltic contractions of the small and large intestine. The amplitude of nonpropulsive, rhythmic, segmental contractions is usually enhanced in these same areas. Within the stomach, a decrease in motility accompanies increased antral tone. Delayed gastric emptying may be produced by coupling this effect with enhanced tone in the first part of the duodenum. Opioids enhance sphincteric tone in the pyloric and anal sphincters and ileocecal valve. Enhanced sphincteric tone, coupled with decreased propulsive activity throughout the bowel, increases transit time. Delay in passage of intestinal contents allows for greater absorption of water, increasing the viscosity and desiccation of bowel contents. All these factors contribute to the production of constipation.

MECHANISM OF ACTION

The exact mechanisms underlying the effects of opioids on bowel motility are unclear. However, opioids appear to have both local and central actions.[82] Opioids affect cholinergic, serotonergic, and enkephalinergic receptors found in the myenteric plexus of the intestine. Neither the administration of ganglionic blocking agents or the removal of the extrinsic innervation of the bowel prevent opioid-induced effects in animal models. When applied to the spinal cord, opioids also decrease peristalsis (see Chs. 11 and 26).[83] Moreover, injection of morphine into the cerebral ventricles inhibits bowel motility. This effect can be abolished by intraventricular administration of naloxone or by vagotomy.[82] Thus, the evidence to date suggests that the decreased bowel motility associated with the use of opioids is both locally and centrally mediated.

Biliary Tract

μ-Agonists produce a marked increase in biliary tract pressure. After the subcutaneous injection of 10 mg morphine, the pressure within the common bile duct may increase 10-fold.[72] Agonist-antagonists produce much less of an increase in biliary pressure than μ-agonists.[84] Nalbuphine has been reported to actively reverse sphincter of Oddi spasm while maintaining pain relief (κ-mediated analgesia).[85]

Cardiovascular Effects

Although opioids are used for anesthesia within the operating room because of their relative cardiovascular and myocardial stability, opioids do produce chronotropic, inotropic, and peripheral vascular changes. Opioids produce a dose-dependent bradycardia caused by central stimulation of the vagal nucleus in the medulla.[86,87] As the bradycardia is vagally mediated, it can be blocked with atropine.[88] Because of its structural resemblance to atropine, meperidine may cause tachycardia (Fig. 8-10).

Except for meperidine, the opioids do not suppress myocardial contractility at clinically useful dosages. The negative inotropic effects of meperidine may be seen at doses as low as 2.0–2.5 mg/kg of meperidine.[89,90] All opioids can produce direct myocardial depression.[89,91,92] However, this effect is not achieved even with very large clinical anesthetic dosages.

Morphine has both a direct effect on vascular smooth muscle and an indirect effect through its release of histamine, thereby producing arteriolar dilation and

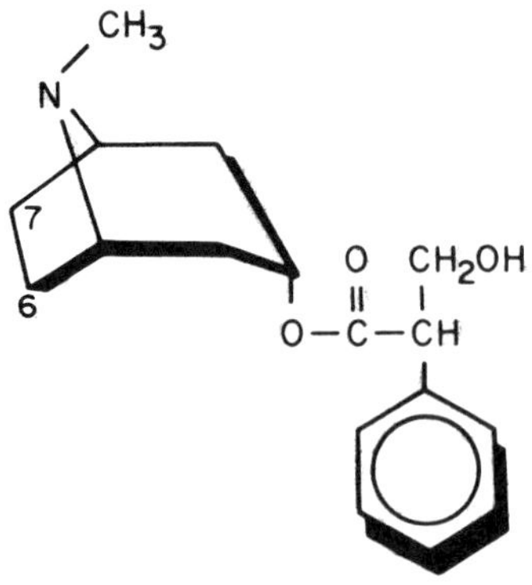

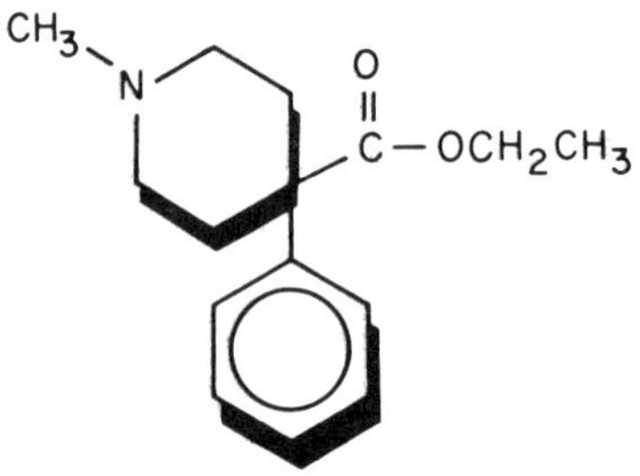

Atropine

Meperidine

Fig. 8-10. At high doses, meperidine may cause tachycardia because of its structural resemblance to atropine.

venodilation.[93–95] The primary mechanism for vasodilation with morphine is believed to be histamine release. Meperidine and codeine also release histamine whereas fentanyl and sufentanil do not.[95,96]

μ-AGONISTS

Alkaloids

Morphine

Morphine (Fig. 8-11) is the prototypic μ-agonist. As previously stated, morphine is an opiate (i.e., an alkaloid derived from the opium poppy). In fact, the opium poppy is still the major source of morphine, as its chemical synthesis is difficult.

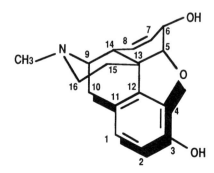

Fig. 8-11. Morphine.

PHARMACOKINETICS

After IV administration, morphine is rapidly distributed to tissues and organs. By 10 minutes, 96–98 percent of the drug is cleared from the plasma.[97] The volume of distribution of morphine is relatively large,[97,98] suggesting extensive tissue uptake. As morphine is hydrophilic, the sequestration probably occurs in nonfat tissues (e.g., skeletal muscle).

Stanski et al[98] reported that peak plasma concentrations were reached 7.5–20 minutes after IM injection. Brunk and Delle[99] reported higher concentrations of morphine 15 minutes to 3 hours after SC or IM administration as compared with IV administration. Thus, morphine is rapidly distributed out of the plasma after IV administration. IM or SC injection creates a depot, which continues to release morphine into the plasma for distribution.

As morphine is so rapidly cleared from the plasma after IV injection, the plasma concentrations do not correlate with the opioid's pharmacologic activity.[100,101] As morphine is hydrophilic, the discrepancy probably relates to a delay in transfer across the blood-brain barrier. Cerebrospinal fluid concentrations of morphine peak 15–30 minutes after an IV injection and decay more slowly than the attendant plasma concentrations.[100] Thus, the analgesic effects of morphine may not be apparent during the time of peak plasma concentrations after IV injection.

METABOLISM: SIGNIFICANCE OF GLUCURONIDE METABOLITES

The principal pathway for metabolism of morphine is glucuronidation in hepatic and extrahepatic sites, particularly, the kidneys.[102] Morphine-3-glucuronide and morphine-6-glucuronide are the major metabolites (Fig. 8-12).[62,103] Morphine-6-glucuronide has significant analgesic activity and may substantially contribute to the analgesic effects of morphine. When administered intracerebrally, morphine-6-glucuronide is 45 times more potent than morphine and four times more potent after SC administration.[104]

Demethylation is a minor pathway for the metabolism of morphine. Only about 5 percent of any morphine dose is demethylated to normorphine.[105] A small amount of codeine may also be formed as part of normal morphine metabolism.

The liver is the principal site of morphine metabolism.[106] Glucuronidation is rarely impaired in hepatic failure,[107] and morphine is well tolerated in patients up to the point of hepatic precoma.[108]

Metabolites of morphine are excreted mainly in the urine, with only 7–10 percent undergoing biliary excretion. Less than 10 percent of morphine is excreted unchanged by the kidneys. The excretion of morphine itself is unimpaired in renal failure.[62,101,109] However, the active metabolite morphine-6-glucuronide can accumulate in patients with decreased renal function and result in prolonged analgesia, sedation, and respiratory depression.[110–114] Thus, it is best to choose other opioids besides morphine as analgesics in patients with impaired renal function.

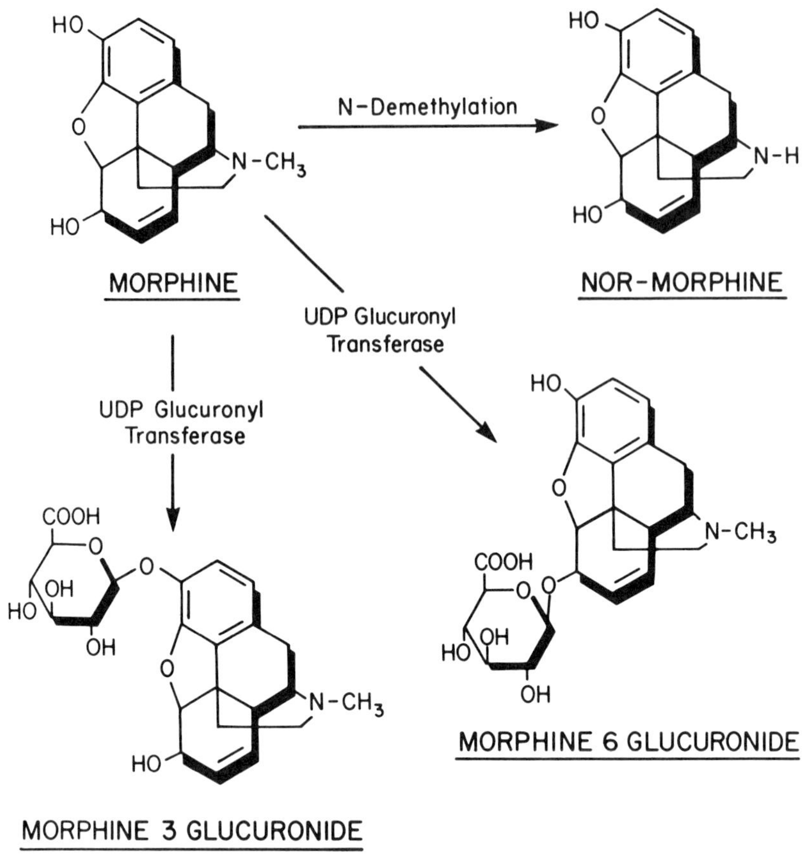

Fig. 8-12. Metabolism of morphine. Morphine-3-glucuronide and morphine-6-glucuronide are major metabolites. Morphine-6-glucuronide possesses significant analgesic activity and may substantially contribute to morphine's analgesic effects. Both metabolites are excreted in the urine, and accumulation may occur after repetitive dosing in patients with renal failure. Demethylation is a minor pathway for morphine metabolism.

PHARMACOLOGIC EFFECTS

As stated previously, morphine is the prototypic opioid; most of its pharmacologic effects have already been discussed in previous sections of this chapter.

CLINICAL USES AND PHARMACEUTICAL PREPARATIONS

Morphine is available as morphine sulfate and morphine hydrochloride. Oral morphine is available as tablets in immediate-release or slow-release preparations or as an elixir. Oral morphine undergoes significant first-pass metabolism. About 30 percent of an orally administered dose reaches the systemic circulation. Despite this, slow-release preparations provide excellent analgesia for moderate to severe chronic pain requiring repetitive dosing. Immediate-release forms

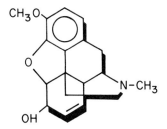

Fig. 8-13. Codeine is the result of substitution of a methyl group on carbon 3 of morphine. Codeine is a naturally occurring alkaloid that has significant efficacy after oral administration because of limitation of first-pass metabolism.

are used to assuage breakthrough pain and provide supplemental analgesia.[115] Rectal suppositories and an injectable form are, of course, available.

Codeine

Codeine is a naturally occurring alkaloid like morphine. Codeine is the result of substitution of a methyl group on carbon 3 of morphine (Fig. 8-13). This substitution limits first-pass hepatic metabolism, conferring good efficacy after oral administration.

PHARMACOKINETICS

After absorption, codeine is metabolized in the liver (largely by demethylation to norcodeine) and excreted by the kidneys. Unlike morphine, it is excreted largely in inactive forms. Approximately 10 percent of a dose of codeine is demethylated to morphine. As codeine has exceptionally low affinity for opioid receptors, the fraction converted to morphine may be responsible for its analgesic properties.[73,116]

PHARMACOLOGIC EFFECTS

Codeine produces mild to moderate analgesia and should not be used in the treatment of severe pain. Similarly, its propensity to produce sedation, nausea, vomiting, constipation, and respiratory depression is limited. While a parenteral form of codeine exists, codeine should not be used intravenously as the histamine-releasing potency of codeine is even greater than that of morphine. The addiction potential of codeine is very low (Table 8-11).

CLINICAL USES AND PHARMACEUTICAL PREPARATIONS

Codeine has excellent antitussive properties at an oral dose as low as 15 mg. Progressively greater cough suppression is seen as the dose is increased to 60 mg.[117] Codeine is most often included in medications for its antitussive properties or is combined with nonopioid analgesics for the relief of mild to moderate pain.[118] Maximal analgesia occurs with 60 mg of codeine, which is equianalgesic to 650 mg of aspirin. When administered intramuscularly, 130 mg codeine is equianalgesic to 10 mg IM morphine.

Semisynthetic Opioids

This group of opioids is composed of drugs that are synthesized by simple chemical modification of the morphine molecule (Fig. 8-2). They do not occur naturally.

Diacetylmorphine (Heroin, Diamorphine)

Diacetylmorphine (Fig. 8-14) is a prodrug that does not bind to opioid receptors and has no analgesic activity itself.[119] It is rapidly hydrolyzed to 6-monoacetylmorphine and morphine. The pharmacologic profile of diacetylmorphines is very similar to that of morphine. It has no clinical advantage over morphine when administered by IM injection or orally.[119,120] It is not known whether there is any real advantage in administration of diacetylmorphine as compared with morphine when administered by the IV, epidural, or subarachnoid routes of administration.[53] Diacetylmorphine has high addiction liability (Table 8-11) and is banned from manufacture and medicinal use in the United States.

Hydromorphone (Dilaudid)

Hydromorphone (Fig. 8-2) is approximately seven to eight times as potent as morphine when administered parenterally. Hydromorphone has a clinical pharmacologic profile similar to that of morphine.[121,122] Despite anecdotal reports of a reduced incidence of nausea, vomiting, respiratory depression, urinary retention, and constipation, there is little evidence to corroborate such claims.[121]

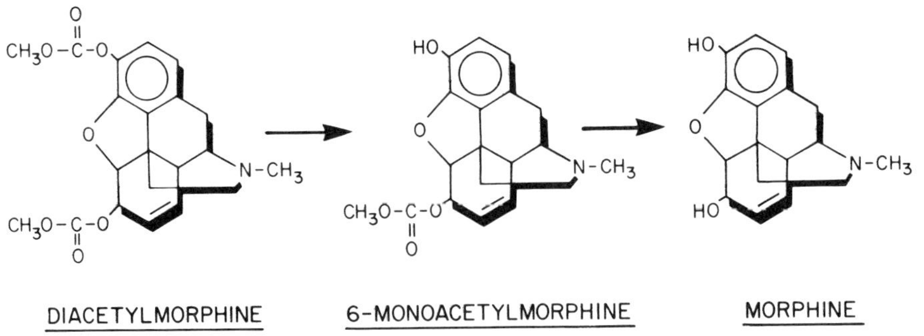

Fig. 8-14. Diacetylmorphine is a prodrug that is rapidly hydrolyzed in the plasma to monoacetylmorphine (analgesically active) and morphine.

PHARMACOKINETICS

Little is known of the pharmacokinetics of hydromorphone despite its wide-spread clinical use for many years.[123] In a recent study,[124] hydromorphone was found to have a rapid distribution phase similar to morphine. About 90 percent was lost from the plasma within 10 minutes. Again similar to morphine, hydromorphone elimination was dependent on tissue uptake with subsequent slow release from tissue to plasma.[124]

CLINICAL USES AND PHARMACEUTICAL PREPARATIONS

Unlike morphine, codeine, and meperidine, hydromorphone has no norhydromorphone metabolites.[116] This characteristic makes hydromorphone particularly useful in patients with renal failure. Otherwise, there is little difference in the pharmacologic profile of hydromorphone as compared with morphine to recommend its superiority.

Hydromorphone is available in 1-, 2-, 3-, and 4-mg tablets. Injectable preparations include concentrations of 1, 2, and 4 mg/ml. A dosage of 1.5 mg IM hydromorphone is equivalent in analgesic potency to 10 mg IM morphine. The duration of analgesia is 3–5 hours. The analgesic potency when administered orally is only about one-fifth that observed after IM injection. Rectal suppositories are available.[125,126]

Oxymorphone (Numorphan)

Oxymorphone is synthesized by addition of a hydroxyl group to carbon 14 of hydromorphone (Fig. 8-2). When administered parenterally, oxymorphone is approximately 10 times as potent as morphine.[127,128] The oral to parenteral potency ratio for oxymorphone itself is 1:6.[128] The clinical pharmacologic profile of oxymorphone is otherwise similar to morphine, except for enhanced addiction liability (similar to heroin[75]) (Table 8-11) and lack of histamine release.[129,130] Despite claims of an increased incidence of nausea and vomiting, there are little data to substantiate these claims.

The structural similarities between oxymorphone and naloxone are of more than passing significance (Fig. 8-15). Naloxone (an opioid antagonist) is the N-allyl ($-CH_2-CH=CH_2$)-substituted analogue of oxymorphone. The structural similarity of these two opioids has been used to study the structure-activity relationships of agonist and antagonist receptor interactions,[131,132] as well as to develop new agonists and antagonists.[133,134]

PHARMACOKINETICS

The pharmacokinetics of oxymorphone have been incompletely studied. Less than 10 percent of a dose is excreted as free oxymorphone in the urine.[135]

CLINICAL USES AND PHARMACEUTICAL PREPARATIONS

Oxymorphone has received extensive study for use via SC-PCA[136] and IV-PCA.[137–139] Because of its potency, short duration of action, and effectiveness when given orally, oxymorphone is under study for use via transdermal prepara-

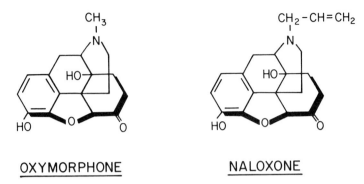

OXYMORPHONE   NALOXONE

Fig. 8-15. Naloxone (an opioid antagonist) is the *N*-allyl-(—CH₂—CH=CH₂)-substituted analogue of the potent μ-agonist oxymorphone.

tions.[140] The usual adult dose of SC or IM oxymorphone is 1–1.5 mg every 4–6 hours. The intravenous dose is 0.5 mg initially.

Oxymorphone is supplied in 1-mg or 1.5-mg/ml ampules. A rectal suppository is also available.[141] Rectal administration is approximately one-tenth as potent as IM administration.[141]

Hydrocodone (Hycodan, Lortab, Vicodin, Tussionex)

The clinical pharmacologic profile of hydrocodone is similar to codeine and has good oral bioavailability (about 50 percent). Hydrocodone is found only in oral preparations in combination with nonopioid analgesics for pain relief. Hydrocodone has excellent antitussive properties (see Table 8-10).

PHARMACOKINETICS

Hydrocodone undergoes *O*-demethylation, *N*-dealkylation, and 6-ketoreduction.[142] Although not definitively proven, hydrocodone may undergo metabolism to hydromorphone in the liver.[143] This may have caused or contributed to two deaths after ingestion of a hydrocodone-containing antitussive.[143]

CLINICAL USES AND PHARMACEUTICAL PREPARATIONS

Hydrocodone is usually found in combination with acetaminophen or acetylsalicylic acid. Such preparations exhibit synergistic analgesia as the analgesia inherent in these preparations is greater than double the dose of each constituent.[144] Side effects are also reduced by these combinations.[144]

Oxycodone (Percocet, Percodan, Roxicet, Roxicodone, Tylox)

Oxycodone has a pharmacologic profile similar to morphine. However, like codeine and hydrocodone, oxycodone has good oral bioavailability, retaining at least one-half of its analgesic activity. Like hydrocodone and codeine, oxycodone is usually admixed with nonopioid analgesics in commercial preparations. Oxycodone is not ordinarily used as an antitussive. Oxycodone has strong abuse potential.[145]

PHARMACOKINETICS

Like most of the other semisynthetic opioids, the pharmacokinetics of oxycodone have been incompletely studied. Oxycodone is metabolized to noroxycodone.[146,147]

CLINICAL USES AND PHARMACEUTICAL PREPARATIONS

Oxycodone's major use in the United States is as an oral analgesic. When given orally, hydrocodone is four times as potent as oxycodone. Parenteral preparations of oxycodone are not available in the United States. A transdermal preparation is under study.[148]

Synthetic Opioids

Levorphanol (Levo-Dromoran)

Levorphanol (Fig. 8-16) is the only commercially available μ-agonist of the morphinan series (Fig. 8-3). The dextrorotatory isomer (dextromethorphan) has antitussive activity equal to codeine but lacks analgesic activity or abuse potential.

Levorphanol has a clinical pharmacologic profile similar to morphine. Levorphanol appears to undergo considerable first-pass metabolism,[149,150] although there is extensive interindividual variability.[150] When given orally, levorphanol has an oral to parenteral potency ratio similar to codeine and oxycodone. Levorphanol is seven times more potent than oral morphine and five times more potent than parenteral morphine (Table 8-8).

PHARMACOKINETICS

Levorphanol has rapid absorption after SC administration. Maximal analgesia occurs at 60–90 minutes. While producing analgesia of a duration similar to morphine after parenteral administration, levorphanol is metabolized less rapidly (half-life, 11 hours).[150] Thus, repeated injections at short time intervals may lead to systemic accumulation.[150]

CLINICAL USE AND PHARMACEUTICAL PREPARATIONS

Levorphanol (Fig. 8-16) is most useful for treatment of chronic pain and has a wide experience in the management of cancer pain.[52,151]

Levorphanol is available as levorphanol tartrate in 2-mg tablets and as an injectable solution in a concentration of 2 mg/ml.

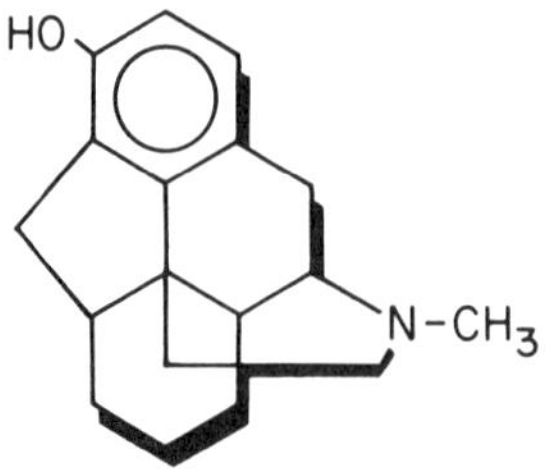

Fig. 8-16. Levorphanol. Only the dextrorotatory isomer has analgesic activity.

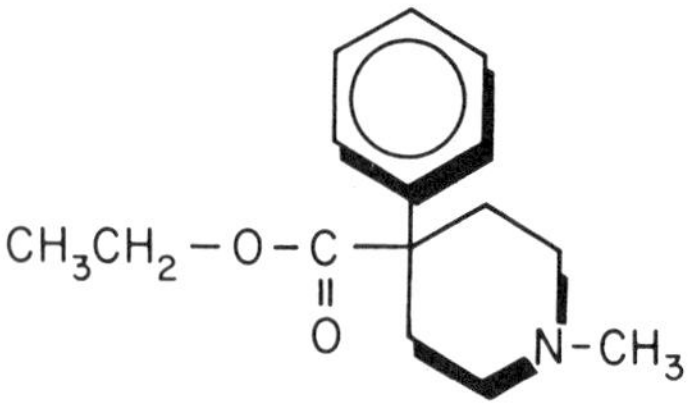

Fig. 8-17. Meperidine.

Meperidine (Demerol)

Meperidine (Fig. 8-17) is a member of the phenylpiperidine series of opioid μ-agonists (Fig. 8-3). The commonly used opioid anesthetics fentanyl (Fig. 8-18), sufentanil (Fig. 8-19), and alfentanil (Fig. 8-20) are all analogues of meperidine.

PHARMACOKINETICS

Oral bioavailability is about 45–75 percent, due to extensive first-pass metabolism in the liver.[152] Meperidine is absorbed slowly after oral administration, with peak plasma concentrations occurring at 2 hours after ingestion.[152]

Absorption from IM depot injection is quite variable, which can lead to erratic and inconsistent analgesia.[54,153]

After IV injection, meperidine is rapidly and extensively distributed to extravascular tissues. Distribution is essentially complete 30–45 minutes after injection. (This is considerably slower than morphine. Distribution is essentially complete in 10 minutes after IV injection of morphine.)

The elimination half-life of meperidine is 3–4.4 hours.[154] About 60 percent of a meperidine dose is bound to plasma protein. This may be of some concern in the elderly where decreased plasma protein binding may manifest as an increased unbound fraction of drug and increased sensitivity to meperidine.[155]

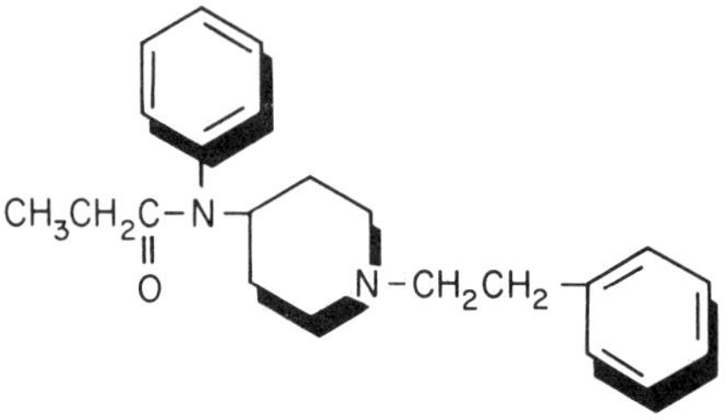

Fig. 8-18. Fentanyl.

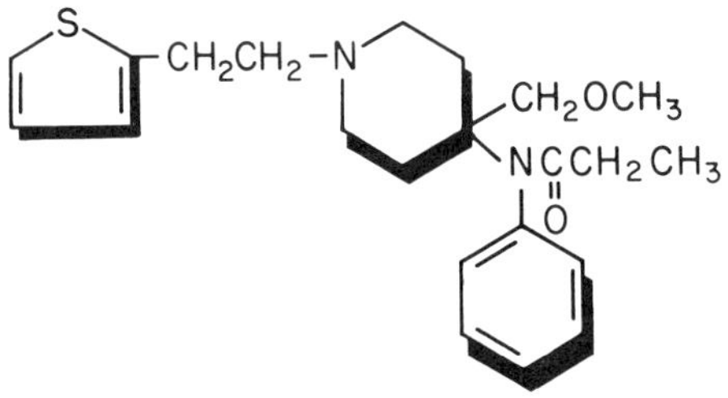

Fig. 8-19. Sufentanil.

METABOLISM: SIGNIFICANCE OF THE NORMEPERIDINE
METABOLITE

Meperidine is extensively metabolized in the liver (Fig. 8-21). Approximately 90 percent of a dose of meperidine undergoes *N*-demethylation to normeperidine and hydrolysis to meperidinic acid.[156,157] Less than 5 percent of meperidine is excreted unchanged in the urine. Normeperidine may subsequently undergo hydrolysis to normeperidinic acid.[152] The acidic metabolites are inactive and are excreted partially unchanged and partially conjugated in the urine.[158]

Urinary excretion of meperidine is pH-dependent.[159] If urinary pH is reduced below 5, as much as 25 percent of the opioid is excreted unchanged in the urine. Speed of elimination of meperidine can therefore be enhanced by acidification of the urine.[159]

Normeperidine has an elimination half-life of 15–40 hours[160] and can be detected in the urine for as long as 3 days after meperidine administration. Normeperidine has CNS stimulant effects, and toxicity may be manifested as myoclonus and seizures.[157,160,161] Thus, administration of meperidine to patients with renal insufficiency may lead to system accumulation and normeperidine toxicity.[160,162] Cirrhosis may cause decreased clearance and persistence of normeperidine in the plasma.[163] Patients with cirrhosis may be relatively protected from normeperidine toxicity because of impaired hepatic function, but the risk of systemic toxicity may still be present with repetitive dosing.[163]

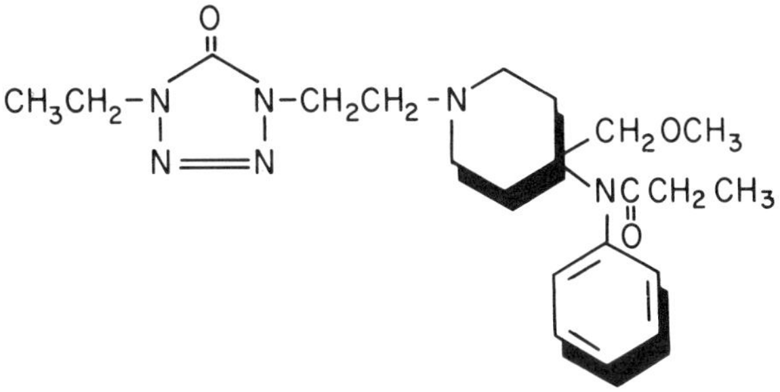

Fig. 8-20. Alfentanil.

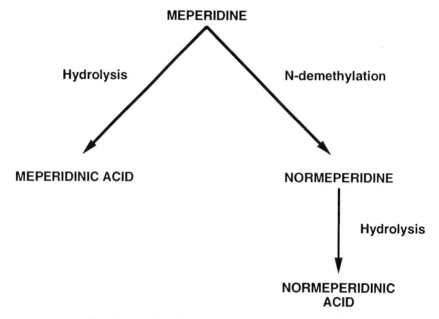

Fig. 8-21. Hepatic metabolism of normeperidine.

PHARMACOLOGIC EFFECTS

Meperidine is approximately one-tenth as potent as morphine when administered orally and seven to 10 times less potent than morphine when administered parenterally.

When administered in analgesic dosages, meperidine has no significant cardiovascular effects. Meperidine, in contrast to morphine and other opioids, rarely causes bradycardia. Because of its modest atropine-like qualities (Fig. 8-10), meperidine may cause tachycardia. When given in large doses, however, meperidine results in reduced myocardial contractility, reduced stroke volume and elevated filling pressures.[89,90] The negative inotropic effects of meperidine may be appreciated at doses as low as 2.0–2.5 mg/kg.[89,90]

Mild antispasmodic properties were first recognized when meperidine was first described by Eisleb and Schaumann in 1939. After equianalgesic doses, meperidine causes less biliary spasm than morphine.[164] As meperidine causes less smooth muscle spasm than other μ-agonists, this property makes meperidine a good choice for patients with renal colic.

Unlike other opioids, meperidine will cause mydriasis rather than miosis, reflecting its modest atropine-like properties.

CLINICAL USES AND PHARMACEUTICAL PREPARATIONS

The IM dose of meperidine used to treat severe pain is 75–100 mg.[165,166] The dose may need to be repeated every 2–4 hours, as the duration of analgesia with meperidine is shorter than with morphine. Meperidine infusions of 0.5–1.5

mg/kg administered as a loading dose over 30–60 minutes followed by a maintenance infusion of 0.25–0.75 mg/min can be used to treat postoperative pain.[167] As explained in Chapter 10, the maintenance infusion will need to be adjusted frequently. Meperidine has been used extensively as an opioid for IV-PCA.[138,168,169]

Meperidine hydrochloride is available for oral use in tablets (50 mg and 100 mg) and as an elixir (50 mg/tsp). Meperidine hydrochloride is available in varying concentrations for parenteral administration.

Fentanyl

Fentanyl (Fig. 8-18) is a cogener of meperidine and a member of the phenylpiperidine series. Fentanyl is 75–125 times more potent than morphine as an analgesic.[170]

PHARMACOKINETICS

Because of its enhanced lipid solubility in comparison with morphine, fentanyl has a rapid onset of action (within 30 seconds) and short duration of action. Because fentanyl is so highly lipid-soluble, it is rapidly and extensively distributed to tissues. High concentrations are rapidly achieved in well-perfused tissue. Termination of the effects of fentanyl is achieved by rapid redistribution to fat and skeletal muscle, with an associated decline in plasma concentrations.[171]

Thus, the short duration of action of a single dose of fentanyl reflects rapid tissue uptake with rapid redistribution and fall of plasma concentrations. With repetitive dosing or continuous infusion of fentanyl, there may be progressive saturation of inactive fat and muscle depots. Systemic accumulation occurs, and the decline in plasma concentration is slower with an associated prolongation of pharmacologic effect. The decline in plasma concentration of fentanyl thus reflects elimination and not distribution.[172]

Fentanyl is metabolized by dealkylation, hydroxylation, and amide hydrolysis to norfentanyl and despropionylnorfentanyl, which are excreted in the bile and urine.[173] Less than 8 percent of a dose of fentanyl is excreted unchanged in the urine. In contradistinction to meperidine, the nor-metabolites of fentanyl are inactive and have no CNS stimulant effects.[173] Thus, fentanyl is a drug of choice for patients with renal disease.[174]

Despite its short duration of action, the elimination half-life of fentanyl is 185–219 minutes and reflects a large volume of distribution (Table 8-7). The large volume of distribution is due to the high lipid solubility of fentanyl. Cirrhosis fails to prolong significantly the elimination half-life.[175] A prolonged elimination half-life is seen in the elderly due to decreased clearance of fentanyl.[176] In the elderly, the volume of distribution is not changed in comparison with younger adults.[176,177] Thus, the effects of fentanyl will be prolonged in the elderly.

PHARMACOLOGIC EFFECTS

Fentanyl is a CNS depressant producing marked analgesia and respiratory depression. Quite interestingly, although a cogener of meperidine, fentanyl has poor hypnotic and sedative activity at low doses (1–2 µg/kg) (Table 8-9). At high doses not used in analgesic practice (50–150 µg/kg), sedation and unconsciousness result.

Although fentanyl is approximately 100 times more potent than morphine when administered parenterally, the same degree of respiratory depression is achieved when both drugs are administered in equianalgesic doses.

In comparison with morphine, administration of fentanyl does not release histamine even at large doses.[95] Bradycardia occurs with fentanyl, although profound bradycardia will only occur with anesthetic doses of fentanyl.[178]

CLINICAL USES AND PHARMACEUTICAL PREPARATIONS

Fentanyl citrate is available for injection in a concentration of 50 µg/ml. Fentanyl is also available as a fixed-dose preparation with droperidol (Innovar), although this combination has little use for postoperative pain management.

There is extensive experience with use of fentanyl via the IV (see Ch. 10), epidural, and subarachnoid routes of administration (see Chs. 11 and 12). The pharmacokinetics of fentanyl after IM injection have not been described.

In the past, fentanyl was not used for oral administration because of its significant first-pass metabolism and poor bioavailability (32 percent).[79] However, a new preparation, oral transmucosal fentanyl citrate (OTFC), has enhanced bioavailability (52 percent).[179] It has been used as a preoperative pediatric sedative[180,181] and as an analgesic for breakthrough pain in cancer patients.[182,183] To date, preparations have ranged in dosage from 10 to 25 µg/kg.[183–186] At these dosages, side effects include mild facial pruritus (65–85 percent), mild generalized pruritus (10–30 percent), and an appreciable incidence of vomiting (30–37 percent).[183–186] While not used for postoperative pain management, as yet, OTFC has proven effective as an adjunctive analgesic and sedative in the emergency room setting.[186] Recently, however, intranasal on-demand administration of fentanyl has been described for the management of postoperative pain.[187]

TRANSDERMAL FENTANYL

The development of the transdermal therapeutic system (TTS) for estrogen, clonidine, and scopalamine fostered interest in the delivery of lipophilic opioids by this system.[188] Fentanyl's lipophilicity and paucity of sedation-related and cardiovascular side effects make it attractive for transdermal delivery.

Four systems have been developed to provide effective transdermal delivery.[189] The TTS-fentanyl patch uses the membrane permeation model (Fig. 8-22). A drug reservoir containing fentanyl is formed from a shallow compartment molded from impermeable laminate. The open surface of the compartment is covered by a microporous rate-limiting membrane. Skin contact is made with

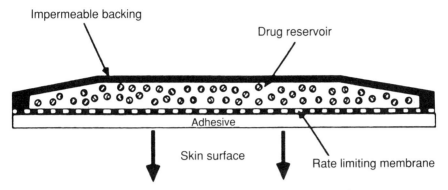

Impermeable backing

Drug reservoir

Adhesive

Skin surface

Rate limiting membrane

Fig. 8-22. Membrane permeation transdermal delivery system. (From Tarver and Stanley,[189] with permission.)

an adhesive polymer coated on the outer surface of the membrane. Large amounts of fentanyl (up to 10 mg) are present in a gel matrix within the reservoir to provide a driving force for diffusion. Increasing dose requirements are obtained by increasing the surface area of the TTS-fentanyl patch and correlate with sustained infusion rates of 25, 50, 75, and 100 μg/h over 3 days.[188]

The major obstacle to diffusion is the strateum corneum, where diffusion occurs primarily via the intracellular lipid medium.[190] The dermis acts as a reservoir that requires filling before sustained systemic absorption. As a depot is established, absorption continues when the patch is removed.[188]

Once the TTS-fentanyl patch is applied, the plasma fentanyl concentration increases over 12–18 hours until a plateau develops. (This corresponds to the formation of a fentanyl reservoir within the dermis.) The plasma fentanyl concentration will remain constant until the patch is discontinued. The plasma concentration will slowly decrease, with an apparent half-life of 15–21 hours (again, corresponding to depletion of the fentanyl depot).[190–192]

In all studies of postoperative pain to date,[191–196] opioid requirements have been reduced by concomitant use of the TTS-fentanyl patch. Side effects have included nausea and vomiting (30–85 percent) and respiratory depression.[191,193–195]

The advantages and disadvantages of the TTS-fentanyl patch are listed in Table 8-12. In our experience at Brigham and Women's Hospital, the inability to titrate dosage is a major drawback of this modality. The effective management of acute pain demands the ability to "titrate" dosage to maximize pain relief. Unfortunately, the TTS-fentanyl patch has the same deficiencies as other fixed-dose systems, effectively rendering it unsuitable for postoperative pain management (in our estimation). However, the true niche for transdermal administration of fentanyl may lie in the treatment of cancer pain. The administration of transdermal fentanyl may be an effective intermediate step for escalation from oral to SC administration.

TABLE 8-12. Advantages and Disadvantages of the TTS-Fentanyl Patch for Postoperative Pain Management

Advantages	Disadvantages
Decreased first-pass metabolism	Inability to "titrate" according to increasing
Stable plasma concentrations	or decreasing analgesic requirements
Improved patient compliance	Preselected dose
Ease of administration	Slow onset
Multiday dosage	Requirement for supplemental analgesics
Administration system does not require	Residual depot after patch removal
needles	Abuse potential
Effective analgesic technique	

Sufentanil

Sufentanil (Fig. 8-19) is a thiamyl analogue of fentanyl and a member of the phenylpiperidine series of synthetic opioids. Sufentanil is five to 10 times more potent than fentanyl, corresponding to the receptor binding affinity of the two opioids.[197]

PHARMACOKINETICS

The high lipid solubility of sufentanil (partition coefficient, 1,250) is consistent with its rapid penetration of the blood-brain barrier and rapid onset of analgesia. The high tissue affinity (consistent with the lipophilicity of the drug) causes rapid distribution. Similar to fentanyl, rapid redistribution to inactive tissue sites (fat, skeletal muscle) terminates the effect of small doses.[198]

Sufentanil is rapidly metabolized by N-dealkylation at the piperidine nitrogen and by O-demethylation.[199] The products of N-dealkylation are inactive. Desmethylsufentanil is produced from O-demethylation and has approximately 10 percent of the activity of sufentanil. Less than 1 percent of a dose of sufentanil is excreted unchanged in the urine.[199]

Sufentanil metabolites are equally excreted in urine and feces. Thirty percent of the excretory products are conjugated, presumably conjugates of desmethylsufentanil. The substantial amount of conjugated metabolite and the production of an active metabolite suggest caution with respect to use in patients with renal disease.[200,201]

The volume of distribution of sufentanil is slightly smaller and the elimination half-life shorter than fentanyl. Sufentanil is extensively protein-bound (90 percent). The clearance of sufentanil is decreased in the elderly, but as the volume of distribution is reduced, elimination half-life is not prolonged.[202] However, a prolonged effect can still occur in elderly patients.[202]

PHARMACOLOGIC EFFECTS

The clinical pharmacologic profile of sufentanil is very similar to fentanyl. Sufentanil is more sedating than fentanyl. Otherwise, sufentanil predictably produces bradycardia, miosis, respiratory depression, nausea and vomiting, and smooth muscle spasm.

Sufentanil citrate is available for injection in a concentration of 50 μg/ml. At present no oral preparation is available. The transdermal administration of sufentanil is under study.[203,204]

There is limited experience with the use of sufentanil for postoperative analgesia. With this in mind, the greatest experience with sufentanil is found with patient-controlled analgesia[205,206] and epidural analgesia.[207,208]

Alfentanil

Alfentanil (Fig. 8-20) is a cogener of fentanyl. Alfentanil is between five and 10 times less potent and has one-third the duration of action of fentanyl.[209]

PHARMACOKINETICS

The salient pharmacokinetic properties of alfentanil that explain its clinical characteristics are its low pH (6.5) and small volume of distribution.[209–211] The onset of analgesia after IV administration of alfentanil is very rapid (1–2 minutes). This can be explained on the basis of its low pKa, such that almost 90 percent of the drug is unionized at pH = 7.4 (Table 8-7). Because of the large ionized fraction, alfentanil rapidly penetrates the blood-brain barrier despite its only moderate lipid solubility.

The volume of distribution of alfentanil is four to five times smaller than that of fentanyl.[209,210] The reduced tissue affinity reflects the lower lipid solubility and greater protein binding of alfentanil.

The short duration of action of alfentanil results from redistribution to inactive tissue sites and hepatic metabolism identical to that described for sufentanil. Less than 1 percent of a dose of alfentanil is recovered unchanged in the urine.

The elimination half-life of alfentanil is 70–98 minutes.[210] The elimination half-life is increased to 219 minutes in patients with cirrhosis.[212] In addition, the unbound fraction of alfentanil is increased in patients with liver disease due to the alteration of protein binding sites.[21] The prolonged elimination half-life and increased free fraction of alfentanil in cirrhotics could result in an exaggerated or prolonged effect of the drug. In patients with renal disease, alfentanil clearance is unaltered. However, the volume of distribution may change depending on alterations in protein binding. Thus, the elimination of alfentanil is unaffected by renal disease, but changes in protein binding may affect drug distribution.

CLINICAL USES AND PHARMACEUTICAL PREPARATIONS

Like sufentanil, alfentanil has been best studied with epidural analgesia[213,214] and IV-PCA.[206,215,216]

Alfentanil's short duration of action may make it unsuitable for delivery via PCA. Its rapid penetration of the blood-brain barrier allows for rapid analgesia.

However, its short duration of action may require excessive demand dosing, with subsequent exhaustion of the patient with the whole process of PCA.[216] Unfortunately, provision of a background infusion to lower patient demand has been unsuccessful in achieving superior analgesia.[215,216]

At the present time, alfentanil is available only for injection in a concentration of 500 μg/ml.

Methadone (Dolphine)

Methadone was originally synthesized by the German pharmaceutical industry during World War II. The two-dimensional structure of methadone does not remotely resemble morphine (Fig. 8-23). However, steric factors force the molecule to simulate a pseudopiperidine ring configuration. (The piperidine ring structure appears to be essential for opioid activity.[72]) The levorotatory isomer is between eight and 50 times more potent than the dextrorotatory isomer and is responsible for the analgesic efficacy of the racemate.[72]

PHARMACOKINETICS

Methadone has good oral bioavailability (41–90 percent).[217,218] Methadone can be detected in the plasma 30 minutes after oral ingestion, and time to peak concentration is approximately 4 hours.[219] The onset of analgesia occurs 30–60 minutes after oral ingestion.

After SC injection, appreciable concentrations of methadone can be found in the plasma within 10 minutes. Peak concentrations occur in the brain 1–2 hours after parenteral administration.[72]

Methadone undergoes extensive biotransformation in the liver via N-demethylation and cyclization to form pyrolidines and pyrroline. The inactive metabolites are excreted in the urine and the bile with small amounts of unchanged drug.[220,221] The excretion of methadone in the urine can be enhanced by acidification of the urine.[222]

Methadone is highly bound to plasma and tissue proteins. After repeated

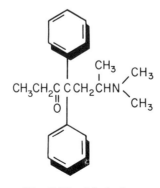

Fig. 8-23. Methadone.

administration or infusion, there is gradual accumulation in tissue. Gradual release from these binding sites maintains plasma concentrations of methadone and explains its slow clearance (Table 8-7).[221,223] After a single IV dose, methadone has an elimination half-life of 14 hours with a secondary half-life of 55 hours (from release of tissue stores).[221] With chronic administration, a single elimination half-life of 22 hours is found.[221]

PHARMACOLOGIC EFFECTS

The clinical pharmacologic profile of methadone is similar to morphine. Despite an initial half-life of 14 hours with acute dosing, the duration of analgesia is 4–6 hours.[224] With repeated usage, cumulative effects are seen (release of methadone from tissue stores). Thus, dosage would need to be adjusted downward or the dosing interval prolonged with chronic oral administration. The oral to parenteral potency ratio for methadone is 1:2.[224]

CLINICAL USES AND PHARMACEUTICAL PREPARATIONS

Methadone is an excellent analgesic and is superb for treatment of chronic pain.[225,226] While there has been some study of the epidural administration of methadone,[227,228] little work has been performed with methadone administered via IV-PCA. In a series of reports, however, Gourlay et al[223,229,230] demonstrated that intermittent IV methadone was very effective in the management of postoperative pain.

Methadone hydrochloride is available in 5-mg and 10-mg tablets and as an oral solution (10 mg/tsp). Methadone hydrochloride is available for injection in a concentration of 10 mg/ml.

Propoxyphene (Darvon, Darvocet, Wygesic)

Propoxyphene (Fig. 8-24) is structurally similar to methadone but is a weak analgesic and is found only in oral preparations. There are four stereoisomers with only the α-racemate having analgesic activity. Unlike methadone, only the dextrorotatory form has analgesic activity.[72]

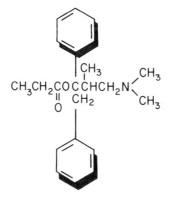

Fig. 8-24. Propoxyphene.

PHARMACOKINETICS

Propoxyphene undergoes extensive first-pass metabolism, and oral bioavailability is limited to between 30 and 70 percent. Metabolism of propoxyphene occurs by demethylation to yield norpropoxyphene, which is slowly excreted in the urine. (The half-life of norpropoxyphene is approximately 23 hours.) The half-life of propoxyphene itself is 14.6 hours. Thus, with repeated dosing the concentration of norpropoxyphene can be four times that of propoxyphene.[231]

CLINICAL USES AND PHARMACEUTICAL PREPARATIONS

The only clinical use of propoxyphene is as a mild oral analgesic. Doses of 90–120 mg propoxyphene are equianalgesic to 60 mg codeine or 600 mg aspirin.[232] Propoxyphene has no antipyretic or anti-inflammatory activity. Its antitussive effects are insignificant.

Propoxyphene hydrochloride is available in 32-mg and 65-mg tablets. Propoxyphene napsylate is available as 100-mg tablets or as a suspension.

OPIOID AGONIST-ANTAGONISTS

The agonist-antagonist opioids can be divided into two groups based on their intrinsic activity (Table 8-5). The mixed agonist-antagonists (although this term is sometimes generically and inclusively used to describe both groups) act simultaneously as an agonist at one receptor and as an antagonist at another. The mixed agonist-antagonists include nalbuphine, pentazocine, and butorphanol. The partial agonists (buprenorphine, dezocine) produce a submaximal response at a particular receptor type (Fig. 8-5). Clinically, these two groups of agents have very similar properties. The clinical properties of the opioid agonist-antagonists and partial agonists are listed in Table 8-13.

Mixed Agonist-Antagonists

Nalbuphine (Nubain)

Nalbuphine (Fig. 8-25) is a semisynthetic mixed agonist-antagonist that is chemically related to oxymorphone and naloxone.[75]

PHARMACOKINETICS

Nalbuphine undergoes extensive first-pass metabolism with an oral bioavailability of approximately 10 percent.[233]

Nalbuphine is metabolized in the liver. An inactive glucuronide conjugate is

---

TABLE 8-13. Clinical Properties of the Opioid Agonist-Antagonists and Partial Agonists

Reduced analgesic efficacy as compared with pure μ-agonists
Both analgesia and respiratory depression exhibit ceiling effects
Antagonist properties may be used to reverse μ-agonist effects (respiratory depression, pruritus, nausea and vomiting) while still preserving analgesia
Dysphoric reactions
Low addiction potential

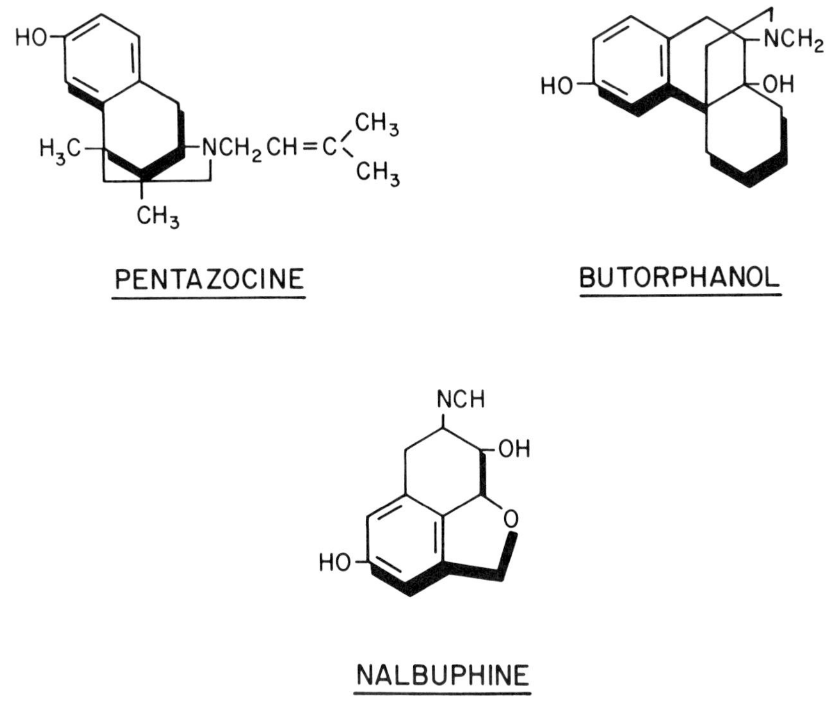

PENTAZOCINE

BUTORPHANOL

NALBUPHINE

Fig. 8-25. Mixed agonist-antagonists.

the major metabolite. Fecal excretion is the primary source of elimination of nalbuphine and its metabolites. Only 7 percent of a single dose of nalbuphine is excreted in the urine as unchanged nalbuphine and metabolites.[233] The elimination half-life of nalbuphine is 3–6 hours.[234]

PHARMACOLOGIC EFFECTS

Nalbuphine is primarily a partial agonist at the κ-receptor. This receptor interaction is responsible for its analgesic properties. Nalbuphine is an antagonist at the μ-receptor.[235]

Nalbuphine produces analgesia comparable with morphine after IM injection (potency ratio 1:1), with a similar time of onset and duration of analgesia. At approximately 0.45 mg/kg, no further analgesia or respiratory depression is attendant to increased dosing.[236]

The analgesic efficacy of subsequently administered μ-agonists may be compromised by nalbuphine. Nalbuphine can also precipitate withdrawal symptoms in individuals who are physically dependent to opioids. However, the μ-antagonist activity of nalbuphine may be used to advantage to reverse the ventilatory depressant effects of μ-agonists while still maintaining analgesia.[237,238] Similarly, nalbuphine can be used to counteract the other physiologic effects of μ-agonists such as pruritus.[239,240]

Sedation is the most common side effect, occurring in about 33 percent of patients. Diaphoresis is also common. The incidence of dysphoria is less than with pentazocine or butorphanol but increases with escalating dose. In contrast to pentazocine and butorphanol, nalbuphine does not increase systemic blood pressure, pulmonary artery pressure, or heart rate.[241]

CLINICAL USES AND PHARMACEUTICAL PREPARATIONS

As stated above, nalbuphine may be very efficacious in reversing the side effects associated with μ-agonists while at the same time preserving analgesia. The experience with nalbuphine for IV-PCA[242,243] and epidural analgesia[244,245] is quite limited. Nalbuphine appears to be an effective agent for administration by IV-PCA but has had poor efficacy when administered epidurally.

With IM or IV administration, the usual adult dose is 10 mg every 3–6 hours. No more than 160 mg should be administered in any 24-hour period.

Nalbuphine hydrochloride is supplied as an injectable solution (10 mg/ml).

Pentazocine (Talwin)

Pentazocine (Fig. 8-25) is a synthetic opioid of the benzomorphan series. The levorotatory isomer of pentazocine is responsible for its analgesic properties.

PHARMACOKINETICS

Pentazocine is well absorbed after oral and parenteral administration. Oral bioavailability is only 20 percent, however, due to extensive first-pass hepatic metabolism.[246] Pentazocine is metabolized by oxidation of terminal methyl groups. Resultant inactive glucuronide conjugates, along with unchanged pentazocine (5–25 percent of the dose), are excreted in the urine. Less than 2 percent of a dose of pentazocine undergoes biliary excretion.[247]

PHARMACOLOGIC EFFECTS

Pentazocine is an agonist at κ-receptors (responsible for analgesia) and at σ-receptors (producing psychotomimetic and dysphoric effects). Pentazocine is one-half to one-third as potent as morphine after parenteral administration. Sedation (a κ-agonist effect) and diaphoresis are common. Hallucinations or psychotomimetic effects ("active thoughts," depersonalization, feelings of impending doom) have been reported, especially at high doses.[248]

Pentazocine produces a similar degree of respiratory depression when compared with equianalgesic dosages of μ-agonists. Pentazocine does exhibit the ceiling effect for respiratory depression and analgesic effect characteristic of the mixed agonist-antagonists. Doses of pentazocine greater than 30 mg do not produce a proportionate increase in respiratory depression. The ceiling effect is achieved at 60 mg in the adult 70-kg human.[249,250]

Pentazocine does not produce hypotension or bradycardia. Increased blood pressure, heart rate, and pulmonary artery pressure have been shown after pentazocine administration.[241,250]

Pentazocine's effect on biliary pressure appears to be milder than that of the μ-agonists.[251,252]

Although abuse potential is low, pentazocine can cause physical dependence and addiction. Its μ-antagonism can precipitate withdrawal in individuals with physical dependence to opioids.

CLINICAL USES AND PHARMACEUTICAL PREPARATIONS

Pentazocine lactate is available for injection in a concentration of 30 mg/ml. Pentazocine hydrochloride is available for oral ingestion compounded with acetylsalicylic acid (12.5 mg pentazocine with 325 mg acetylsalicylic acid) or naloxone (Talwin NX: 50 mg pentazocine hydrochloride with 0.5 mg naloxone.)[72]

The usual adult dose of pentazocine is 30 mg for IM injection and 50 mg every 3–4 hours when administered orally. Fifty mg oral pentazocine is equianalgesic to 60 mg codeine.[72] Pentazocine has been incompletely studied for use via epidural analgesia or administration by IV-PCA.

Butorphanol (Stadol)

Butorphanol (Fig. 8-25) is a synthetic mixed agonist-antagonist of the morphinan series. Compared with pentazocine, the agonist effects of butorphanol are 20 times greater. The antagonist potency is 10–30 times that of pentazocine.[253]

PHARMACOKINETICS

Pharmacokinetic data is sparse for butorphanol. Butorphanol is rapidly and almost completely absorbed after IM injection. The distribution half-life is about 5 minutes, and the terminal distribution half-life is about 160 minutes with a high plasma clearance.[254,255]

Butorphanol is metabolized to hydroxybutorphanol and norbutorphanol. Both metabolites are inactive. Renal excretion accounts for 25 percent of the elimination of butorphanol. Butorphanol is approximately 85 percent bound to plasma proteins.[254,255]

Oral bioavailability is low because of extensive first-pass metabolism.

PHARMACOLOGIC EFFECTS

Butorphanol has low affinity for the μ-receptor (antagonist), moderate affinity for the κ-receptor (producing analgesia), and minimal affinity for the σ-receptor (low incidence of dysphoric reactions).[253] Butorphanol is three to five times more potent an analgesic than morphine.

As with the other mixed agonist-antagonists, sedation and diaphorisis are common. Butorphanol exhibits the ceiling effect for respiratory depression and analgesia characteristic for the mixed agonist-antagonists.[254] Like pentazocine, butorphanol increases systemic blood pressure, heart rate, and pulmonary artery pressure.[241,256] Like pentazocine, the effects of butorphanol on the biliary tract appear milder than those of the μ-agonists.[89]

With respect to analgesia, it is difficult to effectively use a μ-agonist as an analgesic after having received butorphanol. Reversal of respiratory depression as accomplished with nalbuphine has not been reported with butorphanol. However, other μ-agonist-related side effects such as pruritus have been reversed with parenteral administration of butorphanol.[257]

CLINICAL USES AND PHARMACEUTICAL PREPARATIONS

Butorphanol is indicated for moderate to severe pain. The recommended IM dose is 1–2 mg every 3–4 hours; the recommended IV dose is 0.5–2.0 mg every 3–4 hours. Butorphanol is only available for parenteral use in solutions containing 1 or 2 mg/ml.

Butorphanol has been fairly well studied via the epidural route of administration, particularly after cesarean delivery.[258–260] Two milligrams of butorphanol in 10 ml preservative-free normal saline will provide good analgesia. Sedation is associated with epidural butorphanol and is particularly present at higher doses.[258]

Partial Agonists

Buprenorphine (Buprenex)

Buprenorphine (Fig. 8-26) is a semisynthetic opioid derived from the opium alkaloid thebaine.

PHARMACOKINETICS

Buprenorphine is highly lipophilic.[261] As described previously in this chapter, the kinetics of the analgesic response after parenteral administration of buprenorphine are not governed by global pharmacokinetics but rather by the kinetics of receptor dissociation.[41,44] Buprenorphine slowly dissociates from the μ-receptor. This slow receptor dissociation is responsible for buprenorphine's prolonged duration of effect, which would not be predicted from the elimination

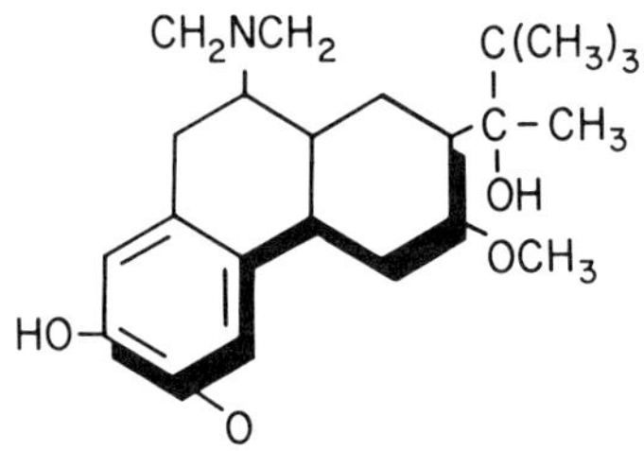

Fig. 8-26. Buprenorphine.

half-life (3–5 hours).[262,263] Thus, there is no direct relationship between plasma concentrations of buprenorphine and its pharmacologic effect.[263]

Buprenorphine is approximately 96 percent bound to plasma proteins.[263]

PHARMACOLOGIC EFFECTS

Buprenorphine is highly potent, with 0.3 mg being equianalgesic to 10 mg of morphine after IM administration. Buprenorphine is a partial agonist at the μ-receptor. However, the affinity of buprenorphine for the μ-receptor is approximately 50 times greater than that of morphine.[264]

The side effects of buprenorphine resemble those of the mixed agonist-antagonists. Sedation or drowsiness occurs in almost 50 percent of patients. The incidence of nausea and vomiting is between 10 and 20 percent.[262] As it is not a σ-receptor agonist, buprenorphine is not associated with psychotomimetic and dysphoric reactions.

A respiratory depressant ceiling effect has been described with buprenorphine. As buprenorphine has great binding affinity for the μ-receptor, respiratory depression may be prolonged.[265,266] Once again because of binding affinity, only high doses of naloxone will reverse the respiratory depressant effects of buprenorphine.[267] Doxapram may be a useful agent to maintain adequate ventilation in patients receiving significant amounts of buprenorphine.[268] Being a partial agonist, however, buprenorphine partially reverses the effects of large doses of μ-agonists and can reverse respiratory depression associated with these opioids.[269]

The cardiovascular effects of buprenorphine are much the same as those of morphine.

CLINICAL USES AND PHARMACEUTICAL PREPARATIONS

Buprenorphine is usually administered IV or IM in recommended doses of 0.3 mg every 6 hours. Parenteral buprenorphine is effective in relieving moderate to severe postoperative pain[270,271] and pain of renal colic, cancer, and myocardial infarction.[271]

Sublingual buprenorphine is available in Europe. Recommended doses are 0.4–0.8 mg. Sublingual "demand" (PCA) buprenorphine has achieved good postoperative analgesia.[272]

Theoretically, buprenorphine would be a poor drug for administration by IV-PCA.[273] Buprenorphine has a slow onset of analgesia. Once analgesia is achieved, it should be protracted because of the μ-receptor binding affinity of buprenorphine. Thus, the latency of response to each dose may lead to overadministration with development of protracted respiratory depression.[273] However, two recent studies find excellent analgesia and minimal respiratory depression associated with buprenorphine administered by IV-PCA.[274,275]

The use of epidural buprenorphine has been described after cesarean delivery[276,277] and for postoperative orthopaedic pain.[261,278] Like nalbuphine and butorphanol, buprenorphine has been used to reverse pruritus associated with

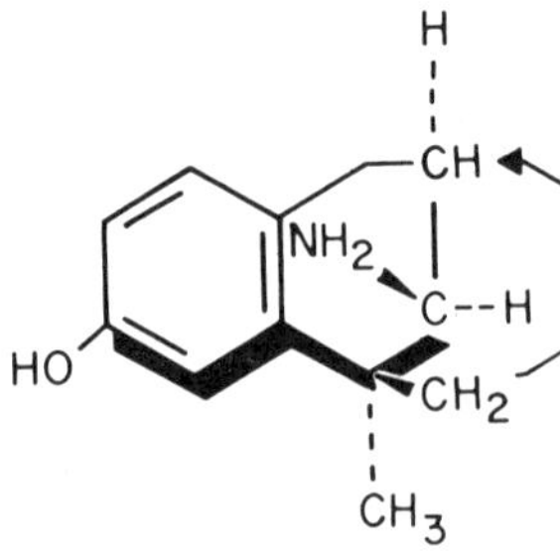

Fig. 8-27. Dezocine.

epidural administration of μ-agonists.[279] A single study examines the use of subarachnoid buprenorphine for analgesia after cesarean delivery.[280]

Buprenorphine hydrochloride is available in solution in a concentration of 0.3 mg/ml.

Dezocine (Dalgan)

Dezocine (Fig. 8-27) is a potent synthetic partial agonist of the morphinan series.

PHARMACOKINETICS

There is only one study of the pharmacokinetics of dezocine in humans.[280] Dezocine has rapid initial distribution followed by slow terminal elimination. Dezocine has a large volume of distribution, indicating extensive tissue uptake. Elimination occurs through a combination of renal excretion of intact drug and hepatic metabolism.[281]

PHARMACOLOGIC EFFECTS

The mechanism of action of dezocine involves partial μ-agonism.[282] Dezocine is a δ-agonist with partial μ-agonism and minimal to no κ-agonist activity, and unlike nalbuphine, pentazocine, and butorphanol, dezocine increases analgesia when administered after μ-agonists.[283] Dezocine is equipotent to morphine after parenteral administration. The analgesic effects of dezocine have been quickly reversed by naloxone in both laboratory and clinical studies.[284,285] (Dezocine does not bind as tightly to μ-receptors as buprenorphine.)

The most common side effects of dezocine are those characteristic of the agonist-antagonists in general: sedation (which may be prolonged), nausea, and vomiting. The sedation produced by 10–15 mg of IM dezocine is maximal at about 1 hour after administration.[286] Although there is one report of a dysphoric reaction after high doses of dezocine,[287] there is little affinity for the σ-receptor.

Respiratory depression associated with increasing doses of dezocine reaches a ceiling.[283,284] Doses higher than 0.3 mg/kg are not associated with increased analgesia or respiratory depression.[288]

At present the cardiovascular effects of dezocine are not fully elucidated. In a single study of patients undergoing cardiac catheterization, dezocine (0.125 mg/kg) resulted in a transient increase in mean pulmonary artery pressure and pulmonary vascular resistance.[289] Dezocine caused no change in heart rate or systemic blood pressure.[288]

The addiction liability of dezocine is thought to be minimal,[289] although there is some controversy about its abuse potential.[290,291] The ability of dezocine to precipitate withdrawal in opioid-dependent patients has not been studied.

CLINICAL USES AND PHARMACEUTICAL PREPARATIONS

Dezocine lactate is available as a solution in a concentration of 5, 10, and 15 mg/ml. Although several clinical trials have been conducted with parenteral administration of dezocine for postoperative analgesia,[292–295] the exact role of dezocine in the armanentarium of postoperative pain management remains to be determined. There is no experience with dezocine via PCA or epidural administration.

ANTAGONISTS

Minor changes in the chemical structure of a μ-agonist can transform the agonist into an antagonist at one or more opioid receptor types.[75] Naloxone is the N-allyl-($-CH_2-CH=CH_2$)-derivative of oxymorphone (Fig. 8-15). Naltrexone possesses cyclopropylmethyl substitution ($-CH_2-\triangleleft$) on the tertiary nitrogen. Other opioid antagonists exist (nalorphine [the first available antagonist],[296] nalmefene,[297] and cholecystokinin[298]) but will not be discussed.

Naloxone and naltrexone are pure antagonists at μ-, κ-, σ-, and δ-receptors. Both naloxone and naltrexone have high affinity for μ-receptors. Their affinity for δ-receptors and κ-receptors is less, but they can still displace agonists from these receptors. Once displaced, naloxone and naltrexone do not activate opioid receptors, thereby producing antagonism.

Parenteral Antagonists

Naloxone (Narcan)

PHARMACOKINETICS

The IV administration of 1–4 μg/kg of naloxone will reverse opioid-induced analgesia and respiratory depression. The duration of action is short (30–45 minutes) and is believed to result from dissociation and rapid removal of naloxone from receptors in the brain.[299] Thus, supplementation of the initial dose of naloxone is usually necessary if sustained antagonism is desired.

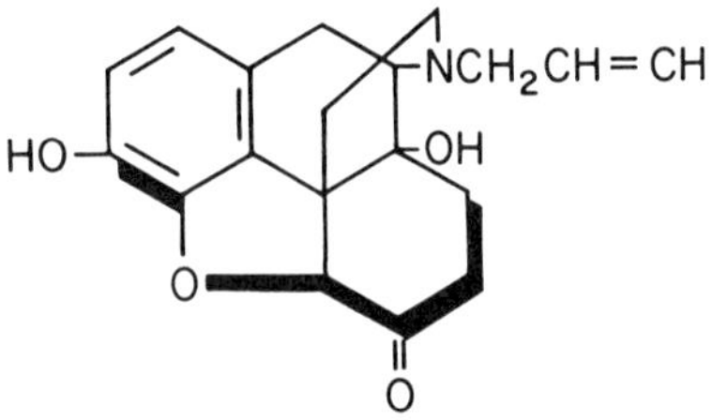

Fig. 8-28. Naloxone.

Naloxone (Fig. 8-28) is primarily metabolized in the liver. The elimination half-life is 64 minutes.[300] Naloxone undergoes extensive first-pass metabolism when administered orally.

PHARMACOLOGIC EFFECTS

For opioids administered by indirect delivery systems (i.e., non-neuraxial) (Table 8-6), naloxone results in antagonism of opioid-induced respiratory depression in association with a concomitant reversal of analgesia. By titration of dosage, it may be possible to obtain partial analgesia with "acceptable" antagonism of respiratory depression. However, nausea, vomiting, and cardiovascular stimulation can still accompany partial reversal of analgesia.

For opioids delivered epidurally, a gradation of effect is seen with increasing doses of naloxone. Naloxone infusions of 5µg/kg/h have been shown not to affect the quality of analgesia of epidural morphine while reversing respiratory depression.[301] An infusion rate of 10 µg/kg/h will affect the quality of analgesia with epidural morphine.[301] Infusion rates of both 5 and 10 µg/kg/h will reverse the analgesia and respiratory depression of patients receiving epidural fentanyl.[302] The reasons for this differential effect between morphine and fentanyl are obscure.

Nausea and vomiting appear to be closely related to the dose and speed of injection of naloxone.[303,304] Administering low doses every 2–3 minutes will reduce the incidence of nausea and vomiting.

Cardiovascular stimulation will occur after administration of naloxone. This will manifest as activation of the sympathetic nervous system: tachycardia, hypertension, pulmonary edema, and cardiac arrhythmias.[305–307]

CLINICAL USES AND PHARMACEUTICAL PREPARATIONS

For the patient with sedation and respiratory depression (rate, <8 breaths/ min), naloxone should be administered intravenously in an initial dose of 10 µg. This dose should be progressively doubled every 2–3 minutes (20–40–80–160, etc.) until arousal and respiratory rate are deemed sufficient. A naloxone infusion or repetitive dosing will then be necessary. For apneic and unarousable patients, 0.4 mg should be administered parenterally, preferably IV.

Naloxone hydrochloride is available in solution in concentrations of 0.02 mg/

ml, 0.4 mg/ml, and 1 mg/ml. An ampule containing 0.4 mg/ml is found most commonly on adult nursing floors.

Oral Antagonists

Naltrexone (Trexan)

Naltrexone, in contradistinction to naloxone, is very effective when given orally and can produce sustained opioid antagonism for as long as 24 hours.[308] It is available in 50-mg tablets. Naltrexone has been used in the treatment of opioid addiction.[308]

CONCLUSION

Opioids, along with local anesthetics and nonsteroidal anti-inflammatory drugs, form the cornerstone of effective pharmacologic management of postoperative pain. The reader, if an anesthesiologist, may wonder about the generous effort spent in this chapter in the discussion of opioids with minimal applicability to parenteral or spinal (epidural and subarachnoid) administration. However, the philosophic tenet of this book is that the practitioner of postoperative pain management (the analgesiologist, if you will) must be a *complete* expert. Postoperative pain management continues after the cessation of sophisticated and invasive techniques. This necessitates a thorough knowledge, and not a circumscribed knowledge, of opioid pharmacology. This chapter is presented in the hopes of providing such a background.

References

1. Tainter ML: Pain. Ann NY Acad Sci 51:3, 1948
2. Macht DI: The history of opium and some of its preparations and alkaloids. JAMA 46:477, 1915
3. Thorpe DH: Opiate structure and activity—a guide to understanding the receptor. Anesth Analg 63:143, 1984
4. Braenden OJ, Eddy NB, Halbach H: Synthetic substances with morphine-like effect; relationship between chemical structure and analgesic action. Bull WHO 13:937, 1955
5. Janssen PAJ: A review of the chemical features associated with strong morphine-like activity. Br J Anaesth 34:260, 1962
6. Beckett AH, Casey AF: Synthetic analgesics, stereochemical considerations. J Pharm Pharmacol 6:986, 1954
7. Fields HL: Central nervous system mechanisms for control of pain transmission. p. 99. In: Pain. McGraw-Hill, New York, 1987
8. Leysen JE, Gommeren W, Niemegeers CJ: [³H]Sufentanil, a superior ligand for mu-opiate receptors: binding properties and regional distribution in rat brain and spinal cord. Eur J Pharmacol 87:209, 1983
9. Kosterlitz HW: Opiate actions in guinea pig ileum and mouse vas deferens. Neurosci Res Program Bull 13:68, 1975
10. Martin WR, Eades CG, Thompson JA et al: The effects of morphine- and nalor-

phine-like drugs in the nondependent and morphine-dependent chronic spinal dog. J Pharmacol Exp Ther 197:517, 1976

11. Gilbert PE, Martin WR: The effects of morphine- and nalorphine-like drugs in the nondependent, morphine-dependent and cyclazocine-dependent spinal dog. J Pharmacol Exp Ther 198:66, 1976

12. Maze M: Clinical implications of membrane receptor function in anesthesia. Anesthesiology 51:160, 1980

13. Vaught JL, Rothman RB, Westfall TC: Mu and delta receptors: their role in analgesia and in the differential effects of opiod peptides on analgesia. Life Sci 30:1443, 1982

14. Pasternack GW, Wood PJ: Multiple mu opiate receptors. Life Sci 38:1889, 1986

15. Pasternack GW: Multiple morphine and enkephalin receptors and the relief of pain. JAMA 259:1362, 1988

16. Goodman RR, Snyder SH, Kuhar MJ et al: Differentiation of delta and mu opiate receptor localizations by light microscopic autoradiography. Proc Natl Acad Sci USA 77:6239, 1988

17. Duka T, Schubert P, Wuster M et al: A selective distribution pattern of different opiate receptors in certain areas of rat brain as revealed by in vitro autoradiography. Neurosci Lett 21:119, 1981

18. Quirion R, Zajac JM, Morgat JL et al: Autoradiographic distribution of mu- and delta-opiate receptors in rat brain using highly selective ligands. Life Sci, suppl.1, 33:227, 1983

19. Wood PL, Richard JW, Thakur M: Mu-opiate isoreceptors: differentiation with kappa agonists. Life Sci 31:2313, 1982

20. Pasternak GW, Childer SR, Snyder SH: Opiate analgesia: evidence for mediation by a subpopulation of opiate receptors. Science 208:514, 1980

21. Nishimura SL, Recht LD, Pasternak GW: Biochemical characterization of high affinity ^{3}H-opioid binding: further evidence for mu_1 sites. Mol Pharmacol 25:29, 1984

22. Pasternak GW, Childer SR, Snyder RH: Naloxazone, a long-acting opiate antagonist: effects in intact animals and on opiate receptor binding in vitro. J Pharmacol Exp Ther 214:455, 1980

23. Yaksh TL: Analgesic actions of intrathecal opiates in cats and primates. Brain Res 153:205, 1978

24. Yaksh TL: In vivo studies on spinal opiate receptor systems mediating antinociception: I. Mu- and delta-receptor profiles in the primate. J Pharmacol Exp Ther 226:303, 1983

25. Yaksh TL, Huang SP, Rudy TA et al: The direct and specific opiate-like effect of met-enkaphalin and analogs on the spinal cord. Neuroscience 2:593, 1977

26. Moulin DE, Max M, Kaiko RF: The analgesic efficacy of intrathecal (IT) [D-Ala^2, D-Leu^5] enkephalin in cancer patients with chronic pain. Pain 23:213, 1985

27. Dickenson AH: A new approach to pain relief? Nature 320:681, 1986

28. Schwartz JC: Metabolism of enkephalins and the inactivating neuropeptidase concept. Trends Neurosci 6:45, 1983

29. Pert CB, Pert A, Chang JK et al: [D-Ala^2]-met-enkephalinamide: a potent, long-lasting synthetic pentapeptide analgesic. Science 194:330, 1974

30. Martin WR: Opioid antagonists. Pharmacol Rev 19:463, 1967

31. Hameroff SR: Opiate receptor pharmacology: mixed agonist-antagonist narcotics. Contemp Anesth Pract 7:27, 1983

32. Freye E: Opioid Agonists Antagonists and Mixed Narcotic Analgesics: Theoretical Background and Considerations for Practical Use. Springer-Verlag, Berlin, 1987

33. Schmidt WK, Tam SW, Shotzberger GS et al: Nalbuphine. Drug Alcohol Depend 14:339, 1985

34. Herz A, Teschemacher HJ: Activities and sites of antinociceptive action of morphine-like analgesics and kinetics of distribution following intravenous intracerebral and intraventricular application. Adv Drug Res 6:79, 1971

35. Simon EJ, Hiller JM: The opiate receptors. Annu Rev Pharmacol Toxicol 18:371, 1978

36. Beaumont A, Hughes J: Biology of opioid peptides. Annu Rev Pharmacol Toxicol 19:245, 1979

37. Snyder SH: Opiate receptors in the brain. N Engl J Med 296:299, 1977

38. Sjöström S, Hartvig P, Persson MP, Tamsen A: Pharmacokinetics of epidural morphine and meperidine in humans. Anesthesiology 67:877, 1987

39. Sjöström S, Tamsen A, Persson MP, Hartvig P: Pharmacokinetics of intrathecal morphine and meperidine in humans. Anesthesiology 67:889, 1987

40. Cousins MJ: Comparative pharmacokinetics of spinal opioids in humans: a step toward determination of relative safety (editorial). Anesthesiology 67:875, 1987

41. Mather LE: Opioid pharmacokinetics in relation to their effects. Anaesth Intensive Care 15:15, 1987

42. Scott JC, Ponganis KV, Stanski DR: EEG quantitation of narcotic effect: the comparative pharmacodynamics of fentanyl and alfentanil. Anesthesiology 62:234, 1985

43. Benson DW, Kaufman JJ, Koski WS: Theoretic significance of pH dependence of narcotics and narcotic antagonists in clinical anesthesia. Anesth Analg 55:253, 1976

44. Mather LE, Owen H: The pharmacology of patient-administered opioids. p. 27. In Ferrante FM, Ostheimer GW, Covino BG (eds): Patient-Controlled Analgesia. Blackwell Scientific, Boston, 1990

45. Hermans B, Gommeren W, DePotter WP, Leysen JE: Interaction of peptides and morphine-like narcotic analgesics with specifically labelled mu- and delta-opiate receptor sites. Arch Int Pharmacodynam 262:317, 1983

46. Mather LE: Clinical pharmacokinetics of fentanyl and its newer derivatives. Clin Pharmokinet 8:422, 1983

47. Boas R, Villager JW: Clinical actions of fentanyl and buprenorphine: the significance of receptor binding. Br J Anaesth 57:192, 1985

48. McQuay HJ, Sullivan AF, Smallman K, Dickenson AH: Intrathecal opioids, potency and lipophilicity. Pain 36:111, 1989

49. Pert CB, Snyder SH: Correlation of opiate receptor affinity with analgesic effects of meperidine homologues. J Med Chem 19:1248, 1976

50. Bullingham RES, McQuay HJ, Moore RA: Clinical pharmacokinetics of narcotic agonists/antagonists. Clin Pharmacokinet 8:322, 1983

51. Hull CJ: General principles of pharmacokinetics. p. 1. In Prys-Roberts D, Hug CC (eds): Pharmacokinetics of Anaesthesia. Blackwell Scientific, Oxford, 1984

52. Foley KM: The treatment of cancer pain. N Engl J Med 313:84, 1985

53. Twycross RG, McQuay HJ: Opioids. p. 686. In Wall PD, Melzack R (eds): Textbook of Pain. 2nd Ed. Churchill Livingstone, Edinburgh, 1989

54. Austin KL, Stapleton JV, Mather LE: Relationship between blood meperidine concentrations and analgesic response: a preliminary report. Anesthesiology 53:460, 1980

55. Lehman KA: Practical experience with demand analgesia for postoperative pain. p. 134. In Harmer M, Rosen M, Vickers MD (eds): Patient Controlled Analgesia. Blackwell Scientific, Oxford, 1985

56. Ferrante FM: Patient-controlled analgesia as a research tool. p. 61. In Ferrante

FM, Ostheimer GW, Covino BG (eds): Patient-Controlled Analgesia. Blackwell Scientific, Boston, 1990

57. Beaver WT, Feise GA: A comparison of the analgesic effect of intramuscular nalbuphine and morphine in patients with postoperative pain. J Pharmacol Exp Ther 204:487, 1978

58. Hew E, Foster K, Gordon R, Hew-Sang E: A comparison of nalbuphine and meperidine in treatment of pain. Can J Anaesth 34:462, 1987

59. Brady MM, Furness G, Fee JPH: A comparison of the analgesic and sedative effects of nalbuphine and morphine following hip replacement, abstracted. Br J Anaesth 58:1332P, 1986

60. Houde RW, Wallenstein SL, Beaver WT: Evaluation of analgesics in patients with cancer pain. p. 59. In Lasagna L (ed): International Encyclopedia of Pharmacology and Therapeutics. Vol 1. Pergammon Press, New York, 1966

61. Inturrisi CE, Foley KM: Narcotic analgesics in the management of pain. p. 257. In Kuhar M, Pasternak G (eds): Analgesics: Neurochemical, Behavioral and Clinical Perspectives. Raven Press, New York, 1984

62. Sawe J, Dahlstöm B, Paalzow L, Rane A: Morphine kinetics in cancer patients. Clin Pharmacol Ther 30:629, 1981

63. Routledge PA, Shand DG: Presystemic drug elimination. Annu Rev Pharmacol Toxicol 19:447, 1979

64. Houde RW, Wallenstein SL, Beaver WT: Clinical measurement of pain. p. 75. In de Stevens G (ed): Analgetics. Academic Press, New York, 1965

65. Twycross RG: The use of narcotic analgesics in terminal illness. J Med Ethics 1: 10, 1975

66. Kaiko RF: Discussion. p. 235. In Foley K, Inturrisi CE (eds): Advances in Pain Research and Therapy. Vol. 8. Raven Press, New York, 1986

67. Urquhart ML, Klapp K, White PF: Patient-controlled analgesia: a comparison of intravenous versus subcutaneous hydromorphone. Anesthesiology 69:428, 1988

68. Mueller RA, Lundberg DBA, Breese GR et al: The neuropharmacology of respiratory control. Pharmacol Rev 34:255, 1982

69. Martin WR: Pharmacology of opioid. Pharmacol Rev 35:283, 1967

70. Bellville JW, Seed JC: The effect of drugs on the respiratory response to carbon dioxide. Anesthesiology 21:727, 1960

71. Eckenoff JE, Oech SR: The effects of narcotics and antagonists upon respiration and circulation in man. Clin Pharmacol Ther 1:483, 1960

72. Jaffe JH, Martin WR: Opioid analgesics and antagonists. p. 491. In Gilman AG, Goodman LS, Rall TW, Murad F (eds): The Pharmacological Basis of Therapeutics. 7th Ed. MacMillan, New York, 1985

73. Kitahata LM, Collins JG, Robinson CJ: Narcotic effects on the nervous system. p. 57. In Kitahata LM, Collins JG (eds): Narcotic Analgesics in Anesthesiology. William & Wilkins, Baltimore, 1982

74. Murphy MR, Hug CC Jr: The enflurance sparing effect of morphine, butorphanol and nalbuphine. Anesthesiology 57:489, 1982

75. Freye E: The various effects caused by opioids. p. 27. In: Opioid Agonists Antagonists and Mixed Narcotic Analgesics: Theoretical Background and Considerations for Practical Use. Springer-Verlag, Berlin, 1987

76. Bovill JG, Sebel PS, Wauquier A et al: Electroencephalographic effects of sufentanil anaesthesia in man. Br J Anaesth 54:45, 1982

77. World Health Organization: Expert committee on drug dependence, 16th report. Technical report series no. 407. World Health Organization, Geneva, 1969

78. Porter J, Jick J: Addiction is rare in patients treated with narcotics. N Engl J Med 302:123, 1980
79. Taub A: Opioid analgesics in the treatment of chronic intractable pain of non-neoplastic origin. p. 199. In Kitahata LM, Collins JD (eds): Narcotic Analgesics in Anesthesiology. William & Wilkins, Baltimore, 1982
80. Portenoy RK, Foley FM: Chronic use of opioid analgesics in non-malignant pain: report of 38 cases. Pain 25:171, 1986
81. Robins LN, Davis DH, Nurco DN: How permanent was Vietnam drug addiction? Am J Pub Health 64:38, 1974
82. Burks TF: Gastrointestinal pharmacology. Annu Rev Pharmacol Toxicol 16:15, 1976
83. Porreca F, Burks TF: The spinal cord as a site of opioid effects on gastrointestinal transit in the mouse. J Pharmacol Exp Ther 227:22, 1983
84. McCammon RL, Stoelting RK, Madura JA: Effects of butorphanol, nalbuphine, and fentanyl on intrabiliary tract dynamics. Anesth Analg 63:139, 1984
85. Humphreys HK, Fleming NW: Opioid-induced spasm of the sphincter of Oddi apparently reversed by nalbuphine. Anesth Analg 74:308, 1992
86. Reitan JA, Stengert KB, Wymore MC et al: Central vagal control of fentanyl induced bradycardia during halothane anesthesia. Anesth Analg 57:31, 1978
87. Laubie M, Schmitt H, Vincent M: Vagal bradycardia produced by microinjections of morphine-like drugs into the nucleus ambiguus in anesthetized dogs. Eur J Pharmacol 59:287, 1979
88. Liu WS, Bidwai AV, Stanley TH et al: Cardiovascular dynamics after large doses of fentanyl and fentanyl plus N₂O in the dog. Anesth Analg 55:168, 1976
89. Strauer BE: Contractile responses to morphine, piritramide, meperidine and fentanyl: a comparative study of effects on the isolated ventricular myocardium. Anesthesiology 37:304, 1972
90. Freye E: Cardiovascular effects of high doses of fentanyl, meperidine and naloxone in dogs. Anesth Analg 53:40, 1974
91. Barash P, Kopriva C, Giles R et al: Global ventricular function and intubation: radionuclear profiles, abstracted. Anesthesiology 53:A109, 1980
92. Goldberg AH, Padget CH: Comparative effects of morphine and fentanyl on isolated heart muscle. Anesth Analg 48:978, 1969
93. Lowenstein E, Whiting RB, Bittar DA: Local and neurally mediated effects of morphine on skeletal muscle vascular resistance. J Pharmacol Exp Ther 180:359, 1972
94. Ward JW, McGrath RL, Weil JV: Effects of morphine on the peripheral vascular response to sympathetic stimulation. Am J Cardiol 29:656, 1972
95. Rosow CE, Moss I, Philbin DM et al: Histamine release during morphine and fentanyl anesthesia. Anesthesiology 56:93 1982
96. Flacke JW, Flacke WE, Boor BC et al: Histamine release by four narcotics: a double-blind study in humans. Anesth Analg 66:723, 1987
97. Murphy MR, Hug CC Jr: Pharmacokinetics of intravenous morphine in patients anesthetized with enflurane-nitrous oxide. Anesthesiology 54:187, 1981
98. Stanski DR, Greenblatt DJ, Lowenstein E: Kinetics of intravenous and intramuscular morphine. Clin Pharmacol Ther 24:52, 1978
99. Brunk SF, Delle M: Morphine metabolism in man. Clin Pharmacol Ther 16:51, 1974
100. Hug CC, Murphy MR, Rigel EP, Olson WA: Pharmacokinetics of morphine injected intravenously into the anesthetized dog. Anesthesiology 54:38, 1981

101. Aitkenhead AR, Vater M, Acholas K et al: Pharmacokinetics of single-dose I.V. morphine in normal volunteers and patients with end-stage renal failure. Br J Anaesth 56:813, 1984

102. Way EL, Adler TK: The pharmacologic implications of the fate of morphine and its surrogates. Pharmacol Rev 12:383, 1960

103. Boerner U, Abbott S, Roe RL: The metabolism of morphine and heroin in man. Drug Metab Rev 4:39, 1975

104. Shimomura K, Kamata O, Ueki S: Analgesic effects of morphine glucuronides. Tohoku J Exp Med 105:45, 1971

105. Brunk SF, Dell M, Wilson MR: Morphine metabolism in man: effect of aspirin. Clin Pharmacol Ther 15:283, 1974

106. Sawe J, Svensson JO, Odar-Cederlof I: Kinetics of morphine in patients with renal failure. Lancet i:211, 1985

107. Patwardhan RV, Johnson RF, Hoyump A et al: Normal metabolism of morphine in cirrhosis. Gastroenterology 81:1006, 1981

108. Laidlaw J, Read AE, Sherlock S: Morphine tolerance in hepatic cirrhosis. Gastroenterology 40:389, 1961

109. Woolner DF, Winter D, Frendin TJ et al: Renal failure does not impair the metabolism of morphine. Br J Clin Pharm 22:55, 1986

110. McQuay HJ, Moore RA: Be aware of renal function when prescribing morphine. Lancet ii:284, 1984

111. Mostert JW, Evers JL, Hobika GH et al: Cardiorespiratory effects of anaesthesia with morphine or fentanyl in chronic renal failure and cerebral toxicity with morphine. Br J Anaesth 43:1053, 1971

112. Don HF, Dieppa RA, Taylor P: Narcotic analgesics in anuric patients. Anesthesiology 42:745, 1975

113. Barnes JN, Goodwin FJ: Dihydrocodeine narcosis in renal failure. Br Med J (Clin Res Ed) 286:438, 1983

114. Redfern N: Dihydrocodeine overdose treated with naloxone infusion. Br Med J (Clin Res Ed) 287:751, 1983

115. Twycross RG, Lack SA: Symptom Control in Far Advanced Cancer: Pain Relief. Pitman, London, 1983

116. Misra AL: Metabolism of opiates. p. 297. In Adler ML, Manara L, Samanin R (eds): Factors Affecting the Action of Narcotics. Raven Press, New York, 1978

117. Sevelius H, McCoy JF, Colmore JP: Dose response to codeine in patients with chronic cough. Clin Pharmacol Ther 12:449, 1971

118. Cooper SA, Beaver WT: A model to evaluate mild analgesics in oral surgery outpatients. Clin Pharmacol Ther 20:241, 1976

119. Inturrisi CE, Max MB, Foley FM: The pharmacokinetics of heroin in patients with chronic pain. N Engl J Med 310:1213, 1984

120. Twycross RG, Wald SJ: Long term use of diamorphine in advanced cancer. p. 653. In Bonica JJ, Albe-Fessard DG (eds): Advances in Pain Research and Therapy. Vol. 1. Raven Press, New York, 1976

121. Mahler DL, Forrest WH, Jr: Relative analgesic potencies of morphine and hydromorphone in postoperative pain. Anesthesiology 42:602, 1975

122. Hanna C, Mazuzan JE Jr, Abajian J, Jr: An evaluation of dihydromorphone in treating postoperative pain. Anesth Analg 41:755, 1962

123. McKenzie R: Pharmacologic developments: nalbuphine hydrochloride and hydromorphone. In Ferrante FM, Ostheimer GW, Covino BG (eds): Patient-Controlled Analgesia. Blackwell Scientific, Boston, 1990

124. Hill HF, Coda BA, Akira T, Schaffer R: Multiple-dose evaluation of intravenous hydromorphone pharmacokinetics in normal human subjects. Anesth Analg 72: 330, 1991

125. Ritschel WA, Parab PV, Denson DD et al: Absolute bioavailability of hydromorphone after peroral and rectal administration in humans: saliva/plasma ratio and clinical effects. J Clin Pharmacol 27:647, 1987

126. Parab PV, Ritschel WA, Coyle DE et al: Pharmacokinetics of hydromorphone after intravenous, peroral and rectal administration to human subjects. Biopharm Drug Dipos 9:187, 1988

127. Sinatra RS, Harrison DM: A comparison of oxymorphone and fentanyl as narcotic supplements in general anesthesia. J Clin Anesth 1:253, 1989

128. Beaver WT, Wallenstein SL, Houde RW, Rogers A: Comparisons of the analgesic effects of oral and intramuscular oxymorphone and of intramuscular oxymorphone and morphine in patients with cancer. J Clin Pharmacol 17:186, 1977

129. Hermens JM, Ebertz JM, Hanifin JM, Hirschman CA: Comparison of histamine release in human mast cells induced by morphine, fentanyl and oxymorphone. Anesthesiology 62:124, 1985

130. Robinson EP, Faggella AM, Henry DP, Russell WP: Comparison of histamine release induced by morphine and oxymorphone administration in dogs. Am J Vet Res 49:1699, 1988

131. Loew GH, Berkowitz DS: Quantum chemical studies at N-substituent variation in the oxymorphone series of opiate narcotics. J Med Chem 21:101, 1978

132. Ronai AZ, Foldes FF, Hahn EF, Fishman J: Orientation of the oxygen atom at C-6 as a determinant of agonistic activity in the oxymorphone series. J Pharmacol Exp Ther 200:496, 1977

133. Hahn EF, Itzhak Y, Nishimura S et al: Irreversible opiate agonists and antagonists. III. Phenylhydrazone derivatives of naloxone and oxymorphone. J Pharmacol Exp Ther 235:846, 1985

134. Botros S, Lipkowski AW, Larson DL et al: Opioid agonist and antagonist activities of peripherally selective derivatives of naltrexamine and oxymorphamine. J Med Chem 32:2068, 1989

135. Cone EJ, Darwin WD, Buchwald WF, Gorodetzky CW: Oxymorphone metabolism and urinary excretion in human, rat, guinea pig, rabbit and dog. Drug Metab Dispos 11:446, 1983

136. White PF: Subcutaneous-PCA: an alternative to IV-PCA for postoperative pain management. Clin J Pain 6:297, 1990

137. Sinatra R, Chung KS, Silverman DG et al: An evaluation of morphine and oxymorphone administered via patient-controlled analgesia (PCA) or PCA plus basal infusion in postcesarean-delivery patients. Anesthesiology 71:502, 1989

138. Sinatra RS, Lodge K, Sibert K et al: A comparison of morphine, meperidine, and oxymorphone as utilized in patient-controlled analgesia following cesarean delivery. Anesthesiology 70:585, 1989

139. Sinatra RS, Harrison DM: Oxymorphone in patient-controlled analgesia. Clin Pharm 8:541, 1989

140. August BJ, Blake JA, Rogers NJ, Hussain MA: Transdermal oxymorphone formulation development and methods for evaluating flux and lag times for two skin permeation-enhancing vehicles. J Pharm Sci 79:1072, 1990

141. Beaver WT, Feise GA: A comparison of the analgesic effect of oxymorphone by rectal suppository and intramuscular injection in patients with postoperative pain. J Clin Pharmacol 17:276, 1977

142. Cone EJ, Darwin WD, Gorodetzky CW, Tan T: Comparative metabolism of hydrocodone in man, rat, guinea pig, rabbit and dog. Drug Metab Dispos 6:488, 1978
143. Park JI, Nakamura GR, Griesemer EC, Noguchi TT: Hydromorphone detected in bile following hydrocodone ingestion. J Forensic Sci 27:223, 1982
144. Beaver WT: Combination analgesics. Am J Med 77:38, 1984
145. Maruta T, Swanson DW, Finlayson RE: Drug abuse and dependency in patients with chronic pain. Mayo Clin Proc 54:241, 1979
146. Poyhia R, Olkkola KT, Seppala T, Kalso E: The pharmacokinetics of oxycodone after intravenous injection in adults. Br J Clin Pharmacol 32:516, 1991
147. Weinstein SH, Gaylord JC: Determination of oxycodone in plasma and identification of a major metabolite. J Pharm Sci 68:527, 1979
148. Tien JH: Transdermal-controlled administration of oxycodone. J Pharm Sci 80: 741, 1991
149. Dixon R, Crews T, Mochacsi E et al: Levorphanol: radioimmunoassay and plasma concentration profiles in dog and man. Res Commun Chem Pathol Pharmacol 29: 535, 1980
150. Dixon R, Crews T, Inturrisi C, Foley K: Levorphanol: pharmacokinetics and steady-state plasma concentrations in patients with pain. Res Commun Chem Pathol Pharmacol 41:3, 1983
151. Portenoy RK, Moulin DE, Rogers A et al: I.V. infusion of opioids for cancer pain: clinical review and guidelines for use. Cancer Treat Rep 70:575, 1986
152. Mather LE, Tucker GT: Systemic availability of orally administered meperidine. Clin Pharmacol Ther 20:535, 1976
153. Austin KL, Stapleton JV, Mather LE: Multiple intramuscular injections: a major source of variability in analgesic response to meperidine. Pain 8:47, 1980
154. Koska AJ, Kramer WG, Romagnoli A et al: Pharmacokinetics of high-dose meperidine in surgical patients. Anesth Analg 60:8, 1981
155. Mather LE, Tucker GT, Pflug AE et al: Meperidine kinetics in man. Clin Pharmacol Ther 17:21, 1975
156. Burns JJ, Berger BL, Lief PA et al: The physiological disposition and fate of meperidine (Demerol) in man and a method for its estimation in plasma. J Pharmacol Exp Ther 16:667, 1979
157. Mather LE, Gourlay GK: Biotransformation of opioids: significance for pain therapy. p. 31. In Nimmo WS, Smith G (eds): Opioid Agonist/Antagonist Drugs in Clinical Practice. Excerpta Medica, Amsterdam, 1984
158. Inturrisi CE, Umans JG: Pethidine and its active metabolite, norpethidine. Clinics Anesthesiol 1:123, 1983
159. Verbeeck RK, Branch RA, Wilkinson GR: Meperidine disposition in man: influence of urinary pH and route of administration. Clin Pharmacol Ther 30:619, 1981
160. Armstrong PJ, Bersten A: Normeperidine toxicity. Anesth Analg 65:536, 1986
161. Kaiko RR, Foley KM, Grabinski et al: Central nervous system excitatory effects of normeperidine in cancer patients. Ann Neurol 13:180, 1983
162. Szeto HH, Inturrisi CE, Houde R et al: Accumulation of normeperidine, an active metabolite of meperidine, in patients with renal failure or cancer. Ann Intern Med 86:738, 1977
163. Pond SM, Tong T, Benowitz NL et al: Presystemic metabolism of meperidine to normeperidine in normal and cirrhotic subjects. Clin Pharmacol Ther 30:183, 1981
164. Radney PA, Brodman E, Mankikar D, Duncalf D: The effect of equi-analgesic doses of fentanyl, morphine, meperidine and pentazocine on common bile duct pressure. Anaesthetist 29:26, 1980

165. Marks RM, Sachar EJ: Undertreatment of medical inpatients with narcotic analgesics. Ann Intern Med 78:173, 1973
166. Lasagna L, Beecher HK: The optimal dose of morphine. JAMA 156:230, 1954
167. Stapleton JV, Austin KL, Mather LE: A pharmacokinetic approach to postoperative pain: continuous infusion of pethidine. Anaesth Intensive Care 7:25, 1979
168. Tamsen A, Hartvig P, Fagerlund C, Dahlström B: Patient-controlled analgesic plasma concentrations of pethidine in postoperative pain. Clin Pharmacokinet 7: 164, 1982
169. Tamsen A, Sakurada T, Wahlström A et al: Postoperative demand for analgesics in relation to individual levels of endorphins and substance P in cerebrospinal fluid. Pain 13:171, 1982
170. Castro J, van de Water A, Wouters L et al: Comparative study of cardiovascular, neurologic and metabolic side effects of eight narcotics in dogs. Acta Anaesthesiol Belg 30:5, 1979
171. Hug CC, Murphy MR: Tissue redistribution of fentanyl and termination of its effects in rats. Anesthesiology 55:369, 1981
172. Murphy MR, Olson WA, Hug CC: Pharmacokinetics of 3H-fentanyl in the dog anesthetized with enflurane. Anesthesiology 50:13, 1979
173. McClain DA, Hugg CC: Intravenous fentanyl kinetics. Clin Pharmacol Ther 22: 106, 1980
174. Corall IM, Moore AR, Strumin L: Plasma concentrations of fentanyl in normal surgical patients and those with severe renal and hepatic disease. Br J Anaesth 52: 101, 1980
175. Haberer JP, Schoeffler P, Couderc E, Duvaldestin P: Fentanyl pharmacokinetics in anesthetized patients with cirrhosis. Br J Anaesth 54:1267, 1982
176. Hudson RJ, Thomson IR, Cannon JE et al: Pharmacokinetics of fentanyl in patients undergoing abdominal aortic surgery. Anesthesiology 64:334, 1986
177. Singleton MA, Rosen JI, Fisher DM: Pharmacokinetics of fentanyl in the elderly. Br J Anaesth 60:619, 1988
178. Bennett GM, Stanley TH: The cardiovascular effects of fentanyl during enflurane anesthesia in man. Anesth Analg 58:179, 1979
179. Streisand JB, Varvel JR, Stanski DR et al: Absorption and bioavailability of oral transmucosal fentanyl citrate. Anesthesiology 75:223, 1991
180. Feld LH, Champeau MW, van Steenis CA, Scott JC: Preanesthetic medication in children: a comparison of oral transmucosal fentanyl citrate versus placebo. Anesthesiology 71:374, 1989
181. Friesen RH, Lockhart CH: Oral transmucosal fentanyl citrate for preanesthetic medication of pediatric day surgery patients with and without droperidol as a prophylactic anti-emetic. Anesthesiology 76:46, 1992
182. Ashburn MA, Fine PG, Stanley TH: Oral transmucosal fentanyl citrate for the treatment of breakthrough cancer pain: a case report. Anesthesiology 71:615, 1989
183. Fine PG, Marcus M, De Boer AJ et al: An open label study of oral transmucosal fentanyl citrate (OTFC) for the treatment of breakthrough cancer pain. Pain 45: 149, 1991
184. Goldstein-Dresner MC, Davis PJ, Kretchman E et al: Double-blind comparison of oral transmucosal fentanyl citrate with oral meperidine, diazepam, and atropine as preanesthetic medication in children with congenital heart disease. Anesthesiology 74:28, 1991
185. Nelson PS, Streisand JB, Mulder SM et al: Comparison of oral transmucosal fentanyl citrate and an oral solution of meperidine, diazepam, and atropine for premedication in children. Anesthesiology 70:616, 1989

186. Lind GH, Marcus MA, Mears SL et al: Oral transmucosal fentanyl citrate for analgesia and sedation in the emergency department. Ann Emerg Med 20:1117, 1991
187. Striebel HW, Koenigs D, Krämer J: Postoperative pain management by intranasal demand-adapted fentanyl titration. Anesthesiology 77:281, 1992
188. Sandler AN: New techniques of opioid administration for the control of acute pain. Anesthesiol Clin North Am 10:271, 1992
189. Tarver SD, Stanley TH: Alternative routes of drug administration and new drug delivery systems. p. 337. In Stoelting RK, Barash P, Gallagher TJ (eds): Advances in Anesthesia. Vol. 7. Year Book Medical, Chicago, 1990
190. Hill HF; Clinical pharmacology of transdermal fentanyl. Eur J Pain 11:81, 1990
191. Caplan RA, Ready LB, Oden RV et al: Transdermal fentanyl for postoperative pain management. A double blind placebo study. JAMA 261:1036, 1989
192. McLeskey CH: Fentanyl TTS for postoperative analgesia. Eur J Pain 11:92, 1990
193. Plezia PM, Linford J, Kramer TH et al: Transdermally administered fentanyl for postoperative pain: a randomized double blind placebo controlled trial, abstracted. Anesthesiology 69:A364, 1988
194. von Bormann B, Ratthey K, Schwetlick G et al: Postoperative schmerztherapie durch transdermales fentanyl. Anasth Intensivther Notfallmed 23:3, 1988
195. Sandler AN, Baxter AD, Norman P et al: A double blind, placebo-controlled trial of transdermal fentanyl for posthysterectomy pain relief. II. Respiratory effects, abstracted. Can J Anaesth 38:A114, 1991
196. Rowbotham DJ, Wyald R, Peacock JE et al: Transdermal fentanyl for the relief of pain after upper abdominal surgery. Br J Anaesth 63:56, 1989
197. Stahl KD, van Bever W, Janssen P, Simon EJ: Receptor affinity and pharmacologic potency of a series of narcotic analgesic, anti-diarrheal and neuroleptic drugs. Eur J Pharmacol 46:199, 1977
198. Bovill JG, Sebel PS, Blackburn CL et al: The pharmacokinetics of sufentanil in surgical patients. Anesthesiology 57:439, 1982
199. Weldon ST, Perry DF, Cork RC, Gandolfi AJ: Detection of picogram levels of sufentanil by capillary gas chromatography. Anesthesiology 63:684, 1985
200. Waggum DC, Cork RC, Weldon ST et al: Postoperative respiratory depression and elevated sufentanil levels in a patient with chronic renal failure. Anesthesiology 63:708, 1985
201. Davis PJ, Stiller RL, Cook DR et al: Pharmacokinetics of sufentanil in adolescent patients with chronic renal failure. Anesth Analg 67:268, 1988
202. Matteo RS, Schwartz AE, Ornstein E et al: Pharmacokinetics of sufentanil in the elderly surgical patient. Can J Anaesth 37:852, 1990
203. Sebel PS, Barrett CW, Kirk CJ, Heykants J: Transdermal absorption of fentanyl and sufentanil in man. Eur J Clin Pharmacol 32:529, 1987
204. Roy SD, Flynn GL: Transdermal delivery of narcotic analgesics: pH, anatomical, and subject influences on cutaneous permeability of fentanyl and sufentanil. Pharm Res 7:842, 1990
205. Lehmann KA, Gerhard A, Horrichs-Haermeyer G et al: Postoperative patient-controlled analgesia with sufentanil: analgesic efficacy and minimum effective concentrations. Acta Anaesthesiol Scand 35:221, 1991
206. Ved SA, Dubois M, Carron H, Lea D: Sufentanil and alfentanil pattern of consumption during patient-controlled analgesia: a comparison with morphine. Clin J Pain, suppl. 1:S63, 1989
207. Graf G, Sinatra R, Chung J et al: Epidural sufentanil for postoperative analgesia:

dose-response in patients recovering from major gynecologic surgery. Anesth Analg 73:405, 1991

208. Dyer RA, Anderson BJ, Michell WL, Hall JM: Postoperative pain control with a continuous infusion of epidural sufentanil in the intensive care unit: a comparison with epidural morphine. Anesth Analg 71:130, 1990

209. Bovill JG, Sebel PS, Blackburn CL, Heykants J: The pharmacokinetics of alfentanil (R39209): a new opioid analgesic. Anesthesiology 57:439, 1982

210. Camu F, Gepts E, Rucquoi M, Heykants J: Pharmacokinetics of alfentanil in man. Anesth Analg 61:657, 1982

211. Stanski DR, Hug CC: Alfentanil—a kinetically predictable narcotic analgesic. Anesthesiology 57:435, 1982

212. Ferrier C, Marty J, Bouffard Y et al: Alfentanil pharmacokinetics in patients with cirrhosis. Anesthesiology 62:480, 1985

213. Camu F, Dubucquoy F: Alfentanil infusion for postoperative pain: a comparison of epidural and intravenous routes. Anesthesiology 75:171, 1991

214. Penon C, Negre I, Ecoffey C et al: Analgesia and ventilatory responses to carbon dioxide after intramuscular and epidural alfentanil. Anesth Analg 67:313, 1988

215. Owen H, Brose WG, Plummer JL, Mather LE; Variables of patient-controlled analgesia. 3. Test of an infusion demand system using alfentanil. Anaesthesia 45: 452, 1990

216. Owen H, Currie JC, Plummer JL: Variation in the blood concentration/analgesic response relationship during patient-controlled analgesia with alfentanil. Anaesth Intensive Care 19:555, 1991

217. Meresaar U, Nilsson MI, Holmstrand J, Änggård E: Single dose pharmacokinetics and bioavailability of methadone in man studied with a stable isotope method. Eur J Clin Pharmacol 20:473, 1981

218. Nilsson MI, Meresaar U, Änggård E: Clinical pharmacokinetics of methadone. Acta Anaesthesiol Scand, suppl. 74:66, 1982

219. Nilsson MI, Änggård E, Holmstrand J, Gunne LM: Pharmacokinetics of methadone during maintenance treatment: adaptive changes during the induction phase. Eur J Clin Pharmacol 22:343, 1982

220. Änggård E, Gunne LM, Holmstrand J et al: Disposition of methadone in methadone maintenance. Clin Pharmacol Ther 17:258, 1975

221. Verebely K, Volavka J, Mulé S et al: Methadone in man: pharmacokinetic and excretion studies in acute and chronic treatment. Clin Pharmacol Ther 18:180, 1975

222. Nilsson MI, Widerlöv E, Meresaar U, Änggård E: Effect of urinary pH on the disposition of methadone in man. Eur J Clin Pharmacol 22:337, 1982

223. Gourlay GK, Wilson PR, Glynn CJ: Pharmacodynamics and pharmacokinetics of methadone during the perioperative period. Anesthesiology 57:458, 1982

224. Beaver WT, Wallenstein SL, Houde RW, Rogers A: A clinical comparison of the analgesic effects of methadone and morphine administered intramuscularly, and of orally and parenterally administered methadone. Clin Pharmacol Ther 8:415, 1967

225. Hansen J, Ginman C, Hartvig P et al: Clinical evaluation of oral methadone in treatment of cancer pain. Acta Anaesthesiol Scand, suppl. 74:124, 1982

226. Ventafridda V, Ripamonti C, Bianchi M et al: A randomized study on oral administration of morphine and methadone in the treatment of cancer pain. J Pain Symptom Manage 1:203, 1986

227. Welch DB, Hrynaszkiewicz A: Postoperative analgesia using epidural methadone. Administration by the lumbar route for thoracic pain relief. Anaesthesia 36:1051, 1981

228. Nyska M, Klin B, Shapira Y et al: Epidural methadone for preoperative analgesia in patients with proximal femoral fractures. Br Med J (Clin Res Ed) 293:1347, 1986

229. Gourlay GK, Willis RJ, Wilson PR: Postoperative pain control with methadone: influence of supplementary methadone doses and blood concentration-response relationships. Anesthesiology 61:19, 1984

230. Gourlay GK, Willis RJ, Lamberty J: A double-blind comparison of the efficacy of methadone and morphine in postoperative pain control. Anesthesiology 64:332, 1986

231. Gram LF, Schou J, Way WL et al: d-Propoxyphene kinetics after single oral and intravenous doses in man. Clin Pharmacol Ther 26:473, 1979

232. Beaver WT: Mild analgesics, a review of their clinical pharmacology (Part II). Am J Med Sci 251:576, 1966

233. Errick JK, Heel RC: Nalbuphine: a preliminary review of its pharmacologic properties and therapeutic efficacy. Drugs 26:191, 1983

234. Lake CL, DiFazio CA, Duckworth EN et al: High performance liquid chromatographic analysis of plasma levels of nalbuphine in cardiac surgical patients. J Chromatogr 233:410, 1982

235. Jansinski DR: Human pharmacology of narcotic antagonists. Br J Clin Pharmacol, suppl. 7:287S, 1979

236. Gal TJ, DiFazio CA, Moscicki J: Analgesic and respiratory depressant activity of nalbuphine: a comparison with morphine. Anesthesiology 57:367, 1982

237. Latasch L, Probst S, Dudziak R: Reversal by nalbuphine of respiratory depression caused by fentanyl. Anesth Analg 63:814, 1984

238. Moldenhauer CC, Roach GW, Finlayson DC et al: Nalbuphine antagonism of ventilatory depression following high-dose fentanyl anesthesia. Anesthesiology 62:647, 1985

239. Davies GG, From R: A blinded study using nalbuphine for prevention of pruritus induced by epidural fentanyl. Anesthesiology 69:763, 1988

240. Henderson SK, Cohen H: Nalbuphine augmentation of analgesia and reversal of side effects following epidural hydromorphone. Anesthesiology 65:216, 1986

241. Lee G, DeMaria A, Amsterdam A et al: Comparative effects of morphine, meperidine and pentazocine on cardiocirculatory dynamics in patients with acute myocardial infarction. Am J Med 60:949, 1976

242. Lehman KA, Tenbuhs B: Patient-controlled analgesia with nalbuphine, a new narcotic agonist-antagonist for the treatment of postoperative pain. Eur J Clin Pharmacol 31:267, 1986

243. Sprigg E, Otton PE: Nalbuphine versus meperidine for postoperative analgesia: a double-blind comparison using patient controlled analgesic technique. Can Anaesth Soc J 30:517, 1983

244. Camann WR, Hurley RH, Gilbertson LI et al: Epidural nalbuphine for analgesia following cesarean delivery: dose-response and effect of local anaesthetic choice. Can J Anaesth 38:728, 1991

245. Baxter AD, Langaniere S, Samson B et al: A dose-response study of nalbuphine for post-thoracotomy epidural analgesia. Can J Anaesth 38:175, 1991

246. Ehrnebo M, Boreus L, Lonroth V: Bioavailability and first pass metabolism of oral pentazocine in man. Clin Pharmacol Ther 22:888, 1972

247. Berkowitz BA, Asling JH, Shnider SM, Way EL: Relationship of pentazocine plasma levels to pharmacologic activity in man. Clin Pharmacol Ther 10:320, 1969

248. Brogden RN, Speight TM, Avery GS: Pentazocine: a review of its pharmacologic properties, therapeutic efficacy, and dependance liability. Drugs 5:6, 1973

249. Lal S, Savidge RS, Chabra GP: Cardiovascular and respiratory effects of morphine and pentazocine in patients with myocardial infarction. Lancet i:379, 1969
250. Schmucker P, VanAckern K, Franke N et al: Hemodynamic and respiratory effects of pentazocine. Studies on surgical cardiac patients. Anaesthesist 29:475, 1980
251. Economou G, Ward-McQuaid JN: A cross-over comparison of the effect of morphine, pethidine and pentazocine on biliary pressure. Gut 12:218, 1971
252. Radnay PA, Brodman E, Manikikar D, Duncalf D: The effect of equianalgesic doses of fentanyl, morphine, meperidine and pentazocine on common bile duct pressures. Br J Clin Pharmacol, suppl. 7:281S, 1979
253. Houde RW: Analgesic effectiveness of the narcotic agonist-antagonists. Br J Clin Pharmacol, suppl. 7:297S, 1979
254. Heel RC, Brogden RN, Speight TM, Avery GS: Butorphanol: a review of its pharmacological properties and therapeutic efficacy. Drugs 16:473, 1978
255. Vandam LD: Butorphanol. N Engl J Med 302:381, 1980
256. Popio KA, Jackson DH, Ross AM et al: Hemodynamic and respiratory effects of morphine and butorphanol. Clin Pharmacol Ther 23:281, 1978
257. Lawhorn CD, McNitt JB, Fibuch EE et al: Epidural morphine with butorphanol for postoperative anaglesia after cesarean delivery. Anesth Analg 72:53, 1991
258. Naulty JS, Weintraub S, McMahon J et al: Epidural butorphanol for post-cesarean delivery pain management, abstracted. Anesthesiology 61:A415, 1984
259. Abboud TK, Moore M, Zhu J: Epidural butorphanol for the relief of postoperative pain after cesarian section, abstracted. Anesthesiology 65:A397, 1986
260. Abboud TK, Moore M, Zhu ZJ et al: Epidural butorphanol or morphine for relief of postcesarean section pain: ventilatory responses to carbon dioxide. Anesth Analg 66:887, 1987
261. Lanz E, Simko G, Theiss D, Glocke MH: Epidural buprenorphine—a double-blind study of postoperative analgesia and side effects. Anesthesiology 41:169, 1974
262. Heel RC, Brogden RN, Speight TM, Avery GS: Buprenorphine: a review of its pharmacological properties and therapeutic efficacy. Drugs 17:81, 1979
263. Bullingham RES, McQuay HJ, Moore A, Bennett MRD: Buprenorphine kinetics. Clin Pharmacol Ther 28:667, 1980
264. Rance MJ: Animal and molecular pharmacology of mixed agonist-antagonist drugs. Br J Clin Pharmacol, suppl. 7:281S, 1979
265. Sekar M, Mimpriss TJ: Buprenorphine, benzodiazepines and prolonged respiratory depression (letter). Anaesthesia 42:567, 1987
266. McQuay HJ, Bullingham RE, Bennett MR, Moore RA: Delayed respiratory depression. A case report and a new hypothesis. Acta Anaesthesiol Belg, suppl. 30:245, 1979
267. Gal TJ: Naloxone reversal of buprenorphine-induced respiratory depression. Clin Pharmacol Ther 45:66, 1989
268. Orwin JM: The effect of doxapram on buprenorphine induced respiratory depression. Acta Anaesthesiol Belg 28:93, 1977
269. Boysen K, Hertel S, Chraemmer-Jorgensen B et al: Buprenorphine antagonism of ventilatory depression following fentanyl anaesthesia. Acta Anaesthesiol Scand 32:490, 1988
270. Budd K: High dose buprenorphine for postoperative analgesia. Anaesthesia 36:900, 1981
271. Albert LH: Newer potent analgesics. Buprenorphine. Ration Drug Ther 16:4, 1982
272. Shah MV, Jones DI, Rosen M: "Patient demand" postoperative analgesia with buprenorphine. Comparison between sublingual and IM buprenorphine. Br J Anaesth 58:508, 1986

273. Hull CJ: The pharmacokinetics of opioid analgesics, with special reference to patient-controlled administration. p. 7. In Harmer M, Rosen M, Vickers MD (eds): Patient-Controlled Analgesia. Blackwell Scientific, Oxford, 1985

274. Lehmann KA, Grond S, Freier J, Zech D: Postoperative pain management and respiratory depression after thoracotomy: a comparison of intramuscular piritramide and intravenous patient-controlled analgesia using fentanyl or buprenorphine. J Clin Anesth 3:194, 1991

275. Ouchi K, Takeda, Matsuno S: Efficacy of patient-controlled analgesia for management of pain after abdominal surgery. Tohoku J Exp Med 165:193, 1991

276. Cohen S, Amar D, Pantuck CB et al: Epidural patient-controlled anaglesia after cesarean section: buprenorphine 0.015% bupivacaine with epinephrine versus fentanyl—0.015% bupivacaine with and without epinephrine. Anesth Analg 74:226, 1992

277. Cohen S, Amar D, Pantuck CB et al: Epidural patient-controlled analgesia after cesarean section: buprenorphine—0.03% vs. fentanyl-bupivacaine 0.03%, abstracted. Anesthesiology 73:A975, 1990

278. Murphy DF, McGrath P, Stritch M: Postoperative analgesia in hip surgery. A controlled comparison of epidural buprenorphine with intramuscular morphine. Anaesthesia 39:181, 1984

279. Keaveny JP, Harper NJ: Treatment of epidural morphine-induced pruritus with buprenorphine (letter). Anaesthesia 44:691, 1989

280. Celleno D, Capogna G: Spinal buprenorphine for postoperative analgesia after cesarean delivery. Acta Anaesthesiol Scand 33:236, 1989

281. Locniskar A, Greenblatt DJ, Zinng MA: Pharmacokinetics of dezocine, a new analgesic: effect of dose and route of administration. Eur J Clin Pharmacol 30:121, 1986

282. Shulman MS: New systemic analgesic agents. Anesthesiol Clin North Am 10:299, 1991

283. Gal TJ, DiFazio CA: Ventilatory and analgesic effects of dezocine in humans. Anesthesiology 61:716, 1984

284. Malis J, Rosenthale ME, Gluckman MI: Animal pharmacology of Wy-16, 225, a new analgesic agent. J Pharmacol Exp Ther 194:488, 1975

285. Vinik HR, McFarland L, Wright D et al: Double-blind postoperative study comparing multiple doses of dezocine (WY 16225) with morphine and placebo, abstracted. Anesthesiology 57:A189, 1982

286. Pandit SK, Kothary SP, Pandit UA et al: Double-blind placebo-controlled comparison of dezocine and morphine for postoperative pain relief. Can Anaesth Soc J 32: 583, 1985

287. Romagnoli A, Keats AS: Ceiling respiratory depression by dezocine. Clin Pharmacol Ther 35:367, 1984

288. Rothbard RL, Schreiner BF, Yu PN: Hemodynamic and respiratory effects of dezocine. Clin Pharmacol Ther 38:84, 1985

289. WHO Technical Report Series 775, Geneva, 1989

290. Jasinski DR, Preston KL: Assessment of dezocine for morphine-like subjective effects and miosis. Clin Pharmacol Ther 38:544, 1985

291. Zacny JP, Lichtor JL, deWit H: Subjective behavioral, and physiologic responses to intravenous dezocine in healthy volunteers. Anesth Analg 74:523, 1992

292. Galloway FM, Farma S: Double-blind comparison of intravenous doses of dezocine, butorphanol and placebo for relief of postoperative pain. Anesth Analg 65:283, 1986

293. Finucane BT, Floyd JB, Petro DJ: Postoperative pain relief: a double-blind comparison of dezocine, butorphanol and placebo. South Med J 79:548, 1986
294. Gravenstein JS: Dezocine for postoperative wound pain. Int J Clin Pharmacol Ther Toxicol 22:502, 1984
295. Camu F, Gepts E: Analgesic properties of dezocine for relief of postoperative pain. Acta Anaesthesiol Belg, suppl. 30:183, 1979
296. Keats AS, Talford J: Subjective effects of nalorphine and nalorphine-morphine combinations in man. J Pharmacol Exp Ther 112:356, 1954
297. Gal TJ, DiFazio CA: Prolonged antagonism of opioid action with intravenous nalmefene in man. Anesthesiology 64:175, 1986
298. Faris PL, Komisaruk BR, Watkins LR, Mayer DJ: Evidence for the neuropeptide cholecystokinin as an antagonist of opiate analgesia. Science 219:310, 1983
299. Ngai SH, Berkowitz BA, Yang YC et al: Pharmacokinetics of naloxone in rats and man. Basis for its potency and short duration of action. Anesthesiology 44:398, 1976
300. Berkowitz BA: Research review. The relationship of pharmacokinetics to pharmacological activity: morphine, methadone and naloxone. Clin Pharmacokinet 1:219, 1976
301. Rawal N, Schött U, Dahlström B et al: Influence of naloxone infusion on analgesia and respiratory depression following epidural morphine. Anesthesiology 64:194, 1986
302. Gueneron JP, Ecoffey CI, Carli P et al: Effects of naloxone infusion on analgesia and respiratory depression after epidural fentanyl. Anesth Analg 67:35, 1988
303. Kripke BJ, Finck AJ, Shah N, Snow JC: Naloxone antagonism after narcotic supplemented-anesthesia. Anesth Analg 55:800, 1976
304. Longnecker DE, Grazis PA, Eggers GWN: Naloxone for antagonism of morphine induced respiratory depression. Anesth Analg 52:447, 1973
305. Flacke JW, Flacke WE, Williams GD: Acute pulmonary edema following naloxone reversal of high-dose morphine anesthesia. Anesthesiology 47:376, 1977
306. Tanaka GY: Hypertensive reaction to naloxone. JAMA 228:25, 1974
307. Michaelis LL, Hickey PR, Clark TA, Dixon WM: Ventricular irritability associated with the use of naloxone. Ann Thorac Surg 18:608, 1974
308. Martin WR, Jasinski DR, Mansky PA: Naltrexone, an antagonist for the treatment of heroin dependence. Arch Gen Psychiatry 28:748, 1973

9

Local Anesthetics

Benjamin G. Covino

Local anesthetics may be defined as pharmacologic agents capable of producing a loss of sensation in a circumscribed area of the body. This localized form of anesthesia is due to an inhibition of excitation at nerve endings or to a blockade of the conduction process in peripheral nervous tissue. Regional anesthesia originated in 1884 when Koller described the topical anesthetic properties of cocaine, an alkaloid that had been isolated from the leaves of the *Erythroxylin coca* bush. Since that time numerous clinical compounds have been synthesized as local anesthetic agents. The agents currently used for regional anesthesia and their primary area of clinical use are listed in Table 9-1.

PHARMACODYNAMIC CONSIDERATIONS

Mechanism of Action

At rest, a negative electric potential of approximately 60–90 mV exists across the nerve membrane (i.e., the resting membrane potential). When a nerve is stimulated, a relatively slow phase of depolarization occurs. During this time, the electric potential within the cells becomes progressively less negative (Fig. 9-1). When the electric potential between the interior and exterior surface of the cell membrane reaches a critical level (i.e., the threshold potential), a rapid phase of depolarization follows. This results in a reversal of the electric potential such that the interior of the cell becomes positively charged with respect to the exterior surface of the membrane. At the peak of the action potential, the interior of the cell has a positive electric potential of approximately 40 mV as compared with the exterior of the cell. The total amplitude of the action poten-

TABLE 9-1. Chemical Structure, Physical-Chemical, Pharmacologic Properties, and Primary Clinical Use of Local Anesthetic Agents

AGENT	CHEMICAL CONFIGURATION (Aromatic Lipophilic — Intermediate Chain — Amine Hydrophilic)	PHYSICOCHEMICAL PROPERTIES				PHARMACOLOGICAL PROPERTIES			
		MOLECULAR WEIGHT BASE	pKa (25°C)	PARTITION COEFFICIENT	% PROTEIN BINDING	ONSET	RELATIVE POTENCY	DURATION	PRIMARY CLINICAL USE
ESTERS									
PROCAINE	$H-N$—C$_6$H$_4$—COOCH$_2$CH$_2$-N(C$_2$H$_5$)(C$_2$H$_5$)	236	8.9	0.02	6	Slow	1	Short	Spinal
TETRACAINE	H$_9$C$_4$N—C$_6$H$_4$—COOCH$_2$CH$_2$-N(CH$_3$)(CH$_3$)	264	8.5	4.1	76	Slow	8	Long	Spinal
CHLOROPROCAINE	H$_2$N—C$_6$H$_3$(Cl)—COOCH$_2$CH$_2$-N(C$_2$H$_5$)(C$_2$H$_5$)	271	8.7	0.14	-	Fast	1	Short	Epidural
AMIDES									
PRILOCAINE	C$_6$H$_4$(CH$_3$)—NHCOCH-N(H)(C$_3$H$_7$)	220	7.9	0.9	55	Fast	2	Moderate	IV Regional
LIDOCAINE	C$_6$H$_3$(CH$_3$)(CH$_3$)—NHCOCH$_2$-N(C$_2$H$_5$)(C$_2$H$_5$)	234	7.9	2.9	64	Fast	2	Moderate	All forms of Regional Anesthesia
MEPIVACAINE	C$_6$H$_3$(CH$_3$)(CH$_3$)—NHCO— piperidine N-CH$_3$	246	7.6	0.8	78	Fast	2	Moderate	Peripheral Nerve Blocks
BUPIVACAINE	C$_6$H$_3$(CH$_3$)(CH$_3$)—NHCO— piperidine N-C$_4$H$_9$	288	8.1	27.5	96	Moderate	8	Long	Epidural and Spinal
ETIDOCAINE	C$_6$H$_3$(CH$_3$)(CH$_3$)—NHCOCH(C$_2$H$_5$)-N(C$_2$H$_5$)(C$_3$H$_7$)	276	7.7	141	94	Fast	6	Long	Epidural

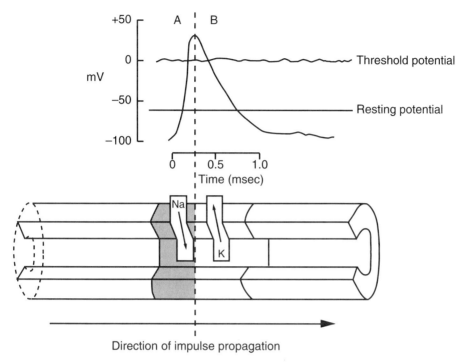

Fig. 9-1. Surface action potential recorded from an isolated nerve (upper figure). *Lower portion* of figure shows sodium channel activation during depolarization phase (upper figure) and potassium channel opening during repolarization phase (upper figure).

tial is approximately 100 mV. When depolarization is complete, the nerve begins to repolarize. The interior of the cell progressively becomes more negative until the resting potential of − 60 to − 90 mV is reestablished. The entire process of depolarization and repolarization occurs within 1 millisecond. Depolarization accounts for 30 percent of the duration of the action potential. The repolarization phase is slower, accounting for the remaining 70 percent of the duration of the action potential.

These electrophysiologic events are dependent on

1. Relative concentration of electrolytes in nerve cytoplasm and extracellular fluid
2. Permeability of the cell membrane to various ions, particularly sodium and potassium

The resting membrane potential is intimately related to the ratio of potassium ions between the inside (K_i) and outside (K_o) of the cell membrane. At rest, a K_i/K_o ratio of approximately 30:1 exists. Because the cell membrane is relatively impermeable to the movement of sodium, this ion does not contribute to the resting membrane potential.

After excitation, the permeability of the cell membrane increases. Sodium ions pass from the exterior to the interior of the nerve cell through the sodium channels. This inward movement of sodium ions accounts for the depolarization phase of the action potential (influx of cations accounting for the positive membrane potential). As the cell becomes maximally depolarized, the permeability of the cell membrane to sodium decreases (sodium inactivation). An increased flow of potassium ions occurs from the interior to the exterior of the cell, resulting in repolarization of the nerve membrane.

The flux of sodium and potassium ions during excitation is a passive phenomenon because these ions are moving down their respective concentration gradients. At the end of the action potential, an excess of sodium ions is present within the cell, and an excess of potassium ions exists outside the nerve cell. Reestablishment of the ionic gradient across the nerve membrane requires energy to extrude sodium ions against a concentration gradient. In addition, potassium ions are believed to be actively transported from the exterior to the interior surface of the nerve membrane. However, potassium ions may also move passively along an electrostatic gradient. The energy required for the active transport of sodium and potassium ions (i.e., the "sodium pump") is derived from the oxidative metabolism of adenosine triphosphate.

After exposure of an isolated nerve to a local anesthetic agent, the membrane resting potential and the threshold potential remain essentially unaltered.[1] The maximum rate of rise of the nerve action potential has been shown to decrease from a control value of 190 V/sec to 120 V/sec after exposure to a solution of 0.005 percent (0.2 mM) lidocaine with no significant change in the rate of repolarization.[1]

Local anesthetic drugs have been shown to decrease the permeability of the nerve membrane to sodium. For example, at a normal sodium concentration of 116 mM, 3.2 mmoles of cocaine produced a 50 percent decrease in the height of the isolated frog sciatic nerve action potential.[2] However, when the sodium concentration was lowered to 12 mmoles in the bathing solution, only 0.15 mmole of cocaine was required to cause a similar reduction in the amplitude of the action potential. Direct sodium and potassium conductance studies have demonstrated a complete loss of sodium currents[3,4] in the presence of 1 mmole of lidocaine. However, 3.5 mmoles of lidocaine caused only a 5 percent decrease in potassium conductance.

Most of the clinically useful local anesthetic preparations are available in the form of solutions of a salt (e.g., lidocaine is usually prepared as an 0.5–2.0 percent solution of lidocaine hydrochloride). In solution, the salts of these local anesthetic compounds exist both in the form of uncharged molecules (B) and as positively charged cations (BH$^+$). The relative proportion between the uncharged base (B) and the charged cation (BH$^+$) depends on the pK$_a$ of the specific chemical compound and the pH of the solution. The relationship between these various factors can be expressed as follows:

$$pH = pK_a - \log \left(\frac{BH^+}{B} \right)$$

Because pK_a is constant for any specific compound, the relative proportion of free base and charged cation will be essentially dependent on the pH of the local anesthetic solution. As the pH of the solution is decreased and H^+ concentration increased, the equilibrium will shift toward the charged cationic form. Conversely, as the pH is increased and H^+ concentration decreased, the equilibrium will be shifted toward the free base form.

Two factors are involved in the action of local anesthetics:

1. Diffusion through the nerve sheath and membrane
2. Binding at some site in the cell membrane

In isolated nerves with an intact epineurium, an increase in the pH of the local anesthetic bathing solution (favoring formation of the base) markedly accelerates the rate of decrease of the height of the surface action potential. In desheathed nerve, however, a less alkaline solution (in which a relatively greater amount of the charged cation is present) results in increased local anesthetic activity. These studies indicate that the uncharged base form is important for optimal penetration of the nerve sheath.[5,6] After diffusion through the epineurium, equilibrium between B and BH^+ is reestablished. At the cell membrane, the charged cation is ultimately responsible for the suppression of electrophysiologic events in peripheral nerve[7] (Fig. 9-2).

The sodium channel is the site at which local anesthetics exert their pharma-

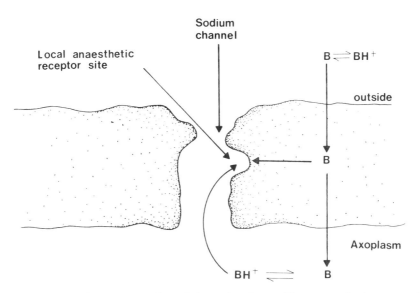

Fig. 9-2. Schematic representation of the active form of local anesthetic responsible for conduction block. Base form (B) is primarily responsible for diffusion through nerve membrane into axoplasm, where it is converted to the cationic form (BH^+). The cationic form is primarily involved in combining with the receptor site within the sodium channel leading to conduction blockade.

cologic action. These agents are believed to combine with a receptor in the sodium channel, such binding ultimately resulting in sodium channel inactivation and conduction blockade.[8] Studies conducted with tertiary amide local anesthetics and quaternary derivatives of lidocaine have revealed that anesthetic potency is enhanced when these compounds are applied to the internal surface of the nerve membrane.[9] Thus, it has been postulated that the conventional local anesthetics, such as lidocaine, enter the sodium channel from the axoplasmic side (Fig. 9-2).

Although the cationic form of local anesthetics is believed to be primarily responsible for conduction blockade by combining with a receptor site in the sodium channel, the uncharged base may also contribute to the action of local anesthetics.[8] The uncharged base may penetrate the lipid portion of the cell membrane and cause conformational change in the lipoprotein matrix. The diameter of the sodium channel decreases, thereby contributing to the inhibition of sodium conductance.

In summary, the sequence of events that results in conduction blockade in peripheral nerves by local anesthetics is as follows:

1. Diffusion of the base form of the local anesthetic molecule across the nerve sheath and nerve membrane
2. Reequilibrium between the base and cationic form of the local anesthetic on the axoplasmic surface of the nerve membrane
3. Penetration into and attachment to a receptor at a site within the sodium channel
4. Blockade of the sodium channel
5. Inhibition of sodium conductance
6. Decrease in the rate and degree of the depolarization phase of the action potential
7. Failure to achieve the threshold potential level
8. Lack of development of a propagated action potential
9. Conduction blockade

STRUCTURE-ACTIVITY RELATIONSHIP

Chemical compounds that demonstrate clinically useful local anesthetic activity possess the following chemical arrangement:

Aromatic portion—Intermediate chain—Amino portion

Alterations in either the aromatic portion, amine portion, or intermediate chain of specific chemical compounds will modify their anesthetic activity. For example, increasing the molecular weight by lengthening the intermediate chain or by adding carbon atoms to the aromatic or amine portion tends to increase intrinsic anesthetic potency until a maximum anesthetic potency is reached.[10] Beyond this point, a further increase in molecular weight results in a decrease in anesthetic activity. The aromatic portion of a local anesthetic molecule is usually responsible for its lipophilic properties, whereas the amine portion is associated with hydrophilicity. Changes in either the aromatic or amine portion will alter the lipid-water distribution coefficient of a specific agent. Chemical modification of either end of the molecule will also affect the protein-binding characteristics, which, in turn, will alter its anesthetic profile. For example, the addition of a butyl group to the aromatic end of the procaine molecule increases lipid solubility and protein binding and results in a compound with greater intrinsic anesthetic potency and a longer duration of anesthetic activity (tetracaine)[11] (Table 9-1). The addition of a butyl group to the amine end of mepivacaine transforms this agent into a compound that is more lipid-soluble and more highly protein-bound and biologically possesses a greater intrinsic potency and longer duration of action (bupivacaine)[12] (Table 9-1). In the case of lidocaine, substitution of a propyl for an ethyl group at the amine end and the addition of an ethyl group to the α-carbon in the intermediate chain yields etidocaine. Etidocaine is more lipid-soluble, more highly protein-bound, and biologically, a local anesthetic agent of greater potency and longer duration.[13]

The clinically useful local anesthetics essentially fall into two chemical categories:

1. Agents with an ester link between the aromatic end of the molecule and the intermediate chain. Procaine, chloroprocaine and tetracaine are examples of *amino-ester* agents
2. Compounds with an amide link between the aromatic portion and the intermediate chain. Lidocaine, mepivacaine, prilocaine, bupivacaine and etidocaine represent *amino-amide* drugs

The basic difference between the ester and amide compounds resides in

1. The manner in which they are metabolized
2. Their allergic potential

The ester agents are hydrolyzed in plasma by pseudocholinesterase, whereas the amide compounds undergo enzymatic degradation in the liver. Para-aminobenzoic acid is one of the metabolites formed from the hydrolysis of ester-type compounds. This substance is capable of inducing allergic-type reactions in a small percentage of patients. The amino-amide agents are not metabolized to para-aminobenzoic acid, and reports of allergic phenomena with these agents are extremely rare.

PHARMACOLOGIC CONSIDERATIONS

The clinically important properties of local anesthetics include potency, speed of onset, duration of anesthetic activity, and differential sensory/motor blockade. The clinical profile of the individual agents is essentially determined by the physicochemical characteristics of the various compounds, which in turn are dependent on their chemical structure. The physicochemical properties that influence anesthetic activity are lipid solubility, protein binding, and pK_a. Minor changes in molecular structure have dramatic effects on these properties (Table 9-1).

Anesthetic Potency

Lipid solubility appears to be the primary determinant of intrinsic anesthetic potency. The nerve membrane is basically a lipoprotein matrix. The axolemma consists of 90 percent lipids and 10 percent proteins. As a result, chemical compounds that are highly lipophilic tend to penetrate the nerve membrane more easily. Fewer molecules are required for conduction blockade, resulting in enhanced potency. In vitro studies on isolated nerves show a correlation between the partition coefficient of local anesthetics and the minimum concentration (C_m) required for conduction blockade.[14,15] For example, among the amino-amides, mepivacaine and prilocaine are the least lipid-soluble and weakest amide agents, whereas etidocaine is the most lipophilic and the most potent local anesthetic (Table 9-1). A similar relationship between lipid solubility and potency exists among the ester-type drugs. Procaine is the least lipid-soluble and the weakest agent, whereas tetracaine is the most lipophilic and the most potent ester-type drug.

Factors other than lipid solubility may also influence anesthetic potency. A comparison of the values of the partition coefficient of the base forms of ester and amide agents and their relative anesthetic potencies indicates that the potency of the amino-esters is greater than that of amino-amides at similar partition coefficient values (Table 9-1). Amino-esters may interact with a greater number of local anesthetic receptor sites, thereby explaining their inherently greater potency.[16]

In vivo studies in humans indicate that the correlation between lipid solubility and anesthetic potency is not as precise as in an isolated nerve. Lidocaine is approximately twice as potent as prilocaine and mepivacaine in an isolated nerve preparation. In humans, however, there is little difference in anesthetic potency among these three agents. Similarly, etidocaine is more potent than bupivacaine in an isolated nerve, whereas etidocaine is clinically less active than bupivacaine.

The difference between the in vitro and in vivo potency of local anesthetics may be related to their vasodilator or tissue redistribution properties. For example, lidocaine causes a greater degree of vasodilation than either mepivacaine or prilocaine, resulting in a more rapid vascular absorption of lidocaine. Fewer lidocaine molecules are available for neural blockade in vivo. The extremely high lipid solubility of etidocaine results in a greater uptake of this agent by adipose tissue in the epidural space. This again results in fewer etidocaine molecules being available for neural blockade as compared with bupivacaine.

Duration of Action

Duration of anesthesia is primarily related to the degree of protein binding of the various local anesthetics. Local anesthetics are believed to combine with a protein receptor located within the sodium channel of the nerve membrane. Chemical compounds that possess a greater affinity for, and bind more firmly to, the receptor site will remain within the channel for a longer period of time. This results in a prolonged duration of conduction blockade. Most of the information regarding the protein binding of local anesthetics has been obtained from studies involving the binding of these agents to plasma proteins. It is assumed that a similar relationship exists between the plasma protein binding of local anesthetics and the degree of binding to membrane proteins.

In vitro studies have demonstrated that local anesthetics that are poorly bound to protein (procaine) are rapidly washed out from isolated nerves, whereas drugs such as tetracaine, bupivacaine, and etidocaine are removed at an extremely slow rate. In vivo studies, including clinical investigations in humans, have confirmed the relationship between protein binding of local anesthetics and their duration of action.[17] For example, procaine produces a duration of brachial plexus blockade of 30–60 minutes, whereas approximately 10 hours of anesthesia have been reported after the use of bupivacaine or etidocaine.[17]

In humans, the duration of anesthesia is markedly influenced by the peripheral vascular effects of the local anesthetic. All local anesthetics except cocaine tend to have a biphasic effect on vascular smooth muscle. At low concentrations these agents tend to cause vasoconstriction, whereas at clinical concentrations, local anesthetics cause vasodilation.[18,19] However, differences exist in the degree of vasodilator activity produced by the various drugs. For example, lidocaine is a more potent vasodilator than mepivacaine or prilocaine. Although there is little apparent difference in the duration of conduction block among these agents in an isolated nerve, the duration of anesthesia produced in vivo by lidocaine is shorter than that of mepivacaine or prilocaine. Addition of a vasoconstrictor drug to these three local anesthetics results in a similar duration of action.

Onset of Action

The onset of conduction block in isolated nerves is primarily determined by the pK_a of the individual agents.[5] The pK_a of a chemical compound is the pH at which the ionized and nonionized forms are present in equal amounts. Because the uncharged form of the local anesthetic is primarily responsible for diffusion across the nerve sheath and nerve membrane, the onset of action will be directly related to the amount of drug that exists in the base form (Table 9-2).

The percentage of a specific local anesthetic present in the base form when injected into tissue at a pH of 7.4 is inversely proportional to the pK_a of that

TABLE 9-2. Relationship of pK$_a$ to Percent Base Form and Time for 50 Percent Conduction Block in Isolated Nerve

Agent	Chemical Class	pK$_a$	% Base at pH 7.5	Onset (min)
Prilocaine	Amino-amide	7.7	35	2–4
Lidocaine	Amino-amide	7.7	35	2–4
Etidocaine	Amino-amide	7.7	35	2–4
Bupivacaine	Amino-amide	8.1	20	5–8
Tetracaine	Amino-ester	8.6	5	10–15
Procaine	Amino-ester	8.9	2	14–18

agent. For example, mepivacaine, lidocaine, prilocaine, and etidocaine possess a pK$_a$ of approximately 7.7. When these agents are injected into tissue at a pH of 7.4, approximately 65 percent of these drugs exist in the ionized form and 35 percent exist in the nonionized base form. However, tetracaine possesses a pK$_a$ of 8.6. Only 5 percent is present in the nonionized form at a tissue pH of 7.4, whereas 95 percent exists in the charged cationic form. The pK$_a$ of bupivacaine is 8.1. Fifteen percent of this agent is present in the nonionized form at a tissue pH of 7.4, and 85 percent exists in the charged cationic form. Therefore, lidocaine, mepivacaine, prilocaine, and etidocaine show a rapid onset of action (low pK$_a$), whereas procaine and tetracaine have a slow onset time (high pK$_a$) (Table 9-2). Bupivacaine occupies an intermediate position in terms of pK$_a$ and latency of block.[20,21]

The onset of conduction blockade in vivo is dependent, in part, on other miscellaneous considerations. The onset of action may be altered by the rate of diffusion through nonnervous tissue. For example, lidocaine and prilocaine possess a similar pK$_a$ and similar onset of action in an isolated nerve. In vivo, however, prilocaine may be somewhat slower in onset than lidocaine. This difference may be related to an enhanced ability of lidocaine to diffuse through nonnervous tissue. More important, however, is the concentration of local anesthetic used. For example, 0.25 percent bupivacaine possesses a rather slow onset of action. However, increasing the concentration to 0.75 percent results in a significant decrease in the latency of anesthetic activity. The rapid onset time of chloroprocaine in vivo may be related, in part, to improved diffusion through nonnervous tissue but also to the use of a 3 percent concentration of this agent. The pK$_a$ of chloroprocaine is approximately 9, and its onset of action in isolated nerves is relatively slow.[22] However, the low systemic toxicity of this agent allows the use of high concentrations. Therefore, the rapid onset time of chloroprocaine in vivo may be related simply to the large number of molecules placed in the vicinity of peripheral nerves.

Differential Sensory/Motor Blockade

One other important clinical consideration is the ability of local anesthetics to cause a differential blockade of sensory and motor fibers. The subarachnoid administration of varying concentrations of procaine has been used to provide a differential blockade of sensory, sympathetic, and motor fibers. However, it has been extremely difficult to produce sensory anesthesia sufficient for surgery without a significant impairment of motor function. Bupivacaine was the first agent to possess a relative specificity for sensory fibers such that adequate sensory analgesia/anesthesia could be achieved without profound inhibition of motor fibers.

Bupivacaine and etidocaine provide an interesting contrast in terms of their differential sensory/motor blocking activity, although they are both potent long-acting agents (Fig. 9-3). Bupivacaine is widely used epidurally for both surgical and obstetric procedures and postoperative pain relief because of its ability to provide adequate sensory analgesia with minimal blockade of motor fibers. This is particularly true when bupivacaine is used as a 0.25 percent or 0.5 percent solution. Thus, the laboring parturient can be rendered pain-free and still be able to move her legs. This is one of the primary reasons why bupivacaine has enjoyed great popularity for continuous epidural blockade during labor. Increasing the concentration of bupivacaine to 0.75 percent will increase the depth of both sensory and motor blockade while also shortening latency and producing a more prolonged duration of anesthesia.[23]

Etidocaine, however, shows little separation of sensory and motor blocking properties (Fig. 9-3).[23] To achieve adequate epidural sensory anesthesia, 1.5 percent concentrations of etidocaine are usually required. At these concentrations, etidocaine has an extremely rapid onset of action and a prolonged duration of anesthesia. However, sensory anesthesia is associated with a profound degree of motor blockade. Thus, etidocaine is a valuable agent, particularly for epidural blockade in surgical situations where optimum muscle relaxation is desirable. Etidocaine demonstrates a rapid onset of action, prolonged duration, and satisfactory quality of anesthesia combined with profound motor blockade. This marked effect on motor function, however, renders etidocaine of limited value for obstetric analgesia and postoperative pain relief.

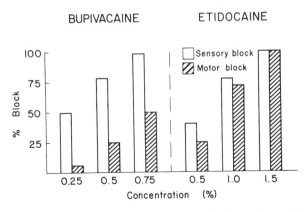

Fig. 9-3. Relative degree of sensory and motor blockade produced by the epidural administration of various concentrations of bupivacaine and etidocaine.

The factors responsible for the differential sensory/motor blockade associated with bupivacaine are not precisely known. Studies on isolated nerves have shown that bupivacaine at low concentrations will initially block unmyelinated C fibers, followed at a later time by a block of myelinated A fibers.[24] However, etidocaine blocks both A and C fibers at approximately the same rate. The slow blockade of A fibers by bupivacaine is believed to be due to the relatively high pK_a of this agent. Fewer uncharged molecules are available to penetrate the diffusion barriers surrounding large A fibers (large degree of myelination and large fiber diameter). In vivo, the combination of the slow diffusion of bupivacaine and its absorption by the vasculature at the site of drug administration may result in smaller numbers of bupivacaine molecules ultimately penetrating the membrane of the large motor A fibers. The numbers may be insufficient to cause conduction blockade. The lack of diffusion barriers around the small sensory C fibers may allow a sufficient number of bupivacaine molecules to reach receptor sites in the C fiber membrane to cause sensory anesthesia. Thus, bupivacaine may possess the optimal pK_a and lipid solubility characteristics required for differential sensory/motor blockade.

In summary, the pharmacologic activity of local anesthetics is primarily related to their physicochemical properties. However, the activity of these agents in vivo may be altered by other factors essentially unrelated to their physicochemical properties. On the basis of anesthetic activity in humans, the various agents may be classified as follows:

1. Agents of low anesthetic potency and short duration of action: procaine and chloroprocaine
2. Agents of intermediate anesthetic potency and duration of action: lidocaine, mepivacaine, and prilocaine
3. Agents of high anesthetic potency and prolonged duration of action: tetracaine, bupivacaine, and etidocaine

In terms of latency, chloroprocaine, lidocaine, mepivacaine, prilocaine, and etidocaine possess a relatively rapid onset of action. Bupivacaine is intermediate in terms of onset of anesthesia, whereas procaine and tetracaine demonstrate a long latency period.

FACTORS INFLUENCING ANESTHETIC ACTIVITY

Although the inherent pharmacologic properties of the various local anesthetics will basically determine their anesthetic profile, other factors may also influence the quality of regional anesthesia. These include

1. Dosage
2. Addition of vasoconstrictor
3. Site of injection

4. Carbonation and pH adjustment
5. Additives
6. Mixtures
7. Pregnancy

Dosage

The mass of administered drug will influence the onset, depth, and duration of anesthesia.[25] As the dosage of local anesthetic is increased, the frequency of satisfactory anesthesia and the duration of anesthesia will increase, and the onset of anesthesia will decrease.

In general, the dosage of administered local anesthetic can be increased by either administering a larger volume or a more concentrated solution. However, in clinical practice an increase in dosage is usually achieved by using a more concentrated solution of the specific agent. For example, increasing the concentration of epidurally administered bupivacaine from 0.125 percent to 0.5 percent (while maintaining the same volume of injectate) resulted in decreased latency, improved incidence of satisfactory analgesia, and increased duration of sensory analgesia.[26] Similarly, an increase in the concentration of epidural bupivacaine in surgical patients from 0.5 percent to 0.75 percent (with a concomitant increase in dosage from approximately 100 mg to 150 mg) produced a more rapid onset and prolonged duration of sensory anesthesia, a greater frequency of satisfactory sensory anesthesia, and an enhanced depth of motor blockade.[23] Prilocaine (600 mg) administered epidurally either as 30 ml of a 2 percent solution or 20 ml of a 3 percent solution showed no difference in onset, adequacy, or duration of anesthesia and onset, depth, or duration of motor blockade.[27]

Such data indicate that dosage rather than volume or concentration of anesthetic solution is the primary determinant of anesthetic activity. The volume of anesthetic solution may influence the spread of anesthesia, however.[28] For example, 30 ml of 1 percent lidocaine administered into the epidural space produced a level of anesthesia that was 4.3 dermatomes higher than that achieved when 10 ml of 3 percent lidocaine was used.[23] Thus, except for the possible effect on the spread of anesthesia, the primary qualities of regional anesthesia, namely, onset, depth, and duration of blockade are related to the mass of drug injected.

Addition of Vasoconstrictors

Vasoconstrictors (particularly epinephrine) are frequently added to local anesthetic solutions to decrease the rate of vascular absorption, allowing more anesthetic molecules to reach the nerve membrane. The depth and duration of anesthesia are thereby improved. Local anesthetic solutions usually contain a 1:200,000 (5 μg/ml) concentration of epinephrine. This concentration of epinephrine has been reported to provide an optimal degree of vasoconstriction when used with lidocaine for epidural or intercostal use.[29] Other vasoconstrictor

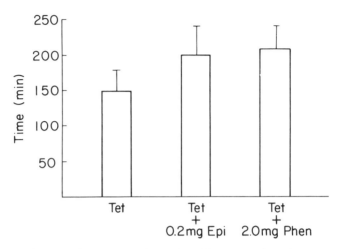

Fig. 9-4. Duration of spinal anesthesia produced by tetracaine alone, tetracaine with 0.2 mg of epinephrine, and tetracaine with 2.0 mg of phenylephrine.

agents such as norepinephrine and phenylephrine have also been added to solutions of local anesthetics. Equipotent concentrations of epinephrine and phenylephrine prolong the duration of spinal anesthesia produced by tetracaine to a similar extent[30] (Fig. 9-4).

The effect of epinephrine on the duration of anesthesia varies as a function of the individual local anesthetic and the site of injection. For example, the duration of action of all agents is prolonged by the addition of epinephrine when used for infiltration anesthesia and peripheral nerve blocks. Epinephrine will also increase the duration of epidural anesthesia when added to procaine, mepivacaine,[31] and lidocaine[32,33] but does not markedly alter the duration of action of epidurally administered prilocaine,[33] bupivacaine,[33,34] or etidocaine.[35] The decreased vasodilator action of prilocaine as compared with lidocaine is responsible for the reduced effect of added epinephrine. The high lipid solubility of bupivacaine and etidocaine may be responsible for the diminished effect of epinephrine. These agents are substantially absorbed by epidural fat and then slowly released, contributing to their prolonged duration of action.[36]

The interaction of epinephrine and the long-acting agents such as bupivacaine is also dependent on the concentration of drug used. For example, in epidural blockade for labor, the frequency and duration of adequate analgesia was improved when epinephrine 1:200,000 was added to 0.125 percent and 0.25 percent bupivacaine.[26] However, the addition of epinephrine to 0.5 and 0.75 percent bupivacaine did not improve the adequacy or prolong the initial regression of epidural sensory anesthesia in obstetric[26] or surgical[35] patients. The intensity but not the duration of motor blockade is enhanced after the epidural administration of epinephrine-containing solutions of bupivacaine and etidocaine.

Epinephrine significantly extends the duration of action of tetracaine in the subarachnoid space.[30] Regression of anesthesia is not markedly enhanced when solutions of lidocaine or bupivacaine with epinephrine are administered. However, anesthesia in the lower thoracic and lumbosacral areas is prolonged. Thus, epinephrine added to spinal solutions of lidocaine and bupivacaine may not significantly prolong the duration of effective surgical anesthesia in the abdominal area but will provide an extended duration of anesthesia in the lower limbs.

Site of Injection

Although local anesthetics are frequently classified as agents of short, moderate, or long duration with a slow or rapid onset of action, these general properties are influenced by the type of anesthetic procedure performed. In general, the most rapid onset but the shortest duration of action occurs after the subarachnoid or subcutaneous administration of local anesthetics.[37] The slowest onset times and the longest durations are observed during the performance of brachial plexus blocks.[37] For example, an agent such as bupivacaine demonstrates an onset time of approximately 5 minutes and a duration of action of approximately 3–4 hours when administered into the subarachnoid space. However, when bupivacaine is administered for brachial plexus blockade, the onset time is approximately 20–30 minutes, whereas the duration of anesthesia averages 10 hours.

Differences in the onset and duration of anesthesia depending on the site of injection are due, in part, to the particular anatomy of the area of injection, the variation of the rate of vascular absorption, and the amount of drug used for various types of regional anesthesia. In the case of spinal anesthesia, the lack of a nerve sheath around the spinal cord and the placement of the local anesthetic solution in the immediate vicinity of the spinal cord are responsible for the rapid onset of action. However, the relatively small amount of drug used for spinal anesthesia probably accounts for the relatively short duration of action associated with this particular technique. In the case of brachial plexus blockade, the onset of anesthesia is slow because the anesthetic agent is usually deposited at some distance from the nerve roots. The drug must then diffuse through various tissue barriers before reaching the nerve membrane. The long duration of brachial plexus blockade is probably related to the decreased rate of vascular absorption from that site and the larger doses of drug commonly used for this technique.

Carbonation and pH Adjustment

Carbon dioxide will enhance the diffusion of local anesthetics through nerve sheaths in isolated nerve preparations, resulting in a more rapid onset (Fig. 9-5) and a decrease in the C_m of local anesthetic required for conduction blockade.[38,39] The enhanced onset and depth of conduction blockade is believed to be due to the diffusion of carbon dioxide through the nerve membrane and a decrease in the axoplasmic pH. The lower pH will increase the intracellular concentration of the active cationic form of the local anesthetic, which binds to

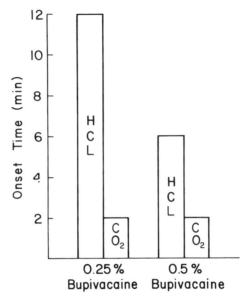

Fig. 9-5. Comparative effect of 0.25 percent and 0.5 percent bupivacaine hydrochloride and bupivacaine carbonate on onset of conduction block in isolated rabbit sciatic nerve.

a receptor in the sodium channel. In addition, the local anesthetic cation does not readily diffuse through membranes. Thus, the drug remains entrapped within the axoplasm, a situation referred to as ion trapping.

Several investigations have demonstrated that lidocaine carbonate solutions produce a more rapid onset of brachial plexus and epidural blockade than the use of lidocaine hydrochloride solutions in humans.[32,40] However, other studies have failed to demonstrate a significantly more rapid onset of action when lidocaine carbonate was compared with lidocaine hydrochloride for epidural blockade.[41] Similarly, bupivacaine carbonate is associated with a more rapid onset of action in humans. However, double-blind studies in which bupivacaine carbonate was compared with bupivacaine hydrochloride for brachial plexus or epidural blockade have failed to confirm these earlier reports.[42,43]

It is not certain whether carbonation of local anesthetic solutions will consistently decrease the latency of conduction blockade in a clinical situation. However, it does appear that carbonated solutions do improve the intensity of sensory anesthesia and motor blockade when administered into the epidural space. The major advantage of these solutions may be in brachial plexus blocks, where a more complete inhibition of conduction in the radial, median, and ulnar nerves has been demonstrated.

Alkalinization of local anesthetic solutions has also been used to decrease the onset of conduction blockade.[44] The addition of sodium bicarbonate will increase the pH of the local anesthetic solution, increasing the amount of drug in the uncharged base form. Thus, the rate of diffusion across the nerve sheath and nerve membrane should be enhanced, resulting in a more rapid onset of anesthesia. Several clinical studies demonstrated that the addition of sodium bicarbonate to solutions of bupivacaine or lidocaine will produce a significant decrease in the latency of brachial plexus and epidural blockade.[44] In addition, the duration of brachial plexus block is prolonged by increasing the pH of bupivacaine.[44]

Additives

Various attempts have been made to prolong the duration of anesthesia by incorporating substances such as dextran into local anesthetic solutions.[45] Discrepancies exist with regard to the effectiveness of dextran in prolonging the duration of regional anesthesia. In one controlled clinical study, prolonged durations of anesthesia were observed in some individual patients, but the mean duration of intercostal neural blockade was not significantly altered when solutions of bupivacaine with and without dextran were compared.[46]

Difference in results obtained by various investigators may be related to the pH of the dextran solution used.[47] Dextran solutions with a pH of 8.0 significantly prolonged the duration of bupivacaine-induced coccygeal nerve blocks in rats. The duration of block was not altered when dextran with a pH of 4.5–5.5 was added to bupivacaine. These results indicated that alkalinization of the anesthetic solution may be responsible for prolonged conduction blockade rather than the dextran itself.[47]

Mixtures

The use of mixtures of local anesthetics for regional anesthesia has become relatively popular in recent years. The basis for this practice is to compensate for the short duration of action of such agents as chloroprocaine or lidocaine and the long latency of such agents as tetracaine and bupivacaine. Mixtures of chloroprocaine and bupivacaine theoretically should offer significant clinical advantages because of the rapid onset and low systemic toxicity of chloroprocaine and the long duration of action of bupivacaine.

It was originally reported that a mixture of chloroprocaine and bupivacaine did result in a short latency and prolonged duration of brachial plexus blockade.[48] However, subsequent studies indicated that the duration of epidural anesthesia produced by a mixture of chloroprocaine and bupivacaine was significantly shorter than that obtained with solutions of bupivacaine alone.[49] Data from isolated nerve studies suggest that a metabolite of chloroprocaine may inhibit the binding of bupivacaine to membrane receptor sites.[50]

At the present time there do not appear to be any clinically significant advantages to the use of mixtures of local anesthetics. Etidocaine and bupivacaine provide clinically acceptable onsets of action and prolonged duration of anesthesia. In addition, the use of catheter techniques makes it possible to administer repeated injections of the rapidly acting agents such as chloroprocaine or lidocaine, which will provide an anesthetic duration of indefinite length.

Pregnancy

It is well known that the spread of epidural or spinal anesthesia is greater in pregnant patients as compared with nonpregnant patients.[51] This exaggerated spread has been attributed to mechanical factors associated with pregnancy. Dilated epidural veins decrease the diameter of the epidural and subarachnoid spaces, resulting in a more extensive longitudinal spread of local anesthetic solution.

Recent studies have suggested that physiologic alterations associated with pregnancy may also play a role in the apparent increase in local anesthetic sensitivity. For example, the spread of epidural anesthesia is similar in patients during the first trimester of pregnancy and in term patients, indicating that mechanical factors alone cannot explain the enhanced spread of anesthesia in parturients.[51] Isolated nerve studies have shown a more rapid onset and an increased sensitivity to local anesthetic-induced conduction blockade in vagus nerves obtained from pregnant rabbits.[52] These results suggest that hormonal changes associated with pregnancy may alter the basic responsiveness of the nerve membrane to local anesthetics. Thus, the drug dosage for any regional anesthetic procedure probably should be reduced during all stages of pregnancy.

PHARMACOKINETIC CONSIDERATIONS

Local anesthetic activity and toxicity are influenced by such factors as systemic absorption from the site of injection, distribution, metabolism, and excretion. The development of specific and sensitive analytic methods for measuring the concentration of local anesthetic drugs in blood and urine (gas chromatography) has resulted in the accumulation of considerable information concerning the pharmacokinetic properties of local anesthetic agents.

Absorption

The systemic absorption of local anesthetics is a function of the site of injection, dosage, addition of a vasoconstrictor agent, and the pharmacologic profile of the agent itself.[29,53,54] A comparison of the peak plasma levels of lidocaine achieved after various regional anesthetic techniques reveals that the highest drug level occurs after intercostal neural blockade.[29,53,54] This is followed in order of decreasing maximum plasma levels by injection into the caudal canal, paracervical area, epidural space, brachial plexus and femoral-sciatic site, sub-

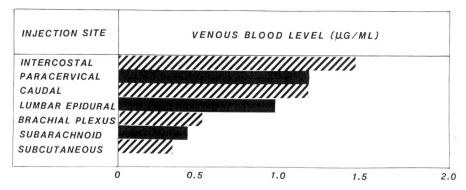

Fig. 9-6. Peak venous blood levels of lidocaine after injection of 100 mg of lidocaine into various anatomic sites.

cutaneous tissue, and the subarachnoid space[29,53–55] (Fig. 9-6). The high plasma levels after intercostal administration may be related to the multiple injections required for intercostal nerve blocks. Local anesthetic solution is exposed to a greater vascular area, resulting in a greater rate and degree of absorption.

This relationship of administration site to rate of absorption is of clinical significance, since use of a fixed dose of a local anesthetic agent may be potentially toxic in one area of administration but not in others. For example, the use of 400 mg of lidocaine without epinephrine for intercostal nerve block results in an average peak venous plasma level of approximately 7 μg/ml.[53,54] This plasma level is sufficient to cause symptoms of CNS toxicity in some patients. This same dose of lidocaine used for brachial plexus block yields a mean maximum blood level of 3.5 μg/ml, which is rarely associated with signs of toxicity.

The absorption and subsequent plasma level of local anesthetics is related to the total dose of drug administered, regardless of the site of administration. For most agents there is a linear relationship between the amount of drug administered and the resultant peak anesthetic plasma level. For example, the mean venous plasma level of lidocaine increased from approximately 1.5 μg/ml to 4 μg/ml as the total dose administered into the lumbar epidural space was increased from 200 to 600 mg.[41] Depending on the site of administration, a plasma level of 0.5–2.0 μg/ml is achieved for each 100 mg of lidocaine or mepivacaine injected.

The peak anesthetic plasma level achieved after regional anesthesia is a function of the total dose of drug administered, irrespective of the concentration or volume of the local anesthetic solution. No significant difference in lidocaine, prilocaine, and etidocaine blood levels are observed after intercostal or epidural administration regardless of alterations in concentration and volume of solutions, provided the total dose remains constant.[53,55,56]

Many commercial local anesthetic solutions contain a vasoconstrictor, usually epinephrine, in concentrations varying from 5–20 μg/ml. The addition of a vasoconstrictor to a local anesthetic solution may prolong the duration of action of certain agents. In addition, epinephrine decreases the rate of absorption

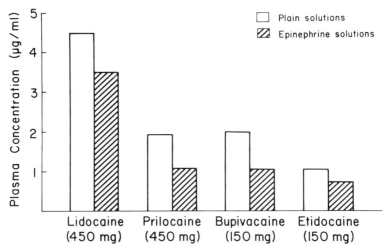

Fig. 9-7. Peak venous plasma concentrations of various local anesthetics administered with and without epinephrine for brachial plexus blockade.

of certain agents from various sites of administration, thereby lowering their potential toxicity (Fig. 9-7). Irrespective of the site of administration, 5 μg/ml of epinephrine (1:200,000) significantly reduces the peak blood levels of lidocaine and mepivacaine.[54,56] However, the peak plasma levels of prilocaine, bupivacaine, and etidocaine are minimally influenced by the addition of a vasoconstrictor substance after epidural administration.[53,55]

The optimal concentration of epinephrine in the lumbar epidural space appears to be 5 μg/ml (1:200,000). Use of a 1:80,000 concentration of epinephrine failed to produce a further reduction in the peak plasma level of lidocaine.[29] Other vasoconstrictor agents, such as phenylephrine and norepinephrine, have been used in combination with local anesthetics. Neither phenylephrine nor norepinephrine in concentrations of 1:20,000 appears to be as effective as epinephrine 1:200,000 in reducing the rate of absorption of lidocaine and mepivacaine.[57,58]

The pharmacologic characteristics of the specific local anesthetic also influence the rate and degree of vascular absorption. A comparison of agents of equivalent anesthetic potency reveals that lidocaine and mepivacaine are absorbed more rapidly after epidural administration than is prilocaine.[59] Bupivacaine is absorbed more rapidly than etidocaine.[55] These rates of absorption (particularly from the epidural space) are probably a reflection of differences in the vasodilator activity and the lipid solubility of these agents. Prilocaine produces less vasodilation than lidocaine. However, etidocaine possesses similar vasodilator activity to bupivacaine. The greater lipid solubility of etidocaine suggests a sequestration of this agent by epidural fat. Such sequestration may be responsible for the decreased rate of absorption and lower peak plasma level after epidural administration.[60]

Distribution

Local anesthetics distribute themselves throughout total body water. The rate of disappearance of local anesthetics from plasma (tissue redistribution), the volume of distribution, and the relative uptake by various tissues are related to the physicochemical properties of the specific agents.

The distribution of local anesthetics can be described by a two- or three-compartment model[61] (Fig. 9-8). The rapid disappearance from blood (α-phase) is related to uptake by rapidly equilibrating tissues (i.e., tissues that have a high vascular perfusion). The slower phase of disappearance from blood (β-phase)

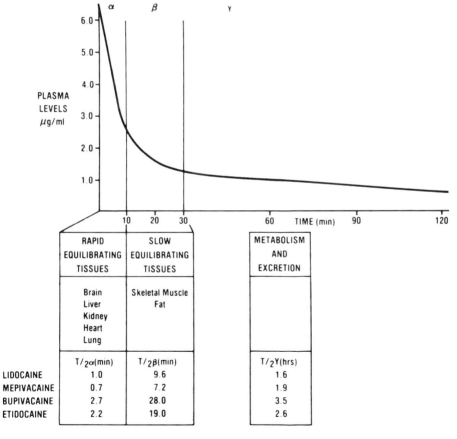

	RAPID EQUILIBRATING TISSUES	SLOW EQUILIBRATING TISSUES	METABOLISM AND EXCRETION
	Brain Liver Kidney Heart Lung	Skeletal Muscle Fat	
	$T/2\alpha$(min)	$T/2\beta$(min)	$T/2\gamma$(hrs)
LIDOCAINE	1.0	9.6	1.6
MEPIVACAINE	0.7	7.2	1.9
BUPIVACAINE	2.7	28.0	3.5
ETIDOCAINE	2.2	19.0	2.6

Fig. 9-8. *Upper portion* shows representative plasma concentration decay curve of a local anesthetic after intravenous injection. α-Phase represents redistribution into rapidly equilibrating tissues. β-Phase represents redistribution into slowly equilibrating tissues and γ-phase represents metabolism and excretion.

is mainly a function of distribution to slowly equilibrating tissues and the metabolism and excretion of the compound. This secondary phase may also be subdivided into a β-phase (distribution to slowly perfused tissue) and a γ-phase (metabolism and excretion).

A comparison of the three amide drugs of similar potency and duration of action (i.e., lidocaine, mepivacaine, and prilocaine) reveals that prilocaine is redistributed at a significantly more rapid rate from blood to tissues than is lidocaine and mepivacaine.[62] The rate of tissue redistribution for these latter two agents is similar. In addition, the β-disappearance phase from blood also occurs more rapidly with prilocaine, suggesting a more rapid rate of metabolism.[59] Differences also exist between the two more potent, longer-acting amide-type local anesthetics. Etidocaine possess a shorter β-half-life than bupivacaine, indicative of a more rapid rate of metabolism.

Local anesthetics are distributed throughout all body tissues, but the relative concentration in different tissues varies.[63,64] In general, the more highly perfused organs such as lung and kidney initially show higher concentrations of local anesthetic than the less well-perfused organs. Over a longer period, however, the highest percentage of an injected dose of a local anesthetic agent is found in skeletal muscle. Although this tissue does not show any particular affinity for this class of drugs, the mass of skeletal muscle makes it the largest reservoir for local anesthetic.

Selected tissue distribution studies have been conducted in humans (Table 9-3). A correlation exists between the degree of plasma protein binding and the plasma/erythrocyte (P/E) ratio of the different agents. Bupivacaine and etidocaine, which have the greatest capacity for plasma protein binding, also have the highest plasma/erythrocyte ratio. However, prilocaine shows the lowest P/E ratio and the lowest level of protein binding. Lidocaine and mepivacaine are intermediate in terms of plasma protein binding and plasma/erythrocyte distribution.[65]

Anesthetic levels in peripheral arteries and veins are also indicative of the distributive properties of the different drugs. For example, simultaneous measurements of samples from the brachial artery and the antecubital vein show a venous-arterial plasma concentration ratio of 0.73 for lidocaine and 0.47 for prilocaine.[64] Thus, the rate of diffusion into muscle is considerably faster for prilocaine than for lidocaine, accounting, in part, for the lower plasma levels observed with prilocaine.

TABLE 9-3. Relationship of Protein Binding Capacity to Plasma/RBC and Fetal/Maternal (U/M) Distribution of Various Local Anesthetic Agents

Agent	Protein Binding Capacity (%)	Plasma/RBC Ratio	U/M Ratio
Prilocaine	55	0.88	1.0–1.18
Lidocaine	64	1.34–2.1	0.52–0.69
Mepivacaine	77	2.6	0.69–0.71
Etidocaine	94	7.5	0.14–0.35
Bupivacaine	95	7.8	0.31–0.44

A specific distribution situation of clinical significance involves the placental transfer of local anesthetics. It is generally accepted that local anesthetics cross the placenta by passive diffusion. However, the rate and degree of diffusion vary significantly among agents and are directly correlated with the degree of maternal plasma protein binding (Table 9-3).[66] Bupivacaine and etidocaine have the lowest value for umbilical vein/maternal blood ratios (UV/M) and are the agents that are most highly protein-bound. Prilocaine shows the highest UV/M ratio and is the least protein-bound. Lidocaine and mepivacaine occupy intermediate positions with regard to their degree of placental transfer and their binding to plasma proteins.

Metabolism and Excretion

The pattern of metabolism of local anesthetics varies according to their chemical classification. Those agents that belong to the ester or procaine-like class undergo hydrolysis in plasma by the enzyme pseudocholinesterase.[67] The rate of metabolism may vary markedly among agents in the same chemical class. Chloroprocaine shows the most rapid rate of hydrolysis (4.7 μmole/ml/h), as compared with a rate of 1.1 μmole/ml/h for procaine and 0.3 μmole/ml/h for tetracaine. With regard to excretion, less than 2 percent of unchanged procaine is found in urine.[68] Approximately 90 percent of para-aminobenzoic acid, the primary metabolite of procaine, appears in urine. However, only 33 percent of diethyaminoethanol, the other major metabolite of procaine, is excreted unchanged.[68]

The local anesthetics that belong to the amide or lidocaine-like series undergo enzymatic degradation, primarily in the liver.[59] Prilocaine undergoes the most rapid rate of hepatic metabolism, whereas the metabolism of bupivacaine appears to be the slowest. Some degradation of the amide-type compounds may take place in tissue other than liver. The formation of certain metabolites has been observed after incubation of prilocaine with kidney slices.

The metabolism of the amide-type agents is more complex than that of the ester drugs. Although many of the metabolites have been identified, the complete metabolic pathways for all the compounds in this class have not been elucidated. Most studies looked at the metabolism of lidocaine. The main pathway of metabolism for this agent in humans involves oxidative de-ethylation of lidocaine to monoethylglycinexylidide, followed by a subsequent hydrolysis of monoethylglycinexylidide to xylidine.[69]

Excretion of the amide-type local anesthetic drugs occurs by way of the kidney. The major portion of the injected agent appears in the urine in the form of various metabolites. Less than 5 percent of the unchanged drug is excreted. The renal clearance of the amide local anesthetic agents appears to be inversely related to their protein binding capacity.[70] Prilocaine, which has a lower protein binding capacity than lidocaine, has a substantially higher clearance value than lidocaine. Renal clearance also is inversely proportional to the pH of urine, suggesting that urinary excretion of these agents occurs by nonionic diffusion.

TOXICOLOGIC CONSIDERATIONS

Local anesthetics are relatively free of side effects if they are administered in an appropriate anatomic location. However, systemic and localized toxic reactions can occur, usually caused by administration of an excessive dose or accidental intravascular or subarachnoid injection. In addition, specific adverse effects are associated with the use of certain agents. Examples of agent-specific adverse effects include allergic reactions to the amino-ester or procaine-like drugs and methemoglobinemia after the use of prilocaine.

Systemic Toxicity

Systemic reactions to local anesthetics primarily involve the central nervous system (CNS) and the cardiovascular system. In general, the CNS is more susceptible to the systemic actions of local anesthetic agents than the cardiovascular system. The dosage and plasma level of local anesthetic required to produce CNS toxicity is usually lower than that which results in circulatory collapse. Although local anesthetic-induced cardiovascular depression occurs less frequently, adverse effects involving the cardiovascular system tend to be more serious and more difficult to manage.

Central Nervous System Toxicity

The initial symptoms of local anesthetic-induced CNS toxicity involve feelings of light-headedness and dizziness, frequently followed by visual and auditory disturbances such as difficulty in focusing and tinnitus. Other subjective CNS symptoms include disorientation and occasional feelings of drowsiness. Objective signs of CNS toxicity are usually excitatory in nature and include shivering, muscular twitching, and tremors, initially involving the muscles of the face and distal extremities. Ultimately, generalized convulsions of a tonic-clonic nature occur. If a sufficiently large dose or a rapid intravenous injection is administered, the initial signs of CNS excitation are rapidly followed by a state of generalized CNS depression. Seizure activity ceases, and respiratory depression and ultimately respiratory arrest may occur. In some patients, CNS depression without a preceding excitatory phase is seen, particularly if other CNS depressant drugs have been administered.

CNS excitation is the result of an initial blockade of inhibitory pathways in the cerebral cortex by local anesthetics.[71] The blockade of inhibitory pathways allows facilatory neurons to function in an unopposed fashion, resulting in an increase in excitatory activity, leading to convulsions. An increase in the dose of administered local anesthetic leads to an inhibition of conduction in both inhibitory and facilatory pathways, resulting in a generalized state of CNS depression.

In general, a correlation exists between the anesthetic potency and intravenous CNS toxicity of various agents.[72] For example, in cats, the dose of procaine required to cause convulsions is approximately seven times greater than the convulsive dose of bupivacaine.[72] However, bupivacaine is also approximately eight times more potent than procaine as a local anesthetic agent. A similar study in dogs indicated that the relative CNS toxicity of bupivacaine, etidocaine, and lidocaine is $4:2:1$, which is similar to the relative potency of these agents for the production of regional anesthesia in humans.[73] Intravenous infusion studies in human volunteers also demonstrated a relationship between the intrinsic anesthetic potency of various agents and the dosage required to induce CNS toxicity.[45,74–76]

The rate of injection and the rapidity with which a particular plasma level is achieved will alter the toxicity of local anesthetic agents. For example, in human volunteers receiving an infusion of etidocaine at 10 mg/min, an average dose of 236 mg of etidocaine and a venous plasma level of 3.0 μg/ml were required before CNS symptoms occurred.[76] When the infusion rate was increased to 20 mg/min, an average of 161 mg of etidocaine and a venous plasma level of approximately 2 μg/ml were required before symptoms of CNS toxicity were evident.[76]

Acid-base status can markedly affect the CNS activity of local anesthetics.[72] In cats, the convulsive threshold of various local anesthetics is inversely related to the arterial PCO_2. A decrease in arterial pH will also decrease the convulsive threshold of these agents. In fact, pH probably exerts a greater influence on the CNS toxicity of local anesthetics than does PCO_2. Respiratory acidosis with a resultant increase in PCO_2 in response to an elevated arterial pH will consistently decrease the convulsive threshold of local anesthetics. However, an increase in PCO_2 in response to an elevated arterial pH (as may occur during metabolic alkalosis) exerts less of an effect on the convulsive threshold.[77]

The potentiating effect of acidosis and/or hypercarbia on the convulsive threshold of local anesthetics may be due to several factors. An elevation of PCO_2 will enhance cerebral blood flow so that more anesthetic agent is delivered to the brain. In addition, diffusion of CO_2 across the nerve membrane in the presence of hypercarbia may result in a fall in intracellular pH. Intracellular acidosis will augment the conversion of the base form of the local anesthetic to the cationic form, resulting in an increase in the intraneuronal level of the active form of the local anesthetic. The cationic form does not diffuse well across the nerve membrane and ion trapping will occur, increasing the apparent CNS toxicity of local anesthetic agents.

Hypercarbia and/or acidosis will also decrease the plasma protein binding of local anesthetics.[78] Therefore, an elevation in PCO_2 or a decrease in pH will increase the proportion of free drug available for diffusion into the brain. However, acidosis will increase the cationic form of the local anesthetic, which should decrease the rate of diffusion.

In summary, local anesthetics can exert marked effects on the CNS. In general, signs of CNS excitation leading to frank convulsions are the most common manifestation of systemic anesthetic toxicity. Excessive doses or rapid intravenous administration of these drugs may also lead to CNS depression and respiratory arrest. In general, the potential CNS toxicity of local anesthetics is correlated with the inherent anesthetic potency of the various agents. However, the toxicity of these agents can be altered by rate of injection, hypercarbia, and acidosis.

Cardiovascular System Toxicity

Local anesthetic agents can exert a direct action both on the heart and peripheral blood vessels.

Direct Cardiac Effects

The primary cardiac electrophysiologic effect of local anesthetics is a decrease in the maximum rate of depolarization due to a decrease in sodium conductance in the fast sodium channels in cardiac membranes. Action potential duration and the effective refractory period are also decreased by local anesthetics. However, the ratio of effective refractory period to action potential duration is increased both in Purkinje fibers and in ventricular muscle.[79]

Qualitative differences may exist between the electrophysiologic effects of various agents. Bupivacaine depresses the rapid phase of depolarization (V_{max}) in Purkinje fibers and ventricular muscle to a greater extent than lidocaine.[80] In addition, the rate of recovery from a steady-state block is slower in bupivacaine-treated papillary muscles as compared with lidocaine. This slow rate of recovery results in an incomplete restoration of V_{max} between action potentials, particularly at high heart rates. In contrast, recovery from lidocaine is complete, even at rapid heart rates. These differential effects of lidocaine and bupivacaine are believed to be responsible for the antiarrhythmic activity of lidocaine and the arrhythmogenic potential of bupivacaine.

Electrophysiologic studies in intact dogs and in humans essentially reflect the findings observed in isolated cardiac tissue.[81,82] As the dose and plasma levels of lidocaine are increased, a prolongation of conduction time occurs within various parts of the heart. These changes are reflected in the electrocardiogram as an increase in the PR interval and QRS duration. Extremely high concentrations of local anesthetics will depress spontaneous pacemaker activity in the sinus node, resulting in sinus bradycardia and sinus arrest.

Local anesthetics also exert profound effects on the mechanical activity of cardiac muscle. All local anesthetics exert a dose-dependent negative inotropic action on isolated cardiac tissue.[83] This depression of cardiac contractility is proportional to the conduction-blocking potency of the various agents in isolated nerves.[83] Thus, the more potent local anesthetics depress cardiac contractility at lower concentrations than the less potent drugs.

In general, local anesthetics can be divided into three groups in terms of their myocardial depressant effect. The more potent agents (i.e., bupivacaine, tetracaine, and etidocaine) depress cardiac contractility at the lowest concentrations. The agents of moderate anesthetic potency (i.e., lidocaine, mepivacaine, and prilocaine) form an intermediate group of compounds in terms of myocardial depression. Finally, procaine and chloroprocaine (the least potent of the

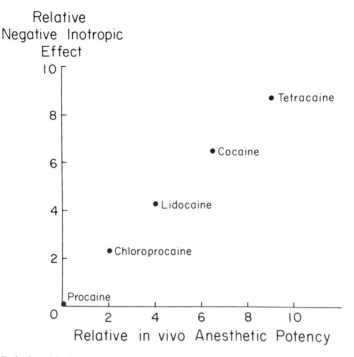

Fig. 9-9. Relationship between the relative negative inotropic effect of various local anesthetics and their relative in vivo anesthetic potency as determined on isolated nerve.

local anesthetics) require the highest concentrations to decrease cardiac contractility.

Studies in intact dogs (in which a strain gauge arch was sutured to the right ventricle) revealed that all evaluated local anesthetics exerted a negative inotropic action.[84] As in the isolated cardiac tissue studies, a relationship existed between the local anesthetic potency of various agents and their relative myocardial depressant effect (Fig. 9-9). For example, tetracaine, which is approximately eight to ten times more potent than procaine as a local anesthetic, was approximately eight times more potent as a depressant of myocardial contractility than procaine.[84] Hemodynamic studies in closed-chest anesthetized dogs showed that tetracaine, etidocaine, and bupivacaine caused a 50 percent decrease in cardiac output at doses of 10–20 mg/kg. Doses of 30–40 mg/kg of lidocaine, mepivacaine, prilocaine, and chloroprocaine were required for a similar decrease in cardiac output. A dose of 100 mg/kg of procaine was needed to reduce cardiac output by 50 percent.[85,86]

The mechanism by which local anesthetics depress myocardial contractility is not precisely known, but may involve an interaction with calcium. Both procaine and tetracaine can increase the release of calcium from isolated skeletal muscle preparations.[87] The ability of tetracaine and procaine to increase the rate of calcium efflux from sartorius muscle was proportional to their local anesthetic activity. A similar displacement of calcium from cardiac muscle should result in a decrease in myocardial contractility. However, studies in the isolated guinea pig heart indicated that an increase in the extracellular concentration of calcium failed to reverse the negative inotropic action of bupivacaine or lidocaine.[88]

Direct Peripheral Vascular Effects

Local anesthetics exert a biphasic effect on peripheral vascular smooth muscle.[89] Direct measurements of the arteriolar diameter in the cremaster muscle of rats revealed that concentrations of lidocaine varying from 10^0 to 10^3 $\mu g/ml$ produced a dose-related state of vasoconstriction varying from 88 to 60 percent of the control vascular diameter.[18] An increase in the concentration of lidocaine to 10^4 $\mu g/ml$ produced approximately a 27 percent increase in arteriolar diameter, indicative of a significant degree of vasodilation. Isolated rat portal vein studies also demonstrated that local anesthetics stimulate spontaneous myogenic contractions and augment basal tone at low concentrations but inhibit myogenic activity at higher concentrations.[89]

In vivo studies also confirmed the biphasic effect of local anesthetics on the peripheral vasculature. Blood flow investigations in animals and humans[90] demonstrated that lower doses of local anesthetics may decrease peripheral arterial flow without any change in blood pressure, indicative of an increase in peripheral vascular resistance. Higher doses of local anesthetics will result in an increased blood flow in peripheral arteries, indicating a state of vasodilation. Cocaine is the only local anesthetic that consistently causes vasoconstriction, because of its ability to inhibit the uptake of norepinephrine by storage granules. The excess concentration of free circulating norepinephrine is responsible for the vasoconstriction associated with the use of cocaine.[91]

Comparison of the peripheral vascular effects of various local anesthetics has failed to demonstrate a good correlation between their relative anesthetic potency and the ability to cause peripheral vasodilation. However, a correlation does exist between the duration of the anesthetic action of these agents and the attendant duration of vasodilation. After intra-arterial injection into the femoral artery of dogs, the peripheral vasodilation associated with lidocaine, mepivacaine, and prilocaine lasts approximately 5 minutes. However, long-acting local anesthetics, such as bupivacaine, etidocaine, and tetracaine, produce a prolonged period of vasodilation.[91,92]

The biphasic peripheral vascular effect of local anesthetics may be related to changes in smooth muscle concentrations of calcium. A competitive antagonism exists between local anesthetic drugs and calcium ions in smooth muscle.[93,94] Local anesthetics may displace calcium from membrane binding sites, resulting in diffusion of this ion into the smooth muscle cytoplasm. Such an increase in cytoplasmic calcium concentration should stimulate the interaction between contractile proteins, leading to an increase in myogenic tone and vasoconstriction. However, as the concentration of local anesthetic at the smooth muscle membrane is increased, the displacement of calcium by these agents will ulti-

TABLE 9-4. Comparative Cardiovascular Collapse (CC)/Convulsive (CNS) Ratio and Cardiac Tissue/Blood Concentration Ratio of Lidocaine, Bupivacaine, and Etidocaine in Adult Sheep

	Lidocaine	Bupivacaine	Etidocaine
CC/CNS dose ratio	7.1 ± 1.1	3.7 ± 0.5	4.4 ± 1.9
CC/CNS blood level ratio	3.6 ± 0.3	1.6 ± 0.1	1.7 ± 0.2
Cardiac tissue	2.0 ± 0.5	3.8 ± 0.6	3.5 ± 0.7

(Data from Morishima et al[98,100])

mately decrease both the cytoplasmic calcium concentration and the interaction between the contractile protein elements of smooth muscle. This will result in a state of muscle relaxation, leading to vasodilation.

COMPARATIVE CARDIOVASCULAR TOXICITY OF LOCAL ANESTHETICS

In general, a direct relationship exists between the anesthetic potency and cardiovascular depressant potential of the various agents. In recent years, the more potent drugs (i.e., bupivacaine and etidocaine) have been reported to cause rapid and profound cardiovascular depression after an accidental intravascular injection in some patients.[95–97] Severe cardiac arrhythmias were observed, and the cardiac depression appeared resistant to various therapeutic modalities. Thus, the more potent and highly lipid-soluble drugs, such as bupivacaine and etidocaine, may be relatively more cardiotoxic than the less potent and less lipid-soluble agents, such as lidocaine.

The cardiotoxicity of the more potent bupivacaine appears to differ from that of lidocaine in the following manner:

1. Ratio of the dosage required for irreversible cardiovascular collapse and the dosage that will produce CNS toxicity (convulsions) (i.e., the CC/CNS ratio) is lower for bupivacaine (and etidocaine) compared with lidocaine[98] (Table 9-4)
2. Ventricular arrhythmias and fatal ventricular fibrillation may occur after the rapid intravenous administration of a large dose of bupivacaine, but not lidocaine[99]
3. The pregnant animal or patient may be more sensitive to the cardiotoxic effects of bupivacaine than the nonpregnant animal or patient[100]
4. Cardiac resuscitation is more difficult after bupivacaine-induced cardiovascular collapse[101–103]
5. Acidosis and hypoxia markedly potentiates the cardiotoxicity of bupivacaine[104]

Miscellaneous Systemic Effects

A variety of miscellaneous systemic actions have been ascribed to local anesthetics. Most of these miscellaneous systemic effects are related to the generalized membrane-stabilizing property of this class of drugs. For example, local anesthetics have been reported to possess neuromuscular blocking, ganglionic blocking, and anticholinergic activity. There is little evidence to suggest that any of these miscellaneous effects are clinically significant under normal conditions.

A unique systemic side effect associated with a specific local anesthetic agent is the formation of methemoglobin after the administration of large doses of prilocaine.[105,106] A dose-response relationship exists between the amount of epidurally administered prilocaine and the degree of methemoglobinemia. In general, a dose of at least 600 mg of prilocaine is required for the development of clinically significant plasma levels of methemoglobin.

The formation of methemoglobin is believed to be related to the chemical structure of prilocaine. The metabolism of this agent in the liver results in the formation of o-toluidine, which is responsible for the oxidation of hemoglobin to methemoglobin.[105] The methemoglobinemia associated with the use of prilocaine is spontaneously reversible or may be treated by the intravenous administration of methylene blue.

Allergic Effects

The amino-ester agents, such as procaine, have been shown to produce allergic reactions. These agents are derivatives of para-aminobenzoic acid, which is known to be allergenic. The amino-amide local anesthetics are not derivatives of para-aminobenzoic acid, and allergic reactions to the amino-amides are extremely rare.[107–109]

Intradermal injections of both amino-ester and amino-amide local anesthetics have been made in patients with and without a presumptive history of local anesthetic allergy.[110] Positive skin reactions were observed in 25 of 60 patients who did not describe any previous allergic symptomatology. In all cases the cutaneous reactions occurred after the injection of an amino-ester agent (i.e., procaine, tetracaine, and chloroprocaine). No cutaneous reactions occurred after the use of the amino-amide agents (i.e., lidocaine, mepivacaine, or prilocaine). Eleven patients who were studied had a history of alleged local anesthetic allergy. Eight of these patients showed a positive skin reaction to procaine, tetracaine, or chloroprocaine. However, no positive cutaneous response was seen after the administration of lidocaine, mepivacaine, or prilocaine. No signs of systemic anaphylaxis occurred in any of the subjects.

Although the amino-amide agents appear to be relatively free from allergic-type reactions, solutions of these agents may contain a preservative, methylparaben, the chemical structure of which is similar to that of para-aminobenzoic acid. Intradermal administration of methylparaben will produce a positive skin reaction.[111]

Local Tissue Toxicity

Local anesthetics that are used clinically rarely produce localized nerve damage. Studies on isolated frog sciatic nerves revealed that the concentrations of procaine, cocaine, tetracaine, and dibucaine required to produce irreversible conduction blockade are far in excess of the concentrations of these agents used clinically.[112] Subarachnoid administration of 4 percent tetracaine caused histopathologic spinal cord changes in rabbits.[113] The maximum concentration of tetracaine employed for spinal anesthesia in humans is 1 percent.

In recent years, prolonged sensory and motor deficits have been reported in some patients after the epidural or subarachnoid injection of large doses of chloroprocaine.[114,115] Studies in animals have proven somewhat contradictory regarding the potential neurotoxicity of chloroprocaine. The etiology of the local neural irritation associated with the use of chloroprocaine solutions is the low pH and presence of the antioxidant sodium bisulfite in these solutions.

Subarachnoid administration of chloroprocaine solutions containing sodium bisulfite has caused paralysis in rabbits.[116] The use of pure solutions of chloroprocaine without sodium bisulfite did not cause paralysis. Administration of sodium bisulfite alone was associated with paralysis.

A detailed study has been conducted on the isolated rabbit vagus nerve to investigate the neurotoxicity of the various components of commercial chloroprocaine solutions.[117] Commercial solutions of 3 percent chloroprocaine contain the local anesthetic itself, 0.2 percent sodium bisulfite, and hydrogen ions that yield a pH of approximately 3.0. Application of commercial 3 percent chloroprocaine to isolated vagus nerves for 30 minutes resulted in irreversible conduction blockade. The use of 3 percent chloroprocaine with sodium bisulfite solution buffered to a pH of 7.0 caused reversible conduction block. A 3 percent chloroprocaine solution with a pH of 3.0 but without sodium bisulfite also resulted in reversible blockade. Application of a 0.2 percent sodium bisulfite solution at a pH of 3.0 resulted in irreversible conduction block, whereas the use of a 0.2 percent sodium bisulfite solution with a pH of 7.0 caused no conduction block. The results of these studies suggest that the combination of a low pH and the presence of sodium bisulfite may be responsible for the neurotoxic reactions observed after the use of large amounts of chloroprocaine solution. Chloroprocaine itself does not appear to be neurotoxic.[117]

Skeletal muscle appears to be more sensitive than other tissues to the local irritant properties of local anesthetics. Histopathologic changes in skeletal muscle have been observed with most of the clinically used local anesthetics.[118,119] In general, the more potent longer-acting agents (i.e., bupivacaine and etidocaine) appear to cause a greater degree of localized skeletal muscle damage than the less potent, shorter-acting agents (i.e., lidocaine and prilocaine). This effect on skeletal muscle is reversible, and muscle regeneration occurs rapidly. Regeneration is complete within 2 weeks after injection of local anesthetics. These histopathologic changes in skeletal muscle have not been correlated with any overt clinical signs of local irritation.

COMPLICATIONS OF REGIONAL ANESTHESIA

Certain regional anesthetic techniques, such as epidural or spinal anesthesia, are associated with sympathetic blockade and can result in profound hypotension. In general, the degree of hypotension is related to the extent of the sympathetic blockade.

Epidural Anesthesia

Cardiovascular alterations after epidural blockade are related to

1. Level of block
2. Drug dosage
3. Specific local anesthetic
4. Addition of vasoconstrictors
5. Blood volume status

Level of Block

Epidural blockade to the T5 dermatomal level or below is not usually accompanied by significant cardiovascular alterations.[120] As the level of anesthesia extends from T5 to T1, a 20 percent fall in blood pressure can be observed. This hypotensive state is related almost exclusively to sympathetic inhibition and peripheral vasodilation below the level of block, resulting in a significant decrease in systemic vascular resistance. Neural blockade at levels of T1 and above can cause a fall in heart rate and cardiac output. The reduction in cardiac output may be related, in part, to inhibition of myocardial sympathetic fibers with decreased cardiac contractility. A decrease in venous return caused by venodilation and expansion of capacitance vessels also contributes to the reduction in cardiac output. (For an extensive discussion of the cardiovascular effects of epidural anesthesia/analgesia, see Chapters 12 and 18.)

Drug Dosage

Relatively large amounts of local anesthetic are required to achieve a satisfactory degree of epidural blockade. Local anesthetic is absorbed rather rapidly from the epidural space, and significant plasma levels may be achieved. The absorbed local anesthetic may produce systemic effects involving the cardiovascular system, as previously discussed. Plasma levels of lidocaine of less than 4 μg/ml after epidural blockade resulted in a slight increase in blood pressure, mainly due to an increased cardiac output.[120] Doses of epidural lidocaine that produced plasma levels in excess of 4 μg/ml resulted in hypotension, caused in part by the negative inotropic and the peripheral vasodilator actions of the drug.

Specific Local Anesthetic

Differences in the onset of epidural anesthesia occur as a function of the specific agent employed. For example, drugs such as chloroprocaine, lidocaine, and etidocaine produce a fairly rapid onset of anesthesia, whereas bupivacaine has been shown to exert a significantly slower onset of action. The more rapidly acting agents produce a more profound degree of hypotension because of the more rapid blockade of sympathetic fibers. In addition, certain agents, such as etidocaine, can penetrate myelinated fibers more readily and may be associated with a more profound degree of sympathetic blockade and hypotension.

Addition of Vasoconstrictors

Epinephrine is frequently added to local anesthetics intended for epidural use to decrease the rate of vascular absorption and prolong the duration of anesthesia. Absorbed epinephrine may produce transient cardiovascular alterations. An exaggerated fall in arterial blood pressure has been reported after the use of epinephrine containing local anesthetics for epidural blockade.[66] The absorbed epinephrine is believed to stimulate β_2-adrenergic receptors in peripheral vascular beds, leading to a state of vasodilation and a fall in diastolic pressure. The β_1-adrenergic receptor stimulating effect of epinephrine results in an increase in heart rate and cardiac output that will counteract the peripheral vasodilator state to some extent. Although absorbed epinephrine may be responsible for the early cardiovascular changes observed after epidural blockade, the more prolonged hypotension seen after epidural anesthesia with epinephrine containing solutions is probably related to the achievement of a more profound degree of sympathetic blockade.

Blood Volume Status

Cardiovascular depression is more severe and more dangerous after the production of epidural anesthesia in hypovolemic patients.[121] Epidural anesthesia in hypovolemic volunteers was associated with profound hypotension caused by peripheral vasodilation and a decrease in cardiac output and heart rate. The addition of epinephrine to the anesthetic solution resulted in a less profound degree of hypotension in these subjects but was unable to prevent a significant fall in blood pressure. The failure of epinephrine to sufficiently increase cardiac output to maintain a normal blood pressure is obviously due to the diminished circulating blood volume.

Spinal Anesthesia

In general, a decrease in blood pressure occurs due to the blockade of sympathetic fibers after the induction of spinal anesthesia. The degree of hypotension is related, almost exclusively, to the extent of sympathetic and sensory blockade. Studies in humans have shown that subarachnoid anesthesia to the T5 level is often associated with hypotension, resulting from a decrease in stroke volume, cardiac output, and peripheral vascular resistance.[122] The decrease in cardiac output and stroke volume is not related to a decrease in myocardial contractility but rather to a decrease in venous return. Placement of patients in a slightly head-down position or the infusion of crystalloid solutions is usually sufficient to reverse the hypotensive state.

Studies in monkeys revealed that the level of sensory anesthesia after the subarachnoid administration of tetracaine is correlated with the degree of hypotension.[123] Anesthesia to the T10 dermatomal level resulted in a fall in blood pressure of approximately 15 percent. This fall in blood pressure was due almost exclusively to a decrease in peripheral vascular resistance, with little change in cardiac output. However, extension of the level of sympathetic and sensory block to the T1 dermatomal level was associated with a 35 percent decrease in blood pressure. This exaggerated state of hypotension was caused, in part, by a decrease in peripheral vascular resistance, but also by a significant reduction in cardiac output.

SPECIFIC LOCAL ANESTHETIC AGENTS

Amino-Ester Agents

Cocaine

Cocaine was the first agent successfully used for the production of clinical local anesthesia. The relatively high potential for systemic toxicity and the addiction liability associated with its use resulted in the abandonment of this agent for most regional anesthetic techniques. However, cocaine is an excellent topical anesthetic and is the only local anesthetic that produces vasoconstriction at clinically useful concentrations. As a result, it is still used to anesthetize and constrict the nasal mucosa before nasotracheal intubation. It is also used frequently by otolaryngologists during nasal surgery because of its topical anesthetic and vasoconstrictor properties.

Procaine

Procaine was the first synthetic local anesthetic introduced into clinical practice. Procaine is a relatively weak local anesthetic with a slow onset and short duration of action. The relatively low potency and rapid plasma hydrolysis of this agent is responsible for the low systemic toxicity of procaine. However, procaine is hydrolyzed to para-aminobenzoic acid, which is responsible for the allergic reactions associated with repeated use. At present, procaine is primarily used for infiltration anesthesia, diagnostic differential spinal blocks, and for obstetric spinal anesthesia.

Chloroprocaine

Chloroprocaine is characterized by a rapid onset of action, a short duration, and low systemic toxicity. Chloroprocaine is primarily used for epidural analgesia and anesthesia in obstetrics because of its rapid onset and low systemic toxicity in mother and fetus. However, frequent injections are required to provide adequate pain relief during labor. Often, epidural analgesia is established in the pregnant patient with chloroprocaine. This is followed by the use of a longer-acting agent, such as bupivacaine. Chloroprocaine is also useful for various regional anesthetic procedures performed in ambulatory surgical patients, when the duration of surgery is not expected to exceed 30–60 minutes.

Some concern exists regarding the potential neurotoxicity of chloroprocaine solutions, due to reports of prolonged sensory and motor deficits after the accidental subarachnoid injection of large doses. These local irritant effects are related to the low pH and sodium bisulfite in chloroprocaine.

Tetracaine

Tetracaine is primarily used for spinal anesthesia. Tetracaine may be used as an isobaric, hypobaric, or hyperbaric solution for spinal blockade, although hyperbaric solutions of tetracaine are probably used most commonly. Tetracaine provides a relatively rapid onset of spinal anesthesia, excellent quality of sensory anesthesia, and a profound block of motor function. Plain solutions of tetracaine provide an average duration of spinal anesthesia of 2–3 hours. Addition of epinephrine can extend the duration of anesthesia to 4–6 hours.

Tetracaine is rarely used for other forms of regional anesthesia because of its extremely slow onset of action and the potential for systemic toxic reactions when larger doses are used. Tetracaine also possesses excellent topical anesthetic properties, and solutions of this agent have been used for endotracheal surface anesthesia. However, the absorption of tetracaine from the tracheobronchial tree is extremely rapid, and several fatalities have been reported after the use of an endotracheal aerosol of tetracaine.

Amino-Amide Agents

Lidocaine

Lidocaine was the first drug of the amino-amide type to be introduced into clinical practice. This agent remains the most versatile and most commonly used local anesthetic because of its inherent potency, rapid onset, moderate duration of action, and topical anesthetic activity. Solutions of lidocaine are available for infiltration, peripheral nerve block, and epidural anesthesia. In addition, hyperbaric 5 percent lidocaine is useful for spinal anesthesia of 30–60 minutes' duration. Lidocaine is also used in ointment, jelly, and viscous and aerosol preparations for a variety of topical anesthetic procedures.

Intravenous lidocaine has also proven of value for certain nonanesthetic indications. This agent has gained wide acceptance as an intravenous drug for the treatment of ventricular arrhythmias. In addition, lidocaine has been used intravenously as an antiepileptic agent, as an analgesic for certain chronic pain states, and as a supplement to general anesthesia.

Mepivacaine

Mepivacaine is similar to lidocaine in terms of its anesthetic profile. Mepivacaine can produce profound depth of anesthesia with a relatively rapid onset and a moderate duration of action. This agent may be used for infiltration, peripheral nerve block, and epidural anesthesia. In some countries, 4 percent hyperbaric solutions of mepivacaine are also available for spinal anesthesia.

Mepivacaine is not effective as a topical anesthetic, and so is less versatile than lidocaine. In addition, the metabolism of mepivacaine is markedly prolonged in the fetus and newborn, making it untenable for obstetric anesthesia. However, in adults, mepivacaine appears to be somewhat less toxic than lidocaine. In addition, the vasodilator activity of mepivacaine is less than that of lidocaine. Thus, mepivacaine provides a somewhat longer duration of anesthesia than lidocaine when the two agents are used without epinephrine.

Prilocaine

The clinical profile of prilocaine is also similar to that of lidocaine. Prilocaine has a relatively rapid onset of action, while providing a moderate duration of anesthesia and a profound depth of conduction blockade. This agent causes significantly less vasodilation than lidocaine and so can be used without epinephrine. In general, the duration of prilocaine without epinephrine is similar to that of lidocaine with epinephrine. Thus, prilocaine is particularly useful in patients in whom epinephrine may be contraindicated. Prilocaine is useful for infiltration, peripheral nerve blockade, and epidural anesthesia.

Prilocaine is the least toxic of the amino-amide local anesthetics. Thus, this agent is particularly useful for intravenous regional anesthesia. CNS toxic effects are rarely seen after tourniquet deflation, even when early accidental release of the tourniquet may occur.

Methemoglobinemia may occur after the use of relatively large doses of prilocaine. This unusual side effect has essentially eliminated the use of this drug in obstetrics, although prilocaine has not been reported to cause any significant adverse effects in mother, fetus, or newborn.

Bupivacaine

Bupivacaine was the first local anesthetic to combine the properties of acceptable onset, long duration of action, profound conduction blockade, and significant separation of sensory anesthesia and motor blockade. This agent is used for various regional anesthetic procedures, including infiltration, peripheral nerve block, and epidural and spinal anesthesia. The average duration of surgical anesthesia of bupivacaine varies from approximately 3–10 hours. Its longest duration of action occurs when major peripheral nerve blocks, such as brachial plexus blockade, are performed.

The major advantage of bupivacaine appears to be in the area of epidural obstetric analgesia for labor. Satisfactory pain relief of 2–3 hours' duration is achieved, significantly decreasing the need for repeated injections in the pregnant patient. Moreover, adequate analgesia is usually achieved without significant motor blockade, such that the patient in labor is able to move her legs. This differential blockade of sensory and motor fibers is also the basis for the widespread use of bupivacaine for postoperative epidural analgesia and for certain chronic pain states.

Etidocaine

Etidocaine is characterized by very rapid onset, prolonged duration of action, and profound sensory and motor blockade. Etidocaine may be used for infiltration, peripheral nerve blockade, and epidural anesthesia. Etidocaine has a significantly more rapid onset of action than bupivacaine. Concentrations of etidocaine required for adequate sensory anesthesia produce profound motor blockade. As a result, etidocaine is primarily useful as an anesthetic for surgical procedures in which muscle relaxation is required. Thus, this agent is of limited use for obstetric epidural analgesia and for postoperative pain relief because it does not provide a differential blockade of sensory and motor fibers.

Miscellaneous

Dibucaine

Dibucaine is used for spinal and topical anesthesia. This agent is available in isobaric, hypobaric, and hyperbaric solutions for spinal anesthesia. Dibucaine is more potent than tetracaine, but the onset of action for these two agents is similar. The duration of spinal anesthesia is slightly longer with dibucaine. The degree of hypotension and the intensity of motor blockade appear to be less in patients receiving subarachnoid dibucaine as compared with patients receiving tetracaine. Spread of sensory anesthesia is similar.

Benzocaine

Benzocaine is used exclusively for topical anesthesia. It is available in a variety of proprietary and nonproprietary preparations. The most common forms used in an operating room setting are as aerosol solutions for endotracheal administration and as ointments for lubrication of endotracheal tubes.

CONCLUSION

Local anesthetics may be classified in three groups, according to their potency and duration of action. Procaine and chloroprocaine are relatively weak agents of short duration. Lidocaine, mepivacaine, and prilocaine are intermediate in terms of potency and duration. Tetracaine, bupivacaine, and etidocaine are potent local anesthetics with a prolonged duration of action. With regard to onset time, chloroprocaine, lidocaine, mepivacaine, prilocaine, and etidocaine have a relatively rapid onset of action. Bupivacaine is intermediate, whereas procaine and tetracaine demonstrate a long latency period. Anesthetic activity is determined primarily by physicochemical factors such as pK_a, lipid solubility, and protein binding. In vivo, the anesthetic properties of the various agents can be modified by the dosage, addition of vasoconstrictors, site of injection, carbonation and pH adjustment, additives, mixtures, and the physiologic status of the patient (i.e., pregnancy).

The toxicity of local anesthetics primarily involves the CNS and the cardio-vascular system. CNS toxicity is characterized by excitation and convulsions. Large doses of local anesthetics may lead to generalized CNS depression. The rapid intravenous administration or injection of large doses of local anesthetics can cause hypotension, bradycardia, and ultimately, cardiac arrest. Certain agents, such as bupivacaine, may also produce ventricular arrhythmias. In general, the potential for CNS and cardiovascular toxicity is related to the anesthetic potency of the various agents. Allergic reactions to local anesthetic agents are primarily limited to the amino-ester drugs, because of the metabolic formation of para-aminobenzoic acid. Methemeglobinemia may occur after the administration of large doses of prilocaine. Complications of regional anesthesia are basically limited to epidural and spinal anesthesia. Hypotension is the most common complication caused by the sympathetic blockade associated with these regional anesthetic procedures.

In general, the local anesthetic agents are very effective and relatively safe drugs when used properly. However, as with any class of drugs, safe and effective regional anesthesia requires a knowledge of the pharmacology and toxicology of the various agents, the ability to perform regional anesthesia properly, and a careful evaluation of the clinical status of the patient.

References

1. Aceves J, Machne X: The action of calcium and of local anesthetics on nerve cells, and their interaction during excitation. J Pharmacol Exp Ther 140:138, 1963
2. Condouris GA: A study of the mechanism of action of cocaine on amphibian peripheral nerve. J Pharmacol Exp Ther 131:243, 1961
3. Taylor RE: Effect of procaine on electrical properties of squid axon membrane. Am J Physiol 196:1071, 1959
4. Hille B: Common mode of action of three agents that decrease the transient change in sodium permeability in nerves. Nature 210:1220, 1966
5. Ritchie JM, Ritchie B, Greengard P: The active structure of local anesthetics. J Pharmacol Exp Ther 150:152, 1965
6. Ritchie JM, Ritchie B, Greengard P: The effect of the nerve sheath on the action of local anesthetics. J Pharmacol Exp Ther 150:160, 1965
7. Strichartz GR, Ritchie JM: The action of local anesthetics on ion channels of excitable tissues. p. 21. In Strichartz GR (ed): Local Anesthetics. Springer-Verlag, Berlin, 1987
8. Butterworth JF 4th, Strichartz GR: Molecular mechanisms of local anesthesia: a review. Anesthesiology 72:711, 1990
9. Narahashi T, Yamada M, Frazier DT: Cationic forms of local anesthetics block action potentials from inside the nerve membrane. Nature 223:748, 1969
10. Takman BH: The chemistry of local anaesthetic agents: classification of blocking agents. Br J Anaesth, suppl. 47:183, 1975
11. Truant AP, Takman B: Differential physical-chemical and neuropharmacologic properties of local anesthetic agents. Anesth Analg 38:478, 1959

12. Tucker GT, Boyes RN, Bridenbaugh PO, Moore DC: Binding of anilide-type local anesthetics in human plasma. I: Relationships between binding, physicochemical properties and anesthetic activity. Anesthesiology 33:287, 1970

13. Boyes RN: Anesthésiques locaux en anesthésie et réanimation. Librairie Arnette, Paris, 1974

14. Gissen AJ, Covino BG, Gregus J: Differential sensitivities of mammalian nerves to local anesthetic drugs. Anesthesiology 53:467, 1980

15. Wildsmith JA, Gissen AJ, Gregus J, Covino BG: Differential nerve blocking activity of amino-ester local anesthetics. Br J Anaesth 57:612, 1985

16. Wildsmith JA, Gissen AJ, Takman B, Covino BG: Differential nerve blockade: esters vs amides and the influence of pK_a. Br J Anaesth 59:379, 1987

17. Covino BG: Pharmacology of local anesthetic agents. Br J Anaesth 58:701, 1986

18. Johns RA, DiFazio CA, Longnecker DE: Lidocaine constricts or dilates rat arterioles in a dose-dependent manner. Anesthesiology 62:141, 1985

19. Johns RA, Seyde WC, DiFazio CA, Longnecker DE: Dose-dependent effects of bupivacaine on rat muscle arterioles. Anesthesiology 65:186, 1986

20. Bridenbaugh PO: Intercostal nerve blockade for the evaluation of local anaesthetic agents. Br J Anaesth, suppl. 47:306, 1975

21. Löfström JB: Ulnar nerve blockade for the evaluation of local anaesthetic agents. Br J Anaesth, suppl. 47:297, 1975

22. Rosenberg PH, Heinonen E, Jansson SE, Gripenberg J: Differential nerve block by bupivacaine and 2-chloroprocaine. An experimental study. Br J Anaesth 52:1183, 1980

23. Scott DB, McClure JH, Giasi RM et al: Effects of concentration of local anaesthetic drugs in extradural block. Br J Anaesth 52:1033, 1980

24. Gissen AJ, Covino BG, Gregus J: Differential sensitivity of fast and slow fibres in mammalian nerve. III. Effect of etidocaine and bupivacaine on fast/slow fibres. Anesth Analg 61:570, 1982

25. Bromage PR: Mechanism of action of extradural analgesia. Br J Anaesth, suppl. 47:199, 1975

26. Littlewood DG, Scott DB, Wilson J, Covino BG: Comparative anaesthetic properties of various local anesthetic agents in extradural block in labour. Br J Anaesth 49:75, 1977

27. Crawford OB: Comparative evaluation in peridural anesthesia of lidocaine, mepivacaine, and L-67, a new local anesthetic agent. Anesthesiology 25:321, 1964

28. Erdimir HA, Soper LE, Sweet RB: Studies of factors affecting peridural anesthesia. Anesth Analg 44:400, 1965

29. Braid DP, Scott DB: The systemic absorption of local analgesic drugs. Br J Anaesth 37:394, 1965

30. Concepcion M, Maddi R, Francis D et al: Vasoconstrictors in spinal anesthesia with tetracaine—a comparison of epinephrine and phenylephrine. Anesth Analg 63:134, 1984

31. Grambling ZW, Ellis RG, Valpitto PP: Clinical experience with mepivacaine (Carbocaine). J Med Assoc Ga 53:16, 1964

32. Bromage PR: A comparison of the hydrochloride and carbon dioxide salts of lidocaine and prilocaine in epidural analgesia. Acta Anaesthesiol Scand, suppl. 16:55, 1965

33. Swerdlow M, Jones R: The duration of action of bupivacaine, prilocaine, and lignocaine. Br J Anaesth 42:335, 1970

34. Kier L: Continuous epidural analgesia in prostatectomy: comparison of bupivacaine with and without adrenaline. Acta Anaesthesiol Scand 18:1, 1974

35. Buckley FP, Littlewood DG, Covino BG, Scott DB: Effects of adrenaline and the concentration of solution on extradural block with etidocaine. Br J Anaesth 50: 171, 1978

36. Sinclair CJ, Scott DB: Comparison of bupivacaine and etidocaine in extradural block. Br J Anaesth 56:147, 1984

37. Covino BG, Bush DF: Clinical evaluation of local anesthetic agents. Br J Anaesth, suppl. 47:289, 1975

38. Gissen AJ, Covino BG, Gregus J: Differential sensitivity of fast and slow fibres in mammalian nerve. IV. Effect of carbonation of local anesthetics. Reg Anesth 10: 68, 1985

39. Catchlove RF: The influence of CO_2 and pH on local anesthetic action. J Pharmacol Exp Ther 181:298, 1972

40. Moore DC, Bromage PR, Gertel M: An evaluation of two new local anesthetics for major conduction blockade. Can Anaesth Soc J 18:339, 1971

41. Morison DH: A double-blind comparison of carbonated lidocaine and lidocaine hydrochloride in epidural anaesthesia. Can Anaesth Soc J 28:387, 1981

42. Brown DT, Morison DH, Covino BG, Scott DB: Comparison of carbonated bupivacaine and bupivacaine hydrochloride for extradural anaesthesia. Br J Anaesth 52: 419, 1980

43. McClure JH, Scott DB: Comparison of bupivacaine hydrochloride and carbonated bupivacaine in brachial plexus block by the interscalene technique. Br J Anaesth 53:523, 1981

44. Hilgier M: Alkalinization of bupivacaine for brachial plexus block. Reg Anesth 10: 59, 1985

45. Loder RE: A local anaesthetic solution with longer action. Lancet ii:346, 1960

46. Bridenbaugh LD: Does the addition of low molecular weight dextran prolong the duration of action of bupivacaine? Reg Anesth 3:6, 1978

47. Rosenblatt RM, Fung DL: Mechanism of dextran prolonging regional anesthesia. Reg Anesth 5:3, 1980

48. Cunningham NL, Kaplan JA: A rapid-onset, long-acting regional anesthetic technique. Anesthesiology 41:509, 1974

49. Cohen SE, Thurlow A: Comparison of a chloropricaine-bupivacaine mixture with chloroprocaine and bupivacaine used individually for obstetric epidural analgesia. Anesthesiology 51:288, 1979

50. Corke BG, Carlson CG, Dettbarn WD: The influence of 2-chloroprocaine on the subsequent analgesic potency of bupivacaine. Anesthesiology 60:25, 1984

51. Fagraeus L, Urban BJ, Bromage PR: Spread of analgesia in early pregnancy. Anesthesiology 58:184, 1983

52. Datta S, Lambert DH, Gregus J et al: Differential sensitivities of mammalian nerve fibers during pregnancy. Anesth Analg 62:1070, 1983

53. Scott DB, Jebson PJ, Braid DP et al: Factors affecting plasma levels of lignocaine and prilocaine. Br J Anaesth 44:1040, 1972

54. Tucker GT, Moore DC, Bridenbaugh PO et al: Systemic absorption of mepivacaine in commonly used regional block procedures. Anesthesiology 37:277, 1972

55. Lund PC, Bush DF, Covino BG: Determinants of etidocaine concentration in the blood. Anesthesiology 42:497, 1975

56. Tucker GT, Mather LE: Pharmacokinetics of local anaesthetic agents. Br J Anaesth, suppl. 47:213, 1975

57. Stanton-Hicks M, Berges PU, Bonica JJ: Circulatory effects of peridural block. IV. Comparison of the effects of epinephrine and phenylephrine. Anesthesiology 39:308, 1973

58. Dhuner KG, Lewis DH: Effect of local anesthetics and vasoconstrictors upon regional blood flow. Acta Anaesthiol Scand, suppl. 23:347, 1966
59. Akerman B, Astrom A, Ross S, Telc A: Studies on the absorption, distribution and metabolism of labelled prilocaine and lidocaine in some animal species. Acta Pharmacol Toxicol (Copenh) 24:389, 1966
60. Scott DB, Jebson PJ, Boyes RN: Pharmacokinetic study of the local anaesthetic bupivacaine (Marcain) and etidocaine (Duranest) in man. Br J Anaesth 45:1010, 1973
61. Tucker GT: Pharmacokinetics of local anaesthetics. Br J Anaesth 58:717, 1986
62. Lund PC, Covino BG: Distribution of local anesthetics in man following peridural anesthesia. J Clin Pharmacol New Drugs 7:324, 1967
63. Katz J: The distribution of ^{14}C-labelled lidocaine injected intravenously in the rat. Anesthesiology 29:249, 1968
64. Englesson S, Eriksson E, Ortengren B, Wahlqvist S: Differences in tolerance to intravenous xylocaine and Citanest. Acta Anaesthesiol Scand, suppl. 16:141, 1965
65. Tucker GT, Boyes RN, Bridenbaugh PO, Moore DC: Binding of anilide-type local anesthetics in human plasma: I. Relationships between binding, physicochemical properties, and anesthetic activity. Anesthesiology 33:287, 1970
66. Covino BG: Comparative clinical pharmacology of local anesthetic agents. Anesthesiology 35:158, 1971
67. Foldes FF, Davidson GM, Duncalf D, Kawabara J: The intravenous toxicity of local anesthetic agents in man. Clin Pharmacol Ther 6:328, 1965
68. Brodie BB, Lief PA, Poet R: The fate of procaine in man following its intravenous administration and methods for the estimation of procaine and diethylaminoethanol. J Pharmacol Exp Ther 94:359, 1948
69. Keenaghan JB, Boyes RN: The tissue distribution, metabolism and excretion of lidocaine in rats, guinea pigs, dogs and man. J Pharmacol Exp Ther 180:454, 1972
70. Eriksson E, Granberg PO: Studies on the renal excretion of Citanest and Xylocaine Acta Anaesthiol Scand, suppl. 16:79, 1965
71. Tanaka K, Yamasaki M: Blocking of cortical inhibitory synapses by intravenous lidocaine. Nature 209:207, 1966
72. Englesson S: The influence of acid-base changes on central nervous system toxicity of local anesthetic agents. I. An experimental study in cats. Acta Anaesthesiol Scand 18:79, 1974
73. Liu PL, Feldman HS, Giasi R et al: Comparative CNS toxicity of lidocaine, etidocaine, bupivacaine and tetracaine in awake dogs following rapid intravenous administration. Anesth Analg 62:375, 1983
74. Usubiaga JE, Wikinski J, Ferrero R et al: Local anesthetic-induced convulsions in man—an electroencephalographic study. Anesth Analg 45:611, 1966
75. Scott DB: Toxicity caused by local anaesthetic drugs (editorial). Br J Anaesth 53:553, 1981
76. Scott DB: Evaluation of clinical tolerance of local anaesthetic agents. Br J Anaesth, suppl. 47:328, 1975
77. Englesson S, Grevsten S: The influence of acid-base changes on central nervous system toxicity of local anaesthetic agents. II. Acta Anaesthesiol Scand 18:88, 1974
78. Burney RG, DiFazio CA, Foster JA: Effects of pH on protein binding of lidocaine. Anesth Analg 57:478, 1978
79. Gettes LS: Physiology and pharmacology of antiarrhythmic drugs. Hosp Pract [Off] 16:89, 1981
80. Clarkson CW, Hondeghem LM: Mechanism for bupivacaine depression of cardiac

conduction: fast block of sodium channels during the action potential with slow recovery from block during diastole. Anesthesiology 62:396, 1985

81. Lieberman NA, Harris RS, Katz RI et al: The effects of lidocaine on the electrical and mechanical activity of the heart. Am J Cardiol 22:375, 1968

82. Sugimoto T, Schaal SF, Dunn NM, Wallace AG: Electrophysiological effects of lidocaine in awake dogs. J Pharmacol Exp Ther 166:146, 1969

83. Block A, Covino BG: Effect of local anesthetic agents on cardiac conduction and contractility. Reg Anesth 6:55, 1982

84. Stewart DM, Rogers WP, Mahaffrey JE et al: Effect of local anesthetics on the cardiovascular system in the dog. Anesthesiology 24:620, 1963

85. Liu PL, Feldman HS, Covino BG et al: Acute cardiovascular toxicity of procaine, chloroprocaine and tetracaine in anesthetized ventilated dogs. Reg Anesth 7:14, 1982

86. Liu PL, Feldman HS, Covino BG et al: Acute cardiovascular toxicity of intravenous amide local anesthetics in anesthetized ventilated dogs. Anesth Analg 61:317, 1982

87. Kuperman AS, Altura BT, Chezar JA: Action of procaine on calcium efflux from frog nerve and muscle. Nature 217:673, 1968

88. Tanz RD, Heskett T, Loehning RW, Fairfax CA: Comparative cardiotoxicity of bupivacaine and lidocaine in the isolated perfused mammalian heart. Anesth Analg 63:549, 1984

89. Blair MR: Cardiovascular pharmacology of local anaesthetics. Br J Anaesth, suppl. 47:247, 1975

90. Jorfeldt L, Löfström B, Pernow B, Wahren J: The effect of mepivacaine and lidocaine on forearm resistance and capacitance vessels in man. Acta Anaesthesiol Scand 14:183, 1970

91. Nishimura N, Morioka T, Sato S, Kuba T: Effects of local anesthetic agents on the peripheral vascular system. Anesth Analg 44:135, 1965

92. Johns RA: Local anesthetics inhibit endothelium-dependent vasodilation. Anesthesiology 70:805, 1989

93. Aberg G, Andersson R: Studies on mechanical actions of mepivacaine (Carbocaine) and its optically active isomers on isolated smooth muscle: role of Ca^{++} and cyclic AMP. Acta Pharmacol Toxicol (Copenh) 31:321, 1972

94. Somlyo AP, Somlyo AV: Vascular smooth muscle. II. Pharmacology of normal and hypotensive vessels. Pharmacol Rev 22:249, 1970

95. Albright GA: Cardiac arrest following regional anesthesia with etidocaine or bupivacaine (editorial). Anesthesiology 51:285, 1979

96. Edde RR, Deutsch S: Cardiac arrest after interscalene brachial plexus block. Anesth Analg 56:446, 1977

97. Prentiss JE: Cardiac arrest following caudal anesthesia. Anesthesiology 50:51, 1979

98. Morishima HO, Pedersen H, Finster M et al: Etidocaine toxicity in the adult, newborn, and fetal sheep. Anesthesiology 58:342, 1983

99. Reiz S, Nath S: Cardiotoxicity of local anaesthetic agents. Br J Anaesth 58:736, 1986

100. Morishima HO, Pedersen H, Finster M et al: Bupivacaine toxicity in pregnant and nonpregnant ewes. Anesthesiology 63:134, 1985

101. Rosen MA, Thigpen JW, Shnider SM et al: Bupivacaine-induced cardiotoxicity in hypoxic and acidotic sheep. Anesth Analg 64:1089, 1985

102. Chadwick HS: Toxicity and resuscitation in lidocaine- or bupivacaine-infused cats. Anesthesiology 63:385, 1985

103. Kasten GW, Martin ST: Bupivacaine cardiovascular toxicity: comparison of treatment with bretylium and lidocaine. Anesth Analg 64:911, 1985

104. Sage DJ, Feldman HS, Arthur GR et al: Influence of lidocaine and bupivacaine on isolated guinea pig atria in the presence of acidosis and hypoxia. Anesth Analg 63: 1, 1984

105. Hjelm M, Holmdahl MH: Biochemical effects of aromatic amines. II. Cyanosis, methemoglobinemia and Heinz-body formation induced by a local anesthetic agent (prilocaine). Acta Anaesthesiol Scand 2:99, 1965

106. Lund PC, Cwik JC: Propitocaine (Citanest) and methemoglobinemia. Anesthesiology 26:569, 1965

107. Brown DT, Beamish D, Wildsmith JA: Allergic reaction to an amide local anesthetic. Br J Anaesth 53:435, 1981

108. Fisher MM, Graham R: Adverse responses to local anaesthetics. Anaesth Intensive Care 12:325, 1984

109. Reynolds F: Allergy reaction to an amide local anaesthetic. Br J Anaesth 53:901, 1981

110. Aldrete JA, Johnson DA: Evaluation of intracutaneous testing for investigation of allergy to local anesthetic agents. Anesth Analg 49:173, 1970

111. Aldrete JA, Johnson DA: Allergy to local anesthetics. JAMA 207:356, 1969

112. Skou JC: Local anesthetics. II. The toxic potencies of some local anesthetics and of butyl alcohol, determined on peripheral nerve. Acta Pharmacol Toxicol (Copenh) 10:292, 1954

113. Adams HJ, Mastri AR, Eicholzer AW, Kilpatrick G: Morphologic effects of intrathecal etidocaine and tetracaine on the rabbit spinal cord. Anesth Analg 53:904, 1974

114. Ravindran RS, Bond VK, Tasch MD et al: Prolonged neural blockade following regional analgesia with 2-chloroprocaine. Anesth Analg 58:447, 1980

115. Reisner LS, Hochman BN, Plumer MH: Persistent neurologic deficit and adhesive arachnoiditis following intrathecal 2-chloroprocaine injection. Anesth Analg 59: 452, 1980

116. Wang BC, Hillman DE, Spielholz NI, Turndorf H: Chronic neurological deficits and Nesacaine-CE—an effect of the anesthetic, 2-chloroprocaine, or the antioxidant, sodium bisulfite? Anesth Analg 63:445, 1984

117. Gissen AJ, Datta S, Lambert D: The chloroprocaine controversy II. Is chloroprocaine neurotoxic? Reg Anesth 9:135, 1984

118. Libelius R, Sonesson B, Stamenovic BA, Thesleff S: Denervation-like changes in skeletal muscle after treatment with a local anesthetic (Marcaine). J Anat 106:297, 1970

119. Moore DC, Spierdijk J, vanKleef JD et al: Chloroprocaine neurotoxicity: four additional cases. Anesth Analg 61:155, 1982

120. Bonica JJ, Berges PU, Morikawa K: Circulatory effects of peridural block. I. Effects of level of analgesia and dose of lidocaine. Anesthesiology 33:619, 1970

121. Bonica JJ, Kennedy WF, Akamatsu TJ, Gerbershagen HU: Circulatory effects of peridural block. III. Effects of acute blood loss. Anesthesiology 36:219, 1972

122. Ward RJ, Bonica JJ, Freund FG, Akamatsu T et al: Epidural and subarachnoid anesthesia: cardiovascular and respiratory effects. JAMA 191:275, 1965

123. Sivarajan M, Amory DW, Lindbloom LE, Schwettmann RS: Systemic and regional blood-flow changes during spinal anesthesia in the rhesus monkey. Anesthesiology 43:78, 1975

10

Patient-Controlled Analgesia: A Conceptual Framework for Analgesic Administration

F. Michael Ferrante

Patient-controlled analgesia (PCA) is commonly (and mistakenly) assumed by the average practitioner to imply the on-demand, intermittent, intravenous (IV) administration of opioids under patient control. Sophisticated infusion device technology with advanced microcircuitry is considered obligatory.

Although this chapter deals mainly with classic intravenous PCA (IV-PCA), it is important to note from the onset that PCA is really a conceptual framework for the administration of analgesics. In a broader sense, the concept of PCA is not restricted to a single class of analgesics or single route or mode of administration (Table 10-1).[1-17] Nor does PCA imply the mandatory presence of sophisticated and expensive pump technology. Any analgesic given by any route (e.g., oral, subcutaneous [SC], or epidural) can be deemed to be PCA if administered on immediate patient demand in plentiful quantities. With this important distinction now made, let us explore the "traditional" system of IV-PCA and its technology.

**TABLE 10-1. PCA: A Conceptual Framework
for Analgesic Administration**[a]

Class of analgesic
  Local anesthetics[1-3]
  Benzodiazepines[4]
  Opioids[5-15]

Route of administration
  Sublingual[5]
  Transbuccal[6]
  Subcutaneous[7,8]
  Intravenous[9-15]
  Epidural[1-3,9,10]

Mode of administration
  Demand dosing[16]
  Constant-rate infusion plus demand dosing[16]
  Infusion-based systems[17]

[a] The concept of PCA is not restricted to a single
class of analgesic or route or mode of administration.

INTRAVENOUS PATIENT-CONTROLLED ANALGESIA

Definition of PCA Modes and Dosing Parameters

The administration of analgesics via PCA has several modes. The most commonly used are *demand dosing* (a dose of fixed size is intermittently self-administered) and *constant-rate infusion plus demand dosing* (a fixed background infusion is supplemented by patient demand). When using a background infusion, it is important to maintain the infusion rate at a minimum in order not to ablate the necessity of patient demand. Otherwise, the risk of respiratory depression is enhanced.[18]

Less commonly available modes of administration include *infusion demand* (in which demands are granted as an infusion) and *variable-rate infusion plus demand dosing* (in which a microprocessor monitors demands and controls the infusion rate accordingly). These modes remain to be studied in detail.[17]

For each mode of PCA, there are basic variables: loading dose, demand dose, lockout interval, background infusion rate, and 1- and 4-hour limits. For the postoperative patient, PCA is preferably implemented in the postanesthesia care unit. The patient is made comfortable by administration of small doses of opioid (*loading doses*). After sufficiently recovering from anesthesia, the patient may initiate demands.

Any opioid can be administered by PCA. Suggested guidelines for the administration of several commonly used opioids via IV-PCA are listed in Table 10-2. The *demand dose* (incremental or PCA dose) is the quantity of analgesic given to the patient on activation of the PCA infuser's demand button. To prevent overdosage by continual demand, all PCA systems use a *lockout interval*. The lockout interval is the length of time between patient demands in which

TABLE 10-2. Guidelines for Opioid Administration via IV-PCA [a]

Drug (concentration)	Demand Dose	Lockout Interval (min)
Morphine (1 mg/ml)	0.5–3.0 mg	5–12
Meperidine (10 mg/ml)	5–30 mg	5–12
Fentanyl (10 μg/ml)	10–20 μg	5–10
Hydromorphone (0.2 mg/ml)	0.1–0.5 mg	5–10
Oxymorphone (0.25 mg/ml)	0.2–0.4 mg	8–10
Methadone (1 mg/ml)	0.5–2.5 mg	8–20
Nalbuphine (1 mg/ml)	1–5 mg	5–10

[a] Analgesic requirements vary widely among patients. Adjustment of dosage because of age, severe disease, or the idiosyncracies of individual drug handling is always necessary.

the infuser will not administer analgesics. Some PCA devices allow determination of *1- and 4-hour limits*. The use of these limits is controversial and has both proponents and detractors.

Unfortunately, the development of guidelines for opioid administration with PCA has been largely empiric. Research into the scientific basis for choice of administration variables for use with each mode of PCA is needed.[19,20]

PCA Infuser Technology

The widespread acceptance of IV-PCA has been due in large measure to the development of sophisticated but "user-friendly" infuser technology. Roe[21] first demonstrated that small IV doses of opioids could provide more effective pain relief than traditional intramuscular (IM) opioid regimens. In his pioneering work on PCA, Sechzer evaluated the analgesic response to small IV doses of opioid given on demand by nursing personnel[22] and subsequently by a programmable mechanical device.[23] However, the widespread, on-demand administration of analgesics by nursing personnel to large numbers of patients would represent an insurmountable logistics problem. Therefore, in the late 1960s prototype demand-analgesia devices were developed. The first widely used PCA infuser (the Cardiff Palliator[24]) was introduced into clinical practice in the United Kingdom in 1976. Since that time, newer infusers have introduced sophisticated computerized programming and fail-safe systems.

From the point of view of the bioengineer, all PCA infusers use negative feedback control technology. In other words, as patients use increasing amounts of analgesic, pain is reduced, and eventually, patients demand less analgesic. This basic tenet is believed to underlie the inherent safety of PCA as an analgesic modality.

The successful management of a PCA service requires the collaborative efforts of anesthesiologists, nurses, pharmacists, and hospital administrators. Thus, choice of an infusion device for a particular institution is best made through the input of these multiple specialties. Several of the commercially available PCA infusers have recently been evaluated with respect to safety, security, and overall ease of use.[25,26] All the devices under study met the accu-

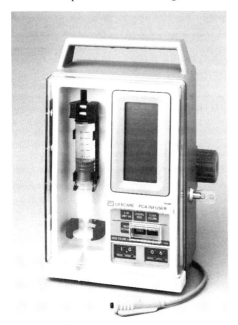 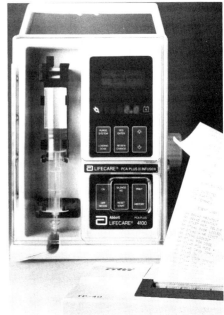

Fig. 10-1. LifeCare PCA Classic (Abbott Laboratories).

Fig. 10-2. LifeCare PCA Plus II (Abbott Laboratories).

racy, electric safety, and performance criteria established by biomedical engineers. Thus, choice of device should be made by a multidisciplinary panel in order to "tailor" the chosen device to the logistic and administrative idiosyncrasies of the particular institution. (Current commercially available PCA infusers are shown in Figs. 10-1 to 10-12.)

Machine-User Interface

A number of points should be addressed during the initial evaluation process (Tables 10-3 and 10-4). Ease of programmability is largely a matter of individual taste, but is the most desirable feature. Earlier devices simply used thumbwheel switches (e.g., Abbott LifeCare PCA Classic) or dials (e.g., Bard PCA I) for programming. Later devices are fully computerized, more difficult to access, but also more versatile (flexible). The mental logic used in programming a PCA infuser can vary from none (e.g., nonprogrammable Baxter PCA Infuser) to direct thumbwheel or dial access, to machine-directed (menu-driven) interactions (e.g., Abbott LifeCare PCA Plus II and Pancretec Provider, Bard PCA [Harvard PCA], Bard Ambulatory PCA and PCA II, Stratofuse PCA Infuser, Graseby Medical PCA, IVAC PCAinfuser, Pharmacia Deltec CADD-PCA). As clinicians think in milligrams not milliliters, devices allowing such programming are probably preferable.

With respect to ease of ambulation, a small lightweight device worn on the

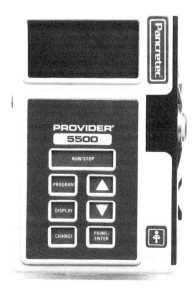

Fig. 10-3. Pancretec Provider 5500 (Abbott Laboratories).

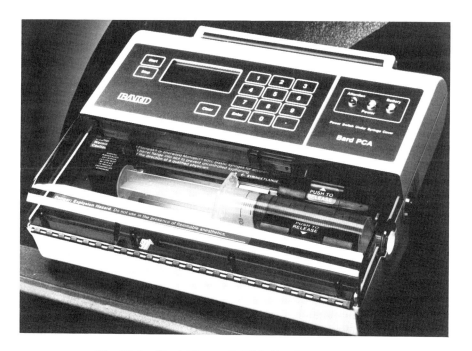

Fig. 10-4. Bard (Harvard) PCA (Bard MedSystems).

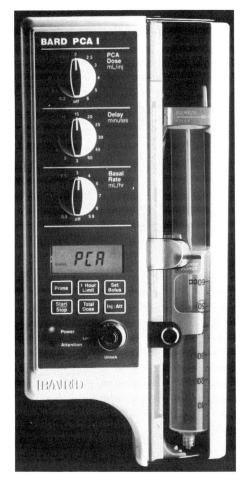

Fig. 10-5. PCA I (Bard MedSystems).

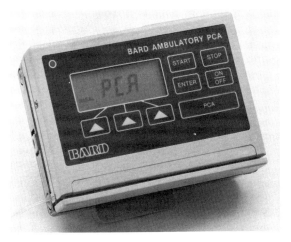

Fig. 10-6. Ambulatory PCA (Bard MedSystems).

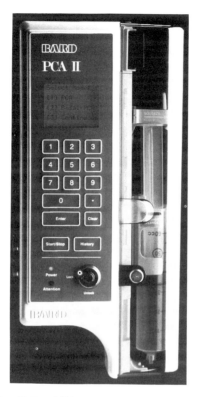

Fig. 10-7. PCA II (Bard MedSystems).

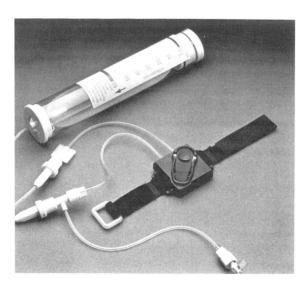

Fig. 10-8. Baxter PCA Infuser (Baxter Healthcare).

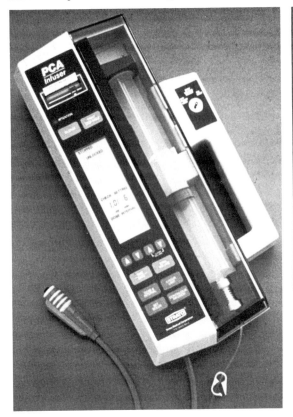

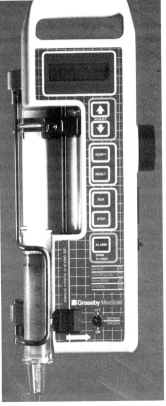

Fig. 10-9. Stratofuse PCA Infuser (Baxter Healthcare).

Fig. 10-10. Graseby Medical PCA (Graseby Medical Ltd).

patient's body or clothing would be optimal. Thus, the Abbott Laboratories Pancretec Provider, the Bard Ambulatory PCA, the Baxter PCA Infuser, and the Pharmacia Deltec CADD-PCA are all suitable for ambulatory use. In the hospital vs. the home care setting, true ease of ambulation may not be of primary concern. The less portable PCA infusers can be affixed to IV poles for ambulation.

Although no infusion device is tamperproof, locked Plexiglass doors, access codes, or both, are a constant design feature. Choice of protection against tampering is largely a matter of individual preference for a particular institution.

Machine Operability

The actual pumping mechanisms of PCA infusers vary from syringe-driven, to rotary and linear peristaltic, to elastomeric pressure mechanisms (Table 10-4).

The Baxter PCA Infuser's elastomeric pressure mechanism is unique. The infuser consists of a lightweight plastic cylinder containing 40 ml of analgesic

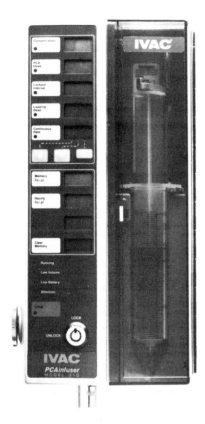

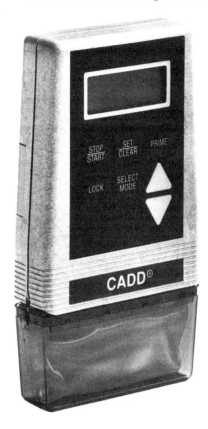

Fig. 10-11. IVAC PCAinfuser 310 (IVAC Corporation).

Fig. 10-12. CADD-PCA 5800 (Pharmacia Deltec).

TABLE 10-3. Points of Concern in Evaluation of PCA Infusers

Machine-user interface
  Programmability
  Flexibility
  Ease of ambulation
  Tamper protection

Machine operability
  Pump mechanism
  Operational modes
  Fail-safe mechanisms
  Alarms and indicators
  Memory
  Mounting
  Disposables
    Reservoir type and capacity
    Infusion tubing

TABLE 10-4. Commercially Available PCA Infusers

Manufacturer and Device	Programming	Pump Mechanism	Infusion Modes	Power Requirements	Printer	Mounting	Retail Cost[a]
Abbott Laboratories							
LifeCare PCA Classic	ml	Syr	D	AC/lead-acid B	None	Pole	$3295
LifeCare PCA Plus II	Both	Syr	D&C	AC/Lead-acid B	External	Pole	$3495
LifeCare Pancretec Provider 5500	Both	RP	D&C	Two 9-V B	None	Amb	$3595
Bard MedSystems Division							
Bard PCA (Harvard PCA)	ml	Syr	D&C	AC/lead-acid B	External	Pole	$3550
PCA I	ml	LP	D&C	Four D-size B	None	Pole	$3295
Ambulatory PCA	Both	Syr	D&C	9-V B	External	Amb	$3095
PCA II	Both	Syr	D&C	AC/Four D-size B	External	Pole	$3795
Baxter Healthcare Corp							
Baxter PCA Infuser	None[b]	Elast P	D	None	None	Wristwatch	$17—watch $21—infuser
Stratofuse PCA Infuser	ml	Syr	D&C	AC/Ni-Cad B	Internal	Pole	$3990
Graseby Medical, Ltd							
Graseby Medical PCA	mg	Syr	D&C	AC/lead-acid B	External	Pole	$3795
IVAC Corporation							
IVAC PCAinfuser 310	mg	Syr	D&C	Four D-size B	None	Pole	$3650
Pharmacia Deltec							
CADD-PCA 5800	Both	LP	D&C	9-V B	None	Amb	$3495

Abbreviations: Amb, ambulatory; B, battery; C, continuous; D, demand; Elast P, elastomeric pressure; LP, linear peristaltic; Ni-Cad, nickel-cadmium; RP, rotary peristaltic; Syr, syringe-driven.
[a] Retail cost as of September 1, 1991.
[b] Fixed dose of 0.5 ml with a lockout of 6 minutes.

within an elastic balloon. With each demand the patient receives 0.5 ml at intervals of 6 minutes or longer. The device is disposable, nonprogrammable, and nonelectronic. The amount of drug delivered with each demand can only be changed by changing the concentration of analgesic in the reservoir. As the balloon reservoir deflates, analgesic solution flows through a small aperture that determines the time required to fill the injection reservoir (6 minutes). The injection reservoir is worn on the wrist. Continuous administration of opioid is impossible with this design. The lack of ability to adjust dosage makes the system less flexible.

Except for the aforementioned Baxter infuser, most newer designs can deliver both demands and background infusions. (The older Abbott LifeCare PCA Classic also cannot deliver background infusions.)

Several other infuser features are worthy of consideration. All PCA infusers have a number of fail-safe mechanisms, alarms, and indicator signals. Some devices possess memory of 24 hours or more. Hard copy may be generated by internal printers (Stratofuse PCA Infuser) or interface with optional external printers. Lastly, disposables (e.g., reservoir type and capacity and infusion sets) are important financial concerns. Cost of disposables may make certain PCA devices unacceptable for particular institutions.

A summary of the features of commercially available PCA infusers is found in Table 10-4.

Safety

The first demonstration of a PCA infuser in the United States occurred in 1984. At the present time, approximately 50,000 devices are in use, with relatively few problems reported. Indeed, such a rapid growth underscores the inherent safety of the modality. The relatively few problems to date can be divided into three groups: (1) adverse reactions and side effects, (2) mechanical problems, and (3) problems at the machine-user interface.

Adverse Reactions and Side Effects

When discussing adverse reactions and side effects, a distinction must be made between complications arising from PCA as a modality itself and the individual drugs being administered. Extensive review of the literature yields few complications inherently associated with PCA as a technique. Problems are attributed to the innate properties of opioids rather than use of the device.[27,28]

Minor side effects include nausea, vomiting, sweating, and pruritus. The incidence of any of these is rarely greater than 10–20 percent. Ileus is also reported. However, it is difficult to distinguish opioid-induced ileus from other contributory variables, such as surgical technique and type of surgery.

In short, there is no evidence to suggest that PCA is associated with a greater incidence of the aforementioned minor side effects. Similarly, there is no evidence to suggest that any particular opioid is associated with a greater or lesser incidence of these side effects.[16]

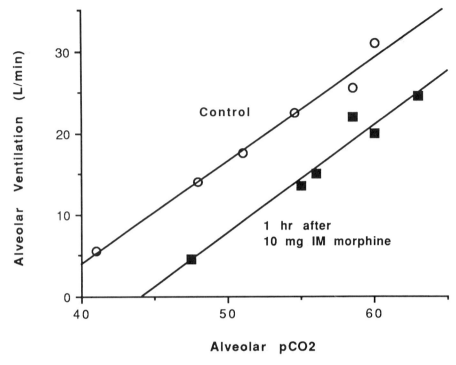

Fig. 10-13. Respiratory response curve obtained before and 1 hour after 10 mg IM morphine. Equianalgesic dosages of opioids produce equivalent changes in the responsiveness of the respiratory center. Therefore, 100 mg IM meperidine, or 1.7 mg IM hydromorphone would produce exactly the same displacement of the CO_2 response curve.

Of course, the clinician's main concern is the avoidance of respiratory depression. The use of opioids by any means carries the risk of respiratory depression.

Opioids cause progressive central respiratory depression manifested as a change in the responsiveness of the respiratory center (displacement of the CO_2 response curve—Fig. 10-13) or change in breathing pattern. Respiratory depression is dose-dependent. Equianalgesic dosages of opioids produce equivalent degrees of respiratory depression.[16,29] Any clinically observed differences are a function of the pharmacokinetics and pharmacodynamics of different opioids.[16,29] Thus, the total equianalgesic dose of opioid over a circumscribed period is much more important than the particular opioid or the technique of PCA in the production of respiratory depression.

It is difficult to contrast the inherent propensity of epidural/subarachnoid opioids vs. IM- or PCA-administered opioids in the production of respiratory depression. Large-scale, well-controlled studies with administration of opioids in equianalgesic dose ranges are needed.

As a first approximation, however, we may obtain useful information from a study by Brose and Cohen.[30] Oxygen saturation was monitored continuously for 24 hours in patients receiving epidural morphine (5 mg) or either IM or PCA meperidine for analgesia after cesarean delivery. PCA patients spent the longest cumulative time with saturations between 91 and 95 percent. However, episodes of severe desaturation (saturation $O_2 < 85$ percent for 30 seconds) occurred in 71 percent of patients in the epidural group, 63 percent in the IM group, and 30 percent in the PCA group. Thus, patients in all three groups were at risk of respiratory depression. However, this was manifested by prolonged periods of mild desaturation with PCA and a high incidence of brief but severe desaturation with epidural and IM opioids.[30]

Mechanical Problems

Most mechanical problems associated with PCA infusers can be subdivided into three areas: (1) "continued delivery or overdelivery," (2) underdelivery, and (3) "siphoning", or "runaway" delivery. Any adverse event associated with the use of a medical device must be reported to the Food and Drug Administration as a Medical Device Report. Examination of these reports shows that very few are truly attributable to mechanical failure.

Reports of "continued" delivery are most often associated with administration of a loading dose through the PCA infuser. Most incidents occur during the first 6–9 months after introduction of PCA into a hospital when the device is still unfamiliar. Such incidents are attributable to misprogramming.

Underdelivery is usually due to appropriate function of the infuser in the face of an alarm condition. When the alarm condition has been corrected (temporary occlusion of an IV line), the interrupted dose is not completed.

"Siphoning", or "runaway" delivery can occur with both glass and plastic reservoir syringes. The use of excessive force in positioning the reservoir syringe can cause a crack in the glass or plastic. Increases in pressure within the syringe can cause the crack to widen. The crack may allow introduction of air causing administration of opioid. In some cases this has lead to constant flow of opioid and respiratory arrest.

Refinements have been made in PCA infuser design to avert the potential for siphoning. These have included addition of antisiphon valves to the intravenous tubing as well as redesign of the syringe mounting. Today, the incidence of siphoning is greatly reduced, but it is still possible with user abuse of the system.

Machine-User Interface

Review of Medical Device Reports reveals that user error was the cause of problems with PCA in 67 percent of cases. Misprogramming, unfortunately, is a recurring theme. Two cases of misprogramming have been reported in the literature.[31]

Despite the best efforts of manufacturers, no device is tamperproof. Access codes to infusers can be memorized by patients. Instruments can be devised by patients to slip behind locked Plexiglas doors to gain access to the dose buttons.

One fatality has been associated with PCA.[32] The reason for the apparent overdose has not yet been explained, but runaway delivery may have occurred.

In summary, PCA infuser technology is safe. The sophistication and safety of PCA infusers are motivating forces in the rapid growth and acceptance of PCA.

The PCA Paradigm

Besides sophisticated infuser technology, the rapid acceptance of PCA is also attributable to the increased awareness that consistent analgesic blood levels cannot be obtained with repetitive IM dosing.[33,34] Analgesia is achieved when the plasma opioid concentration reaches a particular level, dependent on the individual patient (maximum concentration associated with severe pain [MCSP]—Fig. 10-14). For small increases in plasma concentration, a rapid decrease in pain is perceived. Complete pain relief defines the *minimum effective analgesic concentration* (MEAC). For increases in plasma concentration of opioid above MEAC, there is no increased analgesic effect. For small decreases in plasma concentration below MEAC, pain is rapidly appreciated. MEAC exhibits marked interpatient variability, and this may explain the large variability in analgesic requirements among patients.

The relation among opioid concentration, analgesia, and dosing interval defines therapeutic efficacy for a particular method of opioid administration (Fig. 10-15). The attendant plasma concentrations from IM injection are characteristically unpredictable. Within an individual, peak concentration of opioid (C_{max}) can vary twofold with repetitive injections. Time to peak concentration (T_{max}) can vary threefold with repetitive IM injections.[33] There can be a fivefold variation in C_{max} in any given patient population, whereas T_{max} can vary sevenfold.[33] At the same time, plasma concentrations will fluctuate in phase with the dosing interval (Fig. 10-15). It has been calculated that opioid concentrations are in excess of MEAC only 35 percent of the time during any 4-hour dosing interval.

PCA avoids these variable absorption phenomena by allowing on-demand, repetitive dosing with small doses of opioid. When the patient's plasma concentration falls below MEAC, the patient rapidly appreciates pain (steep concentration-analgesic response relation). Thus, PCA is a "flexible" modality, as patients use PCA to "titrate" their plasma concentration of opioid around MEAC. PCA provides more constant plasma levels of opioid[11–13] and more consistent analgesia.[14]

Continuous Infusion Analgesia for Acute Pain Management

From a theoretic standpoint, continuous opioid infusions would at first appear attractive for postoperative pain management. Continuous opioid infusions at a dose above MEAC and below that associated with adverse side effects would abolish the wide swings in analgesia and drug concentration inherent in intermittent IM dosing.

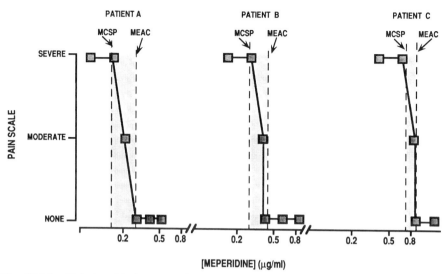

Fig. 10-14. Relationship between the plasma opioid concentration and analgesia. For a minimal increase in opioid concentration above the maximum concentration associated with severe pain (MCSP—first inflection point), there is a rapid decrease in perceived pain. The opioid concentration at which pain reaches its nadir (second inflection point) is called the minimum effective analgesic concentration (MEAC). The area between the MCSP and the MEAC (*shaded*) is called the therapeutic window. The slope of the line between MCSP and MEAC is steep. As little as 0.05 μg/ml of meperidine can determine the presence of severe pain or analgesia. Thus, the opioids as a class of drugs are said to have a "narrow" therapeutic window. (Modified from Austin et al, with permission.[34])

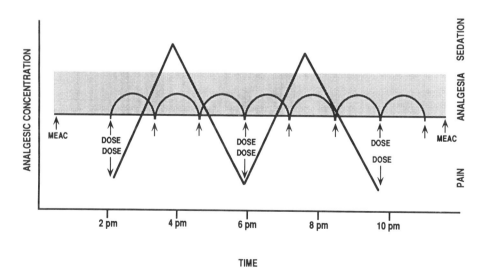

Fig. 10-15. PCA paradigm. The relationship between plasma opioid concentration (ordinate), dosing interval (abscissa), and analgesic effect (*Z* axis), defining therapeutic effectiveness.

Clinical trials comparing intermittent IM dosing and continuous intermittent infusions for acute pain management have demonstrated equivalent or improved analgesia with use of continuous infusions.[35–39] Unlike PCA, however, use of truly "fixed-dose" continuous infusions will not flexibly adapt to the dynamic natural history of postoperative pain, with its temporary flares and rapid diminution over several days. A constant rate infusion of any drug requires 3.3 half-lives to reach 90 percent of the final steady state, and 95 percent of the final steady state is achieved after five half-lives. As most opioids half-lives varying from 2 to 12 hours, a truly constant infusion is impractical, as it is not readily adjustable.

Thus, combinations of one or more loading doses or loading infusions have been used to initiate treatment, with subsequent maintenance through constant infusion. Stapleton et al[39] modeled a "pharmacokinetically optimal" infusion schema based on the well-known kinetics of meperidine. Although this regimen based on average kinetic parameters was successful, steady-state opioid levels can vary twofold because of the normal range of individual drug clearance. Thus, it would be difficult to consistently achieve an ideal opioid concentration that is slightly above MEAC but below a concentration causing side effects in all patients. Indeed, respiratory depression of potentially life-threatening severity has been reported in postoperative patients receiving continuous infusions.[35,40]

In summary, continuous infusions can eliminate the fluctuating levels of analgesia and drug concentration inherent with repetitive IM dosing. Unlike PCA, however, use of a fixed-rate infusion lacks flexibility. Loading doses or loading infusions with repeated rate adjustments are necessary to account for individual variations in pharmacokinetics and pharmacodynamics. Respiratory depression is probably inevitable when the infusion rate is adjusted too infrequently.

Individual Analgesic Requirements

PCA is a dynamic and flexible analgesic modality, allowing patients to "titrate" as little or as much opioid as they desire. Unlike traditional IM administration with its defined dose and dosing interval limitations, PCA can accommodate patients' widely divergent analgesic requirements. Thus, individual differences in analgesic requirements are expressed in individual patterns of analgesic administration. By understanding the pharmacokinetic, pharmacodynamic, and psychological factors affecting analgesic requirements, we can perhaps begin to understand how patients effectively (or ineffectively) use PCA.

Pharmacokinetic Factors

The contribution of pharmacokinetics upon analgesic requirements was studied in a classic series of studies by Tamsen et al.[11–13] The volume of distribution, distribution rate constant, and elimination rate constant for meperidine,[11] ketobemidone,[12] and morphine[13] were studied in patients undergoing laparotomy.

Pharmacokinetic parameters bore no relation to individual hourly analgesic requirements for any opioid. Thus, in patients using PCA, pharmacokinetic variations among patients had no influence on the hourly demand for opioid. However, individual hourly opioid use did correlate with mean plasma opioid concentration and MEAC.

Pharmacodynamic Factors

Exogenously administered opioids produce analgesia by mimicking the actions of endogenous opioids in the central nervous system.[41] A change in opioid receptor numbers or affinity, as well as the discrete levels of endogenous opioids, could influence analgesic requirements.

Work by Tamsen et al[42] explored the possibility that preoperative endogenous opioid levels in the brain, spinal cord, or cerebrospinal fluid (CSF) could affect MEAC, thereby affecting analgesic requirements. Before laparotomy, lumbar puncture was performed. The endogenous opioid content of the CSF sample was determined using a radioreceptor assay. A standardized anesthetic was administered, and patients received meperidine via PCA for postoperative analgesia. While still using PCA, another CSF sample and a sample of central venous blood was obtained 24 hours after laparotomy. The concentration of meperidine was determined in these samples.

A significant inverse relation was discovered between preoperative endogenous opioid content in the CSF and individual postoperative concentrations of meperidine in plasma ($r^2 = .29$, $p < .05$) and in CSF ($r^2 = .43$, $p < .02$) (Fig. 10-16). Stated simply, patients with low preoperative endogenous opioid content in CSF administered more opioid postoperatively via PCA to maintain higher concentrations in the plasma and in the CSF. Likewise, the converse was true.

According to the results of this study, endogenous opioids interact with exogenously administered opioids to influence analgesic demand and MEAC. According to this work by Tamsen et al, individual analgesic demand is determined by an individual's CSF endogenous opioid content. The validity of this assertion has recently been questioned,[43,44] suggesting the need for further research.

Psychological Factors

If neurotransmitter levels were the only determinant of how patients use PCA, PCA would be flawlessly effective in all patients. Patients' use of PCA would be solely mechanistic. Patients would be mechanical automatons, passively responding to CSF opioid levels.

Irrespective of pharmacokinetic and pharmacodynamic considerations, a patient's "decision" to depress the demand button remains paramount. Thus, psychological factors must play an important role in how patients use PCA.

Although illness and pain behaviors have previously been hypothesized to be important in how patients use PCA, two recent studies are the first to really

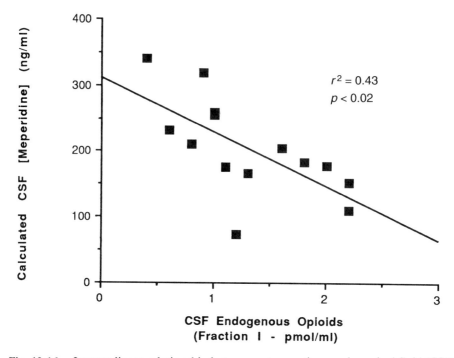

Fig. 10-16. Inverse linear relationship between preoperative cerebrospinal fluid (CSF) levels of endogenous opioids (fraction I) and postoperative analgesic demand (CSF concentration of meperidine) while using PCA. (Modified from Tamsen et al, with permission.[42])

attempt to define their effects.[45,46] Further research is certainly much needed in this area. However, at present it is safe to say that psychometric testing is a viable tool to elucidate factors that affect patients' ability to effectively use PCA.

SUBCUTANEOUS PATIENT-CONTROLLED ANALGESIA

Despite the potential widespread applicability, the subcutaneous route of administration for PCA (SC-PCA) has received attention only recently.[7,8,47] SC-PCA appears to be as equally efficacious as IV-PCA. Patient satisfaction with each modality is also comparable.

To date, hydromorphone,[7] morphine,[8] and oxymorphone[8] have been used via SC-PCA. In all studies the trend was toward higher dose requirements for all drugs as compared with IV-PCA. However, statistical significance was achieved for administration of hydromorphone only.

The reasons for this are somewhat obscure. Certainly, repeated administration of hydromorphone could have produced a "depot" effect caused by delayed absorption.[7] However, the greater bioavailability inherent in the IV route

TABLE 10-5. Guidelines for Opioid Administration via SC-PCA

Drug (concentration)[a]	Demand Dose[a]	Lockout Interval (min)
Morphine (5.0 mg/ml)	0.2 ml = 1 mg	10
Hydromorphone (1.0 mg/ml)	0.2 ml = 0.2 mg	15
Oxymorphone (1.5 mg/ml)	0.2 ml = 0.3 mg	10

[a] As compared with IV-PCA (see Table 10-2), more concentrated solutions and smaller dose volumes are used to minimize the fluid volume administered.
(Data from Urquhart et al[7] and White.[8])

of administration could account for differences in dosage requirement.[7] Unfortunately, pharmacokinetic data for the uptake of hydromorphone from SC tissue are not available. Thus, it is impossible to discern whether the difference in dose requirement for hydromorphone was the result of pharmacokinetic or pharmacodynamic parameters or artifact because of the small number of patients studied so far. Data available to date suggest that a depot effect can occur with highly lipid-soluble opioids. Thus, the less lipid-soluble analgesics (e.g., morphine, oxymorphone) may be preferable for use with SC-PCA.

Suggested dosing parameters for SC-PCA are found in Table 10-5.

Potential complications of SC-PCA include (1) pain secondary to administration of a large volume of fluid to the SC site (see Table 10-5), (2) slow onset of analgesia, (3) delayed respiratory depression caused by a "depot" effect[27] and/or decreased cutaneous blood flow, and (4) infection at the SC site.

In summary, SC-PCA appears to be as efficacious as IV-PCA in the management of postoperative pain. Patient acceptance of SC-PCA is high. Given the potential widespread applicability of SC-PCA, particularly in patients in whom IV access is a problem, more studies of the modality are clearly needed.

PATIENT-CONTROLLED EPIDURAL ANALGESIA

At present, patient-controlled epidural analgesia (PCEA) is a research modality and should be restricted to use under protocol. Opioids[9,10,48] and local anesthetics[1-3] have been used. Both the demand dose[3,9,10,48,49] and continuous infusion plus demand dose[1,2] modes have been used.

In nonobstetric populations, PCEA appears to be "dose-sparing."[9,10,48] With use of PCEA for labor analgesia, there appears to be no dose-sparing effects in comparison with intermittent "top-up" injections.[3] No consensus of opinion exists as to the dose-sparing potential of PCEA in comparison with continuous epidural infusions for labor analgesia.[1,2,49]

A number of important and basic questions regarding PCEA remain to be answered before advocation of its widespread clinical use. With respect to local anesthetics, the volume-concentration relations of the demand dose need to be investigated, as well as the influence of the duration of the lockout interval on local anesthetic and/or opioid analgesic efficacy and toxicity.

Is choice of local anesthetic and/or opioid a concern? The most optimal agents would be of fast onset and intermediate duration. Fast onset is important in order to avoid transiently increased patient demands while adequate analgesia is being achieved. Agents of short analgesic duration could promote a high rate of patient demand and subsequent "exhaustion" of the patient with the analgesic process. Agents of long duration could accumulate, eventually promoting toxicity and untoward side effects. The most optimal local anesthetic or opioid (or combination) for use with PCEA has yet to be elucidated.

Are there any benefits or liabilities to use of particular modes of PCEA administration? With continuous infusion plus demand dose PCEA, as the amount of analgesic supplied by infusion increases, the modality becomes more "physician-controlled" than "patient-controlled."[49] Could this perhaps explain the disparity among various studies with respect to the dose-sparing effects of PCEA?

In clinical trials performed to date, PCEA appears to provide excellent analgesia. According to some researchers, it may also provide the potential for use of lower amounts of analgesic agents. However, no further comment can be made on its widespread applicability until the aforementioned methodologic problems have been investigated.

CONCLUSION

IV-PCA is presently experiencing widespread popularity and growth. The reasons for this are multifactorial but can mainly be attributed to (1) an increased awareness of the inadequacy of traditional IM opioids in the provision of uniformly consistent analgesia, (2) the development of sophisticated, safe, and "user-friendly" infuser technology, and most importantly, (3) the tremendous patient satisfaction with the technique.[50,51] Several basic methodologic questions must be addressed with respect to PCEA before its proper place in the analgesic armamentarium can be determined. As time passes, however, IV-PCA (and, perhaps, SC-PCA) will only continue to supplant IM opioids as the standard analgesic therapy for management of postoperative pain.

References
1. Gambling DR, Yu P, Cole C et al: A comparative study of patient controlled epidural analgesia (PCEA) and continuous infusion epidural analgesia (CIEA) during labour. Can J Anaesth 35:249, 1988
2. Lysak SZ, Eisenach JC, Dobson II CE: Patient-controlled epidural analgesia during labor: a comparison of three solutions with a continuous infusion control. Anesthesiology 72:44, 1990
3. Gambling DR, McMorland GH, Yu P, Laszlo C: Comparison of patient-controlled epidural analgesia and conventional intermittent "top-up" injections during labor. Anesth Analg 70:256, 1990
4. Egan KJ, Ready LB, Nessly M, Greer BE: Self-administration of midazolam for postoperative anxiety: a double-blinded study. Pain 49:3, 1992
5. Shah MV, Jones DI, Rosen M: "Patient demand" postoperative analgesia with

buprenorphine. Comparison between sublingual and IM administration. Br J Anaesth 58:508, 1986

6. Bell MD, Murray GR, Mishra P et al: Buccal morphine—a new route for analgesia? Lancet i:71, 1985

7. Urquhart ML, Klapp K, White PF: Patient-controlled analgesia: a comparison of intravenous versus subcutaneous hydromorphone. Anesthesiology 69:428, 1988

8. White PF: Subcutaneous-PCA: an alternative to IV-PCA for postoperative pain management. Clin J Pain 6:297, 1990

9. Sjöström S, Hartvig D, Tamsen A: Patient-controlled analgesia with extradural morphine or pethidine. Br J Anaesth 60:358, 1988

10. Marlowe S, Engstrom R, White PF: Epidural patient-controlled analgesia (PCA): an alternative to continuous epidural infusions. Pain 37:97, 1989

11. Tamsen A, Hartvig P, Fagerlund C, Dahlström B: Patient-controlled analgesic therapy, Part II: individual analgesic demand and analgesic plasma concentrations of pethidine in postoperative pain. Clin Pharmacokinet 7:164, 1982

12. Tamsen A, Bondesson V, Dahlström B, Hartvig P: Patient-controlled analgesic therapy, Part III: pharmacokinetics and analgesic plasma concentrations of ketobemidone. Clin Pharmacokinet 7:252, 1982

13. Dahlström B, Tamsen A, Paalzow L, Hartvig P: Patient-controlled analgesic therapy, Part IV: pharmacokinetics and analgesic plasma concentration of morphine. Clin Pharmacokinet 7:266, 1982

14. Ferrante FM, Orav EJ, Rocco AG, Gallo J: A statistical model for pain in patient-controlled analgesia and conventional intramuscular opioid regimens. Anesth Analg 67:457, 1988

15. Sinatra R, Chung KS, Silverman DG et al: An evaluation of morphine and oxymorphone administered via patient-controlled analgesia (PCA) or PCA plus basal infusion in postcesarean-delivery patients. Anesthesiology 71:502, 1989

16. Mather LE, Owen H: The pharmacology of patient-administered opioids. p. 27. In Ferrante FM, Ostheimer GW, Covino BG (eds): Patient-Controlled Analgesia. Blackwell Scientific Publications, Boston, 1990

17. Hill HF, Mackie AM, Jacobson RC: Infusion-based patient-controlled analgesia systems. p. 214. In Ferrante FM, Ostheimer GW, Covino BG (eds): Patient-Controlled Analgesia. Blackwell Scientific Publications, Boston, 1990

18. McKenzie R: Patient-controlled analgesia (PCA) (letter). Anesthesiology 69:1027, 1988

19. Owen H, Plummer JL, Armstrong I et al: Variables of patient-controlled analgesia: 1. Bolus size. Anaesthesia 44:7, 1989

20. Owen H, Szekely SM, Plummer JL et al: Variables of patient-controlled analgesia: 2. Concurrent infusion. Anaesthesia 44:11, 1989

21. Roe BB: Are postoperative narcotics necessary? Arch Surg 87:912, 1963

22. Sechzer PH: Objective measurement of pain. Anesthesiology 29:209, 1968

23. Sechzer PH: Studies in pain with the analgesic-demand system. Anesth Analg 50:1, 1971

24. Evans JM, Rosen M, MacCarthy J, Hogg MI: Apparatus for patient-controlled administration of intravenous narcotics during labour. Lancet i:17, 1976

25. Editorial. Patient-controlled analgesia infusion pumps (I). Health Devices 17:137, 1988

26. Editorial. Patient-controlled analgesia infusion pumps (II). Health Devices 17:368, 1988

27. Bahar M, Rosen M, Vickers MD: Self-administered nalbuphine, morphine and pethi-

dine. Comparison, by intravenous route, following cholecystectomy. Anaesthesia 40:529, 1985

28. Bollish SJ, Collins CL, Kirking DM, Bartlett RH: Efficacy of patient-controlled versus conventional analgesia for postoperative pain. Clin Pharm 4:48, 1985

29. Bellville JW, Seed JC: The effects of drugs on the respiratory response to carbon dioxide. Anesthesiology 21:727, 1960

30. Brose WG, Cohen SE: Oxyhemoglobin saturation following cesarean section in patients receiving epidural morphine, PCA or IM meperidine analgesia. Anesthesiology 70:948, 1989

31. White PF: Mishaps with patient-controlled analgesia. Anesthesiology 66:81, 1987

32. Grey TC, Sweeney ES: Patient-controlled analgesia (letter). JAMA 259:2240, 1988

33. Austin KL, Stapleton JV, Mather LE: Multiple intramuscular injections: a major source of variability in analgesic response to meperidine. Pain 8:47, 1980

34. Austin KL, Stapleton JV, Mather LE: Relationship between blood meperidine concentrations and analgesic response: a preliminary report. Anesthesiology 53:460, 1980

35. Church JJ: Continuous narcotic infusions for relief of postoperative pain. Br Med J 1:977, 1979

36. Rutter PC, Murphy F, Dudley HA: Morphine: controlled trial of different methods of administration for postoperative pain relief. Br Med J 280:12, 1980

37. Briggs GG, Berman ML, Lange S et al: Morphine: continuous intravenous infusion versus intramuscular injections for postoperative pain relief. Gynecol Oncol 22:288, 1985

38. Marshall H, Porteous C, McMillan I et al: Relief of pain by infusion of morphine after operation: does tolerance develop? Br Med J [Clin Res] 291:19, 1985

39. Stapleton JV, Austin KL, Mather LE: A pharmacokinetic approach to postoperative pain: continuous infusion of pethidine. Anaesth Intensive Care 7:25, 1979

40. Catling JA, Pinto DM, Jordan C, Jones JG: Respiratory effects of analgesia after cholecystectomy: comparison of continuous and intermittent papaveretum. Br Med J 281:478, 1980

41. Fields HL: Central nervous system mechanisms for control of pain transmission. p. 99. In: Pain. McGraw-Hill, New York, 1987

42. Tamsen A, Sakurada T, Wahlström et al: Postoperative demand for analgesics in relation to individual levels of endorphins and substance P in cerebrospinal fluid. Pain 13:171, 1982

43. Eisenach JC, Dobson II CE, Inturrisi CE et al: Effect of pregnancy and pain on cerebrospinal fluid immunoreactive enkephalins and norepinephrine in healthy humans. Pain 43:149, 1990

44. Ferrante FM: Commentary: patient-controlled analgesia. p. 525. In Max M, Portenoy R, Laska E (eds): The Design of Analgesic Clinical Trials. Advances in Pain Research and Therapy. Vol. 18. Raven Press, New York, 1991

45. Johnson LR, Magnani B, Chan V, Ferrante FM: Modifiers of patient-controlled analgesia efficacy. I: locus of control. Pain 39:17, 1989

46. Gil KM, Ginsberg B, Muir M et al: Patient-controlled analgesia in postoperative pain: the relation of psychological factors to pain and analgesic use. Clin J Pain 6: 137, 1990

47. Taylor E, White PF: Does the anesthetic technique influence the postoperative analgesic requirement? Clin J Pain 7:139, 1991

48. Boudreault D, Brasseur L, Samii K, Lemoing JP: Comparison of continuous epidural bupivacaine infusion plus either continuous epidural infusion or patient-con-

trolled epidural infusion of fentanyl for postoperative analgesia. Anesth Analg 73: 132, 1991

49. Ferrante FM, Lu L, Jamison SB, Datta S: Patient-controlled epidural analgesia: demand dosing. Anesth Analg 73:547, 1991
50. Eisenach JC, Grice SC, Dewan DM: Patient-controlled analgesia following cesarean section: a comparison with epidural and intramuscular narcotics. Anesthesiology 68:444, 1988
51. Harrison DM, Sinatra R, Morgese L, Chung JH: Epidural narcotic and patient-controlled analgesia for post-cesarean section pain relief. Anesthesiology 68:454, 1988

11

Epidural and Subarachnoid Opioids

Timothy R. VadeBoncouer
F. Michael Ferrante

Since the first use of epidural[1] and subarachnoid[2] opioids in 1979, these techniques have become widely accepted for the management of moderate to severe postoperative pain. The ease of application of spinal opioids (encompassing both epidural and subarachnoid delivery) and their relatively high benefit-to-risk ratio (production of maximum analgesia with few side effects) make them ideal for managing postoperative pain. Whether given as a single injection at the time of anesthesia, intermittent injections, or continuous infusions through indwelling epidural catheters, spinal opioids can provide prolonged and intense pain relief.

Unlike local anesthetics, spinal opioids provide analgesia while permitting early ambulation, since motor blockade is not produced. Moreover, their lack of effect on the sympathetic nervous system makes them ideal for pain management in the patient with unstable cardiovascular status. This preferential attenuation of nociception (while preserving normal sympathetic and motor function) permits spinal opioids to be used in a wide range of clinical scenarios without interfering with normal postsurgical convalescence.

This chapter focuses on the clinical use of spinal opioids for postoperative pain management. Side effects and their treatment, as well as recommendations for monitoring patients, are also presented. Coadministration of epidural local anesthetics and opioids is discussed in Chapter 12.

CLINICAL USE OF EPIDURAL OPIOIDS

Mechanism of Action

Segmental analgesia (selective spinally mediated analgesia[3]) occurs through binding of administered agents to receptors in the dorsal horn of the spinal cord.[4,5] This area is richly populated with opioid receptors. (An extensive discussion of the anatomy and physiology of the sensory afferent pain pathways can be found in Chapter 2. Opioid receptors are discussed in Chapter 8.) Production of segmental analgesia requires a minimum concentration of opioid in the cerebrospinal fluid (CSF) and, by inference, in the dorsal horn of the spinal cord segments mediating nociception. This is important to stress, as epidural opioids may produce analgesia despite insignificant amounts of drug in the CSF. This analgesic contribution from systemic drug effects is discussed in detail later. Suffice it to say that true segmental analgesia results from drug effects on the dorsal horn, with little or no contribution from systemic levels of opioid.

Importance of Lipid Solubility

The single physicochemical property of opioids that best predicts their behavior as spinal analgesics is lipid solubility. Although molecular weight,[6] molecular size,[6] and receptor binding affinity[7,8] certainly play a role, lipid solubility[4,9,10] readily predicts how an opioid will behave when given intraspinally. Commonly used epidural opioids are listed in order of increasing lipid solubility in Table 11-1.

When an opioid is delivered to the epidural space, the drug may ultimately be cleared by several routes (Fig. 11-1). Opioids may: (1) bind to extradural fat,[4,7,14] (2) enter the epidural venous system and thus the systemic circulation,[4,9,15] (3) enter the posterior radicular spinal arteries and be delivered directly to the dorsal horn[4,16] (Fig. 11-2), or (4) penetrate the dura through diffusion across the arachnoid granulations and enter the CSF[4,16] (Fig. 11-2).

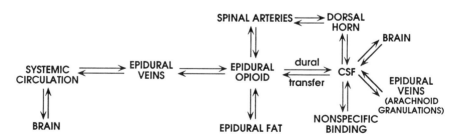

Fig. 11-1. Possible routes of opioid absorption after epidural administration. Distribution depends primarily on lipid solubility. Opioids gain access to the CSF by diffusion across arachnoid granulations in the dural cuff region. Clearance of opioid from CSF occurs primarily at arachnoid granulation/epidural vein complexes. Note that spinal arteries provide rapid access to the dorsal horn.

TABLE 11-1. Commonly Used Epidural Opioids

Drug	Lipid Solubility[a]	Bolus Dose	Onset (min)	Duration (h)	Comments
Morphine	1	2–5 mg	30–60	6–24	Because of spread in CSF, preferred for extensive incisions and when injection site is distant from cord segments mediating nociception
Diamorphine	10	4–6 mg	5	10–12	
Meperidine	30	50–100 mg	5–10	6–8	
Methadone	100	1–10 mg	10	6–10	May accumulate in blood with repetitive dosing[4,11,12]
Fentanyl	800	50–100 μg	5	4–6	Not recommended when incision is extensive or injection site is distant from cord segments mediating nociception
Sufentanil	1,500	10–60 μg	5	2–4	Higher doses may produce excessive sedation or respiratory depression, presumably because of vascular uptake[13]

[a] Octanol/pH 7.4 buffer partition coefficient relative to morphine.

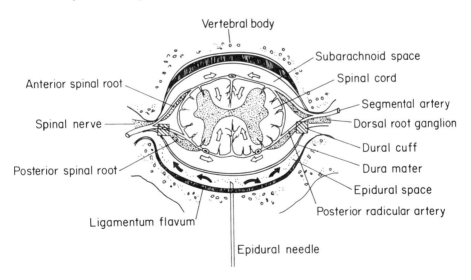

Fig. 11-2. Lipid-soluble epidural opioids may gain rapid access to the CSF by diffusion across the arachnoid granulations in the dural cuff region. The spread of opioids in the epidural space is denoted by *black arrows*. Spread within the CSF and spinal cord is depicted by *white arrows*. Lipid-soluble opioids may also be rapidly absorbed into the posterior radicular artery (a branch of the spinal segmental artery). Branches of the posterior radicular artery directly supply the dorsal horn.

Highly lipid-soluble drugs (e.g., fentanyl) are avidly absorbed by epidural fat and blood vessels.[4,7,14] Drug binding to epidural fat will decrease its availability for diffusion into the CSF through the arachnoid granulations in the dural cuff region (see Ch. 5). Such binding is unpredictable, however, as epidural fat content varies widely among patients.

Diffusion of opioid into epidural veins will result in systemic opioid levels with attendant effects[4,9,15] (Fig. 11-3). If entry into the circulation is substantial and prolonged, clinical analgesia may result more from systemic (supraspinal) than spinal (segmental) effects (see below).

Uptake of opioid by local spinal cord arterial flow may hasten drug delivery to the dorsal horn.[4,16] This feature, along with rapid transfer of drug through arachnoid granulations,[4,16] may explain the rapid onset of analgesia seen with highly lipid-soluble epidural opioids (Fig. 11-2).

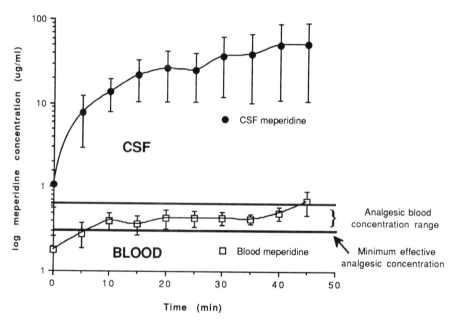

Fig. 11-3. CSF and central venous blood concentrations of meperidine (mean ± standard error) after epidural injection of 100 mg of meperidine ($N = 8$). (The minimum effective analgesic concentration [within the blood] and the range of analgesic blood concentrations were separately determined after intravenous injection of 100 mg meperidine.) Analgesia was related to CSF concentration, in that patients having a high CSF/blood concentration ratio also had complete analgesia. The rapid rise in CSF meperidine concentration in the first 5 minutes after epidural injection also coincided with the onset of analgesia. For most patients receiving epidural meperidine, the analgesic blood concentration range associated with intravenous injection (0.2–0.7 µg/ml) was achieved within 20 minutes. However, one patient never achieved an analgesic blood meperidine concentration at all during the study period, despite excellent analgesia. Thus, the major analgesic effect after epidural injection of a lipophilic opioid is spinally mediated, but vascular absorption may be significant. (Data from Glynn et al.[16])

TABLE 11-2. Clinical Characteristics of Epidural Opioids (After Single Injection)

	Lipid-soluble Agents (prototype = fentanyl)	Hydrophilic Agents (prototype = morphine)
Onset of analgesia	Rapid	Slow
Duration of analgesia	Short	Prolonged
Respiratory depression	Early (systemic uptake)	Late (rostral flow)

Although dural transfer may or may not be increased as lipid solubility increases, it is at the very least inefficient and unpredictable for the highly lipophilic opioids because of the aforementioned factors. Hydrophilic drugs, such as morphine, may have more predictable and efficient dural transfer because they are not well absorbed by epidural fat or blood vessels.[6]

Once opioid has gained access to CSF, it may remain there or bind to spinal cord tissue. Binding to opioid receptors occurs in Rexed's laminae I, II (substantia gelatinosa), and V. Nonspecific binding occurs in the lipid-rich tracts capping the dorsal horn.[17] Sequestration of drug in the CSF would be most likely to occur with the relatively lipid-insoluble (hydrophilic) opioids (i.e., morphine).[9,15,18] Accumulation of opioid in the CSF leads to two well-recognized clinical features of spinal morphine: long duration of analgesia, and predilection for rostral flow within the CSF.[9,15,18]

How, then, does lipid solubility predict the clinical behavior of spinal opioids? Let us review several of the clinical features associated with the use of lipid-soluble and hydrophilic agents (Table 11-2; Figs. 11-4 and 11-5).

Onset of Analgesia

Lipid soluble agents quickly gain access to the dorsal horn via the arachnoid granulations and spinal cord arterial blood flow, resulting in rapid onset of analgesia[9,16,19] (Fig. 11–2). Hydrophilic opioids, although efficiently transferred across the dura, do so slowly and hence produce analgesia more slowly.[9,19]

Duration of Analgesia

Removal of opioid from the dorsal horn primarily occurs through local spinal cord blood flow, including uptake into epidural veins in close proximity to the arachnoid granulations. Highly lipid-soluble agents are rapidly absorbed into blood vessels from receptor sites, and analgesic duration is short.[4,9,16,19] Hydrophilic opioids, which preferentially distribute into the aqueous CSF milieu, diffuse poorly into blood vessels. Moreover, a depot of drug remains in the CSF for long periods with hydrophilic opioids, maintaining opioid receptor binding. Thus, analgesia is prolonged.[9,15,18,19]

Rostrad Migration in CSF

The hydrophilic opioids, essentially sequestered in the CSF, are available to move rostrally via CSF bulk flow[9,15,18,19] (Fig. 11-6). As successively larger rostral concentrations of opioid are achieved, analgesia is extended to include

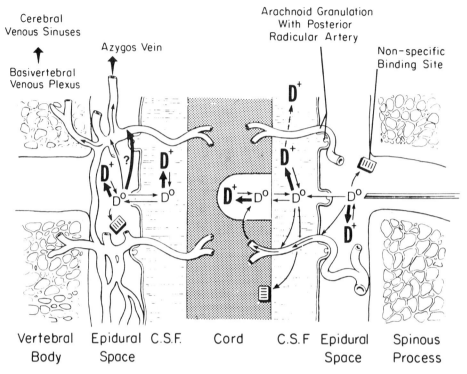

Fig. 11-4. Pharmacokinetic model for epidural injection of a hydrophilic opioid (morphine). D^0 = neutral form of drug able to diffuse through membranes; D^+ = ionized hydrophilic form of drug. After epidural injection of a highly ionized and hydrophilic opioid, only low concentrations of the lipid-soluble neutral form will be present in the epidural space. Thus, diffusion across the arachnoid granulations or into spinal arteries will be slow (slow onset of analgesia). Once within the CSF, most of the opioid will be present in the ionized form, thus presenting a small concentration gradient for diffusion to receptors in the cord or egress into blood vessels from occupied receptors (long duration of analgesia). The high concentration of ionized hydrophilic drug within the CSF will move rostrally with CSF flow (extension of analgesia over a wide number of dermatomes). If significant concentrations of opioid reach the rostroventral medulla, nausea, vomiting, and delayed respiratory depression may result. (Modified from Cousins et al,[4] with permission.)

higher and higher dermatomes.[15,20–26] When significant concentrations of opioid reach the brain stem, respiratory depression and vomiting may occur as a result of direct interaction with centers in the medulla.

Lipid-soluble drugs do not flow rostrad in the CSF to any significant degree, as they are absorbed into lipids close to the site of injection[4,7,14] (see below). Thus, opioid-related side effects are unlikely to be related to rostral CSF drug movement. Side effects can occur, however, when epidural opioid delivery is substantial and excessive, resulting in significant systemic levels of drug.

Tables 11-1 and 11-2 outline the clinical profile of hydrophilic and lipophilic opioids after a single epidural injection.

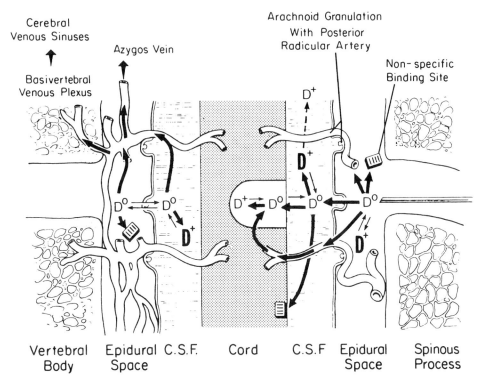

Cerebral Venous Sinuses

Azygos Vein

Arachnoid Granulation With Posterior Radicular Artery

Non-specific Binding Site

Basivertebral Venous Plexus

D^+

D^+

$D^+ \rightleftarrows D^0 \leftarrow D^0 \leftarrow D^0$

$D^0 \leftarrow D^0$

D^+

D^+

| Vertebral Body | Epidural Space | C.S.F. | Cord | C.S.F | Epidural Space | Spinous Process |

Fig. 11-5. Pharmacokinetic model for epidural injection of a lipophilic opioid (e.g., meperidine or fentanyl). D^0 = neutral form of drug able to diffuse through membranes; D^+ = ionized hydrophilic form of drug. After epidural injection of a mostly ionized lipophilic opioid, low concentrations of the neutral form will rapidly diffuse through the arachnoid granulations into CSF, into spinal radicular arteries and thereby to the dorsal horn, and into epidural veins (rapid onset of analgesia). Because of brisk spinal artery flow and slow epidural venous flow, transfer of drug to the spinal cord will occur while the concentration gradient is high (rapid onset of analgesia). Significant vascular absorption into epidural veins will rapidly reduce the concentration gradient (short duration of analgesia, potential early respiratory depression). Diffusion of opioid from receptors into the venous system will be equally as rapid (short duration of analgesia, potential early respiratory depression). As these opioids are lipophilic, there will be significant binding to fat and other nonspecific (nonreceptor) sites. For all the aforementioned reasons, the amount of ionized species (D^+) available to flow rostrally in the CSF will be insignificant (no potential for delayed respiratory depression). (Modified from Cousins et al,[4] with permission.)

Site of Injection

A general guideline for management of continuous epidural opioids (either single injection or infusion) is to place the catheter at the interspace crossed by the middle dermatome of the surgical incision. This permits craniocaudad spread of drug in such a manner as to optimize analgesia and minimize side effects. The highly lipid-soluble opioids, with their limited ability to spread

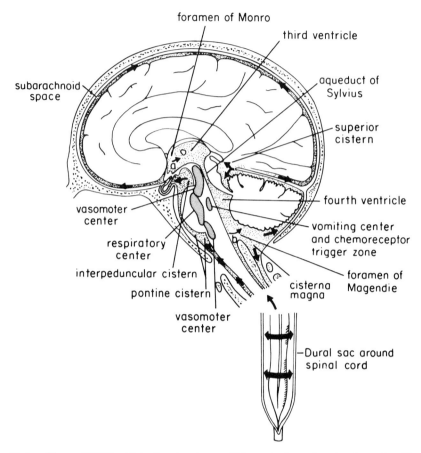

Fig. 11-6. Flow of CSF within the dural sac of the spinal cord and subarachnoid cisterns. CSF is an ultrafiltrate of the plasma produced by the choroid plexuses of the lateral, third, and fourth ventricles. CSF may enter the third ventricle from the lateral ventricle through the foramen of Monro. From the fourth ventricle, CSF enters the cisterna magna through the foramen of Magendie. Subsequent flow through the subarachnoid space is as shown. Flow of CSF within higher centers is rapid. Rostral flow of CSF from the dural sac around the spinal cord is slow. Thus, several hours will be required in order to achieve a significant concentration of a hydrophilic opioid at the respiratory center, vomiting center, or chemoreceptor trigger zones.

in the CSF, are most dependent on catheter location for optimal segmental effect.[27–32] The hydrophilic agents, which readily spread in the CSF, are much less dependent on injection site[21–26] (Fig. 11-7).

Morphine administered in the lumbar epidural space can produce analgesia in dermatomes far removed from the initial site of injection.[21–26] Fromme and colleagues[24] compared the analgesic efficacy of thoracic and lumbar epidural morphine in post-thoracotomy patients. Both groups obtained excellent analgesia while receiving identical low morphine doses. Sullivan and Cherry[25] re-

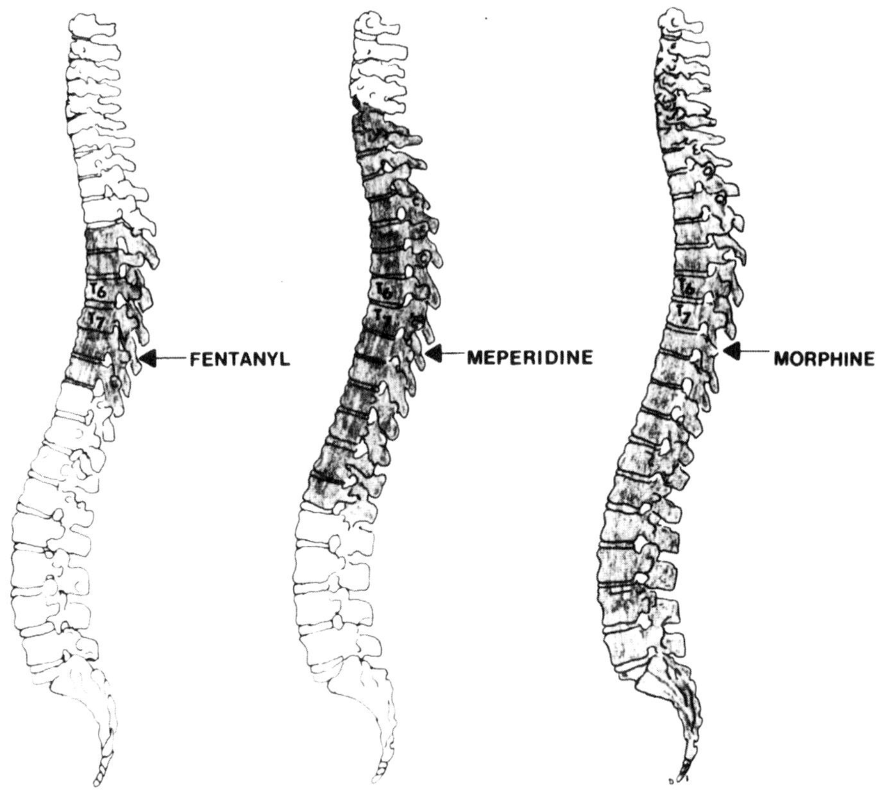

Fig. 11-7. Relation of segmental analgesia to opioid lipophilicity. For purposes of illustration, opioids are administered through the T6-T7 interspace. Fentanyl is the prototypic lipid-soluble opioid. Fentanyl is avidly absorbed into lipid stores because of its inherent lipophilicity. Thus, fentanyl produces a narrow band of true segmental analgesia (*shaded area*) Morphine, however, is relatively insoluble in lipids. Morphine's inherent hydrophilicity allows rostral migration in the CSF and a wide band of effective analgesia (*shaded area*). Meperidine has intermediate lipophilicity with respect to fentanyl and morphine. Thus, the degree of segmental analgesia is intermediate between fentanyl and morphine.

ported on the use of lumbar epidural morphine for treatment of painful invasive facial malignancy. Both of these reports are consistent with the extensive spread of morphine throughout the CSF, producing analgesia in dermatomes distant from the site of injection. Finally, Sjöström et al[26] studied patients who had undergone major abdominal surgery. When these patients were allowed to self-administer epidural morphine through a low thoracic or lumbar catheter (T10–L3), they achieved excellent pain relief from an average of only 0.5 mg/h of morphine. This resulted in plasma morphine levels well below those reported elsewhere for systemic (supraspinal) analgesia, indicating a spinally mediated mechanism for pain relief. Excellent analgesia occurred despite catheter location near the caudad end of an extensive abdominal surgical incision.

Controversy exists as to the ability of the more lipid-soluble opioids to produce segmental spinal analgesia (without a significant supraspinal contribution) when administered to the neuraxis distant to the cord segments mediating nociception. Bodily et al[27] reported lower hourly fentanyl requirements and better pain scores in post-thoracotomy patients receiving thoracic epidural fentanyl, as compared with a group receiving lumbar epidural fentanyl. Badner and colleagues[28] were able to provide analgesia after thoracotomy by using lumbar epidural fentanyl infusions. However, when pain scores were lowest, systemic fentanyl levels were within the range reported for systemic analgesia. Another study reported successful thoracic analgesia when large doses (200 μg) of fentanyl were given through a lumbar epidural catheter every 3–4 hours.[29] The authors reported an alarmingly high incidence of sedation (90 percent) after each dose. Unfortunately, systemic fentanyl levels were not measured.

The controversy over the use of epidural fentanyl for segmental analgesia has been recently extended to include other situations, in particular those where the surgical incision is small and/or the catheter location along the neuraxis is close to the spinal cord segments receiving nociceptive input. Glass et al[30] compared patient-controlled intravenous fentanyl to patient-controlled lumbar epidural fentanyl for treatment of pain after lower abdominal or lower extremity surgery using a double-blind cross-over protocol. The two groups had comparable pain relief and plasma fentanyl levels during therapy. A similar result was noted in another study comparing infusions of intravenous and epidural fentanyl for analgesia after cesarean delivery.[31] Quality of analgesia, plasma fentanyl levels, and incidence of side effects were similar in both groups by the twelfth hour of therapy. Lastly, Loper and colleagues[32] compared continuous infusions of intravenous and epidural fentanyl for treating the pain of knee arthrotomy using a double-blind protocol. They also found no differences in pain scores or systemic fentanyl levels between the two groups.

What conclusions can be drawn from these reports? Clearly, the use of lumbar epidural fentanyl (and, by inference, all highly lipid-soluble opioids) cannot be recommended for the treatment of upper abdominal and thoracic pain.[27,29] High systemic fentanyl levels may result.[28,31,32] Pain relief is incomplete, and this technique appears to have no advantages over intravenous fentanyl.[31,32] Ever more suspect is the use of epidural fentanyl for large incisions (e.g., thoracoabdominal incisions), regardless of catheter location or site of injection. Lipid-soluble drugs have limited ability to spread in the CSF and thus may not reach the appropriate spinal cord segments to produce analgesia.[4,7,14] Because systemic fentanyl levels may be substantial even when opioid is administered close to the appropriate spinal cord segments,[32] this argument is sound. Epidural fentanyl is probably best used when the catheter location along the neuraxis is close to the spinal cord segments receiving nociceptive input and the surgical incision is limited.

As long as fentanyl doses are not excessive, side effects are minimal and pain relief is substantial. Thus, there is no good reason to discontinue epidural fentanyl use for pain management. However, the bulk of recent clinical evidence suggests that excellent segmental analgesia without systemic effects may be very difficult to obtain with fentanyl.[27-32] As described by Dickenson et al,[17] avid absorption of lipid-soluble opioids by blood vessels, fat, and lipid-rich fiber tracts in the spinal cord probably contribute to the unreliable delivery of these agents to their sites of action.

Intermittent Injections versus Continuous Infusions

Epidural opioids can be delivered as intermittent injections or continuous epidural infusions. Intermittent injection therapy is technically simpler, as no special equipment is required. Morphine, with its long duration of action, is the ideal agent for intermittent injection because the need for reinjection should be infrequent.[33,34] Initially, smaller doses of morphine should be used to allow determination of a reliable analgesic dose for achieving good pain relief with few side effects. Small dose increments can be given if the initial dose is inadequate. Even though dosing intervals should theoretically be infrequent with morphine, it may be logistically prohibitive for personnel to simultaneously attend to many patients on an acute pain service using this approach. Ready and colleagues[35] effectively used this technique by permitting nursing staff to reinject epidural opioids when pain recurred. Extensive nursing education is obviously required.

Lipid-soluble opioids have much shorter durations of action than morphine.[4,9,16,19] Intermittent injection therapy with these agents can pose severe logistics problems because of the necessity of frequent reinjection. When extended pain relief is desired, these agents can be given as a continuous epidural infusion in an attempt to minimize the need for reinjection.[28,31,32,36-39] Specific infusion rates are recommended to minimize the likelihood of significant systemic opioid levels and attendant effects (Table 11-3). It must be remembered that the low risk of late respiratory depression with lipid-soluble drugs is applicable only after a single injection, as systemic levels may be significant during infusion.[28,31,32]

Continuous infusions of epidural morphine have also been used.[42,43] Because a single initial injection of 4–5 mg of morphine may produce prolonged analge-

TABLE 11-3. Commonly Used Epidural Opioid Infusions[a]

Drug	Usual Infusion Rate (mg/h)	Comments
Morphine	0.2–1.0	May produce excessive CSF levels; lowest effective rates should be used after a loading injection
Meperidine	10–25	Rates greater than 20 mg/h may produce significant systemic levels and sedation; prolonged therapy may result in accumulation of normeperidine with risk of myoclonus and seizures[40,41]
Fentanyl	0.03–0.1	Rates greater than 0.1 mg/h may produce significant systemic levels; contribution of systemic level to analgesia may be significant[31,32]; requires catheter site close to cord segments mediating nociception.

[a] Preparation of the actual epidural solutions of opioid, with and without local anesthetic, is described in Chapter 12.

sia,[44] infusion rates should be low. Higher rates may be associated with increased risk of delayed side effects, since this agent may accumulate and migrate rostrally in the CSF. Suffice it to say that, because of its low lipid solubility, epidural morphine is perhaps best used via intermittent injection.

Table 11-3 summarizes commonly used epidural opioid infusion protocols for a few select agents, with suggestions for minimizing opioid-related side effects.

Clinical Practice at Brigham and Women's Hospital

Tables 11-1 through 11-3 summarize the clinical profile of several epidural opioids when given as either a single injection or as a continuous infusion.

In our practice in a large university-based acute pain service, we commonly use three opioids: fentanyl, meperidine, and morphine for general use (Fig. 11-2). These agents have widely different lipid solubilities and, thus, different clinical utility. Fentanyl is used for incisions confined to a few dermatomal levels, as long as the epidural catheter is close to the spinal segments mediating nociception. For more extensive incisions, with an optimally positioned catheter, meperidine is used instead of fentanyl. Meperidine, although about 30 times more lipid-soluble than morphine, is also about 30 times less lipid-soluble than fentanyl (Table 11-1). Theoretically, this may result in more extensive spread in the CSF and a greater area of segmental analgesia as compared with fentanyl. Thus, meperidine may be a useful alternative to fentanyl. Although controlled studies documenting better CSF spread than fentanyl are lacking, epidural meperidine has been shown to provide good pain relief after abdominal surgery (i.e., extensive incisions) without resulting in excessive blood meperidine levels.[26] Meperidine is used frequently at Brigham and Women's Hospital for epidural analgesia, alone or with local anesthetics, and we have found it to be useful in situations where fentanyl proved unsatisfactory.

When surgical incisions are very large or the catheter site is far removed from the cord segments mediating nociception, or more lipid-soluble agents are ineffective or result in systemic side effects, morphine would seem to be the ideal epidural agent. This is not to suggest that morphine cannot be used as the drug of choice in most cases. On the contrary, the analgesic reliability and predictable duration of action make morphine the standard to which other epidural opioids are compared. The tendency of morphine to spread in the CSF is both its greatest attribute (more extensive analgesia) and the source of greatest concern (respiratory depression).

When morphine is used via a thoracic catheter, it is prudent to give smaller doses than ordinarily administered through a lumbar catheter. Although opioid can reach the brain stem in either case, greater concentrations of morphine may reach the brain stem sooner if excessive doses are given in the thoracic area.[45]

Indications for Use

Epidural opioids are indicated for the relief of moderate to severe postoperative pain. The use of drugs that spread extensively throughout the CSF permits treatment of pain of nearly any source. As a practical concern, however, operations below the head, neck, and upper extremities would appear most amenable to this modality.

Abdominal and thoracic operations have a long history of successful management with spinal opioids.[16,36,46,47] Pain relief is usually complete at rest, with minor discomfort discernible by patients during vigorous maneuvers (e.g., coughing, ambulation, physical therapy).

In our experience, pain relief after some orthopaedic procedures (e.g., joint replacement) may be incomplete with spinal opioids alone. This may be accentuated by concomitant physical therapy of the affected part.

Contraindications

The following are contraindications to the use of epidural opioid analgesia[35]:

1. Any contraindication to epidural catheter insertion
2. History of adverse reactions to opioid medications
3. Presence of dural puncture[48,49] (a relative contraindication—see below)
4. Central sleep apnea (see below)
5. Lack of familiarity of technique by patient caretakers

Dural puncture, either accidental during performance of epidural catheter insertion or occurring during laminectomy, is a relative contraindication to subsequent epidural opioid therapy.[48,49] Since effective subarachnoid doses of opioid are usually much smaller than epidural doses, it may be impossible to predict how much epidural drug reaches the CSF in the case of a dural rent. Moreover, because the sequelae of excess subarachnoid opioid administration may be life-threatening, it is probably best to avoid epidural opioids in this circumstance.

The use of epidural opioids is controversial in patients with chronic lung disease (COPD) and sleep apnea.[50,51] The advantages of affording excellent analgesia must be weighed against the risks of further possible elevations of arterial PCO_2. These patients should not necessarily be denied the benefits of epidural opioids, however. Use of low doses of opioid with minimal side effects and profound analgesia may be preferable to the high doses of opioid required by more conventional parenteral analgesic regimens. In either case, a high degree of vigilance (frequent observation, intensive respiratory monitoring) must be maintained.

Epidural morphine has been used successfully in a patient with obstructive sleep apnea.[50] Central sleep apnea, however, may be a relative contraindication to epidural opioid use. A case of respiratory arrest following epidural morphine has been reported in such a patient.[51] Central apnea differs from obstructive apnea in that patients exhibit extreme abnormalities of breathing rhythmicity in the respiratory centers of the brain. Rostrad CSF spread of opioid to the brain stem may result in severe respiratory compromise.[51]

CLINICAL USE OF SUBARACHNOID OPIOIDS

The previous discussions have focused primarily on epidural administration of opioids. When protracted postoperative analgesia is desired, epidural administration is preferred, since indwelling epidural catheters permit continuous or repeated opioid therapy. Direct instillation of opioid into the CSF (subarachnoid delivery) also produces potent analgesia.[2,3,18,52] In general, segmental analgesia via subarachnoid administration requires smaller doses.[18,53,54] Competition for drug absorption by epidural fat and blood vessels is avoided, as the drug is delivered directly to the CSF.[18,55] Onset of analgesia is usually faster.[55]

Despite slightly faster onset times with use of subarachnoid opioids, most other factors determining clinical action are as previously described for epidural opioids. Thus, lipid solubility is paramount in determining extent and duration of analgesia.[7,10,56] Because indwelling subarachnoid catheters are not clinically popular (and the Food and Drug Administration has issued a safety alert for microcatheters as of May 1992), it follows that only subarachnoid morphine will reliably produce prolonged pain relief from a single injection. As with epidural delivery, subarachnoid morphine may produce analgesia of up to 24-hours' duration.[53,54,56,57]

Most clinical experience with subarachnoid opioids has been with morphine. Doses of 0.2–1.0 mg produce reliable, long-lasting analgesia.[52–58] These doses are about one-fifth that of effective epidural morphine doses. This indicates a fairly reliable dural transfer fraction of 20 percent when morphine is administered epidurally. Because of competitive binding with fat, blood vessels, and nonspecific binding sites, reliable dural transfer fractions for the lipid-soluble opioids are difficult to predict.[59] Moreover, nonspecific binding of lipid-soluble opioids to fatty fiber tracts of the spinal cord may make even direct subarachnoid dose requirements of these agents uncertain.[17] A wide range of subarachnoid fentanyl doses ($6.25-50\mu g$) will provide similar degrees of analgesia.[60]

Subarachnoid opioids are usually administered as a single injection at the time of establishment of spinal anesthesia for surgery. Since subarachnoid catheters for continuous postoperative pain relief are unpopular (secondary to *alleged* risks of meningitis and nerve root trauma[61]), extension of analgesia beyond the usual duration of action of the drug will require repetitive dural puncture. This would be prohibitive on a busy pain service. Morphine is the subarachnoid opioid of choice for prolonged periods of pain relief (up to 24 hours).[53,54,56,57]

Table 11-4 summarizes commonly used dosing regimens for subarachnoid administration of opioids. It should be noted that very low doses of subarachnoid morphine (0.1 mg) are effective for analgesia after cesarean delivery.[58] It may be prudent to adjust doses downward in this population in order to minimize side effects.

SIDE EFFECTS OF SPINAL OPIOIDS

Possible side effects of spinal opioid therapy are listed in Table 11-5. Their cause, incidence, and treatment are discussed below. The incidence of side effects is probably no different between the epidural and subarachnoid routes of administration when reasonable doses are used.[66]

TABLE 11-4. Commonly Used Subarachnoid Opioids

Drug	Dose	Onset (min)	Duration (h)	Comments
Morphine	0.1–0.75 mg	15–30	10–30	Doses >0.5 mg may produce high incidence of side effects[62–64]; lower doses may be efficacious after cesarean delivery[58]
Meperidine	10–30 mg	5	10–30	High doses have been used for surgical anesthesia[65]
Fentanyl	10–50 μg	5	4–6	Higher doses may not prolong or intensify analgesia[60]
Diamorphine	1–2 mg	5	10–20	

Respiratory Depression

The most-feared side effect of spinal opioid therapy, and certainly the most potentially threatening to patient well-being, is respiratory depression. This occurs as a result of drug delivery to respiratory control centers located in the brain stem. Delivery occurs via (1) rostrad migration in CSF bulk flow (Fig.11-6), and/or (2) absorption into the circulation and subsequent delivery via cerebral blood flow. After a single epidural[9,67–68] or subarachnoid injection,[10,70–72] the former mechanism results in delayed respiratory depression and the latter in early respiratory depression.[4,9,10,45] The "delay" occurs as a result of the time necessary for opioid to ascend in the CSF and interact with brain stem opioid receptors in the respiratory center.

The incidence of respiratory depression after spinal opioid administration is unknown, probably reflecting the widely different criteria used to characterize its occurrence. A decrease in respiratory rate (usually below 8–10 breaths per minute) is most commonly used to denote the presence of respiratory depression. Ready argued that respiratory rate alone is an unreliable predictor of changes in respiratory drive during spinal opioid therapy.[35,73] Similarly, changes in arterial PCO_2 and tidal volume may not accurately predict the presence of respiratory depression.[35] These uncertainties have led to a lack of consistent standards for the monitoring of patients receiving spinal opioids.

After a single injection of spinal opioid, both lipid-soluble and hydrophilic

TABLE 11-5. Side Effects of Spinal Opioids

Common
 Mild pruritus
 Urinary retention
 Mild respiratory depression
 Nausea and/or vomiting
Uncommon
 Severe pruritis
 Severe respiratory depression
 Activation of herpes labialis
 Vertigo-like symptoms
 Nystagmus

agents can produce an early phase of respiratory depression (within 2 hours).[4,9,10,45] The mechanism is no different from that observed after a parenteral injection of the same opioid: vascular uptake of the drug and subsequent systemic delivery to the brain.[73] After this early phase, the lipid-soluble drugs are usually without further respiratory effect, reflecting their limited tendency to migrate rostrad in the CSF. Morphine, with its poor lipid solubility, is the prototypic agent producing delayed respiratory depression.[67-69] This effect may persist for up to 24 hours after the initial dose.[73] Persistent respiratory compromise beyond this period has not been reported for a single injection.

Controlled studies of the respiratory effects of various continuous epidural opioid infusions are lacking. In our experience, continuous epidural opioid infusions may produce respiratory depression at any time during therapy. Persistent elevations of systemic opioid levels (most likely with lipophilic drugs) and/or CSF opioid levels (most likely with hydrophilic drugs) are the cause.

Regardless of which spinal opioid is used, the risk of development of respiratory depression appears to be enhanced by several factors (Table 11-6). These include concomitant use of systemic opioids[46,62,74,75] and/or sedatives[4] and advanced patient age.[45,76] Dose adjustment in the elderly and avoidance of large doses of perioperative systemic opioids and long-acting sedatives would seem prudent.

Mild elevations of arterial PCO_2 (45–50 mmHg) or modest declines in respiratory rate (8–10 breaths per minute) in otherwise healthy patients require no intervention other than continued observation. Immediate treatment is indicated when changes in these parameters are severe. Equipment necessary for assisted ventilation must be available. Naloxone will specifically reverse the respiratory effects of spinal opioids and may be life-saving. In an apneic patient, an intravenous dose of 0.4 mg usually restores spontaneous ventilation. If respiratory depression is less severe (e.g., 4–8 breaths per minute), small increments of naloxone (0.04 mg) can be given. In either case, repeated doses of naloxone may be necessary due to its short half-life,[77] or a continuous intravenous infusion may be started (5 μg/kg/h).[78] If respiratory depression requires naloxone for treatment, the patient should be observed in a monitored setting (intermediate care or intensive care unit).

The concomitant effects of naloxone administration on spinal opioid analgesia have been incompletely studied. Naloxone infusions of 5 μg/kg/h have not affected the quality of epidural morphine analgesia, while being sufficient to re-

TABLE 11-6. Factors Enhancing Risk of Development of Respiratory Depression

Factor	Reference
Concomitant use of parenteral opioids	46, 62, 74, 75
Concomitant use of CNS depressants	4
Advanced age	45, 76
Increased thoracoabdominal pressure ("grunting," painful respiration or artificial respiration)	63
Inadvertent dural puncture	48, 49
Lack of tolerance for opioids	72

verse respiratory depression.[78] An infusion rate of 10 μg/kg/h has been shown to affect the quality of epidural morphine analgesia.[78] Infusion rates of both 5 and 10 μ/kg/h have been shown to reverse respiratory depression and affect the quality of analgesia in patients receiving epidural fentanyl.[79]

Nausea

Nausea and/or vomiting are caused by rostrad flow of opioid in CSF[80] or systemic transport[81–83] of significant opioid levels to the vomiting center and the chemoreceptor trigger zone in the medulla. An early report by Bromage et al[80] documented a 50 percent incidence of nausea or vomiting in human volunteers after epidural injection of morphine. More recently, Ready et al[84] reported an incidence of 29 percent in postoperative patients receiving intermittent injections of epidural morphine. The epidural use of lipid-soluble opioids, however, may be associated with a greatly reduced incidence of nausea and vomiting.[81–83]

Nausea caused by spinal opioids can be treated with antiemetic drugs. Metoclopramide, droperidol, or prochlorperazine may all be useful. Recently, transdermal scopalamine has been shown to be effective in reducing the incidence of nausea after epidural morphine.[85,86] Scopalamine patches can be applied before opioid therapy is begun.

Intravenous naloxone can be used when nausea is severe or intractable. Small incremental doses of naloxone (0.04–0.1 mg) are administered in an attempt to preserve analgesia (especially with lipid-soluble opioids). Such practice is theoretically sound, as CSF opioid concentrations in the brain stem are presumably much lower than at the site of administration in the lumbar or thoracic space. Thus, nausea may be more easily antagonized with small doses of naloxone. If nausea is persistent or recurrent, an intravenous naloxone infusion may be beneficial (1 μ/kg/h, increase rate to effect).

Prophylactic oral naltrexone (a long-acting opioid antagonist) holds promise as a novel means of limiting epidural opioid-related side effects. In a recent study, naltrexone reduced the incidence of side effects with minimal impact on analgesic efficacy. Statistical significance was not achieved, however, presumably due to the small number of patients in the study.[87]

Low doses of the agonist-antagonist drugs butorphanol[88,89] (0.25–0.5 mg) or nalbuphine[90,91] (1–3 mg) may also reverse nausea and other μ-receptor effects (e.g., pruritus, respiratory depression)

Pruritus

Pruritus is a very common side effect of spinal opioid therapy. Fortunately, spinal opioid-induced pruritus is rarely severe and rarely requires treatment.[92] Its incidence may be as high as 50 percent. The possible spinal cord mechanisms involved in the production of spinal opioid-induced pruritus have been reviewed by Ballantyne et al.[93] Histamine release plays a negligible role in the production of spinal opioid-induced pruritus.[93]

Antihistaminics in our experience, however, can be used to treat mild pruritus, despite the negligible role of histamine in the pathogenesis of pruritus. Severe itching may require incremental intravenous naloxone therapy, as described above. Likewise, small doses of butorphanol[88] and nalbuphine[90] may be effective.

Urinary Retention

Urinary retention is a well-recognized side effect of spinal opioid therapy. Its incidence is unknown, but retention is found more commonly in volunteers than in postsurgical patients.[92] The mechanisms for spinal opioid-mediated urinary retention have been elegantly elucidated by Durant and Yaksh.[94] Subarachnoid morphine inhibits volume-induced bladder contractions and blocks the vesicle-somatic reflex necessary for external sphincter relaxation.[94]

Bladder catheterization may be required in patients receiving spinal opioids. Naloxone administration may also be effective, but dose requirements may be sufficiently high so as to reverse analgesia. A more desirable drug treatment for urinary retention is obviously needed. Spinal opioid-mediated urinary dysfunction may be attenuated by β-adrenergic and dopaminergic agonists and α-adrenergic antagonists, as reported in recent animal studies.[94] Validation in human subjects awaits further research.

Activation of Latent Herpes Simplex Labialis

Herpes labialis infection (the cold sore) has occasionally been reported to recur with the use of epidural morphine analgesia after cesarean delivery.[95,96] A recent study in parturients has removed confounding variables and more definitively implicated spinal morphine use as the cause.[97] Reactivation of the virus has not been reported in nonobstetric populations receiving spinal morphine. Reactivation of genital herpes infection has not been documented.

The incidence of reactivation in the study of Crone et al[97] was approximately 15 percent. Approximately 65 percent of the patients receiving spinal morphine had positive herpes serology (i.e., the potential for reactivation). Despite a similar incidence of positive serology in the control group (analgesia with parenteral opioids), none of these patients had reactivation of herpes labialis. Further work is needed to determine if risk of recurrence is indeed as high as 15 percent. More importantly, no neonates born to mothers receiving spinal morphine have been reported to develop herpes infection. Further study is required, since viral screening for this phenomenon has not been heretofore performed in such infants.

Inhibition of Gastrointestinal Function

Thorén et al[98] reported delayed gastric emptying and delayed orocecal and small intestinal transit times in volunteers receiving lumbar epidural morphine. However, after abdominal surgery, systemic opioid use in patients resulted in a greater decrease in gastric emptying than did spinal opioid use, despite provision of equivalent analgesia.[99] It has been hypothesized that spinal cord mechanisms are involved in impaired gastrointestinal function after spinal opioid therapy.[100,101]

Spinal opioids may thus delay postoperative recovery of bowel function.[99–101] It should be emphasized, however, that equivalent analgesia with parenteral opioids may result in even greater delay. Epidural local anesthetics, however, improve bowel motility and cause earlier return of intestinal function than both parenteral and spinal opioids.[102] Local anesthetics selectively block sympathetic innervation to the bowel, while leaving parasympathetic function intact. (A more extensive discussion of the effects of epidural anesthesia/analgesia upon gastrointestinal function may be found in Chapter 26.)

Neurologic Effects

Neurologic side effects generally take the form of somnolence and dysphoria.[103] Hyperesthesia has been reported after high doses of spinal morphine.[104] Two cases of vertical nystagmus have been reported during epidural morphine administration.[105,106]

MONITORING

Patients receiving spinal opioids must be monitored in order to detect potentially life-threatening respiratory depression. Controversy exists as to how best to accomplish this goal.

As discussed before, respiratory rate is the most common method for determining respiratory depression. However, respiratory rate alone may be an unreliable marker for the presence of respiratory depression. Changes in tidal volume, arterial PCO_2, and response to hypercarbia may be present despite normal respiratory rates.[15,24] For this reason, some authors favor a more global assessment of respiratory alteration. Ready et al[35,84] persuasively argued for frequent evaluation of ventilation and sedation in patients receiving spinal opioids. The presence of significant amounts of opioid in the CSF around the brain stem is usually heralded by changes in wakefulness as well as respiration. Therefore, frequent nursing assessment of the level of sedation and respiratory rate should be all that is needed for monitoring most healthy patients receiving spinal opioids.

Without requiring respiratory rate (apnea) monitors or admission to intensive care units, the experience of Ready and colleagues[35,84] speaks strongly for the simple vigilance of caretakers in detecting ventilatory compromise. Furthermore, a recent Swedish study documented an extremely low incidence of respiratory depression during spinal opioid therapy (0.09% after epidural morphine, and 0.36% after subarachnoid morphine).[76] Moreover, when respiratory depression did occur, it was nearly always in patients with concomitant risk factors (e.g., advanced age, concomitant opioid and sedative premedication, or ASA class III-IV).

Based on these findings, intensive monitoring (i.e., apnea monitors, intensive care unit admission) for spinal opioid-induced respiratory depression does not seem cost-effective. Moreover, intensive monitoring does not detect the occurrence of respiratory depression any better than simple nursing assessment. Apnea monitors often alarm unnecessarily and may provide a false sense of security. Intensive care unit admission would limit the widespread applicability of spinal opioids due to both cost and space concerns.

Reasonable guidelines for monitoring patients receiving spinal opioids are as follows:

1. Healthy (ASA class I-II) patients do not require anything more than frequent assessment of ventilation and sedation on medical or surgical wards
2. Vigilance should be *increased* (e.g., step-down or intensive care unit, respiratory rate monitor, etc.) whenever the following factors are present:
   a. advanced patient age
   b. sick patient (ASA class III-IV)
   c. extensive surgery (especially of the thorax or upper abdomen)
   d. concomitant use of other opioids or sedatives

These are only suggestions, and must, of course, be placed in the context of specific institutional policies and logistic limitations.

CONCLUSION

At present, spinal opioid therapy is widely used for postoperative analgesia. Much has been learned since the first reports of profound analgesia with subarachnoid morphine. Many questions still remain, however, and form the basis for further exciting clinical research.

References
1. Behar M, Magora F, Olshwang D, Davison JT: Epidural morphine in the treatment of pain. Lancet i:527, 1979
2. Wang, JK, Nauss LA, Thomas JE: Pain relief by intrathecally applied morphine in man. Anesthesiology 50:149, 1979
3. Cousins MJ, Mather LE, Glynn CJ et al: Selective spinal analgesia. Lancet i:1141, 1979
4. Cousins MJ, Cherry DA, Gourlay GK: Acute and chronic pain: use of spinal opioids. p. 955. In Cousins MJ, Bridenbaugh PO (eds): Neural Blockade in Clinical Anesthesia and Management of Pain. 2nd Ed. JB Lippincott, Philadelphia, 1988
5. Yaksh TL, Noveihed R: The physiology and pharmacology of spinal opiates. Annu Rev Pharmacol Toxicol 25:443, 1975
6. Moore RA, Bullingham RES, McQuay HJ et al: Dural permeability to narcotics: in vitro determination and application to extradural administration. Br J Anaesth 54:1117, 1982
7. Mather LE: Clinical pharmacokinetics of fentanyl and its newer derivatives. Clin Pharmcokinet 8:422, 1983
8. Freye E: The mode of action of opioids. p. 15. In: Opioid Agonists Antagonists and Mixed Narcotic Analgesics. Theoretical Background and Considerations for Practical Use. Springer-Verlag, Berlin, 1987

9. Sjöström S, Hartvig P, Persson MP, Tamsen A: Pharmacokinetics of epidural morphine and meperidine in humans. Anesthesiology 67:877, 1987
10. Sjöström S, Tamsen A, Persson MP, Hartvig P: Pharmacokinetics of intrathecal morphine and meperidine in humans. Anesthesiology 67:889, 1987
11. Gourlay GK, Wilson PR, Glynn CJ: Pharmacodynamics and pharmacokinetics of methadone during the perioperative period. Anesthesiology 57:458, 1982
12. Gourlay GK, Willis RJ, Wilson PR: Postoperative pain control with methadone: influence of supplementary methadone doses and blood concentration-response relationships. Anesthesiology 61:19, 1984
13. Cohen SE, Tan S, White PF: Sufentanil analgesia following cesarean section: epidural versus intravenous administration. Anesthesiology 68:129, 1988
14. Andersen HB, Christensen CB, Findlay JW, Jansen JA: Pharmacokinetics of epidural morphine and fentanyl in the goat, abstracted. Pain 19:A564, 1984
15. Gourlay GK, Cherry DA, Cousins MJ: Cephalad migration of morphine in CSF following lumbar epidural administration in patients with cancer pain. Pain 23:317, 1985
16. Glynn CJ, Mather LE, Cousins MJ et al: Peridural meperidine in humans: analgetic response, pharmacokinetics and transmission into CSF. Anesthesiology 55:520, 1981
17. Dickenson AH, Sullivan AF, McQuay HJ: Intrathecal etorphine, fentanyl, and buprenorphine on spinal nociceptive neurones in the rat. Pain 42:227, 1990
18. Nordberg G: Pharmacokinetic aspects of spinal morphine analgesia. Acta Anaesthesiol Scand 79:1, 1984
19. Tamsen A, Sjöström S, Hartvig P et al: CSF and plasma kinetics of morphine and meperidine after epidural administration, abstracted. Anesthesiology 59:A196, 1983
20. Nordberg G, Hedner T, Mellstrand T, Dahlström B: Pharmacokinetic aspects of epidural morphine analgesia. Anesthesiology 58:545, 1983
21. Larsen VH, Iversen AP, Christensen P et al: Postoperative pain treatment after upper abdominal surgery with epidural morphine at thoracic or lumbar level. Acta Anaesthesiol Scand 29:566, 1985
22. Niv D, Rudick V, Golan A, Cháyen MS: Augmentation of bupivacaine analgesia in labor by epidural morphine. Obstet Gynecol 67:206, 1986
23. Jensen PJ, Siem-Jorgensen P, Nielsen TB et al: Epidural morphine by the caudal route for postoperative pain relief. Acta Anaesthesiol Scand 26:511, 1982
24. Fromme GA, Steidl LJ, Danielson DR: Comparison of lumbar and thoracic epidural morphine for relief of postthoracotomy pain. Anesth Analg 64:454, 1985
25. Sullivan SP, Cherry DA: Pain from an invasive facial tumor relieved by lumbar epidural morphine. Anesth Analg 66:777, 1987
26. Sjöström S, Hartvig D, Tamsen A: Patient-controlled analgesia with extradural morphine or pethidine. Br J Anaesth 60:358, 1988
27. Bodily MN, Chamberlain DP, Ramsey DH, Olsson GL: Lumbar versus thoracic epidural catheter for post-thoracotomy analgesia, abstracted. Anesthesiology 7: A1146, 1989
28. Badner NH, Sandler AN, Colmenares ME: Lumbar epidural fentanyl infusions for post-thoracotomy patients, abstracted. Anesthesiology 71:A667, 1989
29. Melendez JA, Cirella VN, Delphin ES: Lumbar epidural fentanyl analgesia after thoracic surgery. Cardiothor Anesth 3:150, 1989
30. Glass PSA, Estok P, Ginsberg B et al: Use of patient-controlled analgesia to compare the efficacy of epidural to intravenous fentanyl administration. Anesth Analg 74:345, 1992

31. Ellis DJ, Millar WL, Reisner LS: A randomized double-blind comparison of epidural versus intravenous fentanyl infusion for analgesia after cesarean section. Anesthesiology 72:981, 1990

32. Loper KA, Ready LB, Downey M et al: Epidural and intravenous fentanyl infusions are clinically equivalent after knee surgery. Anesth Analg 70:72, 1990

33. Modig J, Paalzow L: A comparison of epidural morphine and epidural bupivacaine for postoperative pain relief. Acta Anaesthesiol Scand 25:437, 1981

34. Rawal N, Sjöstrand UH, Dahlström B et al: Epidural morphine for postoperative pain relief: a comparative study with intramuscular narcotic and intercostal nerve block. Anesth Analg 61:93, 1982

35. Ready LB, Oden R, Chadwick HS et al: Development of an anesthesiology-based postoperative pain management service. Anesthesiology 68:100, 1988

36. Welchew EA, Thornton JA: Continuous thoracic epidural fentanyl. Anaesthesia 37:309, 1982

37. Bailey PW, Smith BE: Continuous epidural infusion of fentanyl for post-operative analgesia. Anaesthesia 35:1002, 1980

38. Boudrenult D, Brasseur L, Samii K, Lemoing JP: Comparison of continuous epidural bupivacaine infusion plus either continuous epidural infusion or patient-controlled epidural injection of fentanyl for postoperative analgesia. Anesth Analg 73:132, 1991

39. Chien BB, Burke RG, Hunter DJ: An extensive experience with postoperative pain relief using postoperative fentanyl infusion. Arch Surg 126:692, 1991

40. Hershey LA: Meperidine and central neurotoxicity. Ann Intern Med 98:548, 1983

41. Armstrong PJ, Bersten A: Normeperidine toxicity. Anesth Analg 65:536, 1986

42. El-Baz NM, Faber LP, Jensik RJ: Continuous epidural infusion of morphine for treatment of pain after thoracic surgery. Anesth Analg 63:757, 1984

43. El-Baz NM, Goldin M: Continuous epidural infusion of morphine for pain relief after cardiac operations. J Thorac Cardiovasc Surg 93:878, 1987

44. Allen PD, Walman T, Concepcion M et al: Epidural morphine provides postoperative pain relief in peripheral vascular and orthopedic surgical patients: a dose-response study. Anesth Analg 65:165, 1986

45. Gustafsson LL, Schildt B, Jacobsen KJ: Adverse effects of extradural and intrathecal opiates: report of a nationwide survey in Sweden. Br J Anaesth 54:479, 1982

46. Rawal N, Sjöstrand UH, Dahlström B et al: Postoperative pain relief by epidural morphine. Anesth Analg 60:726, 1981

47. Shulman MS, Sandler AN, Bradley JW et al: Post-thoracotomy pain and pulmonary function following epidural and systemic morphine. Anesthesiology 61:569, 1984

48. Welch DB: Epidural narcotics and dural puncture. Lancet i:55, 1981

49. Brownridge P, Wrobel J, Watt-Smith J: Respiratory depression following accidental subarachnoid pethidine. Anaesth Intensive Care 11:237, 1983

50. Pellecchia DJ, Bretz KA, Barnette RE: Postoperative pain control by means of epidural narcotics in a patient with obstructive sleep apnea. Anesth Analg 66:280, 1987

51. Lamarche Y, Martin R, Reiher J, Blaise G: The sleep apnea syndrome and epidural morphine. Can Anaesth Soc J 33:231, 1986

52. Chauvin M, Samii K, Schermann JM et al: Plasma morphine concentration after intrathecal administration of low doses of morphine. Br J Anaesth 53:1065, 1981

53. Bengtsson M, Löfström JB, Merits H: Postoperative pain relief with intrathecal morphine after major hip surgery. Reg Anesth 8:138, 1983

54. Katz J, Nelson W: Intrathecal morphine for postoperative pain relief. Reg Anesth 6:1, 1981

55. Chauvin M, Samii K, Schermann JM et al: Plasma pharmacokinetics of morphine after IM extradural and intrathecal administration. Br J Anaesth 54:843, 1981
56. Lazorthes Y, Gouarderes GH, Verdie JC et al: Analgesie par injection intrathecale de morphine. Etude pharmacocinetique et application aux douleurs irreductibles. Neurochirurgie 26:159, 1980
57. Nordberg G, Hedner T, Mellstrand T, Dahlström B: Pharmacokinetic aspects of intrathecal morphine analgesia. Anesthesiology 60:448, 1984
58. Abboud TK, Dror A, Mosaad P et al: Mini-dose intrathecal morphine for the relief of post-cesarean section pain: safety, efficacy, and ventilatory responses to carbon dioxide. Anesth Analg 67:137, 1988
59. McQuay HJ, Sullivan AF, Smallman K, Dickenson AH: Intrathecal opioids, potency and lipophilicity. Pain 36:111, 1989
60. Hunt CO, Naulty JS, Bader AM et al: Perioperative analgesia with subarachnoid fentanyl-bupivacaine for cesarean delivery. Anesthesiology 71:535, 1989
61. Hurley RJ, Lambert DH: Continuous spinal anesthesia with a microcatheter technique: preliminary experience. Anesth Analg 70:97, 1990
62. Davies GK, Tolhurst-Cleaver CL, James TL: Respiratory depression after intrathecal narcotics. Anaesthesia 35:1080, 1980
63. Gjessing J, Tomlin PJ: Postoperative pain control with intrathecal morphine. Anaesthesia 36:268, 1981
64. Jacobson L, Chabal C, Brody M: A dose-response study of intrathecal morphine: efficacy, duration, optimal dose and side effects. Anesth Analg 67:1082, 1988
65. Johnson MD, Hurley RJ, Gilbertson LI, Datta S: Continuous microcatheter spinal anesthesia with subarachnoid meperidine for labor and delivery. Anesth Analg 70:658, 1990
66. Chadwick HS, Ready LB: Intrathecal and epidural morphine sulfate for post-cesarean analgesia—a clinical comparison. Anesthesiology 68:925, 1988
67. Bromage PK, Camporesi EM, Durant PA, Nielsen CH: Rostral spread of morphine. Anesthesiology 56:431, 1982
68. Bromage PR, Camporesi E, Leslie J: Epidural narcotics in volunteers. Sensitivity to pain and to carbon dioxide. Pain 9:145, 1980
69. Bromage PR, Joyal AC, Brinney JC: Local anesthetic drugs. Penetration from the spinal extradural space into the neuraxis. Science 140:392, 1963
70. DiChiro G: Movement of cerebrospinal fluid in human beings. Nature 204:290, 1964
71. DiChiro G: Observations on the circulation of the cerebrospinal fluid. Acta Radiol [Diagn] (Stockh) 5:988, 1966
72. Glynn CJ, Mather LE, Cousins MJ et al: Spinal narcotics and respiratory depression. Lancet ii:356, 1979
73. Camporesi EM, Nielsen CH, Bromage PR et al: Ventilatory CO_2 sensitivity after intravenous and epidural morphine in volunteers. Anesth Analg 62:633, 1983
74. Scott DB, McClure J: Selective epidural analgesia. Lancet i:1410, 1979
75. Boas RA: Hazards of epidural morphine. Anaesth Intensive Care 8:377, 1980
76. Rawal N, Arner S, Gustafsson LL, Allvin R: Present state of extradural and intrathecal opioid analgesia in Sweden. A nationwide follow-up survey. Br J Anaesth 59:791, 1987
77. Ngai SH, Berkowitz BA, Yang JC et al: Pharmacokinetics of naloxone in rats and man: basis for its potency and short duration of action. Anesthesiology 44:398, 1976
78. Rawal N, Schött U, Dahlström B et al: Influence of naloxone infusion on analgesia

and respiratory depression following epidural morphine. Anesthesiology 64:194, 1986

79. Gueneron JP, Ecoffey CI, Carli P et al: Effects of naloxone infusion on analgesia and respiratory depression after epidural fentanyl. Anesth Analg 67:35, 1988

80. Bromage PR, Camporesi EM, Durant PA, Nielsen CH: Nonrespiratory side effects of epidural morphine. Anesth Analg 61:490, 1982

81. Brownridge P: Epidural and intrathecal opiates for postoperative pain relief. Anaesthesia 38:74, 1983

82. Donadoni R, Rolly G, Noorduin H, Vanden Bussche G: Epidural sufentanil for postoperative pain relief. Anaesthesia 40:634, 1985

83. Welchew EA: The optimum concentration for epidural fentanyl. Anaesthesia 38:1037, 1983

84. Ready LB, Loper KA, Nessly M, Wild L: Postoperative epidural morphine is safe on surgical wards. Anesthesiology 75:452, 1991

85. Kotelko DM, Rottman RL, Wright WC et al: Transdermal scopalamine decreases nausea and vomiting following cesarean section in patients receiving epidural morphine. Anesthesiology 71:675, 1989

86. Loper KA, Ready LB, Dorman BH: Prophylactic transdermal scopalamine patches reduce nausea in postoperative patients receiving epidural morphine. Anesth Analg 68:144, 1989

87. Abboud TK, Afrasiabi A, Davidson J et al: Prophylactic oral naltrexone with epidural morphine: effect on adverse reactions and ventilatory responses to carbon dioxide. Anesthesiology 72:233, 1990

88. Lawhorn CD, McNitt JD, Fibuch EE et al: Epidural morphine with butorphanol for postoperative analgesia after cesarean delivery. Anesth Analg 72:53, 1991

89. Bowdle TA, Greichen SL, Bjurstrom RL, Schoene RB: Butorphanol improves CO_2 response and ventilation after fentanyl analgesia. Anesth Analg 66:517, 1987

90. Davies GG, From R: A blinded study using nalbuphine for prevention of pruritis induced by epidural fentanyl. Anesthesiology 69:763, 1988

91. Baxter AD, Samson B, Penning J et al: Prevention of epidural morphine-induced respiratory depression with intravenous nalbupine infusion in post-thoracotomy patients. Can J Anaesth 36:503, 1989

92. Bromage PR, Camporesi E, Chestnut D: Epidural narcotics for postoperative analgesia. Anesth Analg 59:473, 1980

93. Ballantyne JC, Loach AB, Carr DB: Itching after epidural and spinal opiates. Pain 33:149, 1988

94. Durant PA, Yaksh TL: Drug effects on urinary bladder tone during spinal morphine-induced inhibition of the micturition reflex in unanesthetized rats. Anesthesiology 68:325, 1988

95. Crone LA, Conly J, Clark K et al: Recurrent herpes simplex virus labialis and the use of epidural morphine in obstetric patients. Anesth Analg 67:318, 1988

96. Gieraerts R, Navalgund A, Vaes L et al: Increased incidence of itching and herpes simplex in patients given epidural morphine after cesarean section. Anesth Analg 66:1321, 1987

97. Crone LA, Conly JM, Storgard C et al: Herpes labialis in parturients receiving epidural morphine following cesarean section. Anesthesiology 73:208, 1990

98. Thorén T, Tanghöj H, Wattwil M, Järnerot G: Epidural morphine delays gastric emptying and small intestinal transit in volunteers. Acta Anaesthesiol Scand 33:174, 1989

99. England DW, Davis IJ, Timmins AE et al: Gastric emptying: a study to compare

the effects of intrathecal morphine and i.m. papaveretum analgesia. Br J Anaesth 59:1403, 1987

100. Bardon T, Ruckebusch Y: Comparative effects of opiate agonists on proximal and distal colonic motility in dogs. Eur J Pharmacol 110:329, 1985

101. Porreca F, Mosberg HI, Hurst R et al: Roles of mu, delta and kappa opioid receptors in spinal and supraspinal mediation of gastrointestinal transit effects and hotplate analgesia in the mouse. J Pharmacol Exp Ther 230:341, 1984

102. Scheinin B, Asantila R, Orko R: The effect of bupivacaine and morphine on pain and bowel function after colonic surgery. Acta Anaesthesiol Scand 31:161, 1987

103. Knill RL, Clement JL, Thompson WR: Epidural morphine causes delayed and prolonged ventilatory depression. Can Anaesth Soc J 28:537, 1981

104. Yaksh TL, Harty GJ, Onotrio BM: High doses of spinal morphine produce a nonopiate receptor-mediated hyperesthesia: clinical and theoretical implications. Anesthesiology 64:590, 1986

105. Fish DJ, Rosen M: Epidural opioids as a cause of vertical nystagmus. Anesthesiology 73:785, 1990

106. Stevens RA, Sharrock NE: Nystagmus following epidural morphine (letter). Anesthesiology 74:390, 1991

12

Epidural Analgesia with Combinations of Local Anesthetics and Opioids

F. Michael Ferrante
Timothy R. VadeBoncouer

BALANCED ANALGESIA

The concept of *balanced analgesia*[1] signifies the administration of agents that selectively affect the physiologic processes involved in nociception: transduction (nonsteroidal anti-inflammatory drugs [NSAIDs],[1-4]) transmission (local anesthetics, peripheral,[5,6] and/or neuraxial[5,7-10]), and modulation (systemic[11] or epidural[7-10] opioids). Such combined or "balanced" analgesic regimens have been shown to almost completely eliminate postoperative pain, not only at "rest" but also during mobilization.[1-3] Furthermore, balanced analgesic techniques offer the tantalizing possibility of shortened convalescence, although the location of surgery and suppression of the neuroendocrine response to pain do impact on time of recovery (see Ch. 4).[6,12] Thus, much is to be gained by the combinational use of analgesics. Because of the tangible and potential benefits of the coadministration of epidural local anesthetics and opioids, combinations of such drugs as part of a balanced analgesic regimen are rapidly becoming the *sine qua non* of effective postoperative analgesic care.

This chapter examines both the laboratory and clinical data supporting this assertion and the clinical characteristics and management of the coadministration of local anesthetics and opioids by epidural infusion. First, however, we begin by discussing the clinical use of epidural local anesthetics alone.

EPIDURAL LOCAL ANESTHETICS

Epidural local anesthetics are capable of maintaining prolonged analgesia in the postoperative period when administered by intermittent injection or continuous infusion. Surgical pain from a variety of sources (the thorax,[13-17] the abdomen,[18-20] the lower extremities[21-23]) is amenable to this analgesic approach.

Bupivacaine is the local anesthetic most often used for postoperative epidural analgesia. Epidural bupivacaine produces neural blockade of long duration,[24] differential blockade of sensory rather than motor fibers,[25] and it possesses relative resistance to tachyphylaxis (in contradistinction to the short-acting amides, lidocaine, prilocaine, and mepivacaine).[26] These properties make bupivacaine the ideal local anesthetic for postoperative epidural analgesia. (This may not be true in the future with the release of the new amide local anesthetic ropivacaine. Ropivacaine has a pharmacologic profile similar to bupivacaine but produces less motor blockade at comparable concentrations.[27,28])

Cardiovascular Effects of Epidural Blockade

At the present level of pharmacologic sophistication, it is impossible to obtain somatic blockade without some degree of sympathetic blockade with epidural anesthesia/analgesia. Most of the important cardiovascular effects of epidural blockade can be discussed in relation to blockade of sympathetic vasoconstrictor fibers (below T4) or blockade of cardiac (cardioaccelerator) sympathetic fibers (T1–T4) (Fig. 12-1). Blockade of cardioaccelerator fibers is more often achieved with thoracic epidural administration of local anesthetics and will be discussed extensively in Chapter 18. The present discussion confines itself to the cardiovascular effects of epidural blockade below T4.

Epidural blockade that is restricted to the low thoracic and lumbar regions (T5–L4) results in "peripheral" vasodilation within the lower limb and pelvis and decreased mean arterial pressure. Pooling of blood in the gut and abdominal viscera will occur if all splanchnic fibers are blocked (T6–L1). Arteriolar vasodilation and pooling of blood in venous capacitance vessels results in increased lower limb blood flow.[29,30] Excessive venodilation can result in decreased venous return, reduced right atrial pressure, and reduced cardiac output.[26]

Compensatory mechanisms set into motion by the decrease in mean arterial pressure are of two types: (1) an increase in efferent sympathetic vasoconstriction above the level of the block, and (2) increased cardioaccelerator fiber activity (T1–T4), resulting in increased heart rate and contractility. Increased efferent sympathetic activity above the level of the block is mediated through the baroreceptor reflex and circulating catecholamines released from the adrenal medulla. Circulating catecholamines may also contribute to the increased inotropy and chronotropy induced by activation of the cardioaccelerator

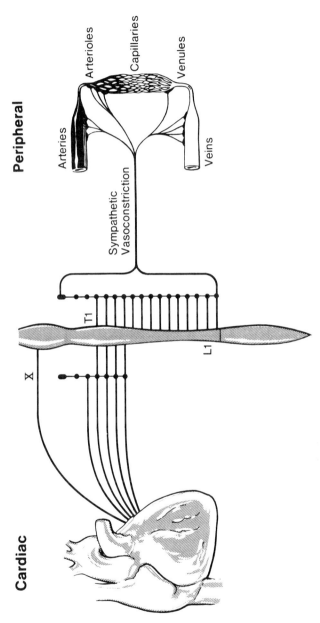

Fig. 12-1. Sympathetic blockade associated with epidural anesthesia/analgesia. Most of the important cardiovascular effects can be related to (1) central blockade of cardiac sympathetic (cardioaccelerator) fibers (T1–T4), or (2) peripheral blockade of sympathetic vasoconstrictor fibers (T1–L2). (From Cousins and Bromage,[26] with permission.)

nerves. If the splanchnic nerves (T6–L1) are completely blocked, no catechols will be released from the adrenal gland.[26]

Thus, the severity of the decline in mean arterial pressure after epidural anesthesia/analgesia results from the interplay of three factors: (1) the relative degree of blockade of peripheral vasoconstrictor fibers, (2) the possible blockade of cardiac sympathetic fibers, and (3) the completeness of blockade of the splanchnic nerves with its attendant effects on adrenal medullary activity and splanchnic vasoconstrictor activity. Certainly hypovolemia, excessive blood loss, loss of cardiovascular compensatory mechanisms for any reason, and the additive cardiovascular effects of sedatives and other analgesics will also be important factors in the potential for production of hypotension.[26]

Intermittent Injections

Intermittent injections of local anesthetic have been used to provide analgesia after a wide variety of surgical procedures. By repeating the injection of local anesthetic through an indwelling catheter, the segmental level of analgesia may be held constant. Bromage[31] calculated segment-time regression curves (Fig. 12-2) for all the commonly used local anesthetics. For the postoperative patient, he advocates timing repeat injection when the sensory level regresses two dermatomal segments. The repeat dose required to maintain segmental analgesia is one-half of the initial dose or less.

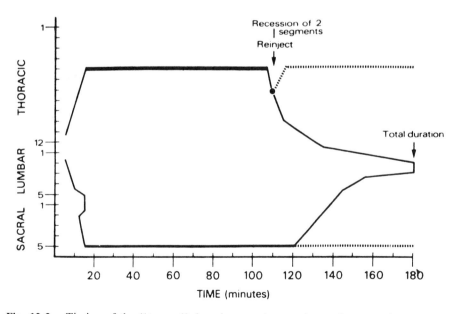

Fig. 12-2. Timing of the "top-up" dose in conscious patients. Segment-time diagram showing spread and regression of analgesia. A stable upper level of analgesia is maintained by injecting one-half of initial dose when upper level of analgesia has regressed two dermatomal segments. (From Bromage,[31] with permission.)

TABLE 12-1. Average Time to Two-Segment Regression for Commonly Used Local Anesthetics and Calculation of the Dosing Interval Between Injections to Maintain Segmental Analgesia in the Patient Under Light General Anesthesia

Local Anesthetic[a]	Average Time to Two-Segment Regression[b] (min)	Standard Deviation	Dosing Interval (min) ($t_{avg} - 1.5_{SD}$)
3% Chloroprocaine	57	7	47
2% Lidocaine	97.5	19	70
2% Prilocaine	97	10	82
3% Prilocaine	99	17	74
0.5% Bupivacaine	196	31	150
0.75% Bupivacaine	201	40	141
1% Etidocaine	170	57	85

[a] All calculations are for local anesthetics administered with 1:200,000 epinephrine.
[b] Time to two-segment regression is defined as the interval of time between complete spread and the regression of analgesia by two dermatomal segments.
(Modified from Bromage,[31] with permission.)

For the unconscious patient under light general anesthesia (when two-segment regression cannot be determined in the individual patient), Bromage advocates timing reinjections by the formula:

$$t_{\text{dosing interval (min)}} = t_{\text{two segment regression (min)}} - 1.5 \text{ (standard deviation)}$$

(see Table 12-1).[31] Such dosing intervals were determined by construction of distribution curves through generation of a large number of segment-time diagrams for individual local anesthetics under standardized conditions. From the distribution curves, the mean duration of time to two-segment regression and the standard deviation of the mean were calculated for predictive purposes (Table 12-1).

The duration of effect of a single injection administered for postoperative analgesia is shorter than that achieved by administration of a similar dose for surgical anesthesia. Moreover, the addition of epinephrine does not produce prolongation of analgesia as during surgery. Adequate analgesia can usually be achieved with 0.25 percent bupivacaine. If the duration of analgesia is too short, however, the concentration of bupivacaine can be increased to 0.375 percent or 0.5 percent.[32]

With repetitive injections, plasma concentrations of local anesthetic will peak 15–20 minutes after each injection. Multiple injections may produce a "sawtooth" plasma concentration curve (Fig. 12-3). If the dosing interval is too short, toxic systemic concentrations of local anesthetics can result (Fig. 12-3).[33]

The drawbacks to use of intermittent injection techniques relate to the attendant side effects, the logistic complexities of frequent administration, and the monitoring requirements necessitated by use of concentrated solutions of local anesthetic. Side effects include the potential for drug accumulation (see above), the enhanced development of tachyphylaxis (in relation to continuous infusions), and hypotension. Hypotension is seen anywhere between 6 percent to 34 percent of the time with intermittent administration.[32] Although compensatory

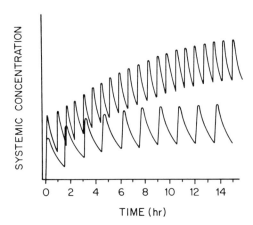

Fig. 12-3. Intermittent epidural injections of local anesthetic will produce a "saw-tooth" plasma concentration curve. If the dosing interval is too short, systemic accumulation of drug and toxicity may occur.

mechanisms attempt to restore mean arterial pressure to preinjection values after each injection, such "roller coaster" cardiovascular effects may make this technique unsuitable for most patients, even in the absence of frank hypotension. Furthermore, each injection has the potential risk of extension of the sympathetic block above T4, with attendant blockade of the cardioaccelerator nerves and its sequelae.

Continuous Infusions

In order to maintain a constant segmental level of analgesia, a continuous epidural infusion must administer local anesthetic to the epidural space at a rate that equals the removal of local anesthetic.[34] The simplicity of this statement does not adequately relate the inherent difficulties in development of pharmacokinetic models for continuous epidural infusions of local anesthetic.[35–37] Similarly, such a simplistic statement does not adequately denote the influence of the phenomenon of tachyphylaxis (see below). A full description of bupivacaine kinetics in the epidural space requires a multiexponential function.[37] However, Denson et al[35,36] demonstrated that safe infusion rates could be predicted by estimation of the total plasma clearance, volume of distribution, and elimination rate of bupivacaine derived from two blood samples.

Early clinical reports suggested that systemic accumulation of bupivacaine was possible if the duration of the epidural infusion was greater than 48 hours.[38,39] However, the pharmacokinetic analyses of Denson et al[35,36] demonstrated that epidural infusions of bupivacaine possess a wide margin of safety. Infusions can be continued for 5 or more days at rates less than 30 mg/h without evidence of systemic accumulation in patients with normal clearances.[35] Infusion rates of up to 30 mg/h did not produce systemic toxicity even when the clearance was reduced by 60 percent. Minor toxicity was observed in patients with renal and hepatic disease at such high infusion rates.[35] Thus, as would be predicted from clinical experience, most patients do not require monitoring of serum bupivacaine concentrations during management of continuous epidural infusions.

The pharmacokinetics of other local anesthetics administered by continuous epidural infusion have not been as rigorously studied. Plasma levels of lidocaine resulting from continuous lumbar epidural infusions were measured by Holmdahl et al[40] and Sjögren and Wright.[41] The incidence of tachyphylaxis and systemic toxicity were significant.[40,41] Most of the other local anesthetics have been inadequately studied or not studied at all. Thus, because of its pharmacokinetically defined safety,[35,36] differential blockade of sensory fibers,[25] and the development of tachyphylaxis[26,40,41] and/or systemic accumulation[40,41] associated with the shorter-acting amides, bupivacaine is the local anesthetic of choice for continuous epidural infusion.[39,42]

Tachyphylaxis

The phenomenon of tachyphylaxis had been mentioned several times in our discussion of epidural local anesthetics. This poorly understood property of prolonged administration of local anesthetics represents the major obstacle to maintenance of continuous analgesia with epidural local anesthetics alone.

Simply stated, tachyphylaxis signifies the development of acute tolerance. A given dose of local anesthetic (whether administered by a single injection or an infusion) becomes less and less effective with repeated use. In clinical practice, this is observed as (1) fewer dermatomes blocked with repeat injections despite administration of identical volumes and identical concentrations of local anesthetic,[43,44] or (2) the regression of a previously stable anesthetic/analgesic dermatomal level during continuous epidural infusion.[45,46]

Natural History

Tachyphylaxis is an irregular phenomenon with respect to the interindividual time of onset after initiation of therapy and the interindividual rate of regression of sensory anesthesia/analgesia.[43] Its development or speed of progression cannot be correlated with gender, weight, height, body surface area, serum albumin concentration, or the duration or site of surgery.[47] However, the duration of sensory anesthesia/analgesia with either intermittent epidural injections[43] or continuous epidural infusions[47] has been shown to be positively correlated with increasing age. Thus, the elderly should be somewhat refractory to the occurrence of tachyphylaxis or somewhat refractory to its speed of development, although this has not been studied outright.

As previously stated, tachyphylaxis has been described after intermittent epidural injections[43,44] and continuous epidural infusions.[45,46] Although the evidence is somewhat obscure, intermittent injections are believed to be associated with a higher incidence of tachyphylaxis than continuous epidural infusions.[32] The volume (i.e., rate) of administration of local anesthetic has been shown to have no effect on the rapidity of regression of sensory anesthesia/analgesia for continuous infusions.[48] The concentration of local anesthetic does appear to be important in the development of tachyphylaxis. Administration of 0.125 percent bupivacaine has been shown to be associated with a lower incidence of tachyphylaxis than higher concentrations.[46,49] This has been demonstrated for both intermittent injections[46] and continuous infusions.[49] In a study by Mogensen et al[49] using continuous epidural infusions of 0.125 percent bupivacaine, the incidence of tachyphylaxis was nil. However, a large proportion of patients developed a unilateral sensory block, which the authors attributed to the total dose of local anesthetic rather than tachyphylaxis per se.

Bupivacaine[44–49] and lidocaine[43,50] are the two local anesthetics that have received the greatest attention in investigations of tachyphylaxis. The use of epidural lidocaine and other short-acting amide local anesthetics is generally believed to be associated with a greater incidence of tachyphylaxis.[26,50] The addition of epinephrine to solutions of short-acting amides prolongs their effect, thereby reducing the incidence of tachyphylaxis.[43]

Mechanism of Tachyphylaxis

The mechanism underlying the phenomenon of tachyphylaxis remains obscure, although various theories have been proposed to explain its occurrence (Table 12-2). Hypotheses as to the mechanism of tachyphylaxis fall into three general categories: (1) *pharmacokinetic*[51] (a reduced concentration of local anesthetic reaches the sodium channel), (2) *pharmacodynamic*[51] (the sodium channel becomes resistant to the same concentration of local anesthetic), and (3) *neuroplastic* (increased nociceptive transmission with enhanced excitability of peripheral nociceptors and dorsal horn neurons overrides neural blockade).[52]

TABLE 12-2. Hypothetical Mechanisms of Tachyphylaxis with Epidural Administration of Local Anesthetic

Hypothesis	Reference
Pharmacokinetic	
Limitation of diffusion by perineural edema	61
Acidification of CSF, epidural space, and neural tissue reduces quantity of lipid-soluble forms	57,59
Enhanced elimination or altered distribution of local anesthetic	60,61
Increased sodium concentration in the epidural space reduces quantity of diffusable anesthetic	54
Pharmacodynamic	
Increased cAMP	62
Neuroplastic	
Increased nociceptive transmission and peripheral and central sensitization of nociceptors	47,52,68

Pharmacokinetic hypotheses imply that tachyphylaxis should only be demonstrable in intact organisms and not in isolated nerve preparations.[53–55]

PHARMACOKINETIC HYPOTHESES

A number of factors have been potentially implicated in reducing the concentration of local anesthetic reaching the axonal membrane.

Perineural Edema. Clinically used concentrations of local anesthetics may cause localized perineural edema in nerves.[56] Such edema would limit intraneuronal diffusion of local anesthetics, thereby promoting tachyphylaxis.[51]

pH. Progressive acidification of cerebrospinal fluid (CSF) and neural tissue may result from repeated injections of commercial (acidic) solutions of local anesthetic.[57] An increase in the hydrogen ion concentration of the epidural space and CSF (i.e., lower pH) would increase the proportion of the charged anionic form of a local anesthetic as compared with the basic nonionized form. As the nonionized form of local anesthetics is the lipid-soluble moiety, less drug would be available for diffusion across nerve membranes at lower pH. The limited buffering capacity of the CSF (and presumably, the epidural space) would make these areas especially vulnerable to progressive acidification.[58]

A more recent study fails to support the acidification hypothesis.[59] Bupivacaine solutions adjusted to pH 4.2 or 6.8 were repetitively injected into a surgically implanted system created to allow in vivo irrigation of rat sciatic nerve. Tachyphylaxis developed at both pH values. Despite a 400-fold difference in hydrogen ion concentration, there was no effect on the development of tachyphylaxis.[59]

Enhanced Elimination or Altered Distribution of Local Anesthetics. Recently, enhanced elimination of bupivacaine from the epidural space has been implicated as an important factor leading to the development of tachyphylaxis.[60] Using a ^{133}Xe clearance technique, Mogensen et al[60] demonstrated that establishment of epidural blockade with 0.5 percent bupivacaine increased epidural blood flow. Epidural blood flow increased further in patients whose sensory level of anesthesia regressed during continuous infusion of bupivacaine. In contrast, patients with a stable level of sensory anesthesia showed no further increase in epidural blood flow.[60] However, increased elimination from the epidural space or altered distribution within the epidural space has been shown to play no role in the development of tachyphylaxis with intermittent injections of lidocaine.[61]

PHARMACODYNAMIC HYPOTHESES

Increased cAMP. A recent in vivo and in vitro study of procaine-induced sciatic nerve block suggests that local anesthetic effects (including tachyphylaxis) may be mediated through interface with adenine and cyclic nucleotides.[62] Both adenine and cyclic nucleotides significantly shortened the duration of nerve block in rats without affecting the frequency, degree of block, or time of onset. A rapid reversal of procaine-induced depression of the action potential was also seen with these nucleotides in isolated nerve preparations.[62] More research is needed to further delineate the role of adenine and cyclic nucleotides in the genesis of tachyphylaxis and other local anesthetic effects.

INCREASED NOCICEPTIVE TRANSMISSION AND NEUROPLASTICITY

The most intriguing hypothesis for the mechanism underlying tachyphylaxis involves the physiology of the nociceptive sensory system.[52] Laboratory experiments have demonstrated increased nociceptive transmission[63–66] and peripheral[63] and central sensitization[63,64] of nociceptors after peripheral trauma (see Ch. 2). Such increased afferent input to the spinal cord can expand the receptive fields of dorsal horn neurons.[65] (Figs. 12-4 and 12-5), as well as induce a progressive "wind-up" of dorsal horn neuronal discharge[66] (Fig. 12-6). Quite interestingly, noxious stimulation of deep somatic structures elicits a greater afferent nociceptive barrage and greater central neuroplastic changes than noxious stimulation of cutaneous structures.[67] By extrapolation, we can hypothesize that noxious stimulation of deeper visceral structures also elicits a greater afferent barrage than cutaneous stimulation.

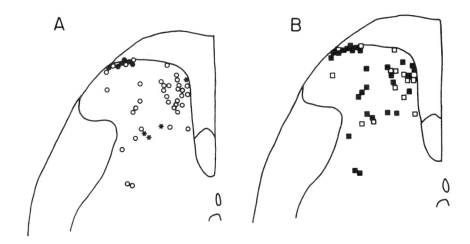

Fig. 12-4. Expansion of receptive fields of dorsal horn neurons. Transverse sections of dorsal horn of the rat spinal cord indicating recording position of 46 neurons. (**A**) Cells that were antidromically activated by stimulation in cervical spinal cord of contralateral dorsolateral funiculus (●) and ventrolateral quadrant (*) with tungsten microelectrodes are shown (dorsal columns sectioned); (○) cells that could not be antidromically stimulated. (**B**) Cells showing either a >50 percent expansion of their receptive fields or increase in their response to a standard pinch or air-jet stimulus after C-fiber conditioning stimulus are indicated (■); (□) cells not sensitized by conditioning input. (From Cook et al,[65] with permission.)

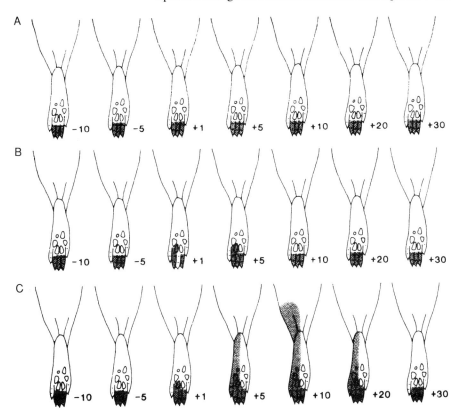

Fig. 12-5. Expansion of receptive fields of dorsal horn neurons. Effect of graded strengths of conditioning stimuli to gastrocnemius-soleus nerve of a rat on size of receptive field of a dorsal horn neuron. *Shaded areas* indicate skin area within which a firm mechanical stimulus elicited a response in the neuron. **(A)** Effect of a stimulus that activates only large myelinated afferents (100 μA, 50 μsec); **(B)** effect of increasing the strength to recruit thin myelinated afferents (500 μA, 50 μsec); **(C)** effect produced when unmyelinated fibers are stimulated (5 mA, 500 μsec). Note expansion of receptive field of the dorsal horn neuron. Number beside each foot in time (min), the conditioning stimulus being applied at time 0 at 1 Hz for 20 sec. (From Cook et al,[65] with permission.)

Similar changes in nociceptive transmission and central hypersensitization should occur in the postoperative period.[68] Such enhanced afferent input and hyperexcitability of dorsal horn neurons would be antagonistic to the neural blocking effect of epidural local anesthetics. Such antagonism would reveal itself as a reduction of sensory analgesia in the rostral part of the neural blockade, where the intensity of blockade and the concentration of bupivacaine are least.[47,52,68] What makes this hypothesis so compelling is its corollary: nociceptive transmission and its attendant neuroplastic changes (and thereby tachyphylaxis itself) could be ablated by combinations of analgesics affecting discrete parts of the nociceptive system (i.e., balanced analgesia).

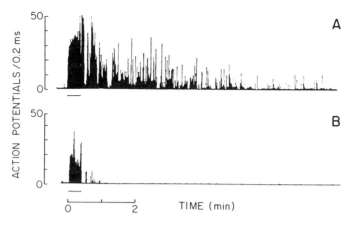

Fig. 12-6. Central hypersensitization or "wind-up." Frequency of discharge evoked in posterior biceps femoris/semitendinous α-motor neurons of the rat by stimulation of a chronically sectioned sciatic nerve for 20 sec at 10 Hz at C-fiber strength. Period of stimulation is denoted by *horizontal lines* under each recording. **(A)** Stimulation of sectioned nerve produces a very long after-discharge (wind-up). **(B)** Stimulation of intact sciatic nerve results in a smaller number of action potentials for a shorter time period. (From Wall and Woolf,[66] with permission.)

CLINICAL PROPERTIES OF COMBINATIONS OF EPIDURAL LOCAL ANESTHETICS AND OPIOIDS

Analgesic Synergy

Analgesic synergy refers to the prolonged and enhanced antinociception associated with coadministration of reduced doses of neuraxial (epidural and subarachnoid) local anesthetics and opioids.[69,70] Such effects have been seen in the laboratory[69,70] as well as clinically.[8,71-73] Recently, a bupivacaine-induced conformational change in spinal opioid receptors was proposed as a possible mechanism underlying analgesic synergy.[70]

The benefits of such synergistic interaction are multiple (Table 12-3): (1) reduction of dosage of individual drugs with a decreased incidence of side effects attributable to opioids and/or local anesthetics (e.g., decreased motor blockade), (2) stable hemodynamics, (3) improved intensity of neural blockade (e.g., inhibition of tachyphylaxis), (4) equivalent or superior analgesia as compared with epidural local anesthetics or opioids alone, (5) prolonged duration of analgesia, and (6) improved functional ability.

Not all studies of the coadministration of epidural local anesthetics and opioids demonstrate analgesic synergy, however. Compared with administration of epidural local anesthetics alone, combinations of epidural local anesthetics and opioids have uniformly been shown to improve analgesic efficacy.[7-10,16,76] In contrast, studies comparing coadministration of epidural local

TABLE 12-3. Clinical Properties of the Coadministration of Neuraxial Local
Anesthetics and Opioids

Property	Reference
Reduction of drug dosage or incidence of side effects	
For opioids	69,70,72
For local anesthetics	74,75
Stable hemodynamics	1,8
Increased intensity of neural blockade	1,9,10
Equivalent or superior analgesia as compared with	
Administration of epidural local anesthetics alone	7–10,16,76
Administration of epidural opioids alone	7,8,16,77–80
Prolonged duration of analgesia	69,71,74
Improved functional ability	1–3

anesthetics and opioids with administration of opioids alone have demonstrated equivalent analgesia.[7,8,16,77–80] However, pain during activity or mobilization was not assessed in any of those studies.

In a double-blind randomized study by Dahl et al,[3] combinations of epidural bupivacaine and morphine were shown to provide superior analgesia as compared with epidural morphine during mobilization after abdominal surgery. Only equivalent analgesia was discernable at rest. In the future, comparisons of different analgesic regimens should include assessment of pain during various activities. Superior analgesic modalities hold the tantalizing prospect of decreased convalescence. Superiority, therefore, should be defined as enhanced analgesia during mobilization: coughing, mobilization from the supine to the sitting position, and ambulation. As defined by Dahl et al,[3] different analgesic modalities may have differential effects on pain at rest and during mobilization.

Inhibition of Tachyphylaxis

The coadministration of epidural local anesthetics with intravenous[81] or epidural[9] opioids (Figs. 12-7 and 12-8) has been shown to either restore a sensory level of anesthesia[81] or prophylax against the occurrence of tachyphylaxis.[9] Although the explanation for this interesting phenomenon is unclear, activation of the descending modulating antinociceptive system is hypothesized to be involved.

Systemic opioids mimic the actions of endogenous opioid peptides in the rostroventral medulla by binding to off-cells and activating the descending modulating system. This mechanism has been shown to contribute to the analgesic effect of systemic morphine in experimental studies.[82,83] Epidural administration of opioids can likewise inhibit tachyphylaxis by this rostral mechanism but also by a direct effect on the spinal cord.[9] Direct application of opioids to the neuraxis may minimize or prevent the sensitization of dorsal horn neurons (central hypersensitization or wind-up), thereby inhibiting the development of tachyphylaxis.[9]

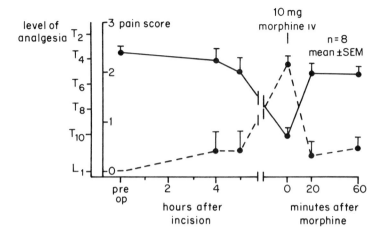

Fig. 12-7. Effect of intravenous morphine on pain and extent of sensory anesthesia/ analgesia during continuous epidural infusion of 0.5 percent bupivacaine (8 ml/h). When the pain score (verbal rating scale from 0 to 4: none, mild, moderate, severe, and unbearable, respectively) increased by two levels or when the rostrad sensory level regressed five dermatomal segments from the initial level, 10 mg of morphine was intravenously administered. Twenty minutes after injection of morphine, pronounced analgesia was achieved, and the sensory level was restored to its initial level. (From Lund et al,[81] with permission.)

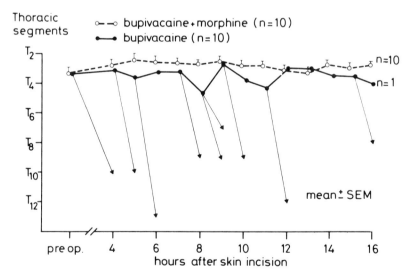

Fig. 12-8. Inhibition of tachyphylaxis by coadministration of epidural local anesthetic and morphine. Patients received either 0.5 percent bupivacaine (8 ml/h) or 0.5 percent bupivacaine (8 ml/h) with 0.5 mg/h of morphine. Patients were removed from the study if the rostrad sensory level regressed five dermatomal segments from original level. Sixteen hours after skin incision, only one patient receiving epidural bupivacaine alone remained in the study. After 16 hours, sensory levels of patients receiving epidural bupivacaine and morphine were not appreciably different from the initial level of sensory anesthesia/analgesia. (From Hjortsø et al,[9] with permission.)

Inhibition of Central Hypersensitization: The Concept of Preemptive Analgesia

As discussed previously, surgical trauma creates a barrage of nociceptive afferent transmission, which may alter the excitability of both peripheral and central neurons.[63-66] Besides the electrophysiologic changes of expansion of receptive fields[65] and progressive "wind-up" of dorsal horn neuronal discharge,[66] postsynaptic morphologic changes have been demonstrated within the spinal cord.[84] These documented electrophysiologic and morphologic changes have fostered the belief that surgical trauma induces neuroplastic changes within the cord. The sequelae of these electrophysiologic and morphologic alterations may long outlast the initial noxious stimulus.[5,15,85]

Enhanced Nociceptive Transmission: The Afferent "Barrage"

Under general anesthesia, the spinal cord is lightly anesthetized and receives massive afferent nociceptive input from the site of surgery. Under regional anesthesia, the spinal cord receives no nociceptive transmission. Prevention of the afferent "barrage" associated with the surgical stimulus may be accomplished by application of regional anesthetic techniques prior to incision. It has been hypothesized that such *preemptive* analgesia can prevent neuroplastic changes within the spinal cord and their attendant physiologic sequelae.

Duration of Effect

It has also been hypothesized that preemptive analgesia may produce prolonged effects that long outlast the initial neural blockade.[86] C-fiber afferent transmission produces prolonged changes in spinal cord excitability.[66,67] In laboratory models, very high doses of opioid are necessary to suppress central hypersensitization once established.[87] However, small doses of opioid administered prior to the barrage of nociceptive transmission can prevent the central hyperexcitability.[87]

Such observations have lead to the surgical incision being viewed as a "priming" mechanism. Once established in a hyperexcitable state, the spinal cord would respond excessively to afferent input. Administration of analgesics prior to the initial noxious stimulus would prevent "priming." The prolonged hyperexcitability of dorsal horn neurons would be prevented.[86] Taken to its extreme conclusion, a single preoperative dose of analgesic could conceivably completely prevent postoperative pain. Unfortunately, many practitioners associate preemptive analgesia with such results by definition.[86]

Clinical Studies

The results of several clinical studies have been invoked to support the concept of preemptive analgesia.[5,85,86]

Tverskoy et al[5] assessed the severity of postoperative pain in patients undergoing inguinal herniorrhaphy with general anesthesia, spinal anesthesia, or preoperative infiltration of the abdominal wall with local anesthetics followed by induction of general anesthesia. The intensity of constant and movement-associated incisional pain was assessed using a visual analogue scale at 24 hour, 48 hour, and 10 days after surgery. Pain was also provoked at the site of incision by pressure applied from an algometer at the same postoperative time intervals.

The use of local anesthetic significantly decreased the intensity of all three types of pain. The effect was most pronounced for constant incisional pain, which completely disappeared by 24 hour after surgery. Cutaneous hyperalgesia as elicited by pressure algometry was still present in the general anesthesia group at 10 days after surgery and almost negligible in the local anesthetic plus general anesthesia patients (Fig. 12-9). The same effect was found in patients receiving spinal anesthesia, although less pronounced.

Tverskoy et al[5] concluded that application of local anesthetics blocked the afferent nociceptive barrage associated with herniorrhaphy. Blockade of this nociceptive input prevented development of central hypersensitization. This was translated into reduced preoperative pain as well as reduced cutaneous hyperalgesia at a time distant from surgery. A single preoperative injection of local anesthetic (irrespective of route of administration) produced measurable physiologic changes as elicited by provocative dolorimetry at a time distant from surgery.

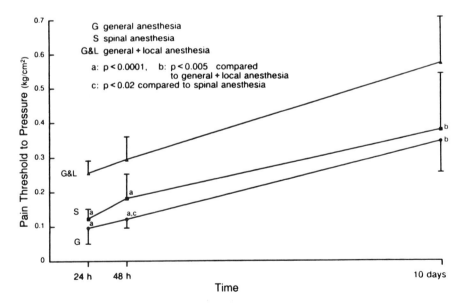

Fig. 12-9. Preemptive analgesia. Postoperative pain thresholds to pressure applied to a surgical wound after three different types of anesthesia. Patients receiving infiltration analgesia before induction and surgical incision had negligible cutaneous hyperalgesia as elicited by pressure algometry 10 days after surgery. Patients receiving general anesthesia still demonstrated significant hyperalgesia. (From Tverskoy et al,[5] with permission.)

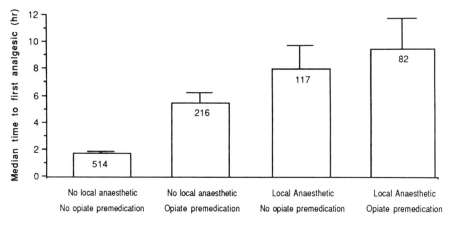

Fig. 12-10. Effect of premedication and regional anesthesia on time to first request for analgesia after elective orthopaedic surgery. Median time to first analgesic (h) is listed by treatment category. *Bars* represent upper 95 percent confidence interval. (From McQuay et al,[88] with permission.)

McQuay et al[88] studied the effects of preoperative opioid premedication and regional anesthesia on the time to first request for postoperative analgesia after elective orthopaedic surgery (Fig. 12-10). If opioid premedication and regional anesthesia were not used, the median time to request for postoperative analgesia was less than 2 hours. Use of opioid premedication and regional anesthesia extended the median time to more than 9 hours. (Please see Fig. 12-10 for the results regarding the remaining study groups.)

McQuay et al[88] drew no conclusions regarding preemptive analgesia from the results of their study. A subsequent editorial by Wall[86] suggested that the results could be explained by prevention (or at least retardation of the development) of central hypersensitization.

A third study deals with the prevention of phantom limb pain by preoperative epidural analgesia with local anesthetics and/or opioids.[85] The results of this study are more closely examined in Chapter 24.

Coadministration of Epidural Local Anesthetics and Opioids

What conclusions regarding preemptive analgesia can be drawn from the literature? First, no current study *definitively* proves its existence in humans. All the current studies have design flaws (most notably, Bach et al[85]; see Ch. 24). Preemptive analgesia has not been studied using a placebo-controlled protocol.[5] Furthermore, McQuay et al never drew conclusions regarding central hypersensitization or preemptive analgesia from the results of their study. In short, although the possibilities attendant to the concept of preemptive analgesia are tantalizing, much further research is necessary to determine whether the concept is clinically viable.

Assuming that preemptive analgesia exists as a phenomenon, do we radically define it as the complete eradication of pain with the single preoperative administration of an analgesic? It is difficult to imagine how the *single* preoperative administration of analgesic could *completely* eradicate pain over several subsequent days. This is especially true during postoperative mobilization of the patient, when afferent nociceptive transmission to the spinal cord is certainly increased. Furthermore, the development of tachyphylaxis during epidural infusions of local anesthetics suggests that continued nociceptive transmission reaches the spinal cord even after the surgical procedure (according to the neuroplasticity hypothesis).

It is perhaps better to state that some benefit does accrue from the preoperative administration of analgesics, particularly regional anesthetics. (This is more in keeping with the extant clinical data.) Such benefits *may* be the result of prevention of neuroplastic changes within the spinal cord. However, such assertions do not obviate the need for continuation of the analgesic (and more importantly, the regional anesthetic/analgesic) into the postoperative period. Thus, continued afferent barrage of the spinal cord may be prevented by extended use of regional anesthesia/analgesia into the postoperative period.

If we adopt this less extreme definition of preemptive analgesia, what is the best method for continued prevention of the afferent barrage of the cord? Balanced analgesic techniques would seem the obvious answer. Balanced analgesic techniques, by definition, affect the physiologic processes involved in nociception: transduction, transmission, and modulation. Thus, the afferent barrage is interdicted at multiple points from its genesis in the periphery to the primary synapse within the dorsal horn. As explained earlier in this chapter, coadministration of epidural local anesthetics and opioids is the "cornerstone" of balanced analgesia.[1-3] Such combinations exhibit analgesic synergy[71-80] but also inhibit tachyphylaxis.[9] As they inhibit tachyphylaxis, such combinations should also inhibit the development of central hypersensitization.[9] Thus, coadministration of epidural local anesthetics and opioids should perhaps be viewed as a continuation of the suppression of central hypersensitization initially achieved through preoperative administration of regional anesthesia. Preemptive analgesia should not be viewed as a static single time point of drug administration but rather conceptualized as part of a dynamic continuing process of suppression of central hypersensitization and neuroplastic changes within the spinal cord.

MANAGEMENT OF EPIDURAL INFUSIONS OF LOCAL ANESTHETIC AND OPIOID: CLINICAL PRACTICE AT BRIGHAM AND WOMEN'S HOSPITAL

As described in the preceding discussion, institution of an epidural infusion of local anesthetic and opioid at Brigham and Women's Hospital is conceived to be a continuation of the suppression of nociceptive transmission and central hypersensitization achieved by intraoperative regional anesthesia. It must be made clear that the postoperative epidural infusion is *not* conceptualized as continuation of an *anesthetic*. Indeed, the motor blockade and dense sensory anesthesia attendant to intraoperative anesthesia are negative factors for effective postoperative management. However, coadministration of epidural local anesthetic and opioid can still achieve its desired effect when viewed as a *regional analgesic* and an integral part of a balanced analgesic technique.

At Brigham and Women's Hospital, 0.125 percent bupivacaine is routinely used with morphine, meperidine, or fentanyl (Tables 12-4 and 12-5). (For open knee surgery, 0.25 percent bupivacaine is the local anesthetic of choice.) The optimal site for epidural catheter insertion is in the interspace crossed by the middle dermatome of the surgical incision. This will theoretically permit spread of the analgesic solution over the appropriate dorsal roots and dorsal root entry zones (dorsal horns) receiving afferent nociceptive transmission. Precise catheter placement may be less of a prerequisite for coadministration of local anesthetic and morphine because of morphine's ability to spread widely in the CSF flow (see Ch. 11).

An infusion of 0.125 percent bupivacaine with meperidine (1.0–2.5 mg/ml) or fentanyl (2.5–5.0 μg/ml) is instituted when the degree of motor blockade has receded to a level of I–II on the Bromage scale.[89] A sufficient level of sensory anesthesia is usually still present, allowing the combinational use of local anesthetic and opioid to retard the rate of sensory level regression (inhibition of tachyphylaxis).[9] Timing the institution of the epidural infusion allows the provision of prolonged profound analgesia.

TABLE 12-4. Combinations of Local Anesthetic and Opioid for Epidural Infusion

Analgesic Solution	Infusion Rate	Comments
Bupivacaine 0.125% + fentanyl 2.5–5 μg/ml	4–15 ml/hr	Infusion should be "tailored" to limit fentanyl administration to no more than 100 μg/h; systemic fentanyl levels may be substantial during infusion (see text); probably not ideal for large incisions or when pain source is far from epidural catheter site
Bupivacaine 0.125% + meperidine 1.0–2.5 mg/ml	4–15 ml/h	Meperidine administration should not exceed 20–25 mg/h to avoid appreciable systemic levels; preferable for larger incisions because of lower lipid solubility
Bupivacaine 0.125% + morphine 0.05–0.1 mg/ml	4–10 ml/h	Preferred for large incisions or when catheter site is distant from pain source; hourly morphine should not exceed 0.5 mg; CSF morphine may become substantial during prolonged therapy
Bupivacaine 0.25% + opioid	4–10 ml/hr	Used primarily for lower extremity pain when early physical therapy is used (e.g., total knee replacement, cruciate ligament repair); significant motor or sensory block during infusion usually warrants change to a lower concentration of bupivacaine

TABLE 12-5. Preparation of Selected Epidural Infusions

B 1/8 D2.5*		D2.5	
0.25% Bupivacaine	100 ml		
PF Meperidine	10 ml (500 mg)	PF Meperidine	10 ml (500 ml)
PFNS	90 ml	PFNS	190 ml
B 1/8 F5*		F5	
0.25% Bupivacaine	100 ml		
Fentanyl	20 ml (1 mg)	Fentanyl	20 ml
PFNS	80 ml	PFNS	180 ml
B 1/8 M0.05*		M0.05	
0.25% Bupivacaine	100 ml		
PF Morphine	10 ml (10 mg)	PF Morphine	10 ml (10 ml)
PFNS	90 ml	PFNS	190 ml

* Epidural solutions may be abbreviated by listing the local anesthetic and/or opioid followed by the respective concentration after each letter. For example:

B 1/8 D2.5 = 0.125% bupivacaine with 2.5 mg of dermerol/ml
F5 = 5 µg of fentanyl/ml
M0.05 = 0.05 mg of morphine/ml

Abbreviations: PF = preservative-free, PFNS = preservative-free normal saline.

As a general guideline, fentanyl is used when the surgical wound is small (covering few dermatomes) and meperidine (as well as morphine) is used for more extensive incisions. This is based on the ability of meperidine to spread more extensively than fentanyl in the CSF as it is considerably less lipid-soluble than fentanyl (30 times less) (see Ch. 11).

Morphine (0.05–0.1 mg/ml) is combined with bupivacaine when maintenance of analgesia is difficult or impossible with meperidine or fentanyl. This is usually manifest as a "never-ending" requirement for "top-up" doses of opioid or local anesthetic. When epidural catheters are far removed from the source of pain (e.g., lumbar catheter for thoracotomy pain), morphine is certainly the preferred opioid. There may be no advantage at all in using bupivacaine in this situation. Morphine in itself may be a sufficient analgesic. Dilute bupivacaine administered in the lumbar epidural space may never physically reach thoracic cord segments.

Troubleshooting

It is not unusual for infusion rates to be adjusted upward during the typical postsurgical course. This may be a result of several factors: tachyphylaxis, leakage of solution out through the tract in the skin, subcutaneous migration of the catheter out of the epidural space, or improper location of the catheter insertion site (Table 12-6). If the need for supplemental top-up injections or adjustment of infusion rates is excessive, consideration must be given to the possibility of a nonfunctional catheter (i.e., a catheter no longer in the epidural space) (Fig. 12-11). The practitioner must be extremely wary before entertaining the possibility of "testing" the catheter with local anesthetic. Prudence and the individual clinical scenario should dictate whether this is warranted (e.g., patient's degree of hydration, availability of resuscitation equipment). Depend-

TABLE 12-6. Common Problems During Epidural Analgesic Therapy

Problem	Solution
Pain despite epidural infusion	Consider verifying catheter position in epidural space by response to local anesthetic injection (2% lidocaine with epinpherine—2–3 ml for high thoracic catheter; 4–7 for lower catheters).
	If no response, replace catheter
	If catheter functional, increase hourly infusion rate.
Continued pain despite infusion rate increases	If catheter working, consider:
	Is catheter in interspace crossed by middle of incision? If not, replace catheter; or
	Change opioid to a more hydrophilic opioid to achieve spread of analgesia over more dermatomes; or
	Increase bupivacaine concentration (from 0.125% to 0.188% or 0.25%).
Patient sedated, sleepy	Is hourly opioid excessive?
	Meperidine, 20–25 mg/h or greater, may produce appreciable systemic levels, sedation. Fentanyl, 100 μg/h or greater may produce appreciable systemic levels, sedation. Morphine, 0.5 mg/h or greater, may produce excessive CSF opioid levels with sedation and respiratory depression.
	If yes:
	Reduce infusion rate or opioid concentration in solution, and Increase vigilance (more frequent respiratory checks, etc.) until symptoms abate.
Catheter insertion site leaking	Inspect site.
	Analgesia adequate? Then continue to follow.
	Analgesia inadequate? Then verify catheter in epidural space; if yes, may have to increase infusion rate to account for losses through leakage.

ing on the individual case, it may be better to reinsert the epidural catheter choosing another insertion site to better approximate spread of analgesic solution to the appropriate cord segments.

If the catheter is deemed to be functional (irrespective of the administration of local anesthetic), tachyphylaxis, leakage of solution, or a less than optimal catheter site location is necessitating the increased dosage requirements. It may be necessary to change the composition of the epidural infusion to prevent opioid-induced side effects. Hourly epidural infusions of meperidine[90] in excess of 25 mg or fentanyl[91] in excess of 100 μg have been shown to produce substantial systemic opioid levels. These levels may be analgesic in themselves or may produce side effects (usually sedation but also nausea, pruritus, and respiratory depression). Escalating epidural infusion rates may only reflect the need for more local anesthetic, and great care should be exercised in limiting systemic opioid concentrations. This may be achieved by simply increasing the infusion rate while decreasing the concentration of opioid and maintaining the concentration of local anesthetic.

Bupivacaine 0.25 percent is used with opioid for analgesia after open knee surgery. This dose (concentration) of local anesthetic allows patients to tolerate

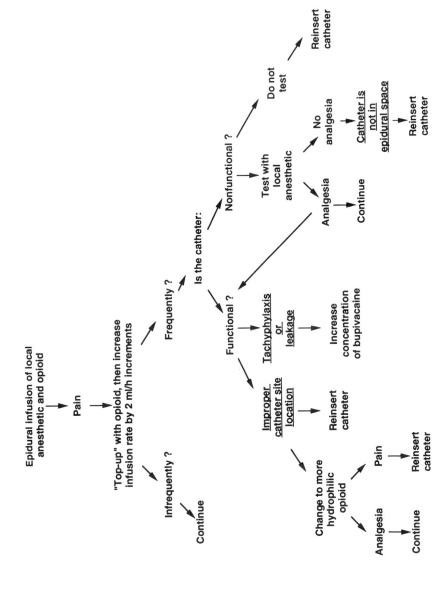

Fig. 12-11. Algorithm for management of frequent complaints of pain with epidural infusions of local anesthetics and opioids.

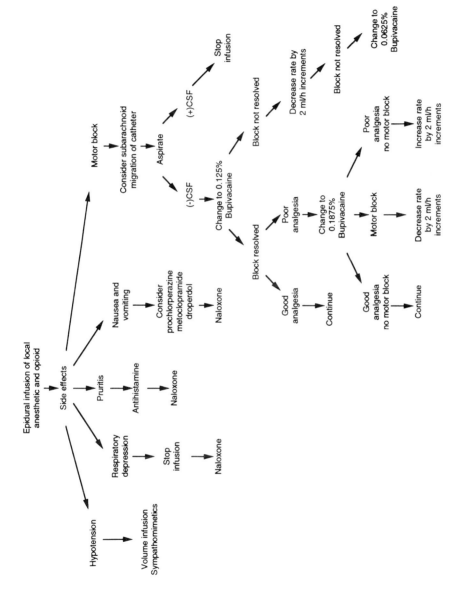

Fig. 12-12. Algorithm for management of side effects and complications of epidural infusions of local anesthetics and opioids.

continuous passive motion of the knee joint without pain in the early postoperative period. If motor blockade or extensive numbness of the legs results during this infusion, the concentration of bupivacaine may be adjusted downward to 0.125 percent or 0.188 percent ($\frac{3}{16}$ percent).

Complications and Side Effects

Whenever local anesthetics and opioids are given epidurally, side effects specific to both agents must be anticipated (Fig. 12-12). Opioid-related effects seem to occur more frequently, perhaps because of the present lack of data demonstrating the optimal dose of opioid for combinational epidural infusion.

Hypotension, numbness, and motor blockade may all occur during coadministration of epidural local anesthetic and opioids. Unless higher bupivacaine concentrations are used or the catheter migrates into the subarachnoid space, these complications are exceedingly unusual, attesting to the essential safety of the technique.

CONCLUSION

This chapter has attempted to provide a rational background for the use of combinational infusions of epidural local anesthetics and opioids. Use of continuous epidural infusions of local anesthetic alone is hampered by the development of tachyphylaxis. The addition of an opioid not only prevents tachyphylaxis, but the combination possesses analgesic synergy. When used as part of a balanced analgesic technique, coadministration of epidural local anesthetics and opioids continue the suppression of central hypersensitization (as well as neuroendocrine responses; see Ch. 4) initially achieved by the intraoperative regional anesthetic. Thus, analgesic care is viewed as a continuum and is not temporally isolated to the postoperative period. The conceptualization of analgesic care as a continuum, the use of balanced analgesic techniques, and the suppression of maladaptive physiologic responses will lead to decreased time of convalescence. The role of combinational administration of epidural local anesthetics and opioids is pivotal in this process.

References
1. Dahl JB, Rosenberg J, Dirkes WE et al: Prevention of postoperative pain by balanced analgesia. Br J Anaesth 64:518, 1990
2. Schulze S, Roikjaer O, Hasselstrøm L et al: Epidural bupivacaine and morphine plus systemic indomethacin eliminates pain but not systemic response and convalescence after cholecystectomy. Surgery 103:321, 1987
3. Dahl JB, Rosenberg J, Hansen BL et al: Differential analgesic effects of low-dose epidural morphine and morphine-bupivacaine at rest and during mobilization after major abdominal surgery. Anesth Analg 74:362, 1992
4. Mogensen T, Vegger P, Jonsson T et al: Systemic piroxicam as an adjunct to combined epidural bupivacaine and morphine for postoperative pain relief—a double-blind study. Anesth Analg 74:366, 1992

5. Tverskoy M, Cozacov C, Ayache M et al: Postoperative pain after inguinal herniorrhaphy with different types of anesthesia. Anesth Analg 70:29, 1990
6. Kehlet H: Surgical stress: the role of pain and analgesia. Br J Anaesth 63:189, 1989
7. Cullen ML, Staren ED, El-Ganzouri A et al: Continuous epidural infusion for analgesia after major abdominal operations: a randomized, prospective, double-blind study. Surgery 98:718, 1985
8. Lee A, Simpson D, Whitfield A, Scott DB: Postoperative analgesia by continuous extradural infusion of bupivacaine and diamorphine. Br J Anaesth 60:845, 1988
9. Hjortsø N-C, Lund C, Mogensen T et al: Epidural morphine improves pain relief and maintains sensory analgesia during continuous epidural bupivacaine after abdominal surgery. Anesth Analg 65:1033, 1986
10. Scott NB, Mogensen T, Bigler D et al: Continuous thoracic extradural 0.5% bupivacaine with or without morphine: effect on quality of blockade, lung function and the surgical stress response. Br J Anaesth 62:253, 1989
11. Møller IV, Dinesen K, Søndergard S et al: Effect of patient-controlled analgesia on plasma catecholamine, cortisol and glucose concentrations after cholecystectomy. Br J Anaesth 61:160, 1988
12. Kehlet H: Modification of responses to surgery by neural blockade: clinical implications. p. 145. In Cousins MJ, Bridenbaugh PO (eds): Neural Blockade in Clinical Anesthesia and Management of Pain. 2nd Ed. Lippincott, Philadelphia, 1988
13. Matthews PJ, Govenden V: Comparison of continuous paravertebral and extradural infusions of bupivacaine for pain relief after thoracotomy. Br J Anaesth 62:204, 1989
14. Griffiths DPG, Diamond AW, Cameron JD: Postoperative extradural analgesia following thoracic surgery: a feasibility study. Br J Anaesth 47:48, 1975
15. Conacher ID, Paes ML, Jacobson L et al: Epidural analgesia following thoracic surgery. A review of two years' experience. Anaesthesia 38:546, 1983
16. Logas WG, El-Baz N, El-Ganzouri A et al: Continuous thoracic epidural analgesia for postoperative pain relief following thoracotomy: a randomized prospective study. Anesthesiology 67:787, 1987
17. James EC, Kolberg HL, Iwen GW, Gellatly TA: Epidural analgesia for post-thoracotomy patients. J Thorac Cardiovasc Surg 82:898, 1981
18. Miller L, Gertel M, Fox GS, MacLean LD: Comparison of effect of narcotic and epidural analgesia on postoperative respiratory function. Am J Surg 131:291, 1976
19. Hendolin H, Lahtinen J, Lansimies E et al: The effect of thoracic epidural analgesia on respiratory function after cholecystectomy. Acta Anaesthesiol Scand 31:645, 1987
20. Hendolin H, Lahtinen J, Lanimies E, Tuppurainen T: The effect of thoracic epidural analgesia on postoperative stress and morbidity. Ann Chir Gynaecol 76:234, 1987
21. Raj PP, Knarr DC, Vigdorth E et al: Comparison of continuous epidural infusion of local anesthetic and administration of systemic narcotics in the management of pain after total knee replacement. Anesth Analg 66:401, 1987
22. Pettine KA, Wedel DJ, Cabanela ME, Weeks JL: The use of epidural bupivacaine following total knee arthroplasty. Orthop Rev 18:894, 1989
23. Ulrich C, Burri C, Worsdorfer O: Continuous passive motion after knee-joint arthrolysis under catheter peridural anesthesia. Arch Orthop Trauma Surg 104:346, 1986
24. Covino BG: Pharmacology of local anaesthetic agents. Br J Anaesth 58:701, 1986
25. Gissen AJ, Covino BG, Gregus J: Differential sensitivity of fast and slow fibers in mammalian nerve. III. Effect of etidocaine and bupivacaine on fast/slow fibers. Anesth Analg 61:570, 1892
26. Cousins MJ, Bromage PR: Epidural neural blockade. p. 253. In Cousins MJ,

Bridenbaugh PO (eds): Neural Blockade in Clinical Anesthesia and Management of Pain. 2nd Ed. JB Lippincott, Philadelphia, 1988

27. Brockway MS, Bannister J, McClure JH et al: Comparison of extradural ropivacaine and bupivacaine. Br J Anaesth 66:31, 1991

28. Concepcion M, Arthur GR, Steele SM et al: A new local anesthetic, ropivacaine. Its epidural effects in humans. Anesth Analg 70:80, 1990

29. Bonica JJ, Berges PU, Morikawa K: Circulatory effects of peridural block. I. Effects of level of analgesia and dose of lidocaine. Anesthesiology 33:619, 1970

30. Shimosato S, Etsten BE: The role of the venous system in cardiocirculatory dynamics during spinal and epidural anesthesia in man. Anesthesiology 30:619, 1969

31. Bromage PR: Continuous epidural analgesia. p. 215. In Epidural Analgesia. WB Saunders, Philadelphia, 1978

32. Raj PP, Denson DD: Prolonged analgesia technique with local anesthetics. p. 687. In Raj PP (ed): Practical Management of Pain. 1st Ed. Year Book, Chicago, 1986

33. Tucker GT, Cooper S, Littlewood D et al: Observed and predicted accumulation of local anaesthetic agents during continuous extradural analgesia. Br J Anaesth 49: 237, 1977

34. Green R, Dawkins CJM: Postoperative analgesia: the use of a continuous drip epidural block. Anaesthesia 21:372, 1967

35. Denson DD, Raj PP, Saldahna F et al: Continuous perineural infusion of bupivacaine for prolonged analgesia: pharmacokinetic considerations. Int J Clin Pharmacol Ther Toxicol 21:591, 1983

36. Denson DD, Thompson GA, Raj PP et al: Continuous perineural infusions of bupivacaine for prolonged analgesia—a rapid two-point method for estimating individual pharmacokinetic parameters. Int J Clin Pharmacol Ther Toxicol 22:512, 1984

37. Ball WD: Unstructured two-point estimation of one-compartment linear pharmacokinetic parameters. J Clin Pharmacol 22:326, 1982

38. Tucker GT, Cooper S, Littlewood D et al: Observed and predicted accumulation of local anaesthetic agents during continuous extradural analgesia. Br J Anaesth 49: 237, 1977

39. Ross RA, Clarke JE, Armitage EN: Postoperative pain prevention by continuous epidural infusion. A study of the clinical effects and the plasma concentrations obtained. Anaesthesia 35:663, 1980

40. Holmdahl MH, Sjögren S, Strom G, Wright B: Clinical aspects of continuous epidural blockade for postoperative pain relief. Upps J Med Sci 77:47, 1972

41. Sjögren S, Wright B: Blood concentration of lidocaine during continuous epidural blockade. Acta Anesthesiol Scand, suppl. 46:51, 1972

42. Scott DB, Schweitzer S, Thorn J: Epidural block in postoperative pain relief. Reg Anesth 7:135, 1982

43. Bromage PR, Pettigrew RT, Crowell DE: Tachyphlaxis in epidural analgesia: 1. Augmentation and decay of local anesthesia. J Clin Pharmacol J New Drugs 9:30, 1969

44. Renck H, Edstrøm H: Thoracic epidural analgesia III. Prolongation in the early postoperative period by intermittent injections of etidocaine with adrenaline. Acta Anesthesiol Scand 20:104, 1976

45. Renck H, Edstrøm H, Kinnberger B, Brandt G: Thoracic epidural analgesia II. Prolongation in the early postoperative period by continuous injection of 1% bupivacaine. Acta Anaesthesiol Scand 20:47, 1976

46. Wüst HJ, Liebau U, Richter O, Strasser K: Tachyphylaxis in continuous epidural anaesthesia with bupivacaine 0.125% and 0.25%. Anasth Intensivther Notf Med 15: 159, 1980

47. Mogensen T, Hjortsø N-C, Bigler D et al: Unpredictability of regression of analgesia during the continuous postoperative extradural infusion of bupivacaine. Br J Anaesth 60:515, 1988

48. Mogensen T, Scott NB, Hjortsø N-C et al: The influence of volume and concentration of bupivacaine on regression of analgesia during continuous postoperative epidural infusion. Reg Anesth 13:122, 1988

49. Mogensen T, Dirkes W, Bigler D et al: No tachypylaxis during postoperative continuous epidural 0.125% bupivacaine infusion. Reg Anesth 13:117, 1988

50. Moir DD, Slater PJ, Thorburn J et al: Extradural analgesia in obstetrics: a controlled trial of carbonated lignocaine and bupivacaine hydrochloride with and without adrenaline. Br J Anaesth 48:129, 1976

51. Tucker GT, Mather LE: Pharmacology of local anaesthetic agents: pharmacokinetics of local anaesthetic agents. Br J Anaesth, suppl. 47:213, 1975

52. Bigler D, Lund C, Mogensen T et al: Tachyphylaxis during postoperative epidural analgesia—new insights (editorial). Acta Anaesthesiol Scand 31;664, 1987

53. Renck H: Tachyphlaxis during postoperative peridural analgesia of long action. p. 188. In Wüst HJ, Zindler M (eds): New Aspects in Regional Anesthesia. Vol. 1. Springer-Verlag, Berlin, 1980

54. Mather LE: Tachyphylaxis in regional anesthesia. Can we reconcile clinical observations and laboratory measurements? p. 3. In Wüst HJ, Stanton-Hicks M (eds): New Aspects in Regional Anesthesia. Vol. 4. Springer-Verlag, Berlin, 1986

55. Lipfert P, Holthusen H, Arndt JO: Tachyphylaxis to local anesthetics does not result from reduced drug effectiveness at the nerve itself. Anesthesiology 70:71, 1989

56. Myers RR, Kalichman MW, Reisner LS, Powell HC: Neurotoxicity of local anesthetics: altered perineurial permeability, edema, and nerve fiber injury. Anesthesiology 64:29, 1986

57. Cohen EN, Levine DA, Collins JE, Gunther RE: The role of pH in the development of tachyphylaxis to local anesthetic agents. Anesthesiology 29:994, 1968

58. Robin ED, Whaley RD, Crump CH et al: Acid-base relations between spinal fluid and arterial blood with special reference to control of ventilation. J Appl Physiol 13:385, 1958

59. Baker CE, Berry RL, Elston RC: Effect of pH of bupivacaine on duration of repeated sciatic nerve blocks in the albino rat. Local anesthetics for neuralgia study group. Anesth Analg 72:773, 1991

60. Mogensen T, Højgaard L, Scott NB et al: Epidural blood flow and regression of sensory analgesia during continuous postoperative epidural infusion of bupivacaine. Anesth Analg 67:809, 1988

61. Mogensen T, Simonsen L, Scott NB et al: Tachyphylaxis associated with repeated epidural injections of lidocaine is not related to changes in distribution or rate of elimination from the epidural space. Anesth Analg 69:180, 1989

62. Kraynack BJ, Gintautas J: Reversal of procaine conduction blockade by adenine nucleotides in vivo and in vitro. Acta Anaesthesiol Scand 26:334, 1982

63. Coderre TJ, Melzack R: Cutaneous hyperalgesia: contributions of the peripheral and central nervous systems to the increase in pain sensitivity after injury. Brain Res 404:95, 1987

64. Woolf CJ: Evidence for a central component of postinjury pain hypersensitivity. Nature 306:686, 1983

65. Cook AJ, Woolf CJ, Wall PD, McMahon SB: Dynamic receptive field plasticity in rat spinal cord dorsal horn following C-primary afferent input. Nature 325:151, 1987

66. Wall PD, Woolf CJ: The brief and prolonged facilitatory effects of unmyelinated

afferent input on the rat spinal cord are independently influenced by peripheral nerve section. Neuroscience 17:1199, 1986

67. Wall PD, Woolf CJ: Muscle but not cutaneous C-afferent input produces prolonged increases in the excitability of the flexion reflex in the rat. J Physiol (Lond) 356:443, 1984

68. Mogensen T, Scott NB, Lund C et al: The roles of acute and chronic pain in regression of sensory analgesia during continuous epidural bupivacaine infusion. Anesth Analg 67:737, 1988

69. Akerman B, Arwestrøm E, Post C: Local anesthetics potentiate spinal morphine antinociception. Anesth Analg 67:943, 1988

70. Tejwani GA, Rattan AK, McDonald JS: Role of spinal opioid receptors in the antinociceptive interactions between intrathecal morphine and bupivacaine. Anesth Analg 74:726, 1992

71. Shapiro LA, Hoffman S, Jedeikin R, Kaplan R: Single-injection epidural anesthesia with bupivacaine and morphine for prostatectomy. Anesth Analg 60:818, 1981

72. Lanz E, Kehrberger E, Theiss D: Epidural morphine: a clinical double-blind study of dosage. Anesth Analg 64:786, 1985

73. Rattan AK, McDonald JS, Tejwani GA: Antinociceptive interactions between morphine and bupivacaine given epidurally, abstracted. Anesthesiology 75:A760, 1991

74. Chestnut DH, Owen CL, Bates JN et al: Continuous infusion epidural analgesia during labor: a randomized double-blind comparison of 0.0625% bupivacaine, 0.0002% fentanyl versus 0.125% bupivacaine. Anesthesiology 68:754, 1988

75. Hunt CO, Naulty JS, Malinow AM et al: Epidural butorphanol-bupivacaine for analgesia during labor and delivery. Anesth Analg 68:323, 1989

76. King MJ, Bowden MI, Cooper GM: Epidural fentanyl and 0.5% bupivacaine for elective cesarean section. Anaesthesia 45:285, 1990

77. Bisgaard C, Mourisden P, Dahl JB: Continuous lumbar epidural bupivacaine plus morphine versus epidural morphine after major abdominal surgery. Eur J Anaesthesiol 7:219, 1990

78. Douglas MJ, McMorland GH, Janzen JA: Influence of bupivacaine as an adjuvant to epidural morphine for analgesia after cesarean section. Anesth Analg 67:1138, 1988

79. Badner NH, Reimer EJ, Komar WE, Moote CA: Low-dose bupivacaine does not improve postoperative epidural fentanyl analgesia in orthopedic patients. Anesth Analg 72:337, 1991

80. Parker RK, Baron M, Helfer DL et al: Use of epidural PCA for post-operative pain management: effect of local anesthetic on the opioid requirement, abstracted. Anesth Analg 70:S297, 1990

81. Lund C, Mogensen T, Hjortsø N-C, Kehlet H: Systemic morphine enhances spread of sensory analgesia during postoperative epidural bupivacaine infusion. Lancet ii: 1156, 1985

82. Fields HL, Vanegas H, Hentall ID, Zorman G: Evidence that disinhibition of brain stem neurones contributes to morphine analgesia. Nature 306:684, 1983

83. Fields HL, Heinricher MM: Anatomy and physiology of a nociceptive modulatory system. Phil Trans R Soc Lond [Biol] 308:361, 1985

84. Sugimoto T, Takemura M, Sakai A, Ishimaru M: Rapid transneuronal destruction following peripheral nerve transection. Pain 30:385, 1987

85. Bach S, Noreng MF, Tjéllden NV: Phantom limb pain in amputees during the first 12 months following limb amputation, after preoperative lumbar epidural blockade. Pain 33:297, 1988

86. Wall PD: The prevention of postoperative pain (editorial). Pain 33:289, 1988
87. Woolf CJ, Wall PD: Morphine-sensitive and morphine-insensitive actions of C-fibre input on the rat spinal cord. Neurosci Lett 64:221, 1986
88. McQuay HJ, Carroll D, Moore RA: Postoperative orthopedic pain—the effect of opiate premedication and local anaesthetic blocks. Pain 33:291, 1988
89. Bromage PR, Camporesi EM, Durant PA, Nielson CH: Influence of epinephrine as an adjuvant to epidural morphine. Anesthesiology 58:257, 1983
90. Sjöström S, Hartvig D, Tamsen A: Patient-controlled analgesia with extradural morphine or pethidine. Br J Anaesth 60:358, 1988
91. Loper KA, Ready LB, Downey M et al: Epidural and intravenous fentanyl infusions are clinically equivalent after knee surgery. Anesth Analg 70:72, 1990

13

Inguinal Paravascular Approach to Lumbar Plexus Analgesia (The "3-in-1" Block)

Leonard J. Lind

Using an inguinal paravascular approach,[1] either femoral nerve block or neural blockade of the complete lumbar plexus may be achieved. Administration of small volumes of local anesthetic within the femoral sheath will remain localized. Anesthesia will only be obtained in the distribution of the femoral nerve. Administration of large volumes of local anesthetic within the femoral sheath will "push" local anesthetic proximally toward the lumbar plexus. Anesthesia may be obtained in the distribution of the femoral, lateral femoral cutaneous, and obturator nerves.

ANATOMY

The lumbar plexus (Fig. 13-1) gives rise to three major branches supplying sensory and motor innervation to the leg: the femoral nerve, the obturator nerve, and the lateral femoral cutaneous nerve.[1] The femoral nerve is the largest constituent of the plexus and is formed from the L2, L3, and L4 nerve roots. This nerve enters the upper anterior thigh under the inguinal ligament (Fig. 13-2) lateral and deep to the femoral artery (which lies in the femoral sheath). Two layers of fascia, the fascia lata and fascia iliaca, lie between the skin and subcutaneous tissue and the femoral nerve (Fig. 13-3).

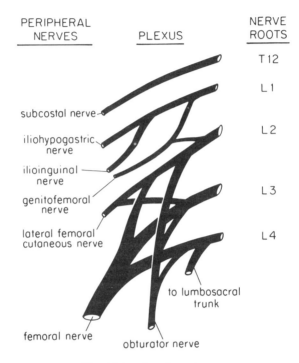

Fig. 13-1. Lumbar plexus.

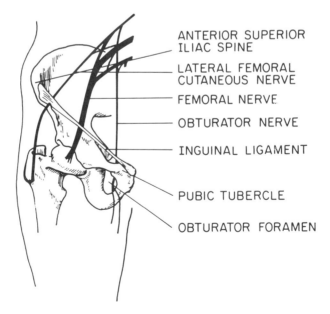

Fig. 13-2. Course of the femoral, lateral femoral cutaneous, and obturator nerves in the pelvis and thigh.

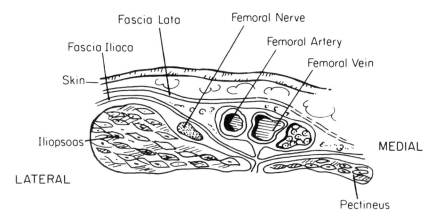

Fig. 13-3. Relationship of the femoral nerve to the femoral artery, fascia lata, and fascia iliaca.

The femoral nerve subsequently divides into anterior and posterior branches. The anterior division supplies cutaneous and deep sensory fibers to the anterior and medial thigh. Motor branches of this division supply the pectineus and sartorius muscles. The posterior division is primarily a motor nerve supplying the quadriceps femoris (rectus femoris, vastus lateralis, vastus intermedius, and vastus medialus muscles). Sensory branches arise to supply the hip and knee joints and the periosteum of the femur. The saphenous nerve, also derived from the posterior division, runs medially along the calf to the level of the ankle. The saphenous nerve innervates the skin of the medial aspect of the lower leg from the upper calf to the medial malleolus.

The lateral femoral cutaneous nerve (composed of the anterior primary divisions of L2 and L3) enters the anterior thigh medial to the anterior superior iliac spine, beneath the most lateral aspect of the inguinal ligament (Fig. 13-2). As this nerve courses toward the lateral thigh, it lies below the fascia lata. This purely sensory nerve supplies cutaneous innervation to the anterior and lateral aspects of the thigh.

Fibers from L2, L3, and L4 join to form the obturator nerve. Passing through the obturator foramen, this nerve leaves the pelvis and enters the medial aspect of the thigh (Fig. 13-2). Anterior branches of the obturator nerve supply the hip joint and skin above the knee along the medial aspect of the thigh. Motor branches arise to the adductor brevis, adductor longus, and gracilis muscles. The posterior division supplies sensory fibers to the knee joint and motor fibers to the obturator externus and adductor magnus muscles.

MECHANISM OF ACTION

Several methods have been described for obtaining a lumbar plexus block: a posterior approach at L3 (psoas sheath block),[2] a posterior approach at L4-L5 (psoas compartment block),[3,4] and the anterior approach or "3-in-1" block (inguinal paravascular technique).[1,5] Both posterior approaches require the use of a nerve stimulator, whereas the anterior approach can be performed without one. Because most postoperative patients are supine and relatively immobile, the anterior approach is the most useful.

Using an inguinal paravascular approach, the degree of completeness of lumbar plexus blockade is really a volume-mediated phenomenon. The femoral nerve itself can be easily blocked at the level of the inguinal ligament with 5–10 ml of local anesthetic solution, thereby providing pain relief after surgery of the anterior thigh and femoral shaft. As increasing volumes of local anesthetic are used, anesthetic is "pushed" proximally within the femoral sheath toward the lumbar plexus. If 20–30 ml is injected, complete lumbar plexus block is obtained. Superior analgesia is provided over the anterior, lateral, and medial aspects of the thigh, the femoral shaft, and the knee.[1]

TECHNIQUE

Inguinal Paravascular Technique

Before skin preparation and draping, the femoral pulse must be palpated 2–3 cm below the inguinal ligament. Abduction of the leg 15°–30° is often helpful in locating the pulse. The skin of the lower abdomen and upper anterior thigh should be cleansed with an alcohol or iodine-containing solution. At this point, an assistant is required to hold and aspirate the syringe containing the local anesthetic and to operate the nerve stimulator (when used). The assistant flushes a length of clear plastic tubing with the local anesthetic of choice and connects it to the needle held by the gloved operator. The type of needle chosen will depend on whether a nerve stimulator is used: a 20-gauge 5-cm intravenous needle/catheter assembly when using a stimulator, or a 20- to 22-gauge needle when a stimulator is not used. The femoral artery is again palpated and the skin is anesthetized 1 cm lateral to the point of maximal arterial pulsation. The needle is inserted lateral to the femoral artery. It is advanced in a slightly cephalad direction while carefully observing for blood return in the clear connecting tubing during repeated aspiration. If the femoral artery is entered, the needle is withdrawn and firm pressure is placed on the puncture site for 5–10 minutes.

When a nerve stimulator is not used, correct needle placement will depend on an appreciation of two distinct losses of resistance ("pops") felt when traversing the fascia lata and fascia iliaca.[5] Paresthesiae are often not obtained with this technique and are not necessary to ensure a successful block. The second "pop" will occur at approximately 2–4 cm below the skin surface at the fascia iliaca. The needle tip is then stabilized by the operator just below this fascial plane. The absence of blood return must be confirmed before injection of the local anesthetic solution and after every 5-ml aliquot. Firm pressure is held below the injection site during the instillation of local anesthetic as advocated by Winnie et al.[1] Such a maneuver is performed in order to promote proximal spread of the solution within the femoral sheath to anesthetize the lumbar plexus.

A peripheral nerve stimulator can be used to guide placement of the needle tip. The characteristics of available stimulators and needles (sheathed or unsheathed) are extensively discussed by Pither et al[6] and will not be reviewed here (see Chapter 14). Quadriceps contraction that persists at 0.7–1 mA of current is evidence of close proximity of the needle tip to the femoral nerve. At this point, 2–3 ml of local anesthetic is injected. If the quadriceps twitch diminishes over 10–15 seconds and no blood is aspirated, needle tip placement is satisfactory. Again, the local anesthetic is administered in 5-ml increments while carefully observing for blood return. If serial injections or the use of a continuous infusion are desired, a catheter can be advanced into the connective tissue sheath surrounding the femoral nerve. Femoral nerve catheters can be problematic because they frequently become dislodged from the femoral sheath with patient movement. Insertion of a catheter mandates use of a nerve stimulator.

Contraindications

There are two absolute contraindications to use of this technique: (1) burn or infection in the region of the femoral triangle, and (2) presence of a vascular graft to the femoral artery near the site of injection.

CLINICAL APPLICATIONS

The "3-in-1" block has only a limited role for intraoperative anesthesia. Even with large volumes of local anesthetic solution (0.3 ml/kg), incomplete lumbar plexus anesthesia may occur, resulting in pain in the medial and lateral aspects of the knee.[2,7] Separate obturator and lateral femoral cutaneous nerve blocks can be performed to enhance sensory anesthesia in these cases.[2,7] Additionally, the use of a thigh tourniquet will often cause discomfort during surgery because of the absence of posterior thigh anesthesia (sciatic nerve). For intraoperative anesthesia, spinal or epidural anesthesia can reliably provide excellent anesthesia of the entire lower extremity.

Femoral nerve block can relieve pain resulting from acute traumatic injuries (fractured femur)[8,9] and operations on the lower extremity (skin grafting from the upper thigh and orthopaedic procedures involving the femur)[10–12] (Table 13-1). Both pediatric and adult patients are suitable candidates.[8–10]

In patients with femoral shaft fractures, coexisting injuries may preclude the

TABLE 13-1. Indications for Femoral Nerve Block

Post-trauma analgesia	Femoral shaft fracture
Surgical anesthesia	Quadriceps muscle biopsy
	Skin graft harvest from anterior thigh
	Knee arthroscopy
Postoperative analgesia	Skin graft from anterior thigh
	Knee arthroscopy
	Knee arthrotomy and menisectomy
	Knee ligament reconstruction
	Total knee replacement

use of opioids before complete neurologic and surgical evaluation. Femoral nerve block with 1–1.5 percent lidocaine and 1/200,000 epinephrine will rapidly produce pain relief and relaxation of the quadriceps muscle. Muscle relaxation and analgesia will facilitate reduction and splinting of the femoral fracture.[4,8] Long-acting local anesthetics (2 mg/kg of 0.5 percent bupivacaine) have also been used in children with femoral fractures.[9] With bupivacaine, the onset of analgesia was 8.0 ± 3.5 minutes, and satisfactory analgesia was present 1–2 hours after injection.[9]

The most common indication for the "3-in-1" block is the treatment of pain after knee surgery (arthroscopy, arthroscopic menisectomy, ligament repair, and total knee replacement). Although analgesia after knee arthrotomy is often obtained with femoral nerve block alone, it is likewise often incomplete, because obturator, lateral femoral cutaneous, and sciatic components are missed. Analgesia after knee arthrotomy is best obtained with lumbar plexus anesthesia/analgesia.[11]

Outpatients can receive a femoral nerve block. These patients, however, must be cautioned to expect quadriceps weakness with inability to fully bear weight for several hours.

For postoperative pain relief, femoral nerve or lumbar plexus block can be performed in the operating room before patient emergence from general anesthesia or in the postanesthesia care unit after general or regional anesthesia.

For knee arthrotomy, lumbar plexus anesthesia should be achieved before commencement of continuous passive motion (CPM) of the lower limb.[12] Bupivacaine is preferred in order to enhance the duration of analgesia.[5,8,12] In a double-blind placebo-controlled study of adult patients, Tierney et al[12] observed excellent analgesia in the early postoperative period (1–2 hours) using 20 ml of 0.25 percent bupivacaine without epinephrine. However, requirement for opioid supplementation did not differ between treatment groups after 3–4 hours. Addition of epinephrine to the local anesthetic solution or the use of 0.35–0.5 percent bupivacaine will provide effective analgesia for at least 4–8 hours.[13,14] Clonidine (150 μg) has been reported to markedly enhance the duration of analgesia when added to 0.35 percent bupivacaine with or without epinephrine.[14]

Continuous administration of local anesthetic through a catheter placed in the connective tissue surrounding the femoral nerve can provide satisfactory postoperative analgesia for extended periods. After total knee replacement, patients receiving 0.25 percent bupivacaine by infusion (7–10 ml/h) had diminished pain (during the first 24 hours) and more rapid progression to complete flexion as compared with controls (receiving only intravenous patient-controlled opioids).[15] However, there was no observed difference in total opioid requirement over the first postoperative day or in pain scores reported during the second day. In this study, incomplete lumbar plexus block was apparently common.[15]

CONCLUSIONS

Further study of the role of lumbar plexus block and femoral nerve sheath catheters for pain control after knee surgery is necessary. It is important to identify patients who may derive benefit from this simple approach to lower extremity analgesia. Small amounts of parenteral or oral analgesics, in addition to blockade of the lumbar plexus or its branches, may provide quite satisfactory results in many patients.

References

1. Winnie AP, Ramamurthy S, Durrani Z: The inguinal paravascular technic of lumbar plexus anesthesia: the "3-in-1" block. Anesth Analg 52:989, 1973

2. Parkinson SK, Mueller JB, Little WL, Bailey SL: Extent of blockade with various approaches to the lumbar plexus. Anesth Analg 68:243, 1989

3. Chayen D, Nathan H, Chayen M: The psoas compartment block. Anesthesiology 45:95, 1976

4. Dalens B, Tanguy A, Vanneuville G: Lumbar plexus block in children: a comparison of two procedures in 50 patients. Anesth Analg 67:750, 1988

5. Khoo ST, Brown TC: Femoral nerve block: the anatomical basis of a single injection technique. Anaesth Intensive Care 11:40, 1983

6. Pither CE, Raj PP, Ford DJ: The use of peripheral nerve stimulators for regional anesthesia. Reg Anesth 10:49, 1985

7. Patel NJ, Flashburg MH, Paskin S, Grossman R: A regional anesthetic technique compared to general anesthesia for outpatient knee arthroscopy. Anesth Analg 65: 185, 1986

8. Berry FR: Analgesia in patients with fractured shaft of femur. Anaesthesia 32:576, 1977

9. Ronchi L, Rosenbaum D, Athouel A et al: Femoral nerve blockade in children using bupivacaine. Anesthesiology 70:622, 1989

10. McNicol LR: Lower limb blocks for children. Lateral cutaneous and femoral nerve blocks for postoperative pain relief in paediatric practice. Anaesthesia 41:27, 1986

11. Rosenblatt RM: Continuous femoral anesthesia for lower extremity surgery. Anesth Analg 59:631, 1980

12. Tierney E, Lewis G, Hurtig JB, Johnson D: Femoral nerve block with bupivacaine 0.25 percent for postoperative analgesia after open knee surgery. Can J Anaesth 34: 455, 1987

13. Bonica JJ, Buckley FP: Regional anesthesia with local anesthetics. p. 1883. In Bonica JJ (ed): The Management of Pain. 2nd Ed. Lea & Febiger, Philadelphia, 1990

14. Goldfarb G, Ang ET, Debaene B et al: Duration of analgesia after femoral nerve block with bupivacaine: effect of clonidine added to the anesthetic solution, abstracted. Anesthesiology 71:A643, 1989

15. Hord AH, Roberson JR, Thompson WF et al: Evaluation of continuous femoral nerve analgesia after primary total knee arthroplasty, abstracted. Anesth Analg 70: S164, 1990

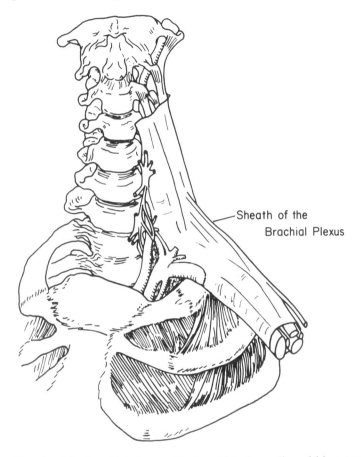

Sheath of the
Brachial Plexus

Fig. 14-1. Sheath of the brachial plexus. The brachial plexus lies within a continuous fascia-enclosed space extending from the cervical transverse processes to several centimeters beyond the axilla. All techniques for blockade of the brachial plexus involve injection and spread of local anesthetic within the fascial sheath.

analgesia may be obtained by insertion of a catheter into this perivascular fascial compartment.

The concept of "sheath anesthesia" is not universally accepted. In 1983, Thompson and Rorie[8] examined the brachial plexus sheath in cadavers using dissection and radiography and in surgical patients with computerized axial tomography. Septae were seen to form separate compartments around the individual nerves of the plexus. Such septae would limit circumferential spread of local anesthetic. Adoption of such a model would envisage the necessity for multiple injections with small volumes of local anesthetic in order to obtain successful neural blockade.[8]

Partridge et al[9] also examined the axillary sheath in cadavers and demonstrated the presence of velamentous septae forming compartments around the various structures inside the sheath. These septae were incomplete, however, and did not limit the spread of solutions injected into the compartment. Immediately after the injection of methylene blue into the axillary sheath, spread was noted around the radial, median, and ulnar nerves. Thus, the presence of septae within the axillary sheath is not a barrier to the spread of local anesthetic administered by a single injection. Multiple injections are not required to provide successful anesthesia. Similarly, these septae do not represent a barrier to the diffusion of local anesthetic as administered by a continuous catheter technique.

Indeed, the use of continuous brachial plexus blockade has been widely reported to provide prolonged surgical anesthesia and effective postoperative analgesia.[10–13] The development of long-acting local anesthetics has greatly reduced the need to use continuous brachial plexus neural blockade for surgical anesthesia. Selander,[14] however, still advocates the use of a catheter technique for surgical procedures. Selander suggested that the need to elicit paresthesiae is abolished by use of this technique. Similarly, the use of epinephrine to prolong the duration of anesthesia is superfluous. In addition, the presence of the catheter allows supplemental injections of local anesthetics when insufficient volume has resulted in incomplete anesthesia.

At the present time, however, the management of postoperative pain is the major indication for continuous brachial plexus blockade. The development of sophisticated surgical techniques for microvascular and reattachment surgery of the upper extremity has increased the demand for continuous techniques. The use of continuous techniques is particularly warranted during the postoperative period in order to provide analgesia, sympathetic blockade, and increased blood flow to the injured extremity.

ANATOMY

The brachial plexus (Figs. 14-2 and 14-3) is formed by the anterior rami of the lower four cervical spinal nerves (C5–C8) and the first thoracic spinal nerve (T1). The plexus receives contributions from C4 in approximately two-thirds of patients and from T2 in more than one-third. The roots emerge from the vertebral foraminae and pass behind the vertebral artery and across the transverse processes of the corresponding cervical vertebrae (Fig. 14-2). After leaving the transverse processes, the roots are directed toward the first rib and join to form the three trunks (Figs. 14-2 and 14-3). The fifth and sixth cervical roots form the superior trunk; the seventh cervical nerve continues as the middle trunk; and finally, the lower trunk is formed by the union of the eighth cervical and the first thoracic nerves (Fig. 14-3).

The trunks pass under the clavicle and over the first rib, and each trunk divides into an anterior and posterior division. As they pass the rib, the divisions join again to form the three cords of the plexus (Fig. 14-3). The lateral cord is formed by the anterior divisions of the superior and middle trunks; the medial cord is the continuation of the anterior division of the lower trunk, and the posterior cord is formed by the union of the three posterior divisions (Table 14-1).

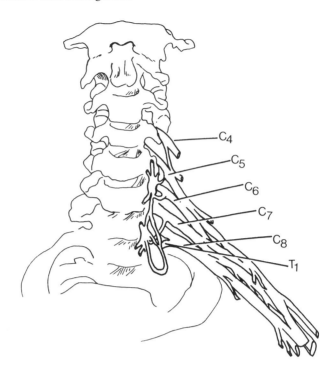

Fig. 14-2. Anatomic diagram of the origin and formation of the brachial plexus.

The cords give off the terminal nerves of the brachial plexus (Table 14-2). The lateral and medial cords give off the lateral and medial heads of the median nerve (Fig. 14-3). These cords then continue as major terminal nerves. The lateral cord becomes the musculocutaneous nerve. The medial cord continues as the ulnar nerve. The posterior cord gives off the axillary nerve and then becomes the radial nerve.

TABLE 14-1. Derivation of the Three Cords of the Brachial Plexus

Lateral cord—anterior divisions of superior and medial trunks (C5–C7)
Medial cord—anterior division of lower trunk (C8–T1)
Posterior cord—posterior divisions of the three trunks (C5–C8–T1)

TABLE 14-2. Terminal Nerves of the Brachial Plexus
(Five Major Nerves)

Lateral cord	(1) Musculocutaneous nerve	
	(2) Lateral head of median nerve	Median nerve
Medial cord	Medial head of median nerve	
	(3) Ulnar nerve	
Posterior cord	(4) Axillary nerve	
	(5) Radial nerve	

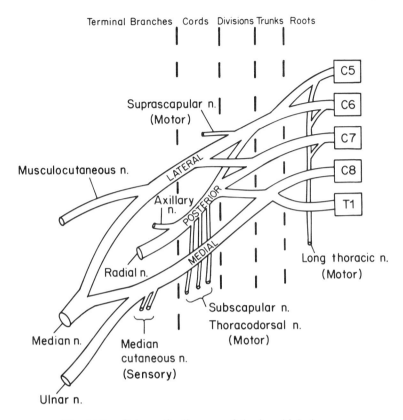

Fig. 14-3. Schematic diagram of the brachial plexus.

Numerous smaller nerves arise from the brachial plexus. With the exception of the suprascapular nerve (C5-C6), which supplies sensory branches to the shoulder joint, all the branches arising from the brachial plexus above the clavicle are motor branches.

Sympathetic Innervation of the Upper Extremity

In addition to knowledge of the formation and distribution of the somatic nerves of the upper extremity (brachial plexus), it is important to understand the sympathetic innervation of the upper extremity. The reader is referred to Chapter 3 for an introduction to the anatomy of the sympathetic nervous system.

The preganglionic sympathetic neurons contributing to the brachial plexus lie within the intermediolateral gray matter of the spinal cord. Segmental contributions arise from as far cephalad as T2 (occasionally from T1) and may extend as far caudad as T8-T9.

Postganglionic contributions to the brachial plexus arise from the inferior cervical ganglion but more commonly from the stellate ganglion (see Ch. 3). Postganglionic sympathetic fibers may also reach the central roots of the brachial plexus from the sympathetic plexus associated with the vertebral artery. After entering the roots, sympathetic fibers travel along with the somatic fibers as they form the trunks, divisions, cords, and terminal nerves of the plexus.

There are two distinct pathways by which sympathetic fibers reach the upper extremity. (1) Sympathetic fibers are carried to peripheral vessels via the somatic nerves of the plexus as described above. Sympathetic vasoconstrictor fibers are then distributed to the distal arterial system of the extremity.[15] (2) More proximally, sympathetic innervation arises from the cervical sympathetic chain and passes directly to the subclavian artery. This sympathetic plexus continues around the vessel and into the arm along the axillary artery. This periarterial sympathetic innervation does not extend beyond the brachial artery.

TECHNIQUE

Continuous brachial plexus catheter techniques can be performed by any of the approaches routinely used for brachial plexus anesthesia. Only the axillary and infraclavicular approaches will be discussed in detail, as these have the greatest applicability for the management of postoperative pain. If the reader requires basic information regarding any of the approaches to brachial plexus anesthesia and analgesia, Winnie's[15] classic text should be consulted.

Continuous brachial plexus catheter techniques can be performed by any of the approaches routinely used for brachial plexus anesthesia. Over-the-needle catheters and catheter-through-needle techniques have been successfully used. Two important considerations common to all approaches merit emphasis: (1) use of a nerve stimulator is mandatory in order to properly identify the plexus, and (2) the fascial sheath must be distended by injection of saline or local anesthetic before advancement of the catheter.

Procedure

Axillary Approach

The axillary approach to continuous brachial plexus blockade is performed after the technique described by Winnie.[15] With the arm at 90° or less, the axillary artery is palpated, and the neurovascular bundle is fixed and occluded distally by the palpating finger (Fig. 14-4). A skin wheal of local anesthetic is raised if a large or blunt needle is to be used. When a blunt needle or an epidural needle is used, the skin should be "nipped" with a sharp 18-gauge needle. Using a blunt needle will facilitate identification of the axillary sheath, as a more characteristic "pop" is appreciated on piercing the sheath (see below).

Continuous brachial plexus anesthesia/analgesia is usually accomplished using commercially available intravenous catheters. The metal introducer of

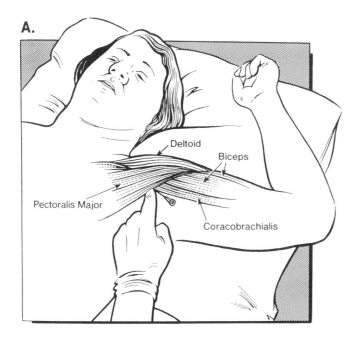

A.

Deltoid

Biceps

Pectoralis Major

Coracobrachialis

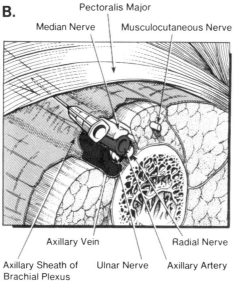

B.

Pectoralis Major

Median Nerve   Musculocutaneous Nerve

Axillary Vein   Radial Nerve

Axillary Sheath of   Ulnar Nerve   Axillary Artery
Brachial Plexus

Fig. 14-4. Axillary approach to the brachial plexus. **(A)** The forefinger palpates the axillary artery, and the needle is inserted tangentially or parallel to the axillary artery. Needle insertion is adjacent to the coracobrachialis and pectoralis major muscles, immediately superior to the tip of the forefinger. A characteristic "click" or "pop" is felt on entrance into the fascial sheath. However, flexion of the fingers with use of the nerve stimulator is the true definitive end point. **(B)** After distention of the sheath with 30–40 ml of local anesthetic, the catheter is advanced into the fascial sheath in much the same way as insertion of an intravenous catheter. (From Bridenbaugh,[31] with permission.)

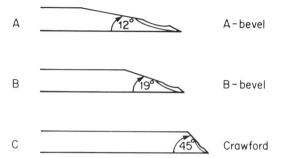

Fig. 14-5. Three types of needle bevels. (**A**) The needle of the typical intravenous catheter has a long sharp bevel (A-bevel). Long bevel needles may be associated with a greater frequency of nerve trauma. (**B**) Bevel of the typical "block needle" or "B-bevel" needle. Its shorter bevel theoretically protects against nerve trauma. (**C**) Bevel of the Crawford point needle. This bevel is short and blunt but only available in the United States with the Crawford epidural needle. Its lack of availability has resulted in the great popularity of B-bevel needles for single injection neural blockade techniques. The ease of insertion of the over-the-needle catheter of the A-bevel needle has lead to its adoption for continuous brachial plexus catheter techniques.

the common intravenous over-the-needle catheter has a sharp long bevel (Fig. 14-5). Long bevel needles may be associated with a greater incidence of neural trauma as compared with short bevel or blunt needles. In addition, penetration of a blood vessel would be easier with this type of needle tip. Hence, this needle must be used carefully.

Insertion of the needle tangentially or parallel to the axillary artery is recommended, and use of a nerve stimulator is mandatory. To provide metal contact with the nerve stimulator, the stylet of a 26-gauge spinal needle is inserted between the plastic cannula and the metal introducer of the typical intravenous over-the-needle catheter[16] (Fig. 14-6). It is preferable to wrap the stylet around the metal introducer several times. An alligator clip is attached to the stylet at one end and to the active electrode of a nerve stimulator at the other end. Over-the-needle catheters with blunt-tipped introducers are available, as mentioned before. These possess a metal hub through which electric contact to the nerve stimulator can be established.

The nerve stimulator is used as described by Raj et al[17] and Galindo.[18] Needle entry into the brachial plexus sheath is denoted by flexion of the fingers at the lowest electric output. Penetration of the fascial sheath is appreciated as a characteristic "pop." However, only flexion of the fingers as elicited by the nerve stimulator should be used as the definitive end point. Two milliliters of local anesthetic are then injected. The muscular response to stimulation (flexion) should be abolished within 30 seconds. The needle with the catheter must then be advanced approximately 0.5 cm to ensure that the catheter has penetrated the sheath. A total volume of 30–40 ml of local anesthetic is injected, with frequent aspiration. After distention of the axillary sheath, the catheter is then inserted in the same way as an intravenous catheter. If verification of the

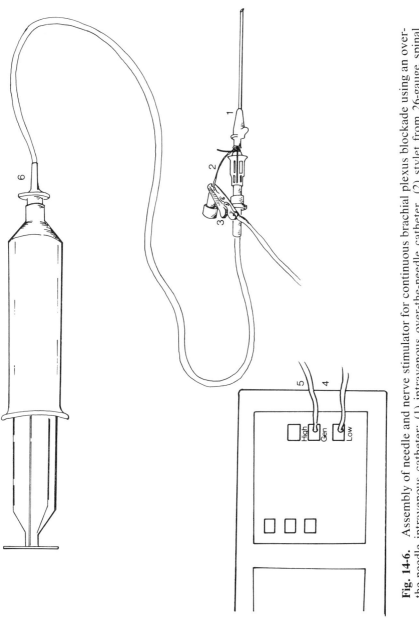

Fig. 14-6. Assembly of needle and nerve stimulator for continuous brachial plexus blockade using an over-the-needle intravenous catheter: (1) intravenous over-the-needle catheter, (2) stylet from 26-gauge spinal needle, (3) alligator clip attached to the stylet and to the low-output terminal of a nerve stimulator, (4) nerve stimulator, (5) ground wire attached to the common port of the nerve stimulator (marked as "Gen" in the diagram) and to the patient, and (6) extension set and syringe for "immobile needle technique."

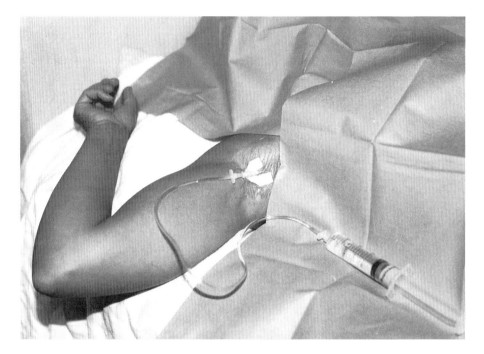

Fig. 14-7. Catheter technique by the axillary approach. An 18-gauge intravenous catheter is sutured and taped securely in place with an adhesive sterile plastic bandage.

catheter position is desired, this could be easily achieved by inserting an arterial line wire (Arrow, Duoflex Spring wire) through the catheter and stimulating at a higher output. The corresponding muscular response should be obtained again.

Once the catheter is in place, two options are available: (1) the catheter can be sutured in place, and an adhesive sterile plastic bandage applied (an extension set is attached for intermittent injection or continuous infusion) (Fig. 14-7), or (2) if an 18-gauge intravenous catheter has been used, a disposable epidural catheter can be inserted through the intravenous catheter. The epidural catheter can then be secured in place.

Several authors have reported variations of the technique as described here for the axillary approach to continuous brachial plexus analgesia.[11,13,14,19,20]

Interscalene Approach

Variations of this approach have been reported by Manriquez and Pallares,[12] Winnie,[21] Rosenblatt and Cress,[22] and Vatashsky and Aronson.[23] It may be difficult to advance a catheter using the interscalene approach, as the needle approaches the brachial plexus perpendicularly (Fig. 14-8). The needle—and, hence, the catheter—will be perpendicular to the neural bundle rather than directed alongside the plexus, making advancement of the catheter problematic.

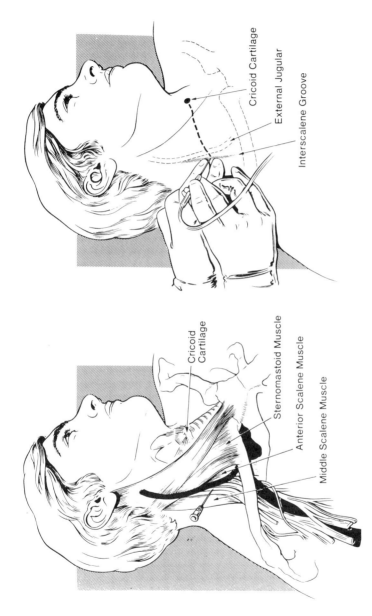

Cricoid Cartilage

External Jugular

Interscalene Groove

Cricoid Cartilage

Sternomastoid Muscle

Anterior Scalene Muscle

Middle Scalene Muscle

Fig. 14-8. Interscalene approach to brachial plexus blockade. The interscalene groove is palpated by rolling the fingers back from the border of the clavicular head of the sternocleidomastoid muscle (at the level of the cricoid cartilage) and over the belly of the anterior scalene muscle to the groove. The needle is inserted into the interscalene groove at the level of the cricoid cartilage. The direction of the needle is mainly inward, 45° caudad and slightly backward. (From Bridenbaugh,[31] with permission.)

A modified Seldinger technique was developed by Rosenblatt and Cress to address this difficulty.[22] The authors localized the brachial plexus with the aid of a nerve stimulator and a 25-gauge needle. The 25-gauge needle was removed and an 18-gauge epidural needle was then inserted. The brachial plexus was again identified with the aid of the nerve stimulator. The sheath was distended with 40 ml of local anesthetic. A guide wire was then introduced through the epidural needle 4 cm distally. Finally, an 18-gauge epidural catheter was inserted, and the wire removed.

Subclavian Perivascular Approach

The subclavian perivascular technique is best performed as described by Winnie and Colins[24] (Fig. 14-9). In this technique, the needle is inserted into the neck musculature approximately 2.5 cm cephalad to the clavicle and advanced directly caudad. To insert a catheter, the needle is inserted higher, in the middle of the interscalene grove. The needle is subsequently directed caudally and laterally, facilitating the catheter insertion along the long axis of the plexus. After distention of the sheath, the catheter is advanced as described in the axillary technique.

Infraclavicular Approach

Dislodgement of catheters because of upper limb mobilization is a frequent problem common to the various approaches of catheter insertion. Advancing the catheter a distance of 5 cm or more into the neurovascular sheath and securing with sutures and adhesive plastic dressing may decrease the frequency of dislodgement. The most common reason for dislodgement of an axillary catheter is motion of the arm. Movement of both the head and arm cause dislodgement when the interscalene or subclavian perivascular routes are used. The best technique to ensure catheter stability is use of the infraclavicular approach for continuous brachial plexus anesthesia/analgesia.

The infraclavicular approach for brachial plexus block was originally described by Brazy et al[25] in 1917. In 1973, Raj et al[26] described a modified infraclavicular approach. In this technique, the patient lies supine with the arm to be blocked abducted at 90° (Fig. 14-10). The head is turned to the opposite side. The clavicle is palpated in its entire length, and the midclavicular point is identified. The point of needle insertion will be 2–2.5 cm below the middle of the clavicle. If a line is drawn from this point to the point where the axillary artery is palpated, this line will closely represent the trajectory of the brachial plexus (Figs. 14-10 and 14-11). A skin wheal of local anesthetic is raised at the point of needle entry.

Raj et al recommended using a 22-gauge 9-cm unsheathed spinal needle. An over-the-needle 5¼-in. catheter may be preferable. As with all continuous techniques, a nerve stimulator is used to identify the plexus. An over-the-needle catheter is itself a sheath, so the tip of the needle becomes a stimulating elec-

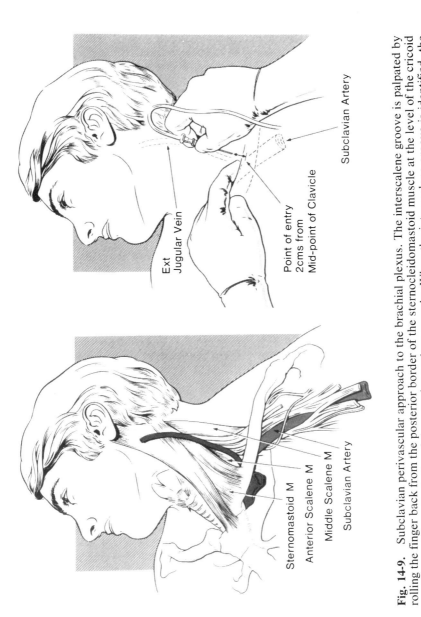

Ext
Jugular Vein

Point of entry
2cms from
Mid-point of Clavicle

Subclavian Artery

Sternomastoid M

Anterior Scalene M

Middle Scalene M

Subclavian Artery

Fig. 14-9. Subclavian perivascular approach to the brachial plexus. The interscalene groove is palpated by rolling the finger back from the posterior border of the sternocleidomastoid muscle at the level of the cricoid cartilage and over the belly of the anterior scalene muscle. When the interscalene groove is identified, the finger is moved inferiorly along the groove as far as possible. The needle is then inserted just above the palpating finger and advanced in a directly caudad direction. (From Bridenbaugh,[31] with permission.)

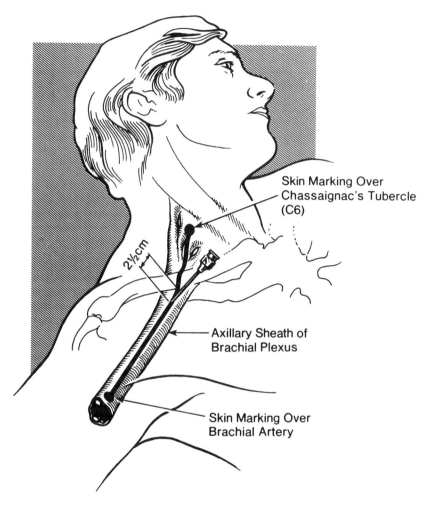

Fig. 14-10. Schematic diagram of the landmarks for infraclavicular brachial plexus block. (From Bridenbaugh,[31] with permission.)

trode. The metallic shaft of the needle is thereby protected (sheathed) and will not cause extraneous muscle contractions.

After injection of local anesthetic into the neurovascular space, the over-the-needle catheter is then simply advanced in the same fashion as an intravenous catheter. It is important not to advance the catheter too far down into the lower part of the axilla. This may lead to incomplete anesthesia or analgesia.

As with any other approach, puncture of blood vessels may occur. Pneumothorax should not occur, as the needle moves laterally, away from the lung and pleura.

Regardless of the approach, the catheter should be sutured in place. Betadine ointment and a sterile plastic adhesive dressing should then be applied (Fig. 14-

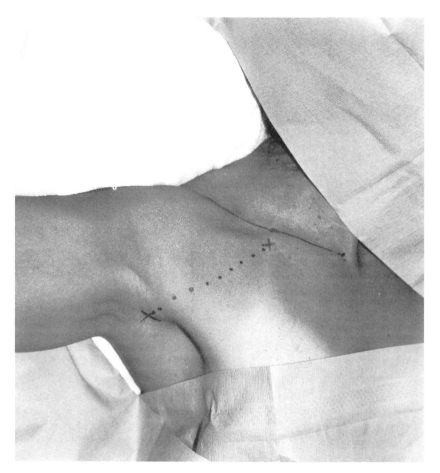

Fig. 14-11. Landmarks for the infraclavicular approach to brachial plexus blockade as seen in a model. The middle of the clavicle is identified and marked. The point of needle insertion will be 2–2.5 cm below the middle of the clavicle. A line representing the direction of needle advancement is drawn from the point of needle insertion to the spot where the axillary artery can first be palpated.

12). An extension set is attached to the catheter and subsequently to an infusion pump, if desired.

Choice and Dosing of Local Anesthetic

Once brachial plexus blockade has been established, continuous analgesia and sympathectomy can be provided by intermittent injections or by continuous infusion. Intermittent injections of 20–30 ml of 0.25 percent or 0.5 percent bupivacaine every 4–6 hours have been reported to provide satisfactory analgesia and successful sympathetic blockade for several days.[12,13] However, a con-

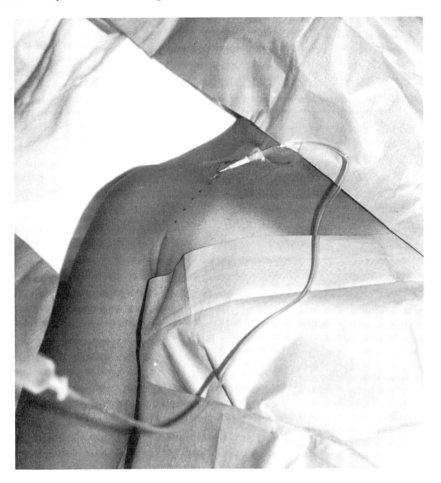

Fig. 14-12. Catheter position after infraclavicular brachial plexus block. The catheter is sutured and secured in place with sterile transparent dressing. An extension set is attached to the catheter.

tinuous infusion of local anesthetic is the method of choice for production of analgesia and sympathetic block. In addition to providing constant and consistent analgesia, it has an added advantage as the infusion system will have to be manipulated (changed) once a day at most. This may minimize the potential for contamination and drug administration errors, which may occur with repeated injections.

The optimal dose of local anesthetic for continuous infusion has not been definitively determined. Protocols for continuous brachial plexus infusion are derived from a number of case reports and small studies (Table 14-3). Haynsworth et al[13] used an initial infusion of 0.125 percent bupivacaine at 5 ml/h. The infusion rate was gradually increased to 7–10 ml/h, and the bupivacaine concentration was increased to 0.25 percent in order to provide satisfac-

TABLE 14-3. Mode of Injection and Dosage of Brachial Plexus Catheters

Author	Approach	Intermittent	Continuous	Bupivacaine (%)	Infusion Rate
Tuominen et al[10]	Axillary		√	0.25	10 ml/h
Gaumann et al[11]	Axillary		√	0.125	7 ml/h
Manriquez and Pallares[12]	Interscalene	√			20 ml q 3 h
Haynsworth et al[13]	Axillary		√	0.125[a]	5 ml/h[a]
				0.25	7–10 ml/h
Rosenblatt et al[19]	Axillary		√	0.25	10 ml/h
Sada et al[20]	Axillary	√		0.5	10 ml q 3 h
Rosenblatt and Cress[22]	Interscalene		√	0.25	10 ml/h

[a] Satisfactory analgesia and sympathectomy were not achieved with 0.125% bupivacaine, necessitating use of a higher concentration at greater infusion rates.

tory analgesia and sympathectomy. Rosenblatt and Cress[19,22] reported the use of continuous infusions through the interscalene and axillary approaches. With both approaches, 0.25 percent bupivacaine at 10 ml/h produced satisfactory results. At Brigham and Women's Hospital, it is our experience that an infusion of 0.25 percent bupivacaine at rates of 8–12 ml/h will result in excellent analgesia and sympathectomy. Use of this concentration and infusion rate, however, may affect motor function of the arm.

Indwelling brachial plexus catheters have remained in place for as short a period as 17 hours[10] to as long as 11.5 days.[12] There are no reports in the literature of local or systemic infection associated with the use of continuous brachial plexus catheters. A number of studies have reported the results of culture of the catheter tip after its removal.[10–13] A direct relation between duration of use and culture positivity has not been established.

CLINICAL APPLICATIONS

Continuous brachial plexus blockade is often used to provide analgesia and sympathectomy and to improve blood flow when vascular insufficiency occurs. It has been used to treat vascular insufficiency caused by intravascular injection of drugs,[12,13] traumatic hand or digit amputation,[19] and prolonged and extensive upper extremity surgery.[10,20,27] In addition, continuous brachial plexus blockade can be used in the treatment of early reflex sympathetic dystrophy. This technique can be used in all age groups including children.

Uninterrupted analgesia through continuous neural blockade may have significant and beneficial psychological effects in patients with traumatic injuries. Postoperative anxiety can potentiate pain.[28] The uniform analgesia and anesthesia produced by a continuous technique will prevent anxiety. This would be particularly significant in patients with traumatic injuries, whose sense of body image may now be altered. Rosenblatt et al's report of traumatic hand injury in a 15-year-old carpenter's apprentice clearly demonstrates the physical and psychological benefits of this technique.[19]

COMPLICATIONS

Complications similar to those associated with traditional brachial plexus block can be expected. The following discussion therefore focuses on potential complications more specific to use of the continuous technique.

Local Anesthetic Toxicity

Several authors have reported the plasma concentrations of bupivacaine attendant to continuous brachial plexus infusions. Haynsworth et al[13] measured plasma concentrations of local anesthetic on the eighth, ninth, and tenth days of a continuous infusion of 0.125 percent bupivacaine. The levels reported were 0.24, 0.40, and 0.54 μg/ml, respectively. (Such concentrations are well below the toxic level of 4 μg/ml for bupivacaine.) Other studies, however, reported significantly greater plasma levels during continuous infusions. Whereas Tuominen et al[10] reported a mean level of 1.03 μ/ml after only 16 hours of infusion, Rosenblatt et al[19] reported a gradual increase in plasma concentrations over time, with bupivacaine concentrations greater than 1 μg/ml after 48 hours. Both authors infused 0.25 percent bupivacaine at a rate of 10 ml/h. Thus, systemic drug accumulation may occur when the rate of infusion exceeds the clearance of local anesthetic by metabolism and excretion. Potential systemic toxicity must be considered if long-term continuous infusions are to be used.

Nerve Damage

The effects of prolonged exposure of peripheral nerves to local anesthetics are unknown, although several studies have looked at the potential neurotoxicity of local anesthetics.

Barsa et al[29] investigated the neurotoxicity of several local anesthetics. The carotid sheaths of rabbits (containing the vagus nerve) were exposed and completely submerged in differing local anesthetic solutions for approximately 45–55 minutes. Exposure to 3 percent 2-chloroprocaine produced pinpoint petechiae in surrounding tissues. Such changes appeared early during treatment and gradually increased in size. These hemorrhages also occurred with 2-chloroprocaine when the pH was neutralized to 6.8–7.2 or when a mixture of 1.5 percent 2-chloroprocaine and 0.375 percent bupivacaine was used. Addition of epinephrine enhanced the production of petechiae. These changes suggest an effect on blood vessels and/or red cells. Pinpoint hemorrhages were not observed with the other local anesthetics studied (2 percent lidocaine and 0.75 percent bupivacaine).

Nerve conduction and histopathologic studies were then carried out 10–12 days after exposure to local anestics. C-fiber conduction was absent or impaired in most preparations treated with 3 percent 2-chloroprocaine. Nerves treated with either lidocaine or bupivacaine showed normal impulse conduction. In addition, histologic studies revealed marked epineural and perineural fibrosis and axonal degeneration in nerves exposed to 2-chloroprocaine. These histologic abnormalities were absent or insignificant in nerves exposed to lidocaine or bupivacaine.

Myers et al[30] used the rat sciatic nerve to study the potential neurotoxicity of local anesthetics applied to an intact nerve bundle. The effects of 3 percent 2-chloroprocaine, 1 percent tetracaine, 2 percent lidocaine, and 0.75 percent bupivacaine were studied. The direct application of 2-chloroprocaine and tetracaine to the sciatic nerve produced endoneurial edema, resulting in an increased endoneurial pressure. Perineural permeability was also increased by these two local anesthetics. In addition, endoneurial fibrosis, Schwann cell injury, and axonal dystrophy were also significant. The edema produced by tetracaine and 2-chloroprocaine was present in all parts of the nerve. Lidocaine and bupivacaine resulted in occasional edema, limited to some parts of the nerve. The edema produced by the two amino-ester local anesthetics was significantly greater than that produced by the two amino-amide agents.

Both studies suggested that clinically used local anesthetics can produce neurotoxic injury. The results of these two investigations suggested that amino-ester local anesthetics may be significantly more neurotoxic than amino-amide agents.

CONCLUSION

In summary, continuous brachial plexus blockade is a valuable technique for prolonged surgery of the upper extremity, provision of continuous postoperative analgesia, and production of sympathectomy leading to increased blood flow of the upper extremity.

Bupivacaine in concentrations of 0.125–0.25 percent is recommended for continuous infusion at a rate of 7–10 ml/h. The maximum safe duration of use of an indwelling brachial plexus catheter without fear of infection is undetermined.

Finally, although the technique has been described for many years, its use has been only sporadically reported. In recent years, continuous brachial plexus anesthesia/analgesia has become more widely used. Further studies are needed on the relation between infusion rate and local anesthetic plasma levels, duration of safe treatment without fear of infection, and the long-term effects of local anesthetic infusions on peripheral nerves.

ACKNOWLEDGMENTS

The author thanks Ellen M. Silvius, R.N., for her photographic services.

References
1. Koller C: On the use of cocaine for producing anesthesia of the eye. Lancet ii:990, 1884
2. Halsted WS: Surgical Papers, by William Steward Halstead. Vol. 1. Johns Hopkins Press, Baltimore, 1925

3. Kulenkampff D: Anesthesia of the brachial plexus (German). Zentralbl Chir 38:1337, 1911

4. Hirschel G: Anesthesia of the brachial plexus for operations on the upper extremity (German). Munchen Med Wochenschr 58:1555, 1911

5. Etienne J: Regional anesthesia: its application in the surgical treatment of cancer of the breast (French). Doctoral Thesis, Faculte de Medicine de Paris, 1925

6. Ansbro FP: Method of continuous brachial plexus block. Am J Surg 71:716, 1946

7. Winnie AP, Radonjic R, Akkineni SR, Durrani Z: Factors influencing distribution of local anesthetic injected into the brachial plexus sheath. Anesth Analg 58:225, 1979

8. Thompson GE, Rorie DK: Functional anatomy of the brachial plexis sheaths. Anesthesiology 59:117, 1983

9. Partridge BL, Katz J, Benirschke K: Functional anatomy of the brachial plexus sheath: implications for anesthesia. Anesthesiology 66:743, 1987

10. Tuominen M, Rosenberg PH, Kalso E: Blood levels of bupivacaine after single dose, supplementary dose and during continuous infusion in axillary plexus block. Acta Anaesthesiol Scand 27:303, 1983

11. Gaumann DM, Lennon RL, Wedel DJ: Continuous axillary block for postoperative pain management. Reg Anesth 13:77, 1988

12. Manriquez RG, Pallares V: Continuous brachial plexus block for prolonged sympathectomy and control of pain. Anesth Analg 57:128, 1978

13. Haynsworth RF, Heavner JE, Racz GB: Continuous brachial plexus blockade using an axillary catheter for treatment of accidental intra-arterial injections. Reg Anesth 10:187, 1985

14. Selander D: Catheter technique in axillary plexus block. Presentation of a new method. Acta Anaesthesiol Scand 21:324, 1977

15. Winnie AP: Plexus Anesthesia. Perivascular Techniques of Brachial Plexus Block. WB Saunders, Philadelphia, 1983

16. Hymes JA: A simple, inexpensive needle assembly for peripheral nerve stimulation and neural blockade. Anesthesiology 10:197, 1985

17. Raj P, Rosenblatt R, Montgomergy SJ: Use of the nerve stimulator for peripheral blocks. Reg Anesth 5:14, 1980

18. Galindo A: Electrical localization of peripheral nerves: instrumentation and clinical experience, abstracted. Reg Anesth 8:49, 1983

19. Rosenblatt R, Pepitone-Rockwell F, McKillop MJ: Continuous axillary analgesia for traumatic hand injury. Anesthesiology 51:565, 1979

20. Sada T, Kobayashi T, Murakami S: Continuous axillary brachial plexus block. Can Anaesth Soc J 30:201, 1983

21. Winnie AP: Interscalene brachial plexus block. Anesth Analg 49:455, 1970

22. Rosenblatt RM, Cress JC: Modified Seldinger technique for continuous interscalene brachial plexus block. Reg Anesth 6:82, 1981

23. Vatashsky E, Aronson HB: Continuous interscalene brachial plexus block for surgical operations on the hand (letter). Anesthesiology 53:356, 1980

24. Winnie AP, Colins VG: The subclavian perivascular technique of brachial plexus anesthesia. Anesthesiology 25:353, 1964

25. Bazy L, Pauchet V, Sourdat P, Laboure J: Anesthie Regionale. WB Saunders, Philadelphia, 1917

26. Raj P, Montgomergy SJ, Nettles D, Jenkins MT: Infraclavicular brachial plexus block—a new approach. Anesth Analg 52:897, 1973

27. DeKrey JA, Schroeder CF, Buechel DR: Continuous brachial plexus block. Anesthesiology 30:332, 1969

28. Chapman CR, Cox GB: Determinants of Anxiety in Elective Surgery Patients. In Spielberger CB (ed): Stress and Anxiety. Vol. 4. John Wiley and Sons, New York, 1978
29. Barsa J, Batra M, Fink BR, Sumi SM: A comparative in vivo study of local neurotoxicity of lidocaine, bupivacaine, 2-chloroprocaine, and a mixture of 2-chloroprocaine and bupivacaine. Anesth Analg 61:961, 1982
30. Myers RR, Kalichman MW, Reisner LS, Powell HC: Neurotoxicity of local anesthetics: altered perineurial permeability, edema, and nerve fiber injury. Anesthesiology 64:29, 1986
31. Bridenbaugh LD: The upper extremity: somatic blockade. p. 387. In Cousins MJ, Bridenbaugh PO (eds): Neural Blockade in Clinical Anesthesia and Management of Pain. 2nd Ed. JB Lippincott, Philadelphia, 1988

15

Continuous Intercostal Nerve Block

Vincent W. S. Chan

Conventional intercostal nerve block [the injection of 3–5 ml of local anesthetic into individual intercostal spaces at multiple levels (Fig. 15-1)] is highly effective in the treatment of somatic pain involving the chest and abdominal walls.[1-4] The associated beneficial effects on pulmonary function are well documented.[5-9] However, the use of conventional intercostal nerve block is limited by the relatively short duration of local anesthetic effect. To achieve long-lasting analgesia, repetitive procedures are necessary. Each series of injections is accompanied by the discomfort of multiple needle insertions and the repeated risk of pneumothorax.

To overcome these problems, the technique of continuous intercostal nerve block was introduced by O'Kelly and Garry[10] in 1981. Repeated injection of a large volume of local anesthetic (10–20 ml) through an indwelling catheter located in a single intercostal space can provide continuous analgesia over a large number of thoracic dermatomes. Despite its effectiveness in treating pain of the chest and abdominal walls, continuous intercostal nerve block has unfortunately, and undeservedly, remained unpopular.

ANATOMY

Of the 31 pairs of spinal nerves leaving the vertebral canal through the intervertebral foraminae, 12 emerge at the thoracic level with the corresponding ribs. Each thoracic spinal nerve is formed by the union of two roots: a ganglion-containing dorsal root carrying sensory afferent fibers and a ventral root carry-

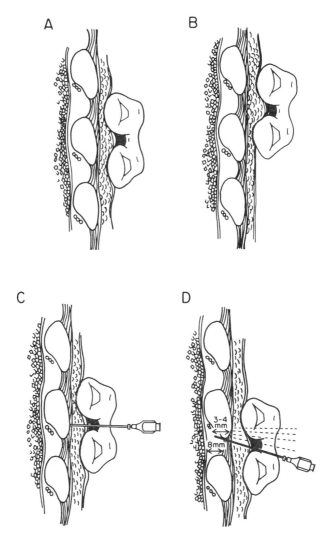

Fig. 15-1. Conventional intercostal nerve block. Rigorous technical discipline during performance of conventional intercostal nerve block will lower the incidence of pneumothorax. Injections are performed at the angle of the rib as the anteroposterior width of the intercostal space is largest at this site (approximately 8 mm). (**A**) Two fingers are initially placed in adjacent intercostal spaces, straddling the rib. (**B**) The skin of the inferior intercostal space is pulled cephalad, and the rib is palpated beneath the inferior finger. (**C**) A small-gauge needle is inserted onto the rib. (**D**) The needle is withdrawn, and tension on the skin is lessened. The needle is repetitively withdrawn and reinserted, using the rib as a landmark. With each withdrawal of the needle, tension on the skin is further reduced. Gradually, the inferior finger will be seen to move back toward its original position. Eventually, the needle will "walk off" the inferior border of the rib. At this point it should be advanced 3–4 mm, and injection of local anesthetic should be performed. Unlike the continuous intercostal technique, multiple needle insertions will be necessary to achieve a band of sensory anesthesia.

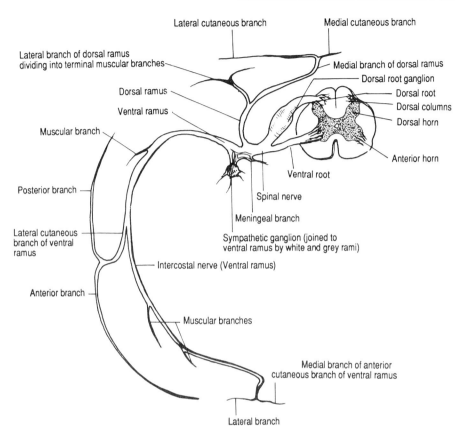

Lateral cutaneous branch

Medial cutaneous branch

Lateral branch of dorsal ramus
dividing into terminal muscular branches

Medial branch of dorsal ramus

Dorsal root ganglion

Dorsal ramus

Dorsal root

Ventral ramus

Dorsal columns

Dorsal horn

Muscular branch

Anterior horn

Posterior branch

Ventral root

Spinal nerve

Meningeal branch

Lateral cutaneous
branch of ventral
ramus

Sympathetic ganglion (joined to
ventral ramus by white and grey rami)

Intercostal nerve (Ventral ramus)

Anterior branch

Muscular branches

Medial branch of anterior
cutaneous branch of ventral ramus

Lateral branch

Fig. 15-2. Origin and distribution of a typical spinal nerve.

ing motor efferent fibers (Fig. 15-2). Each spinal nerve divides into two rami in the paravertebral space. An anatomic description of the paravertebral space may be found in Figure 15-3. The dorsal ramus sends off cutaneous and muscular branches to innervate axial muscles (e.g., erector spinae), the scapula, and the skin of the back (Fig. 15-2). At the origin of each ventral ramus, preganglionic sympathetic fibers leave as the white ramus communicantes to enter the thoracic sympathetic trunk (Fig. 15-2). Postganglionic fibers return as the gray ramus communicantes. The thoracic ventral ramus subsequently courses anteriorly along the inferior border of the corresponding rib, innervating the skin and muscles of the chest wall.

Intercostal nerves are, in actuality, the 12 thoracic ventral rami. The twelfth intercostal nerve lies below the twelfth rib and is sometimes (and more appropriately) called the subcostal nerve. The intercostal nerves supply postganglionic sympathetic innervation as well as sensory and motor innervation to most parts of the chest and abdominal walls.

The intercostal nerves lie in the subcostal grooves of the corresponding ribs along with the intercostal vessels (artery and vein), sandwiched between muscle layers (Figs. 15-4 and 15-5). Each intercostal nerve gives off cutaneous and muscular branches. The two major cutaneous branches are: (1) the anterior cutaneous branch, supplying the thoracic and abdominal walls anteriorly in the midline (Fig. 15-4), and (2) the lateral cutaneous branch (originating at the midaxillary region), which subdivides into anterior and posterior branches to innervate most of the chest and abdominal walls. The cutaneous branches of the ventral ramus, together with those of the dorsal ramus at the corresponding level, provide segmental innervation to an entire skin strip in the form of a dermatome.

In clinical practice, it is important to recognize that blockade of an intercostal nerve is complete only if it is performed proximal to the origin of the lateral cutaneous branch (e.g., at the angle of the rib). As there is extensive collateral linkage among intercostal nerves, total sensory anesthesia along a single dermatome can only be achieved when the two other adjacent intercostal nerves

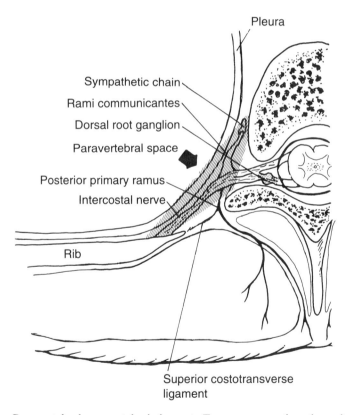

Fig. 15-3. Paravertebral space *(shaded area)*. Transverse section through a typical thoracic vertebra. The paravertebral space is a triangular-shaped space. The posterior wall is formed by the superior costotransverse ligament, running from the lower border of the transverse process above to the upper border of the rib below. Anterolaterally the space is defined by the parietal pleura. The medial wall is formed by the posterolateral aspect of the vertebral body and the intervertebral foramen and its contents.

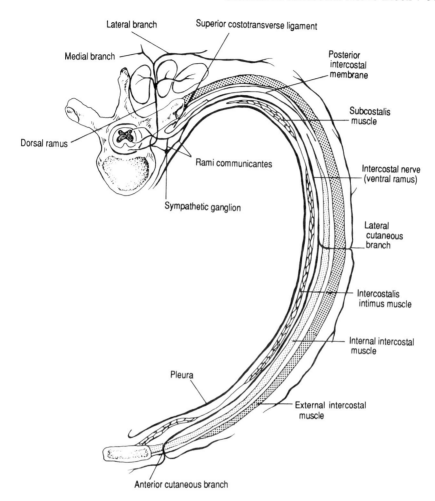

Lateral branch

Superior costotransverse ligament

Medial branch

Posterior
intercostal
membrane

Dorsal ramus

Subcostalis
muscle

Rami communicantes

Intercostal nerve
(ventral ramus)

Sympathetic ganglion

Lateral
cutaneous
branch

Intercostalis
intimus muscle

Internal intercostal
muscle

Pleura

External intercostal
muscle

Anterior cutaneous branch

Fig. 15-4. Course of a typical intercostal nerve. Muscular and the collateral branches are not shown. Note that through its entire course, the intercostal nerve is sandwiched between two muscles anteriorly, or a muscle and an aponeurosis (the posterior intercostal membrane) in its posterior aspect.

are also blocked (blockade of three nerves in total). Also, incisional pain in the paraspinal region or in the periscapular region (e.g., a posterolateral thoracotomy incision) will not be completely alleviated by intercostal nerve blocks. These areas are predominantly innervated by the thoracic dorsal rami. For midline incisions, bilateral intercostal nerve blocks will be necessary, as there is a significant contribution to skin innervation from the contralateral intercostal nerves.

The muscular branches of the intercostal nerves not only provide motor innervation but also sensory innervation to muscles, ligaments, joints, bones, and fascia. Branches of the first two intercostal nerves supply the upper limbs in

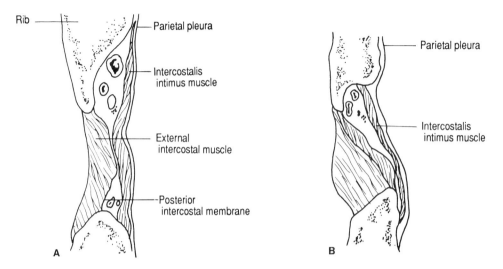

Rib — Parietal pleura — Intercostalis intimus muscle — External intercostal muscle — Posterior intercostal membrane — Parietal pleura — Intercostalis intimus muscle

A B

Fig. 15-5. (A) Posterior and (B) lateral sections through the sixth intercostal space.

addition to the upper trunk. As the third to sixth intercostal nerves supply the intrinsic thoracic muscles and the seventh to eleventh intercostal nerves supply the abdominal muscles and fascia, somatic incisional pain in these areas can be blocked by anesthesia of the appropriate nerves. However, intercostal nerve block will not relieve visceral pain.

For the technique of intercostal nerve block, the angle of a rib (which is 7–8 cm from the posterior midline) is often chosen as the landmark for needle entry. Nunn and Slavin[11] described the posterior intercostal space at this site in detail (Fig. 15-5). At the angle of the rib, the posterior intercostal space is a fat-filled triangular area with an average cross-sectional area of 0.75 cm^2 at the sixth interspace. It contains the intercostal vein, artery, and nerve, usually oriented in that order, proceeding from superior to inferior.[11]

The intercostal nerve trunk, often running as several separate bundles in the subcostal groove, is sandwiched between muscle layers (Figs. 15-4 and 15-5). Local anesthetic injection into the posterior intercostal space at the angle of the rib requires needle penetration of the external intercostal muscle and then the posterior (internal) intercostal membrane. The posterior intercostal membrane is actually an aponeurosis derived from the internal intercostal muscle. From within, the intercostal nerve is separated from the pleura by the intercostalis intimus (innermost intercostal) muscle.

It is important to realize that the distance from the posterior aspect of a rib to the parietal pleura is 8 mm on the average. To avoid pleural puncture and pneumothorax, the tip of a needle should be advanced no more than 3–4 mm beyond the inferior border of the rib, leaving a margin of safety of 4–5 mm. Equally important, the posterior intercostal membrane is impermeable to local anesthetic. Neural blockade will not occur if the needle fails to penetrate this membrane.

MECHANISMS OF ACTION

Using the technique of continuous intercostal nerve block, anesthesia and analgesia can be achieved over several dermatomal segments after injection of local anesthetic into a single posterior intercostal space. Local anesthetic may spread away from the site of injection into (1) the subpleural space[11,12] (Figs. 15-6 and 15-7), (2) the paravertebral space, by communication with the intercostal space[10,12–14] (Fig. 15-8), and (c) eventually the epidural space (Fig. 15-8).[15] Spread of local anesthetic to all these locations has been shown in both humans and cadavers using India ink, radiopaque dye, and radionuclides (Table 15-1).

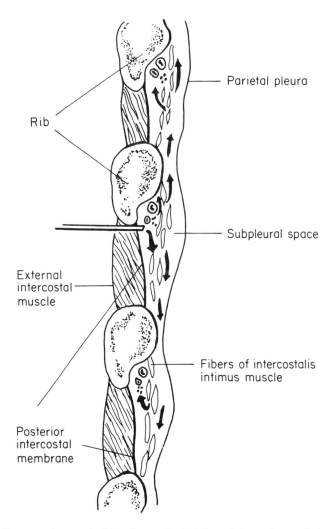

Fig. 15-6. Pattern of spread of local anesthetic injected 3 mm beyond the lower edge of the rib.

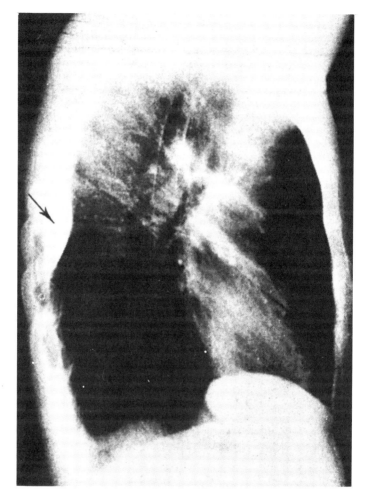

Fig. 15-7. Lateral roentgenogram of the chest after injection of 20 ml of local anesthetic and radiopaque dye. Spread of local anesthetic and radiopaque dye in the subpleural space is denoted by the bulging of the pleura away from the ribs and into the lung parenchyma. Note the spread of contrast over several thoracic segments. (From Crossley and Hosie,[16] with permission.)

Although there is no direct communication between intercostal spaces, local anesthetic deposited in one posterior intercostal space can pass onto other adjacent spaces by way of the subpleural space (Figs. 15-6 and 15-7). As the pleura is not firmly attached to the ribs, injection of a large volume of local anesthetic is free to pass over the internal aspect of the ribs above and below (Fig. 15-6). The intercostalis intimus muscle is a rather flimsy structure and provides no barrier to diffusion. The spread of local anesthetic into the subpleural space in a cephalad-caudad orientation is a volume-mediated phenomenon. Injection of small amounts of local anesthetic (5 ml), as in conventional intercostal nerve blocks, will not spread to adjacent intercostal spaces.[13]

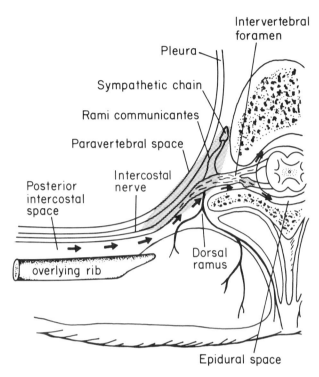

Fig. 15-8. Transverse section through a typical thoracic vertebra at the level of the intervertebral foramen. *Shaded area* represents the paravertebral space. *Arrows* show the potential route of spread of local anesthetic from the intercostal space to the paravertebral space, and eventually, the epidural space.

TABLE 15-1. Mechanisms of Action (Local Anesthetic Spread)

Author	Years	Nature of Study (N)	Nature of Injectate (ml)	Sites of Spread	Extent of Spread
Nunn and Slavin[11]	1980	Cadaver (6)	India ink (3)	Subpleural + paravertebral	Several intercostal spaces
O'Kelly and Garry[10]	1981	Human (1)	Radiopaque contrast dye (10)	Subpleural + paravertebral	5 Spaces
Murphy[12]	1984	Cadaver (12)	India ink (20)	Subpleural + paravertebral	2 Spaces in $\frac{1}{12}$ 3 Spaces in $\frac{7}{12}$ >5 Spaces $\frac{4}{12}$
Middaugh et al[15]	1985	Human (1)	Radioactive technetium (DTPA)	Epidural + paravertebral	10 Spaces bilaterally
Mowbray et al[13]	1987	Human (21)	Methylene blue	Paravertebral	2–3 Spaces after 10 ml injection 2–5 Spaces after 20 ml
Crossley and Hosie[16]	1987	Human (10)	Radiopaque dye (20)	Subpleural + paravertebral	3–4 Spaces

Anatomically, the posterior intercostal space communicates medially with the paravertebral space (Figs. 15-3 and 15-8). From the paravertebral space, communication with the epidural space is possible through the intervertebral foraminae (Figs. 15-3 and 15-8). After a large volume injection, local anesthetic may track medially to reach the paravertebral space and, eventually, the epidural space.[15]

TECHNIQUE

Positioning and Landmarks

Continuous intercostal nerve block can be performed in the sitting position or in the lateral decubitus position, with the side to be blocked uppermost. If this procedure is performed at the end of surgery when the patient is still anesthetized, the lateral decubitus position is preferred for obvious reasons. Patient positioning is also governed, to some extent, by the operator's preference. Performance of this block with the patient lying prone has not been described in the literature. In the author's opinion, this is a feasible option. Although not clearly defined, gravity may play a role in the spread of local anesthetic. A sitting position may promote caudad spread, and a lateral decubitus position may facilitate spread medially to the paravertebral space.

As explained in the anatomy section, the landmark for needle and catheter insertion is the angle of a rib. The angle of the rib lies 7–8 cm from the posterior midline. At this site, the intercostal space has its largest anteroposterior width (an average of 8 mm from the posterior intercostal membrane to the parietal pleura). Thus, performance of the technique at the angle of the rib should minimize the risk of pneumothorax.

Identification of the ribs and palpation of the angles may be difficult at times, especially in obese patients. Because ribs in the axilla are more superficial, retrograde palpation toward the posterior midline is often very helpful. Location of a rib can also be assisted by surface anatomy, using the inferior angle of the scapula as a guide (T7 level). To approach the upper ribs, raising the ipsilateral arm above the head will retract the scapula laterally and facilitate exposure.

The choice of an intercostal space for needle and catheter placement is dependent on the focus of the painful stimulus. Ideally, local anesthetic should be deposited at the center of the desired band of analgesia (e.g., at the dermatome in the center of the surgical incision).

Procedure

Intravenous access should be established before performing the block, and sedation may be given as necessary. With the patient sitting upright and both arms stabilized on a supporting table, the site of needle entry overlying the rib is identified by palpation. The area is prepped with antiseptic solution and draped to allow a sterile field. A skin wheal is raised at the site by injecting 1 percent lidocaine through a small-gauge needle. A skin nick is made with an 18-gauge needle to allow easier insertion of a 16- to 18-gauge epidural needle. Blunt forceful puncture can thereby be avoided.

After making contact with the rib, the epidural needle is walked down the inferior margin of the rib to reach its inferior border and advanced 3–4 mm beyond this point. At times, the sensation of a "give" or "pop" is felt, indicating penetration of the posterior intercostal membrane. However, this give or pop can be subtle. Also, there is no true loss of resistance to saline or air as is appreciated when traversing the ligamentum flavum during performance of epidural analgesia.

The needle bevel is then rotated medially before the stylet is removed. An empty syringe is then attached to the needle hub and used to check for blood and air by aspiration. After a negative aspiration test, a conventional 20-gauge epidural catheter is threaded 3–5 cm medially into the posterior intercostal space toward the midline. The epidural needle is then withdrawn, leaving behind an indwelling intercostal catheter (Fig. 15-9). The intercostal catheter should be securely taped to the skin so that the chance of dislodgment is minimized.

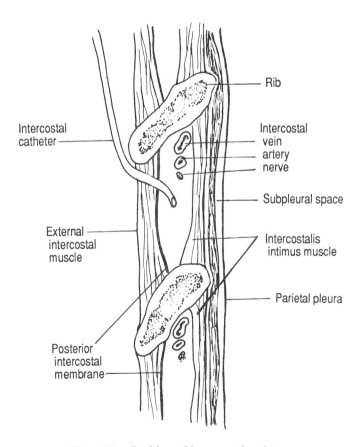

Fig. 15-9. Position of intercostal catheter.

Potential Technical Difficulties

When blood is detected on needle aspiration, intercostal vascular puncture is likely. It is best to repeat the procedure at an adjacent site. If a true loss of resistance is detected, the pleural space has been entered. One is left with two options: to insert a catheter and thereby convert the technique to interpleural regional analgesia (see Ch. 16), or to simply withdraw the needle and repeat the procedure. In either case, it is prudent to radiologically assess the extent of any potential pneumothorax and to treat appropriately.

If difficulty with catheter advancement is encountered, the epidural needle is withdrawn and redirected medially at a 60° angle from the skin surface rather than perpendicularly. Needle insertion at such an acute angle can facilitate catheter threading toward the midline.

However, if a catheter can be easily advanced beyond 3–5 cm, interpleural catheterization should be highly suspected.

Variations of the Technique

For thoracotomy incisions, intercostal catheterization can be accomplished under direct vision at the end of surgery before chest wall closure. If an intrathoracic approach is used, the parietal pleura is peeled back to place the catheter into the subpleural space and subsequently into the posterior intercostal space through the flimsy intercostalis intimus muscle.

Use of other catheters besides a conventional epidural catheter or catheters has also been described.[17-22]

Choice and Dosing of Local Anesthetic

As with conventional intercostal nerve block, bupivacaine with or without epinephrine has been used in most instances. As systemic absorption of local anesthetic is greater after intercostal nerve block in comparison with other regional anesthetic procedures,[23] it is advisable to limit the amount of bupivacaine to 100 mg per injection. Addition of epinephrine (1/200,000) can further restrict the rise in systemic bupivacaine level. In one study, nontoxic mean cumulative serum bupivacaine concentrations of 1.19 ± 0.18 μg/ml were found after four doses of 100 mg over 24 hours.[17]

At present, the optimal dose, concentration, or volume of bupivacaine to be used per injection for continuous intercostal nerve block has not been determined. Whether 20 ml of 0.5 percent bupivacaine or 40 ml of 0.25 percent bupivacaine results in better local anesthetic spread and analgesic efficacy has yet to be determined.

Dosing Interval

Most experience with continuous intercostal nerve block has been with on-demand, intermittent injections (Table 15-2). After an injection of 100 mg of bupivacaine (without epinephrine), analgesia for fractured ribs lasts for 7–13 hours.[10,15] The duration of analgesia for subcostal surgical incisions is approximately 6–7 hours (Table 15-2).[19] For solutions containing bupivacaine with epinephrine, the duration of analgesia is likely to be longer. Prolonged use (up to 6 days) has been found to be safe, without clinical evidence of local anesthetic toxicity (Table 15-2).[10,14]

Continuous infusion protocols have also been developed. Safran et al[24] used 1 percent lidocaine at 1 mg/kg/h after a loading dose of 3 mg/kg of 1.5 percent lidocaine with epinephrine 1/160,000. Maximum concentration of serum lidocaine after the loading dose was 1.9 ± 0.7 μg/ml. Lidocaine serum concentrations averaged 4.8 ± 0.9 μg/ml under steady-state conditions.

Sabanathan et al[14,25] reported the use of continuous infusions of 0.5 percent bupivacaine for post-thoracotomy pain. Patients were initially injected with 10–20 ml of 0.5 percent bupivacaine and started on infusions of 5–10 ml/h. Using this technique, a large proportion of patients required no opioid supplementation at all.

CLINICAL APPLICATIONS

With the exception of minor chest or abdominal wall incisions, continuous intercostal nerve block should not be used as the sole anesthetic technique for surgery.

Effective alleviation of pain has been reported after fractured ribs,[10,15,26,27] flail chest, thoracotomy,[13,14,17,20–22,24,25] sternotomy (with double catheters),[28] and cholecystectomy.[19,29] Its use in acute herpes zoster or postherpetic neuralgia has not been studied (Table 15-2).

COMPLICATIONS

Inadequate Analgesia

Inadequate analgesia is most likely related to technical failure of catheter placement. Local anesthetic deposited in the intercostal muscle or superficial to the posterior intercostal membrane will always result in inadequate analgesia.

Local anesthetic tachyphylaxis may occur. Tachyphylaxis is usually seen between 24 and 48 hours after initiation of therapy. Continued shortening of the duration of analgesia and the need for frequent top-up doses may lead to termination of therapy in anticipation of potential local anesthetic toxicity.

Pneumothorax

The incidence of clinically significant pneumothorax with this technique is unknown. Puncture of the parietal pleura was found in 42 percent of specimens in a cadaver study[12] and in 14 percent in one clinical study.[13] However, Murphy[29] did not detect pneumothorax in 25 cholecystectomy patients.

TABLE 15-2. Reports of Analgesia Using Continuous Nerve Block

Author	Year	Origin of Pain	Drug Dose	Extent of Analgesia	Duration of Analgesia (h)	Remarks
O'Kelly and Garry[10]	1981	Fractured ribs	Bupivacaine 0.5% plain 20 ml (intermittent injection)	T4–T9	7–8	Use for 6 days No supplemental opioid Improvement in PaO_2 and coughing
Murphy[27]	1983	Fractured ribs	Bupivacaine 0.5% plain 20 ml (intermittent injection)	?	8–12 (up to 10–24)	Analgesia but lack of pinprick anesthesia Tachyphylaxis may occur
Middaugh et al[15]	1985	Fractured ribs	Bupivacaine 0.5% with epinephrine 20 ml (intermittent injection)	Bilateral analgesia T1–T10 on left T2–L1 on right	7	Epidural spread
Lyles et al[26]	1986	Fractured ribs	Bupivacaine 0.5% plain 20 ml (intermittent injection)	?	9–13	Use up to 4 days Improvement in spirometric volumes
Olivet et al[21]	1980	Thoracotomy	Bupivacaine 0.5% with epinephrine 4 ml into each of 4 catheters (intermittent injection)	?	6	Use up to 3 days
Mowbray et al[13]	1987	Thoracotomy Sternotomy	Bupivacaine 0.25% plain 20 ml (intermittent injection)	2–5 dermatomes	?	High rate of technical failure (48%)
Baxter et al[28]	1987	Sternotomy for cardiac surgery	Bupivacaine 0.25% plain 20 ml into each of 2 catheters (intermittent injection)	?	10 (range 6–24)	Bilateral catheters Use for 2 days No significant improvement in pulmonary function or rate of complications

Reference	Year	Operation	Drug/dose	Dermatomes	Duration	Comments
Sabanathan et al[14]	1988	Thoracotomy	Bupivacaine 0.5% plain 10 ml bolus + 5–7 ml/h infusion	?	Continuous	Use for 5 days 93% required no opioid supplementation over 24 h
Chan et al[17]	1989	Thoracotomy	Bupivacaine 0.5% with epinephrine 10 ml into each of 2 catheters (intermittent injection)	?	≥6	Nontoxic cumulative serum bupivacaine level after 400 mg over 24 h
Kolvenbach et al[20]	1989	Thoracotomy	Bupivacaine 0.5% plain 5 ml into each of 3 adjacent catheters	?	5.5	Use for 3 days No significant difference in rate of pulmonary complications or duration of hospital stay when compared with control group
Sabanathan et al[25]	1990	Thoracotomy	Bupivacaine 0.5% plain 20 ml bolus + 5–10 ml/h infusion	?	Continuous	Improvement in pulmonary function when compared with control group 59% required no opioid supplementation
Safran et al[24]	1990	Thoracotomy	Lidocaine 1.5% with epinephrine 3 mg/kg as bolus + lidocaine 1% plain at 1 mg/kg/h infusion	7 dermatomes	Continuous	Nontoxic cumulative lidocaine level after 24-h infusion
Murphy[29]	1983	Cholecystectomy	Bupivacaine 0.5% plain 20 ml	?	7	Use for 2 days Improvement in peak expiratory flow
Kirno and Lindell[19]	1983	Cholecystectomy	Bupivacaine 0.5% plain 20 ml	?	9.2	Failure rate 12.5%

Vascular Damage

There is a single report of a massive flank hematoma in a patient after cardiac surgery. The patient received bilateral intercostal catheters after reversal of heparinization.[28] As a large hematoma from intercostal vascular bleeding can potentially collapse a lung, the use of continuous intercostal nerve block is contraindicated in patients with a bleeding diathesis.

Local Anesthetic Toxicity

Local anesthetic toxicity can result from systemic absorption or accidental intravascular injection. Although safe clinical use has been reported for up to 6 days,[10] it is unknown as to whether progressive cumulative systemic absorption can occur after prolonged infusions or repetitive injections. Inadvertent intravascular injection may also occur through catheter migration into an intercostal vessel.

Nerve Damage

Neuralgia after continuous intercostal nerve block has not been reported.

CONCLUSION

In summary, continuous intercostal nerve block is easy to perform, has potential complications similar to conventional intercostal nerve block, and relieves patients of the need for multiple needle insertions and the repeated risk of pneumothorax. In view of its consistent and predictable efficacy, the popularity of this technique should only increase.

References
1. Cronin KD, Davies MJ: Intercostal block for postoperative pain relief. Anaesth Intensive Care 4:259, 1976
2. Bridenbaugh PO, DuPen SL, Moore DC et al: Postoperative intercostal nerve block analgesia versus narcotic analgesia. Anesth Analg 52:81, 1973
3. Engberg G: Single-dose intercostal nerve blocks with etidocaine for pain relief after upper abdominal surgery. Acta Anaesthesiol Scand, suppl. 60:43, 1975
4. Moore DC: Intercostal nerve block for postoperative somatic pain following surgery of the thorax and upper abdomen. Br J Anaesth, suppl. 47:284, 1975
5. Bergh N, Dottore B, Axison L et al: Effects of intercostal blockade on lung function after thoracotomy. Acta Anaesthesiol Scand, suppl. 24:85, 1966
6. Engberg G, Wiklund L: Pulmonary complications after upper abdominal surgery: their prevention with intercostal blocks. Acta Anaesthesiol Scand 32:1, 1988
7. Hecker BR, Bjurstrom R, Schoene RB: Effect of intercostal nerve blockade on respiratory mechanics and CO_2 chemosensitivity at rest and exercise. Anesthesiology 70:13, 1989
8. Faust RJ, Nauss LA: Post-thoracotomy intercostal block: comparison of its effect

on pulmonary function with those of intramuscular meperidine. Anesth Analg 55: 542, 1976

9. Toledo-Pereyra LH, DeMeester T: Prospective randomized evaluation of intrathoracic intercostal nerve block with bupivacaine on postoperative ventilatory function. Ann Thorac Surg 27:203, 1979

10. O'Kelly E, Garry B: Continuous pain relief for multiple fractured ribs. Br J Anaesth 53:989, 1981

11. Nunn JF, Slavin G: Posterior intercostal nerve block for pain relief after cholecystectomy. Anatomical basis and efficacy. Br J Anaesth 52:253, 1980

12. Murphy DF: Continuous intercostal nerve blockade. An anatomical study to elucidate its mode of action. Br J Anaesth 56:627, 1984

13. Mowbray A, Wong KKS, Murray JM: Intercostal catheterisation. An alternative approach to the paravertebral space. Anaesthesia 42:958, 1987

14. Sabanathan S, Smith PJ, Pradhan GN et al: Continuous intercostal nerve block for pain relief after thoracotomy. Ann Thorac Surg 46:425, 1988

15. Middaugh RE, Menk EJ, Reynolds WJ et al: Epidural block using large volumes of local anesthetic solution for intercostal nerve block. Anesthesiology 63:214, 1985

16. Crossley AW, Hosie HE: Radiographic study of intercostal nerve blockade in healthy volunteers. Br J Anaesth 59:149, 1987

17. Chan VWS, Chung F, Cheng DCH et al: Analgesic effect of continuous intercostal nerve block following thoracotomy, abstracted. Anesth Analg 68:S50, 1989

18. Ishizuka E, Iwasaki A, Okutsu Y, Kobayaski T: Continuous intercostal nerve block for pain relief after lumbar incision. J Urol 122:506, 1979

19. Kirno K, Lindell K: Intercostal nerve blockade (letter). Br J Anaesth 58:246, 1986

20. Kolvenbach H, Lauven PM, Schneider B, Kunath U: Repetitive intercostal nerve block via catheter for postoperative pain relief after thoracotomy. Thorac Cardiovasc Surg 37:273, 1989

21. Olivet RT, Nauss LA, Payne WS: A technique for continuous intercostal nerve block analgesia following thoracotomy. J Thorac Cardiovasc Surg 80:308, 1980

22. Restelli L, Movilia P, Bossi L, Caironi C: Management of pain after thoracotomy: a technique of multiple intercostal nerve blocks (letter). Anesthesiology 61:353, 1984

23. Moore DC, Mather LE, Bridenbaugh LD et al: Arterial and venous plasma levels of bupivacaine following peripheral nerve blocks. Anesth Analg 55:763, 1976

24. Safran D, Kuhlman G, Orhant EE et al: Continuous intercostal blockade with lidocaine after thoracic surgery. Clinical and pharmacokinetic study. Anesth Analg 70: 345, 1990

25. Sabanathan S, Mearns AJ, Bickford Smith PJ et al: Efficacy of continuous extrapleural intercostal nerve block on post-thoracotomy pain and pulmonary mechanics. Br J Surg 77:221, 1990

26. Lyles R Jr, Skurdal D, Stene J, Jaberi M: Continuous intercostal catheter techniques for treatment of post-traumatic thoracic pain, abstracted. Anesthesiology 65:A205, 1986

27. Murphy DF: Continuous intercostal nerve blockade for fractured ribs and postoperative analgesia. Description of a new technique. Reg Anesth 8:151, 1983

28. Baxter AD, Jennings FO, Harris RS et al: Continuous intercostal blockade after cardiac surgery. Br J Anaesth 59:162, 1987

29. Murphy DF: Continuous intercostal nerve blockade for pain relief after cholecystectomy. Br J Anaesth 55:521, 1983

16

Interpleural Regional Analgesia

Timothy R. VadeBoncouer

In 1984, Reiestad and Strømskag reported on the use of local anesthetics instilled into the thoracic cavity for postoperative pain management.[1] This intra- or interpleural technique (see below) resulted in profound, long-lasting pain relief after mastectomy, nephrectomy, and cholecystectomy. Numerous studies have been published since the original work of Reiestad and Strømskag, documenting new uses for the technique and several of its limitations.

Interpleural regional analgesia has gained widespread acceptance as a useful tool for pain management. However, several controversies surrounding the technique still exist, including what to actually call it.

ANATOMY

The thoracic cavity is lined by the parietal and visceral pleura. The parietal pleura is actually an embryologically derived reflection of the visceral pleura. Viewed embryologically, local anesthetic is placed *within* the pleural sac, and intrapleural regional analgesia would appear to be the proper name. Viewed anatomically, the technique involves percutaneous introduction of a catheter into the thoracic cavity *between* the visceral and parietal pleura. Thus, *interpleural regional analgesia* would appear to be the more proper name.[2] To date, there is no consensus regarding correct nomenclature.

A thorough knowledge of the anatomy of the thoracic cage is necessary to understand the proposed mechanism of action of interpleural regional analgesia.

The reader is referred to the preceding chapter, in which the anatomy of the thoracic wall is extensively reviewed.

MECHANISM OF ANALGESIA

Multidermatomal intercostal neural blockade is believed to be the mechanism underlying interpleural analgesia. Such a proposed mechanism can be reconciled with the classic clinical observations found during interpleural analgesia: (1) unilateral sensory anesthesia to pinprick, (2) sensory blockade (analgesia) of insufficient intensity to provide surgical anesthesia, and (3) unilateral sympathetic blockade (hypotension is not observed).

Although unequivocal evidence in humans is lacking, multidermatomal intercostal neural blockade with interpleural regional analgesia has been substantiated in a canine model.[3] Using alterations in somatosensory evoked responses as a marker for neural blockade, interpleural injection of local anesthetic resulted in intercostal neural blockade without spinal, epidural, or cerebral effects.

After interpleural injection, local anesthetic may gain access to intercostal nerves through three possible routes. (1) Near the posterior midline, the intercostal nerves are separated from the thoracic cavity by only the parietal pleura and a thin layer of connective tissue (Fig. 16-1). In the upper intercostal spaces, this "naked" area (i.e., denuded of the intercostalis intimus muscle) extends further laterally toward the angle of the rib (Fig. 16-2).[4] It is likely that these sections of the posterior thorax represent the primary route of access to the intercostal nerves for production of interpleural analgesia.[2,3] Diffusion of local anesthetic through the pleura would be brisk because of the paucity of diffusion barriers. This would explain the typical rapid onset of analgesia after interpleural injection. (2) This same area of the thoracic wall abuts the paravertebral space (Fig. 16-1). The importance of the paravertebral space as a means of drug access to the intercostal nerves has been implicated in at least two studies.[3,5] (3) As described previously in Chapter 15, the intercostalis intimus muscle is a flimsy structure composed of separate fascicles.[4] Local anesthetic may readily diffuse through this muscle to reach the subpleural space (see Ch. 15).

Neural blockade with interpleural regional analgesia is strongly dependent on gravity. Local anesthetic will accumulate in the most dependent areas of the thorax, regardless of patient position (e.g., supine, prone, upright)[3,5] (Fig. 16-3). Such distribution after injection has been substantiated in dogs using somatosensory evoked responses[3] and in humans using computerized tomography[6] (Fig. 16-4).

The paravertebrally located sympathetic chain and the splanchnic nerves (see Ch. 3 for discussion of anatomy) are anatomically positioned within the hemithorax such that they can be affected by interpleural local anesthetic. Despite the fact that hypotension has not been described,[7,8] (unilateral) sympathetic blockade can be significant, as there are several reports of Horner's syndrome resulting from interpleural injection.[7,9,10] Furthermore, interpleural

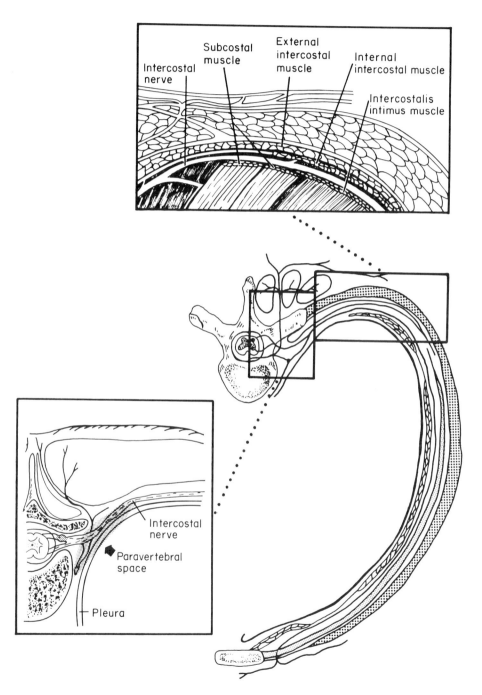

Subcostal muscle

External intercostal muscle

Internal intercostal muscle

Intercostal nerve

Intercostalis intimus muscle

Intercostal nerve

Paravertebral space

Pleura

Fig. 16-1. Course of an intercostal nerve. Just medial to the angle of the rib, the intercostal nerve is separated from the thoracic cavity by only the parietal pleura. Interpleural local anesthetic likely gains access to intercostal nerves in this region.

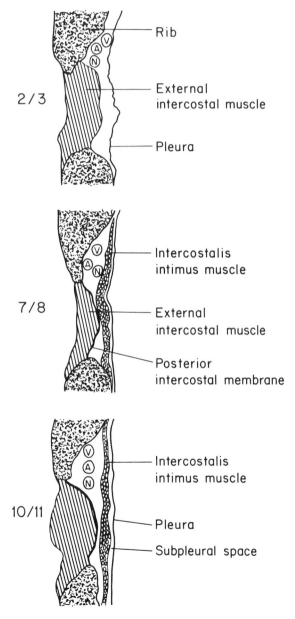

Fig. 16-2. In the upper intercostal spaces, the intercostalis intimus muscle is poorly developed. Thus, intercostal nerves are separated from the thoracic cavity by only the parietal pleura in this region. (Numbers at left refer to the interspace between the corresponding ribs.) V, vein; A, artery; N, nerve.

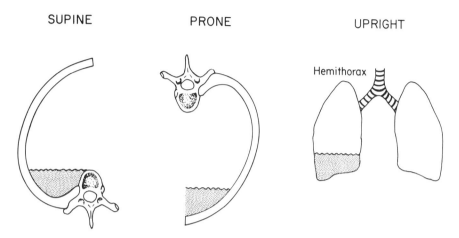

SUPINE   PRONE   UPRIGHT

Hemithorax

Fig. 16-3. Effect of gravity on distribution of interpleural local anesthetic. Local anesthetic will accumulate in the most dependent areas of the thorax, regardless of body position (i.e., supine, prone, or upright).

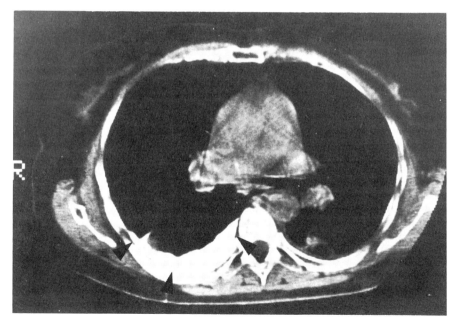

Fig. 16-4. CT scan of human thorax showing distribution of local anesthetic/contrast (*black arrowheads*) after interpleural injection in supine position. Note proximity to the paravertebral region of the pleura where intercostal nerves are most accessible to interpleural local anesthetic. (From Strømskag et al,[6] with permission.)

regional analgesia can be used to treat sympathetically mediated pain[11] and pain of visceral origin.[12,13]

TECHNIQUE

Two of the great advantages of interpleural analgesia are its technical simplicity (ease of performance) and widespread applicability. Interpleural catheters may be placed in awake and anesthetized patients, with patients breathing spontaneously or mechanically ventilated. Because interpleural regional analgesia is used nearly exclusively for pain of a continuous nature, it requires an indwelling catheter for ease of administration. Single injection techniques are rarely, if ever, performed.

Positioning and Landmarks

The patient is placed in the lateral decubitus position with the side to be injected uppermost. The thorax is cleansed with a bactericidal solution. The sixth, seventh, or eighth ribs are palpated, and a skin wheal is raised over the chosen rib with local anesthetic. Deep infiltration with local anesthetic is then performed, serving primarily as a means to locate the rib before advancement of the epidural needle.

Needle insertion has been described in the posterior midclavicular line (as in the original description of the technique by Reiestad and Strømskag[1]), and the anterior,[14,15] middle,[16-18] and posterior[19] axillary lines. Because the aforementioned canine studies suggest that position is important only at the time of interpleural injection,[4] the site of epidural needle insertion is largely a matter of preference.

Procedure

Before needle insertion, a decision must be made as to the visual end point to be used to determine entry into the interpleural space. All techniques used to identify the interpleural space make use of the pressure difference between atmospheric pressure and intrathoracic pressure.[1] Three options are available (Fig. 16-5). These include (1) a "hanging-drop" technique,[20] (2) the "falling column" technique[21] (a syringe sleeve without the plunger is attached to the needle and filled with 2 or 3 ml of saline; the needle is advanced until the saline is pulled into the interpleural space by negative interpleural pressure on entry), or (3) the original end point of Reiestad and Strømskag[1] (a well-lubricated syringe containing 2 or 3 cc of air is attached to the epidural needle; once again, the needle is advanced until the plunger of the syringe is pulled forward by negative pressure on entry into the interpleural space).

After local infiltration and choice of visual end point, an epidural needle is advanced inward until the rib is contacted. The needle (or needle-syringe assembly) is then "walked off" the superior margin of the rib and advanced inward. Puncture of the parietal pleura is usually perceived as a distinct "pop," and this is followed by entry of the air or saline into the interpleural space.

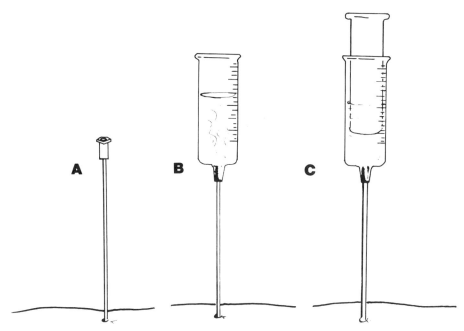

Fig. 16-5. Three techniques for interpleural catheter placement. (A) Needle is filled with saline (the hanging-drop technique). (B) Syringe sleeve is filled with saline (the falling column technique). (C) Air is placed in syringe-sleeve assembly (the original technique of Reiestad and Strømskag[1]). The hanging-drop and falling column techniques would appear to be most effective in locating the interpleural space, as the plunger may "stick" to the sleeve in technique C, thereby increasing the likelihood of pneumothorax.

Passive air or saline movement into the chest is the requisite sign of accurate needle placement. Catheters should not be threaded through the needle unless this end point is reached. It must be stressed that the technique of Reiestad and Strømskag[1] is *not* a loss of resistance technique. Loss of resistance techniques[22] may result in catheter placement within the subpleural space or the lung parenchyma and will not be discussed here.

Once the interpleural space has been located with the epidural needle, an epidural catheter should be threaded into the thorax. The catheter should be inserted 5–6 cm beyond the needle tip. This distance appears to be both safe and effective. No study has defined a rationale for insertion of longer lengths of catheter, and one study documented placement within the lung parenchyma when excessive lengths (30 cm) were used.[23] In any case, there should be no appreciable resistance to threading the catheter through the needle if the needle tip is in the interpleural space. If any resistance to catheter insertion is encountered, the needle and catheter should be withdrawn as a unit. Interpleural placement can then be reattempted.

The puncture site on the skin is covered with a sterile dressing, and the catheter is connected to an injection port adapter. The adapter site should be secured to the upper anterior chest, so that it is easily located for reinjection.

Most commonly, interpleural catheters are intermittently injected with 20–30 ml of 0.5 percent bupivacaine with epinephrine (although other concentrations, local anesthetics, and injectate volumes have been used—see below). Onset of analgesia is rapid and usually complete within 30 minutes. Maintaining the patient in the supine position or in a semilateral position with the surgical site uppermost should ensure adequate access of local anesthetic to the intercostal nerves. As with any catheter, negative aspiration of blood or fluid is required before injection. It is not unusual to aspirate a small amount of air (2–5 cc) through the interpleural catheter. This small volume represents the air entrained during catheter insertion. If air aspiration is excessive, the possibility of lung puncture and pneumothorax should be considered.

Choice and Dosing of Local Anesthetic

Concentration of Bupivacaine

Nearly all clinical reports of interpleural analgesia have used bupivacaine as the local anesthetic. Concentrations of 0.25–0.75 percent bupivacaine have all been reported to be effective.[1,18,24,25] In one study,[25] duration of analgesia after a single 20-ml interpleural injection was longest for 0.5 percent bupivacaine, intermediate for 0.375 percent bupivacaine, and least for 0.25 percent bupivacaine. Thus, duration of analgesia would appear to be directly proportional to the amount of bupivacaine administered per standardized injection volume (i.e., concentration). However, these differences were not statistically significant because of the wide range in duration of analgesia per injection (2–18 hours).[25]

Therefore, there appears to be no advantage in using 0.75 percent bupivacaine in terms of duration of analgesia. The risk of excessive systemic bupivacaine levels with use of 0.75 percent bupivacaine is significant. Furthermore, the potential duration of analgesia with use of lower concentrations of bupivacaine is too long to justify obtaining a *possibly* slightly increased duration of analgesia with the more concentrated solution. One clinical report[26] using 0.75 percent bupivacaine for bilateral interpleural analgesia (30 ml per hemithorax) documented excessive blood bupivacaine concentrations (≥ 4 μg/ml) in the first 30 minutes after injection. Frank local anesthetic toxicity was seen in two of five patients. Based on these limited reports,[25,26] 0.75 percent bupivacaine cannot be recommended for routine interpleural use.

However, concentrations of 0.25–0.5 percent bupivacaine have an extensive record of safety and efficacy in an injection volume of 20–30 ml. Blood levels are nearly always below the toxic threshold,[25] and reports of toxicity with use of these concentrations of bupivacaine are rare.

Volume of Injection

The most commonly used volume of bupivacaine for injection is 20 ml, which reliably produces analgesia throughout the thoracic dermatomes. Injection volumes as low as 10 ml[18] and high as 30 ml[24] have also been successfully used.

It would seem reasonable that a larger volume of local anesthetic would spread more effectively over the pleural surface, increasing both the area and density of analgesia. Indeed, a canine study documented a more profound and extensive area of intercostal nerve block when comparing 10 ml versus 20 ml of 0.5 percent bupivacaine.[27]

However, it would seem prudent to inject the smallest volume of drug that provides a reasonable duration of analgesia (3–6 hours), given the potential risk of systemic toxicity. This would permit a reasonable dosing schedule without increased risk of excessive blood levels of local anesthetic. Twenty milliliters of bupivacaine appears to be adequate in most cases.

Other Local Anesthetics

Although lidocaine[14,28] and etidocaine[29] have both been reported to be efficacious, studies of local anesthetics other than bupivacaine for interpleural analgesia are few. When a dose of 1 mg/kg of lidocaine in a 30-ml injection volume was given for thoracic trauma, analgesia lasted about 3 hours. This dosage regimen produced drowsiness in some individuals despite low maximum blood lidocaine concentrations.[28] Another study[14] documented successful use of a continuous interpleural infusion of lidocaine for rib fractures. The infusion rate was 2.2 mg/min (i.e., 8 ml/h of 1.6 percent lidocaine), a rate commonly used intravascularly to treat cardiac arrhythmias. In this single patient, effective analgesia without toxicity was demonstrated.

Etidocaine has theoretic advantages for interpleural administration: large volume of distribution, rapid plasma clearance, and greater uptake into lung parenchyma than bupivacaine, all of which decrease the likelihood of systemic toxicity.[29] Etidocaine has been shown to provide effective interpleural analgesia in children and adolescents after pectus repair or chest trauma.[29] Analgesia lasted 5–12 hours (mean, 8 hours) after a single injection of 0.3 mg/kg of 1 percent etidocaine. No local anesthetic toxicity was reported. Given the theoretic advantages and these preliminary results, more extensive trials of etidocaine in adult patients are warranted.

Epinephrine

Epinephrine is commonly used with interpleural administration of local anesthetics in an attempt to minimize systemic toxicity. In theory, epinephrine may produce local vasoconstriction and impede the rapid uptake of local anesthetic by the richly vascularized pleural membrane. Although this effect has been well documented for other nerve blocks, the data for interpleural injection remain controversial.

An early report by Denson et al[30] in monkeys showed no difference in the rate or extent of absorption of interpleural bupivacaine, regardless of the presence or absence of epinephrine. Time to maximum blood bupivacaine concentration was approximately 5 minutes in both groups. No significant differences were observed in maximum blood bupivacaine concentrations.

A clinical study in humans using 0.5 percent bupivacaine with or without epinephrine for post-thoracotomy pain demonstrated significantly lower maximum blood bupivacaine concentrations in the epinephrine group.[31] Mean concentrations in both groups, however, were below the reported toxic level of 4.0 µg/ml. These authors also reported a significantly faster time to peak concentration in the plain bupivacaine group.

The controversy over whether to use epinephrine with interpleural local anesthetic is unresolved. However, based on the extensive clinical experience and low incidence of systemic toxicity with this combination, it is probably best to use epinephrine-containing solutions for interpleural regional analgesia.

Dosing Interval

Intermittent Injections

The initial description of the technique by Reiestad and Strømskag[1] indicated that analgesia from a single injection of 20 ml of 0.5 percent bupivacaine with epinephrine lasted about 10 hours (range, 6–27 hours). Subsequent studies have failed to reproduce these results. Brismar et al[18] found analgesia to be of 2–3 hours' duration after 20 ml of 0.25 percent bupivacaine and 3–5 hours after the same volume of 0.5 percent bupivacaine. In this study, patients frequently requested interpleural injections within 3–4 hours of the previous injection. A similar finding was demonstrated in a study by VadeBoncouer et al.[16] These authors used morphine administered by intravenous patient-controlled analgesia (IV-PCA) as a measure of the intensity of analgesia after interpleural bupivacaine. Patients typically stopped administering morphine for approximately 3 hours after an interpleural injection. Morphine use then gradually increased. By the sixth hour after interpleural injection, patient-controlled morphine administration was similar to morphine requirements before interpleural injection.

Although some patients may obtain a very long duration of analgesia after a single interpleural injection, this appears to be the exception rather than the rule. Significant pain, necessitating reinjection, should be anticipated within 4–6 hours.[16,18,32] Such an injection schedule may be prohibitive on a busy pain service, so alternative analgesic modalities should be made available to patients receiving interpleural regional analgesia. Intravenous PCA with opioids appears to be the optimal choice.[18] There is no contraindication to administration of opioids in patients receiving interpleural local anesthetics. Furthermore, the inherent flexibility of patient-controlled opioid administration is ideal in view of the wide variability in analgesic duration seen after interpleural injection. However, there may be periods just before reinjection when patients may experience significant discomfort despite provision of IV-PCA. This is due to the waning intercostal nerve block. Such "peak and trough" effects have motivated the investigation of continuous interpleural infusions as an alternative to intermittent injection therapy.

Continuous Interpleural Infusions

There is a paucity of reports on continuous interpleural infusions in the literature, most likely because it is by no means a well-accepted technique. Many aspects of the technique remain unstudied, including a lack of consensus regarding its ultimate efficacy.

Rocco et al[33] first reported the use of continuous interpleural infusions in patients sustaining multiple rib fractures. After an initial 20-ml injection of 0.5 percent bupivacaine, a continuous infusion of 5–10 ml/h of 0.25 percent or 0.5 percent bupivacaine was begun. Only the 0.5 percent solution resulted in complete analgesia, although significant but incomplete analgesia was observed with infusions of 0.25 percent bupivacaine. Infusions were continued for 5–10 days. No adverse effects were noted, but bupivacaine blood levels beyond the first several hours of therapy were not reported.

Continuous interpleural lidocaine has been used for 9 days in a single patient with rib fractures.[14] Lidocaine was infused at a rate not greater than 2.2 mg/min (8 ml/h of 1.6 percent lidocaine). This rate was chosen because it is commonly used intravenously to treat cardiac arrhythmias without producing systemic toxicity. Lidocaine serum concentrations were monitored frequently and not allowed to exceed 5 μg/ml.

Scott and colleagues[19] compared continuous interpleural 0.5 percent bupivacaine (20-ml loading dose followed by 10 ml/h) to continuous thoracic epidural 0.5 percent bupivacaine (9-ml loading dose followed by 5 ml/h). Both groups had significant but incomplete analgesia, and the analgesic superiority of either technique was not established. Infusions were only continued for 8 hours after a single injection, and bupivacaine blood levels during this period were not excessive.

Other reports have described successful use of continuous interpleural bupivacaine in a lactating woman[34] and in children after thoracotomy.[35] The latter study demonstrated excellent analgesia, high blood bupivacaine concentrations (>2 μg/ml), and no signs of cardiovascular or central nervous system toxicity. It is interesting to note that epinephrine was used in the continuous infusion, and abnormalities of heart rate or blood pressure were not noted during the study.

Rosenberg et al,[36] however, were unable to achieve good analgesia with continuous interpleural infusions in thoracotomy patients. All patients received an initial injection of 0.5 percent bupivacaine based on body weight. Within 1 hour, 0.25 percent bupivacaine was infused at a rate of 5–10 ml/h. Analgesia was uniformly poor. The unsatisfactory analgesia was attributed to loss of bupivacaine through thoracostomy tube drainage and poor interpleural distribution of bupivacaine (by movement of an operated lung or lack thereof.)[36] Other authors[37] confirmed the failure of continuous interpleural infusions for post-thoracotomy pain.

Thus, before general recommendations can be given, much further research is needed.

Many questions still remain regarding a number of important aspects of interpleural regional analgesia: the choice of local anesthetic, the optimal injectate volume, the efficacy of epinephrine in reducing systemic toxicity, the appropriate injection interval, and the use of continuous interpleural infusions. The findings of pertinent studies defining several of the controversies surrounding interpleural analgesia are presented in Table 16-1. Given these controversies, a protocol for intermittent dosing of interpleural catheters is presented in Table

TABLE 16-1. Studies Defining the Controversies Regarding Interpleural Regional Analgesia

Author	Year	Origin of Pain	Drug Dose	Duration of Analgesia (h)	Remarks
Choice of local anesthetic					
Reiestad and Strømskag[1]	1986	Cholecystectomy Nephrectomy Mastectomy	20 ml of 0.5% bupivacaine with epinephrine (intermittent injections)	10 (range, 6–26)	The original paper defining the technique; choice of bupivacaine, 0.5% concentration, use of epinephrine, and 20-ml injection volume became the standard because of the influence of this study
Strømskag et al[25]	1988	Cholecystectomy	20 ml of 0.25% bupivacaine 20 ml of 0.375% bupivacaine 20 ml of 0.5% bupivacaine (All with 1:200,000 epinephrine) (single injection)	4.33 6 7.75	First attempt to compare attendant effects of different concentrations of bupivacaine; toxic systemic levels not achieved with any concentration of bupivacaine; wide range in duration of analgesia obscured differences among groups
El-Naggar et al[26]	1988	Midline abdominal incisions	Bilateral catheters 20 ml of 0.5% bupivacaine (each side) 20 ml of 0.75% bupivacaine (each side)		First use of bilateral catheters; 0.5% bupivacaine ineffective for midline incisions; 30-ml injection volume caused toxicity in 40% of patients
Brismar et al[18]	1987	Cholecystectomy	10 and 20 ml of 0.25% bupivacaine 10 and 20 ml of 0.5% bupivacaine (All with 1:200,000 epinephrine) (intermittent injections)	3–5, irrespective of study group	No significant difference in analgesia among groups; no toxic systemic levels but wide interindividual variation in systemic concentrations; 10-ml injection volume suggested as optimal

Author	Year	Model/Condition	Protocol	Duration	Comments
Seltzer et al[17]	1987	Cholecystectomy	30 ml of 0.5% bupivacaine with 1:100,000 epinephrine (intermittent injections)	Range 4.5–11.2	Pharmacokinetic study; one of 11 patients had a convulsion
VadeBoncouer et al[27]	1990	Canine model	10 ml of 0.5% bupivacaine 20 ml of 0.5% bupivacaine (No epinephrine) (single injection)		Larger injection volume produced more intense and widespread intercostal nerve block
Epinephrine					
Denson et al[30]	1988	Primate model	Crossover protocol 20 ml of 0.5% bupivacaine with and without 1:200,000 epinephrine (single injection)		Pharmacokinetic study; no difference in pharmacokinetic analyses irrespective of presence or absence of epinephrine
Kambam et al.[31]	1989	Thoracotomy	20 ml of 0.5% bupivacaine with and without 1:200,000 epinephrine (single injection)		Significant decrease in peak plasma concentration of bupivacaine with use of epinephrine
Continuous interpleural infusions					
Rocco et al[33]	1987	Rib fractures	20 ml of 0.5% bupivacaine followed by 0.25% or 0.5% bupivacaine at 5–10 ml/h	Continuous for 5–10 days	No toxic systemic concentrations despite prolonged use; more widespread and intense analgesia with infusions of 0.5% bupivacaine
Rosenberg et al[36]	1987	Thoracotomy	Initial injection of 0.5% bupivacaine based on body weight followed by infusion of 5–10 ml/h	Continuous for 48 h	Poor analgesia attributed to uneven spread of anesthetic because of removal of lung parenchyma and loss of anesthetic through thoracostomy tube drainage
Pond et al[14]	1989	Rib fractures	Infusion of 8 ml/h of 1.6% lidocaine; infusion rate adjusted to maintain serum lidocaine concentration <5 µg/ml	Continuous for 9 days	
Scott et al[19]	1989	Cholecystectomy	20-ml injection of 0.5% bupivacaine followed by 10 ml/h	Continuous for 8 h	Significant but incomplete analgesia

TABLE 16-2. Protocol for Intermittent Dosing of Interpleural Catheters

Insert epidural needle at sixth, seventh, or eighth ribs at midaxillary line or more posteriorly
Avoid loss of resistance techniques for location of interpleural space
Thread no more than 5 or 6 cm of catheter into the chest
Secure catheter with sterile transparent dressing
Inject catheter with 10–20 ml of 0.25% or 0.5% bupivacaine with epinephrine
Use least amount of local anesthetic that provides 4–6 h of analgesia
Position patient in supine or semilateral position (painful side uppermost) during injection
Observe patient for at least 30 min after injection for signs of local anesthetic toxicity
Provide availability of other forms of analgesia (i.e., PCA)
Redose catheter every 4–6 h

16-2. Despite the quandaries, interpleural regional analgesia can be very effective.

CLINICAL APPLICATIONS

Interpleural analgesia is an effective method of postoperative pain management after unilateral surgical incisions in the chest and/or abdomen (Table 16-3). Because interpleural local anesthetics may produce neural blockade from the first through twelfth thoracic intercostal nerves, it follows that the technique will be effective for somatic pain in these dermatomes.

Cholecystectomy,[1,15–19,25] mastectomy,[1] and nephrectomy[1] are the surgical procedures most effectively treated with interpleural analgesia. In all these situations, the surgical wound extends through several of the middle or lower thoracic dermatomes. Pain relief is usually profound, permitting effective coughing and deep breathing.

The pain of fractured ribs is particularly amenable to interpleural regional analgesia.[28,33] Pain relief is associated with a dramatic improvement in the hypercarbia and hypoxemia resulting from splinting and hypoventilation.[33]

Pain relief with interpleural local anesthetics after thoracotomy may be equiv-

TABLE 16-3. Clinical Applications of Interpleural Regional Analgesia

Thorax
    Chest wall operations (e.g., rib section)[a]
    Pectus repair
    Mastectomy or other breast procedures

Abdomen
    Cholecystectomy
    Splenectomy
    Nephrectomy

Nonsurgical
    Rib fracture

[a] This does *not* include thoracotomy. The results of interpleural regional analgesia are equivocal or unsatisfactory after thoracotomy.

TABLE 16-4. Rationale for Failure of Interpleural Regional Analgesia After Thoracotomy

Loss of local anesthetic through thoracostomy tube drainage

Diffusion barriers to local anesthetic
  Pleural and chest wall edema
  Extravasated tissue fluid

Dilution and protein binding of local anesthetic by collections of blood and serum

Rapid systemic absorption of local anesthetic through depleuralized areas

Change in distribution of local anesthetic
  Uneven spread
  Channeling of flow

Sequestration of interpleural local anesthetic by restricted motion of operated lung (or lack thereof)

ocal or unsatisfactory. Numerous reports have documented inadequate analgesia in this circumstance.[5,36,37] Adequate analgesia has been reported[31] but appears to be the exception rather than the rule. The reasons for the lack of efficacy are multifactorial[38] (Table 16-4).

Midline abdominal incisions receive bilateral innervation and require bilateral interpleural catheters for management. Although reports of successful analgesia with bilateral interpleural catheters do exist,[26,39] the requirement for frequent administration of large doses of local anesthetic and the attendant risk of toxicity preclude easy applicability. Interpleural analgesia cannot be routinely recommended for midline abdominal incisions.

COMPLICATIONS

The chief complications of interpleural analgesia are pneumothorax and local anesthetic toxicity. Other unusual effects may also result from the presence of local anesthetic in the chest cavity.

Pneumothorax

As discussed previously, the risk of pneumothorax with interpleural catheter placement should be low if loss of resistance techniques are avoided. Overall, the frequency of pneumothorax with interpleural regional analgesia is 2 percent.[7] Studies documenting alarmingly high rates of pneumothorax used either a loss of resistance technique for needle insertion[22] or excessive lengths of interpleural catheter insertion.[23]

Clinically significant pneumothorax (i.e., dyspnea, shortness of breath, diminished breath sounds) should be distinguished from that resulting from the entrainment of small volumes of air (3–5 cc) during catheter insertion. In the latter instance, although a small amount of air may be evident on a chest roentgenogram, the pneumothorax is typically without symptomatology and is harmlessly absorbed. Symptomatic pneumothorax will almost always be the result of unintentional lung trauma during catheter insertion.

If dyspnea, shortness of breath, or decreased breath sounds are detected after interpleural catheter placement, pneumothorax should be suspected and the appropriate measures instituted. Aspiration of air through the interpleural catheter may be diagnostic. Tube thoracostomy may be required if symptoms are severe or tension pneumothorax develops.

Local Anesthetic Toxicity

The possibility of local anesthetic toxicity should always be anticipated with use of interpleural regional analgesia. The necessity for administration of large doses of local anesthetic with frequent reinjection places the patient at risk for ever increasing systemic levels of local anesthetic. Because nearly all reports document maximum blood concentrations within 30 minutes of injection,[5,25,26,30,31] patients should not be left unattended during this time. All patients should be questioned for symptoms of dysgeusia, circumoral numbness, light-headedness, and tinnitus.

Pleural Effusions

Iatrogenic pleural effusions from interpleural regional analgesia occur with an incidence of 0.4 percent.[7] Such effusions may resorb spontaneously or progress to pleural infection.

Horner's Syndrome

As previously stated, unilateral Horner's syndrome may result during interpleural regional analgesia.[7,9,10] Production of Horner's syndrome may be more likely to occur when patients are positioned head down and slightly lateral at the time of injection. This body position would optimize local anesthetic spread to the sympathetic chain. Patients merely need reassurance if Horner's syndrome occurs.

Phrenic Nerve Block

A recent study documented bilateral phrenic nerve block and subsequent paradoxical motion of the abdomen during interpleural regional analgesia in a canine model.[40] Although never clinically reported in humans, bilateral phrenic nerve block with the potential for respiratory compromise is clearly a concern if bilateral interpleural catheters are used.[39,41,42]

**TABLE 16-5. Contraindications to
Interpleural Regional Analgesia**

Presence of
  Pleural effusion
  Pleural fibrosis
  Pleural inflammation (e.g., recent pneumonia)
  Lung-pleural adhesions (e.g., lung malignancy)
  Empyema
  Anticoagulation or bleeding diathesis

CONTRAINDICATIONS

Contradindications to interpleural catheter placement are those conditions that make the risk of lung puncture and/or local anesthetic toxicity unacceptably high (Table 16-5).

Pulmonary malignancy, pleural fibrosis, and extensive or chronic pulmonary disease may result in pleural-parenchymal adhesions. This could make correct location of the interpleural space impossible, with a high likelihood of lung puncture and resultant pneumothorax.[22]

Patients with recent pneumonia, empyema, or known pleuritis should not receive interpleural analgesia. An inflamed vascular pleura may be expected to absorb local anesthetic avidly, resulting in the rapid attainment of a high local anesthetic concentration in the blood. The risk of systemic toxicity may be great in this scenario. An early report of convulsions after interpleural bupivacaine documented a resolving pneumonia and suspected pleuritis as factors contributing to this complication.[17]

Contraindications to regional anesthesia are, in general, contraindications to interpleural analgesia. These include the presence of a bleeding diathesis and sepsis.

CONCLUSION

Interpleural regional analgesia is an innovative new modality for the management of pain. It is not a panacea. Interpleural regional analgesia clearly has limitations in a number of clinical settings, and many basic questions still remain regarding the optimal methods for performance of the technique. Interpleural regional analgesia can, however, provide profound pain relief in the appropriate setting. In those instances in which epidural management is impossible or unacceptable, interpleural analgesia may provide an effective alternative. The simplicity of its application and the attendant patient satisfaction with the technique make it a desirable adjunct to the more traditional forms of regional anesthesia/analgesia.

References
1. Reiestad F, Strømskag KE: Interpleural catheter in the management of postoperative pain. A preliminary report. Reg Anesth 11:89, 1986
2. Covino BG: Interpleural regional analgesia (editorial). Anesth Analg 67:427, 1988

3. Riegler FX, VadeBoncouer TR, Pelligrino DA: Interpleural anesthetics in the dog: differential somatic neural blockade. Anesthesiology 71:744, 1989

4. Nunn JF, Slavin G: Posterior intercostal nerve block for pain relief after cholecystectomy. Anatomical basis and efficacy. Br J Anaesth 52:253, 1980

5. Ferrante FM, Chan VWS, Arthur GR, Rocco AG: Interpleural analgesia after thoracotomy. Anesth Analg 72:105, 1991

6. Strømskag KE, Hauge O, Steen PA: Distribution of local anesthetics injected into the interpleural space, studied by computerized tomography. Acta Anesthesiol Scand 34:323, 1990

7. Strømskag KE, Minor B, Steen PA: Side effects and complications related to interpleural analgesia: an update. Acta Anaesthesiol Scand 34:473, 1990

8. Strømskag KE, Pillgram-Larsen J, Reiestad F, Steen PA: Hemodynamic effects of interpleural analgesia in pigs. Acta Anaesthesiol Scand 34:342, 1990

9. Sihota MK, Holmblad BR: Horner's syndrome after intrapleural analgesia with bupivacaine for postherpatic neuralgia. Acta Anaesthesiol Scand 32:593, 1988

10. Parkinson SK, Mueller JB, Rich TJ, Little WL: Unilateral Horner's syndrome associated with interpleural catheter injection of local anesthetic. Anesth Analg 68:61, 1989

11. Reiestad F, McIlvaine WB, Kvalheim L et al: Interpleural analgesia in treatment of upper extremity reflex sympathetic dystrophy. Anesth Analg 69:671, 1989

12. Durrani Z, Winnie AP, Ikuta P: Interpleural catheter analgesia for pancreatic pain. Anesth Analg 67:479, 1988

13. Reiestad F, McIlvaine WB, Kvalheim L et al: Successful treatment of chronic pancreatitis pain with interpleural analgesia. Can J Anaesth 36:713, 1989

14. Pond WW, Somerville GM, Thong SH et al: Pain of delayed traumatic splenic rupture masked by interpleural lidocaine. Anesthesiology 70:154, 1989

15. Laurito CE, Kirz LI, VadeBoncouer TR et al: Continuous infusion of interpleural bupivacaine maintains effective analgesia after cholecystectomy. Anesth Analg 72:516, 1991

16. VadeBoncouer TR, Riegler FX, Gautt RS, Weinberg GL: A randomized, double-blind comparison of the effects of interpleural bupivacaine and saline on morphine requirements and pumonary function after cholecystectomy. Anesthesiology 71:339, 1989

17. Seltzer JL, Larijani GE, Goldberg ME, Marr AT: Intrapleural bupivacaine—a kinetic and dynamic evaluation. Anesthesiology 67:798, 1987

18. Brismar B, Pettersson N, Tokics L et al: Postoperative analgesia with intrapleural administration of bupivacaine-adrenaline. Acta Anaesthesiol Scand 31:515, 1987

19. Scott NB, Mogensen T, Bigler D, Kehlet H: Comparison of the effects of continuous intrapleural vs. epidural administration of 0.5% bupivacaine on pain, metabolic response and pulmonary function following cholecystectomy. Acta Anaesthesiol Scand 33:535, 1989

20. Squier RC, Morrow JS, Roman R: Hanging-drop technique for interpleural analgesia (letter). Anesthesiology 70:882, 1989

21. Ben-David B, Lee E: The falling column: a new technique for interpleural catheter placement (letter). Anesth Analg 71:212, 1990

22. Symreng T, Gomez MN, Johnson B, et al: Intrapleural bupivacaine—technical considerations and intraoperative use. J Cardiothorac Anesth 3:139, 1989

23. Gomez MN, Symreng T, Johnson B et al: Intrapleural bupivacaine for intraoperative analgesia—a dangerous technique?, abstracted. Anesth Analg 67:S78, 1988

24. El-Naggar MA, Schaberg FJ Jr, Phillips MR: Intrapleural regional analgesia for pain management in cholecystectomy. Arch Surg 124:568, 1989

25. Strømskag KE, Reiestad F, Holmqvist ELO, Ogenstad S: Intrapleural administration of 0.25%, 0.375%, and 0.5% bupivacaine with epinephrine after cholecystectomy. Anesth Analg 67:430, 1988

26. El-Naggar MA, Bennett B, Raad C, Yogaratnam G: Bilateral intrapleural intercostal nerve block, abstracted. Anesth Analg 67:S57, 1988

27. VadeBoncouer TR, Riegler FX, Pelligrino DA: The effects of two different volumes of 0.5% bupivacaine in a canine model of interpleural analgesia. Reg Anesth 15:67, 1990

28. Carli PA, Mazoit X, Zetlaoui J, Lambert Y: Intrapleural administration of lidocaine for treatment of post traumatic thoracic pain, abstracted. Anesthesiology 67:A241, 1987

29. Queen JS, Kahana MD, DiFazio CA et al: An evaluation of interpleural analgesia with etidocaine in children, abstracted. Anesth Analg 68:S228, 1989

30. Denson D, Sehlhorst CS, Schultz REG et al: Pharmacokinetics of intrapleural bupivacaine: effects of epinephrine, abstracted. Reg Anesth, suppl. 13(1S):47, 1988

31. Kambam JR, Hammon J, Parris WCV, Lupinetti FM: Intrapleural analgesia for postthoracotomy pain and blood levels of bupivacaine following interpleural injection. Can J Anaesth 36:106, 1989

32. Frank ED, McKay W, Rocco A, Gallo JP: Interpleural bupivacaine for postoperative analgesia following cholecystectomy: a randomized prospective study. Reg Anesth 15:26, 1990

33. Rocco A, Reiestad F, Gudman J, McKay W: Intrapleural administration of local anesthetics for pain relief in patients with multiple rib fractures. Preliminary report. Reg Anesth 12:10, 1987

34. Baker PA, Schroeder D: Interpleural bupivacaine for postoperative pain during lactation. Anesth Analg 69:400, 1989

35. McIlvaine WB, Knox RF, Fennessey PV, Goldstein M: Continuous infusion of bupivacaine via intrapleural catheter for analgesia after thoracotomy in children. Anesthesiology 69:261, 1988

36. Rosenberg PH, Scheinin BM-A, Lepäntalo MJA, Lindfors O: Continuous intrapleural infusion of bupivacaine for analgesia after thoracotomy. Anesthesiology 67:811, 1987

37. El-Baz N, Faber LP, Ivankovich AD: Intrapleural infusion of local anesthetic: A word of caution (letter). Anesthesiology 68:809, 1988

38. El-Baz N: The experts opine. Interpleural analgesia: advantages and limitations in comparison to thoracic epidural analgesia (editorial). Survey Anesthesiol 23:193, 1989

39. Aquilar JL, Montero A, Lopez FV, Llamazares JF: Bilateral interpleural injection of local anesthetics. Reg Anesth 14:93, 1989

40. Kowalski S, Bradley B, Greengrass R et al: The effects of interpleural bupivacaine (0.5%) on canine diaphragmatic function, abstracted. Anesthesiology 73:A1191, 1990

41. Redick LF: Is phrenic nerve block possible with interpleural analgesia? (letter). Reg Anesth 15:44, 1990

42. Aquilar J, Montero A, Lopez FV, Llamazares JF: Intrapleural analgesia and phrenic nerve palsy (letter). Reg Anesth 15:45, 1990

17

Continuous Thoracic Paravertebral Block

Vincent W. S. Chan
F. Michael Ferrante

The technique of thoracic paravertebral neural blockade was first introduced by Kappis[1] in 1919. However, reports of its use were infrequent over the next several decades.[2,3] In 1979, interest in this technique was revitalized by Eason and Wyatt,[4] who described the anatomy of the paravertebral space in detail. Because of the fear of potential complications (i.e., pneumothorax), the popularity of thoracic paravertebral block for postoperative analgesia still remains somewhat limited. Unfortunately, the description of this technique has even been omitted from some regional anesthesia textbooks.

ANATOMY

As the name implies, the *thoracic paravertebral space* is a narrow triangular space just lateral to the vertebral column (Fig. 17-1). The thoracic paravertebral space is wedge-shaped, bounded posteriorly by the superior costotransverse ligament, anterolaterally by the parietal pleura, and superiorly and inferiorly by the heads and necks of the adjoining ribs (Fig. 17-1). The base of this space is formed by the vertebral body and the intervertebral foramen. Medially, the paravertebral space communicates with the epidural space through the intervertebral foramen. Laterally, it is in continuity with the intercostal space.

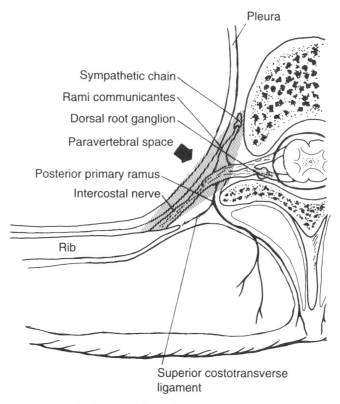

Fig. 17-1. The paravertebral space (*shaded triangle*). Transverse section at the level of the intervertebral foramen.

The thoracic spinal nerves divide into dorsal and ventral rami within the paravertebral space shortly after emerging from the intervertebral foraminae (Figs. 17-1 and 17-2). Within this space, the sympathetic fibers of the ventral rami enter the sympathetic trunk via the preganglionic white rami communicantes and the postganglionic gray rami communicantes. In essence, local anesthetic injection into the paravertebral space will achieve motor, sensory, and unilateral sympathetic blockade.

Safe access of the thoracic paravertebral space relies on proper identification of two anatomic landmarks: the spinous processes and the transverse processes of two adjacent thoracic vertebrae. Because of the downward inclination of a thoracic vertebral spinous process, its tip usually lies adjacent to the transverse processes of the vertebra immediately below (Figs. 17-3 and 17-4). For example, the tip of the spinous process of T6 lies at the level of the transverse processes of T7. The transverse processes are usually located approximately 3 cm lateral to the tip of the spinous process in the midline. The typical thoracic transverse process is short, with a distance of only 2–4 cm separating the vertebral body from the head of the respective rib. The superior costotransverse ligament

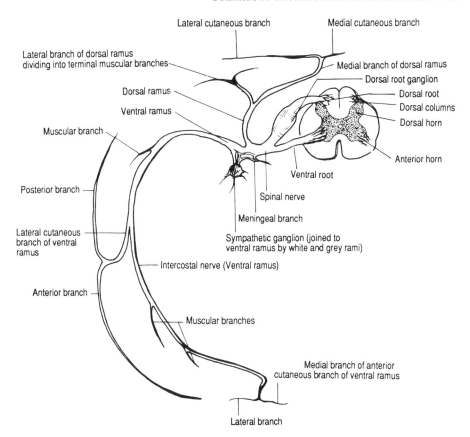

Fig. 17-2. Origin and distribution of a typical spinal nerve.

courses obliquely and downward from the superior transverse processes to the heads of ribs below (Fig. 17-5). (An inferior costotransverse ligament connects the transverse processes to their respective ribs at the same thoracic level [Fig. 17-5].)

Location of the transverse process or the head of a rib with an epidural needle and subsequently "walking off" to traverse the superior costotransverse ligament is the essence of performance of thoracic paravertebral neural blockade. As the epidural needle passes into the loose adipose tissue of the paravertebral space through the superior costotransverse ligament, a loss of resistance to saline or air can be appreciated, similar to that used to identify the epidural space.

MECHANISMS OF ACTION

The paravertebral space is contiguous with the intercostal and epidural spaces (Fig. 17-6). Thus, anesthesia and analgesia can be obtained over several dermatomes by local anesthetic spread: (1) laterally along the intercostal space,

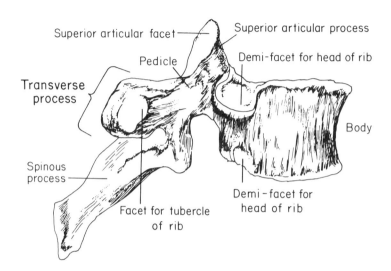

Fig. 17-3. Typical midthoracic vertebra. Right lateral aspect.

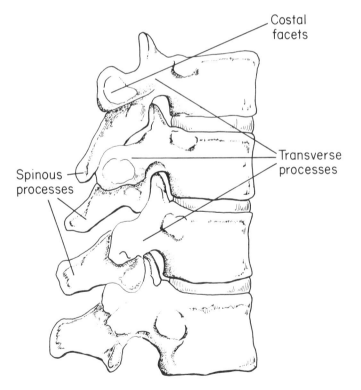

Fig. 17-4. Articulating thoracic vertebrae, Right lateral aspect. Because of the downward inclination of a thoracic vertebral spinous process, its tip lies adjacent to the transverse processes of the immediately caudad vertebra.

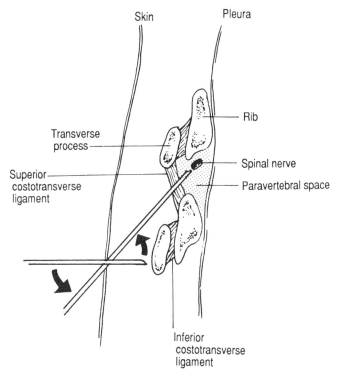

Skin   Pleura

Rib

Transverse
process

Spinal nerve

Superior
costotransverse
ligament

Paravertebral space

Inferior
costotransverse
ligament

Fig. 17-5. Longitudinal section. Proper direction of epidural needle insertion. The epidural needle is "walked off" the rib or transverse process in a cephalad direction to pierce the superior costotransverse ligament.

and subsequently through the subpleural space (see Ch. 15), (2) cephalad and caudad within the paravertebral space (Fig. 17-7), (3) medially to the epidural space, and (4) through a combination of the above.[5–9] Thus, the anatomic spread of local anesthetic injected into the paravertebral space is often unpredictable. Epidural spread of varying degrees was reported in 70 percent of patients in a study by Purcell-Jones et al,[8] whereas spread was restricted to the paravertebral space in only 18 percent of patients.

The potential epidural spread of local anesthetic after paravertebral injection is of more than passing significance. The sensory anesthesia/analgesia of "pure" paravertebral neural blockade is unilateral, whereas that of epidural blockade is bilateral. With pure paravertebral neural blockade, only unilateral sympathetic block is produced. Thus, the risk of hypotension (a potential complication of thoracic epidural anesthesia) should be significantly reduced.[4] However, the potential for hypotension does exist because of the possible epidural spread of local anesthetic after paravertebral injection.[8,9]

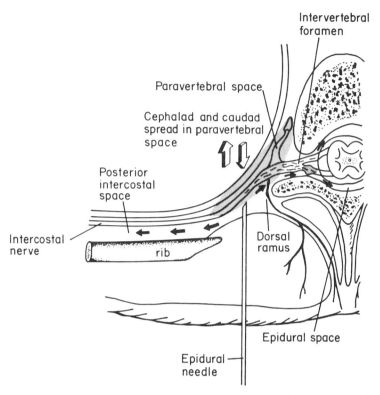

Intervertebral foramen

Paravertebral space

Cephalad and caudad spread in paravertebral space

Posterior intercostal space

Intercostal nerve

rib

Dorsal ramus

Epidural space

Epidural needle

Fig. 17-6. The paravertebral space is contiguous with the intercostal and epidural spaces. Thus, local anesthetic may spread laterally to the intercostal space, cephalad and caudad in the paravertebral space, and medially to the epidural space.

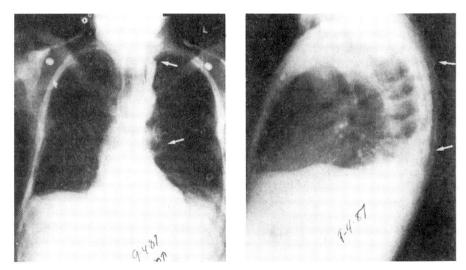

Fig. 17-7. Chest roentgenogram (posteroanterior and lateral views) demonstrating extent of spread of 6 ml of contrast (*arrows*) injected into the paravertebral space. Note that local anesthetic is confined to the paravertebral space. (From Johnson et al,[6] with permission.)

TECHNIQUE

Positioning and Landmarks

Thoracic paravertebral block can be performed sitting upright or in a lateral decubitus position with the hemithorax to be injected uppermost. Intravenous access is established before needle insertion, and sedation may be provided as necessary. The spinous process palpable at the desired thoracic level is chosen as a landmark. (As stated previously, this is actually the spinous process of the next most cephalad thoracic vertebra above the desired level of the needle insertion.) The point of needle entry is marked (3 cm lateral to the midline spinous process).

Procedure

The area is prepared and draped in a sterile manner, and a skin wheal is raised with 1 percent lidocaine at the proposed site of needle entry. After local infiltration, a 22-gauge 4-cm finder needle is introduced perpendicular to the skin in all planes, and contact is made with the transverse process or the head of the rib. Bony contact is often made at a depth of 2–3 cm in an average individual. In obese patients, this distance can be up to 6 cm.

With the direction and depth of penetration in mind, a 16- to 18-gauge epidural needle is now inserted perpendicular to the skin in all planes. Once bony contact is made, the needle stylet is withdrawn, and an air- or saline-filled glass syringe is attached. The epidural needle is directed cephalad to "walk off" the upper border of the transverse process or rib. A loss of resistance will be appreciated as the needle penetrates the superior costotransverse ligament (Figs. 17-5 and 17-8). On entry into the paravertebral space, aspiration is performed to test for air, blood, and/or cerebrospinal fluid (CSF). If blood is encountered on aspiration, the epidural needle is removed, and placement is reattempted. After negative aspiration, a 20-gauge epidural catheter can be advanced 2–3 cm into the paravertebral space. The epidural needle is then withdrawn, and the indwelling paravertebral catheter is securely taped to the skin surface to avoid dislodgement.

Variations of the Technique

The thoracic paravertebral block has been performed in a number of different ways, with the point of epidural needle insertion varying from 3–5 cm from the midline, the angle of needle insertion varying from 45°–90°, and the needle passing above or below the rib or transverse process.[4]

The technique of Eason and Wyatt[4] described in this chapter minimizes the chance of pneumothorax. Older techniques[2] advocated "walking" caudad off the rib or transverse process. As can be seen in Figure 17-9, the distance from the superior costotransverse ligament to the pleura when walking caudad (line CD) is much smaller than the distance to the pleura when walking cephalad (line

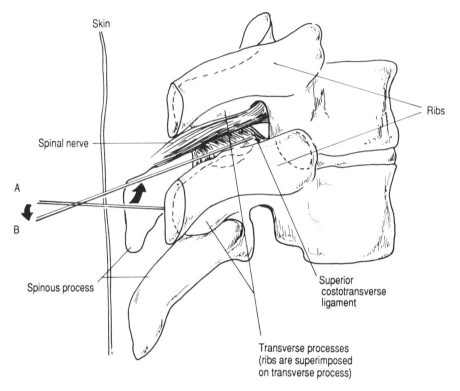

Skin

Ribs

Spinal nerve

A

B

Spinous process

Superior
costotransverse
ligament

Transverse processes
(ribs are superimposed
on transverse process)

Fig. 17-8. Direction of epidural needle. (A) The needle strikes the transverse process or rib. (B) The needle is then angled cephalad to pass through the superior costotransverse ligament.

AB). Thus, the cephalad approach should be preferentially used to minimize the risk of pneumothorax with this technique.

In the case of thoracotomy, a similar percutaneous technique can be used under direct vision while the chest is still open. Proper placement of the paravertebral catheter can be verified visually, by palpation, or by injected dye (which will enhance the success rate).[10,11] Double-catheter techniques to provide analgesia for both the incision *and* the thoracostomy tube site have also been advocated to obtain complete postoperative analgesia.[4]

Choice and Dosing Interval of Local Anesthetic

Long-acting bupivacaine has been used in most clinical studies. Before injection, catheter aspiration is mandatory to test for air, blood, or CSF. After a test dose of 3 ml, local anesthetic should be administered in titrated doses over 5–10 minutes. Commonly used doses are 20–30 ml of 0.25 percent or 10–20 ml of 0.5 percent bupivacaine. Generally speaking, at least four dermatomes will be

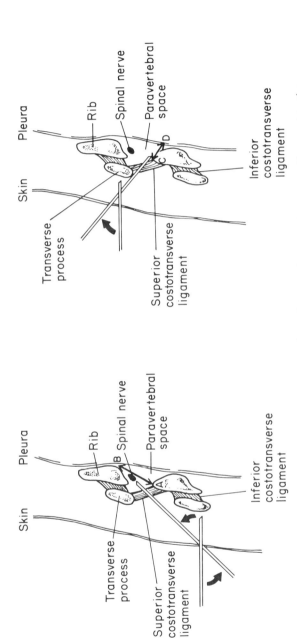

Fig. 17-9. Variations of technique. The distance from the superior costotransverse ligament to the pleura is smaller when "walking" caudad (line CD) than when "walking" cephalad (line AB). Thus, walking cephalad off the rib or transverse process minimizes the risk of pneumothorax.

anesthetized by a single 15-ml injection.[4] Analgesic duration is highly variable (anywhere from 1 to 10 hours after 20–25 ml of 0.5 percent bupivacaine).[12,13] The effect of epinephrine on the duration of analgesia has not been studied. (See Table 17-1 for a compilation of previously used dosing regimens and their effects.)

Maintenance of analgesia can be achieved by repeated injections or by continuous infusion.[14–16] A continuous infusion of 0.5 percent bupivacaine at 5 ml/h was found to be inadequate for postcholecystectomy pain in one study.[16] However, an infusion of 0.25 percent bupivacaine at 5 ml/h over 4 days was sufficient to completely ablate the pain of acute herpes zoster.[6]

At present, neither the optimal dose, volume, or concentration of local anesthetic for a single injection has been determined. Similarly, no data exist as to the range of safe and/or effective infusion rates for continuous delivery. Consideration of potential local anesthetic toxicity will determine the maximal single and cumulative (24-hour) dose. However, data on systemic bupivacaine absorption from the paravertebral space are lacking.

CLINICAL APPLICATIONS

Knowledge of anatomic landmarks and boundaries provides essential clinical information and prevents potential complications when performing thoracic paravertebral block. As shown in Figure 17-1, only a narrow gap exists between the superior costotransverse ligament and the parietal pleura at the lateral margin of the paravertebral space. Therefore, a needle directed laterally is likely to puncture the pleura. Conversely, a needle directed medially may enter the epidural space through an intervertebral foramen, resulting in dural puncture.

Indications for use of thoracic paravertebral neural blockade are similar to that of continuous intercostal nerve block. Paravertebral nerve block provides analgesia after cholecystectomy,[12] thoracotomy,[11,14] and rib fractures.[13] It has also been used effectively to treat the neuralgia of acute herpes zoster.[6,17]

COMPLICATIONS

Pneumothorax

Pneumothorax is a potentially life-threatening complication. The incidence of pleural puncture has been found to vary from 0.5 percent[15] to 20 percent.[5] Such a wide variation in incidence may directly reflect operator experience. Performance of thoracic paravertebral block is obviously safest in post-thoracotomy patients with thoracostomy tubes.

Dural Puncture

Dural puncture and subarachnoid injection resulting in total spinal anesthesia are potential complications. Postural headache resembling that of postdural puncture headache has been reported.[18]

TABLE 17-1. Reports of Analgesia Using Thoracic Paravertebral/Neural Blockade

Author	Year	Origin of Pain	Drug Dose	Extent of Analgesia	Duration of Analgesia (h)	Remarks
Gilbert and Hultman[13]	1989	Trauma	Bupivacaine 0.5% plain 25 ml (intermittent injection)	8 dermatomes	9.9	30% Incidence of contralateral anesthesia; 10% incidence of hypotension
Conacher and Kokri[5]	1987	Thoracotomy	Bupivacaine 0.25% plain 20–30 ml (single injection)	3–8 dermatomes	?	Evidence of intercostal paravertebral, and epidural spread of contrast
Purcell-Jones and Justins[9]	1988	Thoracotomy	Bupivacaine 0.5% plain 5 ml (single injection)	"Widespread"	?	No contralateral anesthesia; 9% incidence of hypotension; 70% epidural spread; 20% spread confined to paravertebral space; no pneumothorax despite "walking" caudad during technique
Matthews and Govenden[14]	1989	Thoracotomy	Bupivacaine 0.25% plain bolus ± 3–10 ml/h infusion	8 dermatomes	Continuous	No contralateral anesthesia or hypotension; continuous infusion for 24 h
Giesecke et al[12]	1988	Cholecystectomy	Bupivacaine 20 ml (concentration and amount [mg] unknown)	?	1–6	Attenuation of surgical stress response
Bigler et al[16]	1989	Cholecystectomy	Bupivacaine 0.5% plain bolus ± 5 ml/h	7 dermatomes	Continuous	30% Incidence of contralateral anesthesia; continuous infusion for 8 h
Eason and Wyatt[4]	1979	Multiple sources	Bupivacaine 0.375% plain 15 ml (intermittent injection)	At least 4 dermatomes	?	100% Unilateral anesthesia; no hypotension
Purcell-Jones et al[8]	1989	Chronic pain	Bupivacaine 0.75% plain 5 ml	1–10 dermatomes		70% Epidural spread, 18% spread confined to paravertebral space; 7% contralateral anesthesia; extent of sensory anesthesia dependent on anatomic location of spread; greater extent with epidural spread

Hypotension

As previously stated, unilateral sympathetic blockade does not usually lead to hypotension. Compared with thoracic epidural blockade, the incidence of hypotension with thoracic paravertebral block should be substantially lower.[4] However, as the possibility of spread of local anesthetic to the contiguous epidural space does exist, the risk of hypotension after performance of thoracic paravertebral neural blockade is real.[8,9]

Vascular Damage

Accidental venous cannulation has been reported with this technique,[4,16] although significant bleeding from vascular laceration has not been reported.

Nerve Damage

As with continuous intercostal neural blockade, damage to the intercostal nerves is a potential complication but has never been reported.

CONCLUSION

Continuous thoracic paravertebral neural blockade can provide excellent and predictable analgesia. Similar to continuous intercostal neural blockade, many practitioners have avoided this technique, perhaps because of the potential for pneumothorax. A large study comparing the incidences of complications attendant on performance of continuous intercostal, interpleural, continuous paravertebral, and thoracic epidural techniques is certainly warranted.

References
1. Kappis M: Burns' Beitz. Klin Chir 115:161, 1919
2. Moore DC: Paravertebral thoracic somatic nerve block. p. 200. In: Regional Block. 4th Ed. Charles C Thomas, Springfield, IL, 1953
3. Shaw W, Hollis N: Medial approach for paravertebral somatic nerve block. JAMA 148:742, 1952
4. Eason MJ, Wyatt R: Paravertebral thoracic block—a reappraisal. Anaesthesia 34: 638, 1979
5. Conacher ID, Kokri M: Postoperative paravertebral blocks for thoracic surgery. A radiological appraisal. Br J Anaesth 59:155, 1987
6. Johnson LR, Rocco AG, Ferrante FM: Continuous subpleural-paravertebral block in acute thoracic herpes zoster. Anesth Analg 67:1105, 1988
7. Conacher ID: Resin injection of thoracic paravertebral spaces. Br J Anaesth 61:657, 1988
8. Purcell-Jones G, Pither CE, Justin DM: Paravertebral somatic nerve block: a clinical, radiographic, and computed tomographic study in chronic pain patients. Anesth Analg 68:32, 1989

9. Purcell-Jones G, Justins DM: Postoperative paravertebral blocks for thoracic surgery (letter). Br J Anaesth 61:369, 1988
10. Berrisford RG, Sabanathan SS: Direct access to the paravertebral space at thoracotomy (letter). Ann Thorac Surg 49:854, 1990
11. Govenden V, Matthews P: Percutaneous placement of paravertebral catheters during thoracotomy (letter). Anaesthesia 43:256, 1988
12. Giesecke K, Hamberger B, Järnberg PO, Klingstedt C: Paravertebral block during cholecystectomy: effects on circulatory and hormonal responses. Br J Anaesth 61:652, 1988
13. Gilbert J, Hultman J: Thoracic paravertebral block: a method of pain control. Acta Anaesthesiol Scand 33:142, 1989
14. Matthews PJ, Govenden V: Comparison of continuous paravertebral and extradural infusions of bupivacaine for pain relief after thoracotomy. Br J Anaesth 62:204, 1989
15. McKnight CK, Marshall M: Monoplatythela and paravertebral block (letter). Anaesthesia 39:1147, 1984
16. Bigler D, Dirkes W, Hansen R et al: Effects of thoracic paravertebral block with bupivacaine versus combined thoracic epidural block with bupivacaine and morphine on pain and pulmonary function after cholecystectomy. Acta Anaesthesiol Scand 33:561, 1989
17. Findley T, Patzer R: The treatment of herpes zoster by paravertebral procaine block. JAMA 128:1217, 1945
18. Sharrock NE: Postural headache following thoracic somatic paravertebral nerve block. Anesthesiology 52:360, 1980

18

Thoracic Epidural Analgesia

Simon C. Body

The insertion of midthoracic epidural catheters for neural blockade or the administration of opioids has historically been regarded as more difficult than that of lumbar placement. Trepidation with respect to performance of this technique is based on the fear of potential spinal cord injury, the anatomic differences between lumbar and midthoracic vertebral morphology, and the potential physiologic derangements resultant from administration of midthoracic local anesthetics and opioids. There is justification for avoidance of a cavalier attitude toward thoracic epidural analgesia, but fear or awe of this technique is unreasonable.

ANATOMY

A complete discussion of the anatomy of the vertebral column can be found in Chapter 5. This chapter will confine itself to the important distinctions in the bony and soft tissue anatomy of the midthoracic and lumbar spine.[1,2]

The midthoracic spinous processes have a 45° caudad angulation with a narrow interspace between each spinous process (Figs. 18-1 and 18-3). In addition, the thoracic interlaminar foraminae are crescent-shaped and considerably smaller than their counterparts in the lumbar spine, each measuring approximately 15 mm × 5 mm (Fig. 18-2). The ligamentum flavum covering the interlaminar foraminae is thinner in the thoracic spine. Thus, the tactile sensation of passage of an epidural needle through the ligamentum flavum will be less easily appreciated. As a result of the 45° angulation of the spinous processes, the depth of insertion of the epidural needle is deeper than that commonly encountered during performance of lumbar epidural analgesia.[1,2]

417

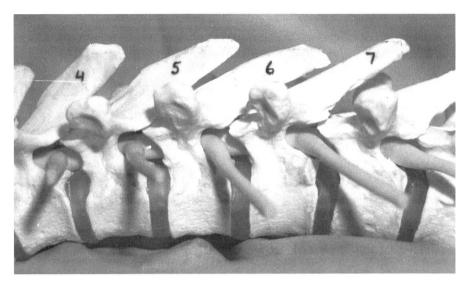

Fig. 18-1. Lateral view of the midthoracic spine. Numbers denote the spinous processes of the respective thoracic vertebrae. Note the narrow interspinous space between each spinous process.

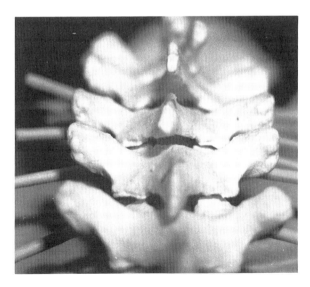

Fig. 18-2. Midthoracic spine from the midline position. Note the crescent-shaped interlaminar foraminae. Also note the difference in size of the midthoracic interlaminar foraminae when compared with the view from the paramedian position (Fig. 18-4).

**TABLE 18-1. Anatomic Differences Between the
Thoracic and Lumbar Spine**

45° Caudad angulation of the thoracic spinous processes (Fig. 18-1)
Less robust thoracic ligamentum flavum (poorer tactile sensation)
Narrower thoracic epidural space
Narrower thoracic nerve root foraminae
Narrower thoracic interlaminar foraminae (Fig. 18-2)
Less well-defined and narrower thoracic interspinous ligaments
Larger thoracic laminae (Fig. 18-3)

The salient anatomic differences between thoracic and lumbar vertebral morphology are summarized in Table 18-1. These differences form the anatomic basis for the distinctions between lumbar and midthoracic epidural technique.

TECHNIQUE

The three-dimensional spatial anatomy of the thoracic spine should be studied intensively before the inexperienced practitioner attempts to perform thoracic epidural analgesia. An inexperienced practitioner should be supervised until *both* teacher and student are comfortable with the pupil's facility with the technique.

Monitoring and Preparation

Patients receiving thoracic epidural analgesia should be monitored with electrocardiogram (ECG), blood pressure cuff, and pulse oximeter (if sedated). The patient should receive supplemental oxygen irrespective of whether sedation is used or not. Intravenous access is mandatory, and resuscitation equipment and drugs must be close by.

The use of sedation is preferable in patients receiving thoracic epidural analgesia to increase patient acceptance and cooperation. Judicious "titration" of an opioid and benzodiazepine is advisable. The patient should not be overly sedated, but able to answer questions and perform commands. Such a degree of sedation will enable the patient to communicate the sensation of a paresthesia, if necessary. The performance of midthoracic epidural technique in anesthetized or unconscious patients is strongly discouraged, as the perception of paresthesiae cannot be communicated. In the rare event that epidural analgesia must be performed in an anesthetized patient, placement of the catheter should be undertaken by the most experienced practitioner available.

Positioning and Landmarks

The patient is positioned in a moderate knee-chest and lateral decubitus position. Some practitioners prefer the upright (sitting) position, especially in obese patients. This position requires the presence of an assistant to hold the patient, however. In addition, the sitting position is associated with a significant incidence of postural hypotension, especially in sedated patients.

The back should be prepared and draped in the usual manner and the surface anatomy palpated. The two procedural techniques for thoracic epidural analgesia differ at this point and will be described separately.

Procedure

As most practitioners use a loss of resistance technique to determine entry into the epidural space, the initial description of the paramedian and midline approaches will use this technique. Other techniques for verification of entry into the epidural space will be discussed subsequently.

Paramedian Approach

Some authors consider the paramedian approach to be the preferred technique for midthoracic epidural insertion because of the caudad angulation of the spinous processes and the narrow interlaminar foraminae. The difficulty of epidural needle entry into the narrow crescent shape of the thoracic interlaminar foraminae is readily apparent in Figures 18-2 and 18-4. Even in the lumbar

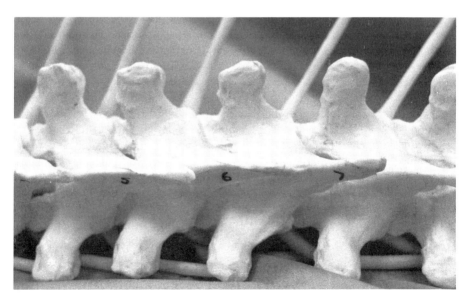

Fig. 18-3. Midline view of the midthoracic spine. Numbers denote the spinous processes of the respective thoracic vertebrae. Note the narrow spinous processes and wide laminae.

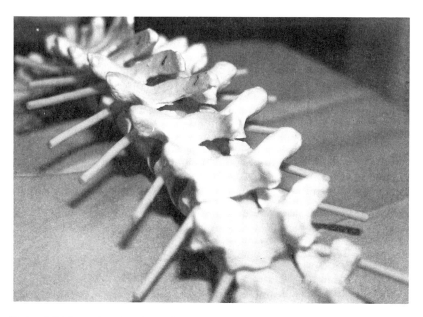

Fig. 18-4. Midthoracic spine from the paramedian position. Note the crescent shape of the interlaminar foramine. Also note the difference in size of the midthoracic interlaminar foraminae when compared with the view from the midline position (Fig. 18-2).

space, the paramedian approach has been associated with a lower incidence of technical difficulties.[3] The paramedian technique allows the ligamentum flavum to be approached at a more acute angle and completely avoids the frequently calcified and cystic interspinous ligament.

The major drawback to use of the paramedian approach is that most clinicians do not practice this technique in the lumbar spine and therefore feel uncomfortable using this technique in the thoracic spine. It is recommended that the paramedian approach be practiced extensively in the lumbar spine before use of the technique in the thoracic spine.

A skin wheal of local anesthetic is raised at a point approximately 1–1.5 cm lateral to the middle of the chosen interspace (Fig. 18-5). Using a long 23-gauge or 21-gauge needle, the paraspinous muscle, fascia, and periosteum of the lamina are infiltrated with local anesthetic by insertion of the needle perpendicular to the plane of the skin. An epidural needle is then inserted perpendicular to the plane of the skin and directed inward until the lamina is encountered (Figs. 18-6 and 18-7). This depth is noted. The needle is then withdrawn 1 cm and redirected in a medial and rostral manner and readvanced. One or two further adjustments of needle direction are commonly needed. When lamina is not encountered, the stylet of the needle is withdrawn and an air- or saline-filled syringe is attached to the needle (Fig. 18-8). The ligamentum flavum will be appreciated when the needle is inserted approximately 0.5–1.5 cm beyond the distance at which the lamina was previously encountered (Fig. 18-9). A very

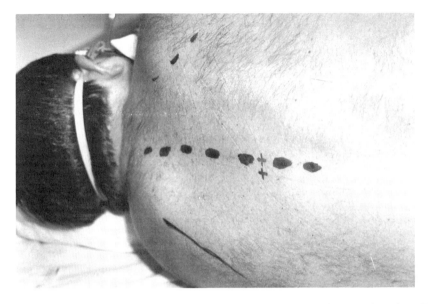

Fig. 18-5. Skin markings of a paramedian approach to the midthoracic spine. The midline, oblong, dark markings represent the palpable tips of the spinous processes. A " + " is made at the middle of the chosen interspace. Another " + " is made 1–1.5 cm lateral to it, and a skin wheal of local anesthetic is raised.

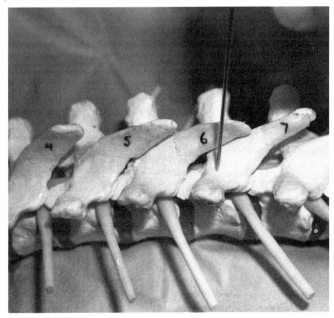

Fig. 18-6. Method of approach of an epidural needle to the lamina from the paramedian position. The epidural needle is inserted perpendicular to the plane of the skin. The needle is directed inward until the lamina is encountered.

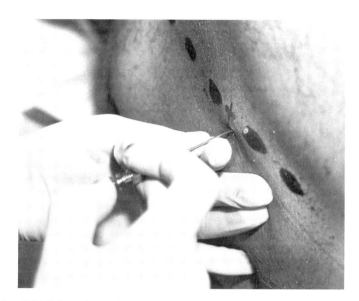

Fig. 18-7. Initial insertion of an epidural needle for a paramedian approach to the midthoracic spine. Note the perpendicular insertion of the needle to the plane of the skin.

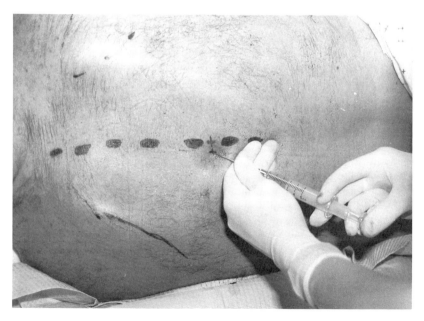

Fig. 18-8. Paramedian approach to the midthoracic epidural space after "walking off" the lamina. An air- or saline-filled syringe can be used for the loss of resistance technique as demonstrated here. Note the 20° angulation to the midline plane and the 45° angulation to the cross-sectional plane.

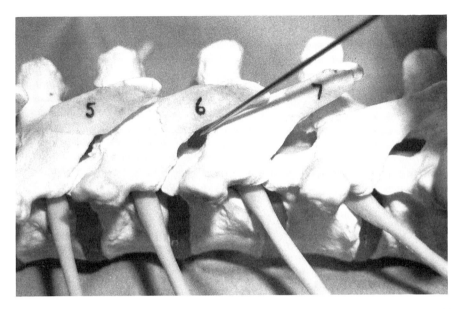

Fig. 18-9. Paramedian approach to the midthoracic epidural space after "walking off" the lamina. Note the ability to easily approach the interlaminar space from the paramedian position even when the interspinous space is narrowed.

careful and controlled approach is made to the epidural space. The epidural needle is advanced until a loss of resistance is appreciated. The final angle of the needle after insertion is usually $20° \pm 5°$ from the perpendicular to the midline plane and $45° \pm 10°$ from the cross-sectional plane. The distance of insertion from skin to thoracic epidural space is 7 ± 2 cm on the average (Fig. 18-10).

Midline Approach

The midline approach is sometimes more difficult to perform and prone to false losses of resistance. Nevertheless, for the practitioner skilled in only the midline approach, it is the preferred technique.

A skin wheal of local anesthetic is raised in the center of the proposed interspace of insertion (Fig. 18-11). The epidural needle is inserted at an angle of 45° to the cross-sectional plane and advanced approximately 3 cm until it is firmly felt to be within the supraspinous and interspinous ligaments (Figs. 18-12 and 18-13). The stylet is then removed and an air- or saline-filled syringe is attached to the epidural needle. The needle is advanced in a very careful and controlled manner until the epidural space is encountered and a loss of resistance is appreciated (Figs. 18-14 and 18-15). If bone is encountered, it is usually best to redirect the needle rostrally.

Occasionally, a loss of resistance is encountered at a shallow depth. This

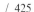

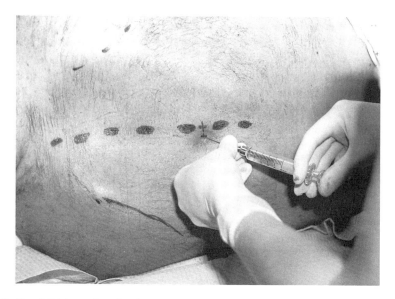

Fig. 18-10. Midthoracic spine from the paramedian position. Note that the final angulation of the needle after insertion is usually 20° ± 5° from the perpendicular to the midline plane and 45° ± 10° from the cross-sectional plane.

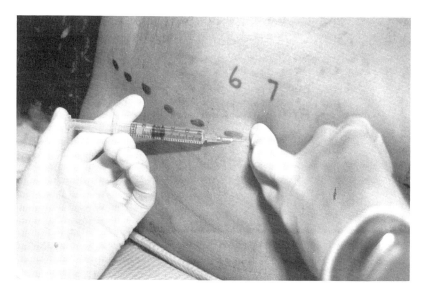

Fig. 18-11. Midline approach to the midthoracic spine for thoracic epidural analgesia. A skin wheal of local anesthetic is raised in the middle of the proposed interspace of needle insertion. Oblong, dark markings represent the palpable tips of the spinous processes. Numbers denote the spinous processes of the respective vertebrae.

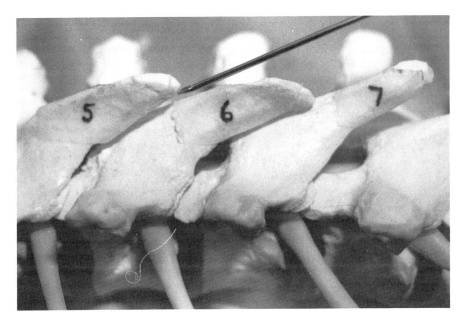

Fig. 18-12. Initial insertion of the epidural needle from the midline position. Note the 45° angulation of the epidural needle to the cross-sectional plane.

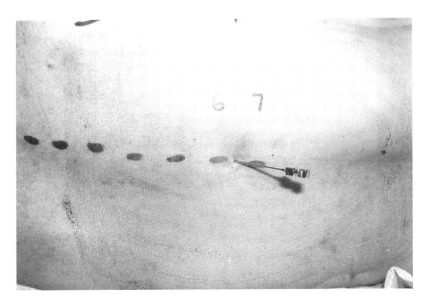

Fig. 18-13. Insertion of the epidural needle for a midline approach to the midthoracic spine. Note the 45° angulation of the epidural needle to the cross-sectional plane.

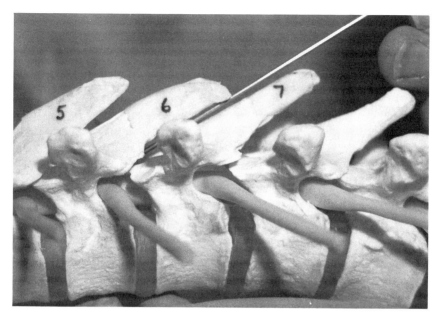

Fig. 18-14. Final position of the epidural needle when inserted from the midline position. Numbers represent the spinous processes of respective vertebrae. Note the 45° angulation of the epidural needle to the cross-sectional plane. Also note the narrow interspinous spaces.

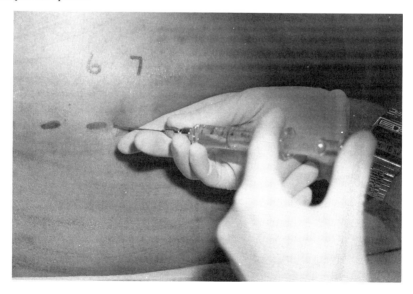

Fig. 18-15. Insertion of the epidural needle for a midline approach to the midthoracic spine. Note the 45° angulation of the epidural needle to the cross-sectional plane and the careful, controlled approach to the epidural space. An air- or saline-filled syringe can be used for the loss of resistance technique as demonstrated here.

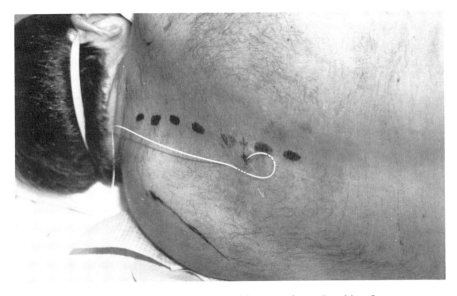

Fig. 18-16. Fixation of the catheter to the skin away from the side of surgery.

denotes that the needle tip has left the midline and has become paramedian. The epidural needle should be withdrawn and repositioned.

At this point, a catheter may now be threaded into the epidural space (5 cm). After insertion, the entry site should be cleaned of blood. The catheter should be looped away from the operative side and dressed with a sterile occlusive dressing. It is usually easier to tape the catheter over the shoulder, on the side contralateral to the site of surgery (Figs. 18-16 and 18-17).

Verification of Entry into the Epidural Space

Although most practitioners use loss of resistance to determine entry into the epidural space, a number of other techniques are available.[4]

Loss of Resistance

The loss of resistance technique was first described by Sicard and Forestier[5] in 1921 and then again by Dogliotti[6] in 1933. The technique relies on the high-compliance, low-resistance physical properties of the epidural space.[7] There is no advantage to the use of air versus fluid for loss of resistance, as there appears to be no difference in the rate of dural puncture between the two media.[8]

There is some debate about whether constant or intermittent pressure should be kept on the plunger of the syringe, especially when using a paramedian approach. When using a paramedian approach, intermittent rather than constant pressure on the plunger of the syringe will provide the best "feel" of loss of

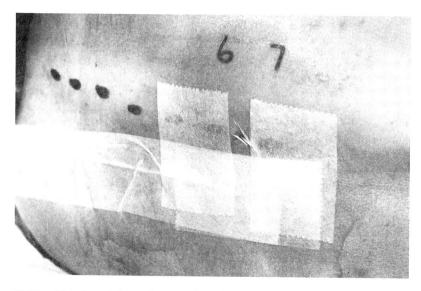

Fig. 18-17. Fixation of the catheter to the skin away from the side of surgery. Note the clear dressing over the insertion site.

resistance, as paraspinous muscle and tissue have a higher compliance and lower opening pressure than the interspinous ligament. As a result, constant pressure on the plunger can overcome the opening pressure of paraspinous muscle and mimic a loss of resistance. By tapping on the plunger of the syringe, the tissue compliance and opening pressure of muscle and epidural space can be differentiated. When using a midline approach, the interspinous ligament has a low compliance and high opening pressure. Thus, constant pressure on the syringe will not give a false loss of resistance.

Hanging Drop

The hanging-drop technique relies on the difference in pressure between atmospheric pressure and the negative pressure of the epidural space. A drop of saline or local anesthetic is placed in the hub of the epidural needle. The fluid is drawn into the barrel of the needle by the negative pressure of the epidural space on entry. The technique was first described by Gutierrez[9] in 1933.

The presence of a negative pressure within the thoracic epidural space was first described by Janzen[10] in 1926. The origin of the negative epidural pressure has been clearly established after some debate in the early literature. The negative pressure of the interpleural space is transmitted by way of the paravertebral space, intervertebral foraminae, and epidural veins to the epidural space.[11]

Mean interpleural pressure in normal subjects varies over the entire respiratory cycle, depending on the position of the patient and the site of measurement in the interpleural space. In some individuals with severe lung disease, a negative epidural pressure is not a certainty, especially if the expiratory period is prolonged. In the lumbar epidural space there is a less negative or even positive pressure in the epidural space. The negative interpleural pressure is not well transmitted to the lumbar epidural space, and not even conveyed at all to the sacral epidural space.

Although some authors have claimed a single figure for epidural pressure, this is not the case, as the epidural pressure will vary with the phase of the respiratory cycle, the patient's position, and the site of measurement. In addition, a significant proportion of patients (approximately 25 percent) do not have a markedly negative midthoracic epidural pressure, which may make the hanging-drop technique difficult.[12,13] The range of midthoracic epidural pressure is -6 to -16 cmH$_2$O with a mean of -10 cmH$_2$O.[13,14]

Ligamentum Flavum Sensation

The tactile sensation of passage through the ligamentum flavum is not always a reliable indicator of entrance into the thoracic epidural space, even to the experienced practitioner. Although a palpable click or the tactile sensation of passage through the ligament can be felt in most patients, there is a significant number of patients in whom this does not occur. As a result, reliance on the "feel" of the ligamentum flavum increases the risk of dural puncture and potential cord injury. Tactile sensation of the ligamentum flavum can only be used as a minor adjunctive sign of entry into the epidural space.

Ease of Catheter Insertion

The ease of catheter insertion is a reliable sign of entry into the thoracic epidural space. The presence of minor or major obstructions to passage is very indicative of misplacement of the catheter. The catheter and needle should be withdrawn as a unit, and the procedure should be attempted again. The intervertebral foraminae are small in the midthoracic space and usually do not allow the catheter to pass out into the paravertebral space. As a result, the practitioner should have no qualms about threading the catheter up to 5 cm. Threading the catheter a shorter distance than 5 cm may result in a higher incidence of catheter dislodgment during the postoperative period.

Physiologic Responses

There are isolated reports of hemodynamic and respiratory changes associated with the injection of fluid into the thoracic epidural space. These changes include bradycardia,[15] tachycardia,[12] and tachypnea.[12] The etiology of these physiologic responses is unclear, but they probably represent painful or reflex events resulting from temporarily increased epidural pressure. Such physiologic responses are unreliable as indicators of entrance into the epidural space and cannot be used as confirmatory signs.

Choice and Dosing of Analgesics

A test dose of local anesthetic (with or without epinephrine) should always be administered to obtain a sensory block of the thoracic dermatomes, thereby demonstrating successful technique. The usual test dose for the average adult patient is 4 ml of 2 percent lidocaine given in two divided doses over 10 minutes. Such a test dose results in a sensory block covering approximately six dermatomes. All patients with thoracic epidural catheters at the Brigham and Women's Hospital receive a test dose irrespective of whether the catheter will eventually be used for the administration of opioids, local anesthetics, or both. Lidocaine is the most useful local anesthetic for test-dosing because of its rapid onset.

The use of epidural opioids was discussed in Chapter 11, and the reader is referred to that source for an exhaustive discussion of the topic. Suffice it to say that dosage guidelines are similar for lumbar and thoracic analgesia, except for the administration of morphine. When morphine is administered for thoracic epidural analgesia, it is prudent to give smaller doses than ordinarily administered in the lumbar space. Although opioid can reach the brain stem in either case, greater concentrations of morphine may reach the brain stem sooner after thoracic epidural administration. Thus, use of excessive doses of morphine for thoracic epidural analgesia carries an increased risk of delayed respiratory depression.[16,17]

Great fear has been associated with the use of local anesthetics in the midthoracic space because of the potential for profound hypotension.[18] This potential is heightened by certain surgeons' desire for post-thoracotomy patients to be maintained in a relatively hypovolemic state, due to the fear of post-thoracotomy pulmonary edema.[19,20] The intermittent administration of local anesthetics is associated with a high incidence of hypotension.[18] Administration of local anesthetics by continuous infusion, however, is associated with a much-reduced incidence, although the possibility of hypotension is still present.[21]

In the experience of the Acute Pain Service at Brigham and Women's Hospital, the vast majority of patients receiving thoracic epidural analgesia will *not* be made hypotensive by a test dose of 2 percent lidocaine and institution of an infusion of a dilute concentration of bupivacaine and opioid. Of course, vigilance should always be maintained and appropriate measures instituted if hypotension occurs. Guidelines for dosing and management of thoracic epidural catheters are found in Table 18-2.

As administration of local anesthetics in the midthoracic epidural space can have profound physiologic effects, the cardiovascular responses to such administration will be reviewed.

**TABLE 18-2. Dosage Guidelines for Thoracic
Epidural Analgesia**

Test dose
  2 ml of 2% lidocaine × 2 at 5-min intervals
Opioids
  Intermittent injection
    Fentanyl 50–100 μg in 10 ml preservative-free saline[a]
    Meperidine 30–100 mg[a]
    Morphine 1–2 mg
  Infusion[b]
    Fentanyl 30–100 μg/h
    Meperidine 10–25 mg/h
Local anesthetic and opioid
  Infusion[b]
    0.125% Bupivacaine with 5 μg/ml fentanyl at 3–7 ml/h
    0.125% Bupivacaine with 2.5 mg/ml meperidine at 3–7 ml/h
"Rescue" for breakthrough pain
  Increase infusion rate after
    Fentanyl 50–100 μg in 10 ml preservative-free saline[a]
    Meperidine 30–50 mg
    2 ml of 2% lidocaine × 1 or × 2 at 5-min intervals
    Ketorolac 60 IM or IV, then 30 mg IM or IV q 6 h

  [a] Diluent volume affects time of onset and duration of analgesia with a single injection of epidural fentanyl.[22] Administration of fentanyl in a volume of 10 ml will optimize time of onset and duration of analgesia.[22] No such effect has been described for meperidine or morphine, though meperidine is usually administered in a volume of 10 ml.

  [b] The use of continuous infusions of morphine into the thoracic epidural space is not suggested. Excessive administration of morphine in the thoracic epidural space enhances the risk of late respiratory depression.[16,17]

CARDIOVASCULAR EFFECTS OF THORACIC EPIDURAL ANALGESIA WITH LOCAL ANESTHETICS

Reduction in Mean Arterial Pressure

The cardiovascular changes seen with the administration of midthoracic epidural local anesthetics (signifying the conduction blockade of *anesthesia*, not merely *analgesia*) are manifested as a reduction in arterial pressure. The etiology of such changes are twofold: (1) sensory anesthesia results in reduced nociceptive input to thalamocortical projection pathways that synapse in brain stem autonomic centers (see Ch. 2), and (2) sympathetic peripheral deafferentation results from loss of sympathetic outflow to the heart and the adrenal medulla, and from peripheral vasodilation (caused by loss of vascular sympathetic efferents). Quantitatively, however, the decreased inotropism from loss of cardiac sympathetic outflow is of greater import than vasodilatory effects. This can be explained by the segmental distribution of the thoracolumbar outflow. (See Ch. 3 for a detailed discussion of the autonomic nervous system.)

**TABLE 18-3. Segmental Distribution of
the Thoracolumbar Outflow**

Head, neck, upper limbs	T1–T4
Heart, lungs	T1–T4
Upper GI tract	T5–T10
Lower GI tract	T10–L2
Adrenal medulla	T8–T12
Lower limbs	T12–L2

Table 18-3 details the segmental distribution of the sympathetic nerves of the thoracolumbar outflow. Cardiac sympathetic innervation originates in the intermediolateral gray matter from T1 to T4. Innervation of the adrenal medulla originates in spinal cord segments T8–T12. Midthoracic epidural anesthesia results in decreased or ablated sympathetic outflow to the adrenal medulla, with a decrease in circulating levels of catecholamines.

Vasodilation of the lower gut (and splanchnic vascular beds) requires neural blockade extending from spinal cord segments T10–L2. Vasodilation of the lower limbs requires blockade extending from T12–L2. Such a segmental distribution of anesthesia is not usually achieved with thoracic epidural anesthesia. Thus, arteriolar dilation and venodilation of the aforementioned areas is not as great as that achieved by lumbar epidural anesthesia. In addition, midthoracic epidural anesthesia leaves the sympathetic outflow intact below the level of neural blockade, allowing vasoconstriction in vascular beds supplied by spinal cord segments below the block.[23–28]

With respect to neural blockade of more cephalad spinal cord segments, blockade from T1 to T5 is achieved (or at least partially achieved) with thoracic epidural anesthesia. Such segmental blockade will result in (1) unchanged systemic vascular resistance, (2) little change in heart rate (despite blockade of cardioaccelerator nerves), and (3) a fall in mean arterial pressure caused by reduction of cardiac output (decreased inotropism despite a rise in central venous pressure).[23–28]

Thus, the predominant cardiovascular effect of thoracic epidural blockade is a decrease in inotropism rather than a decrease in systemic vascular resistance. Splanchnic vasodilatory capacity is maintained while cardiac output is concomitantly reduced because of the blockade of cardioaccelerator nerves. This is in direct contrast to lumbar epidural anesthesia, in which systemic vascular resistance decreases due to intense arteriolar dilation and venodilation (see Chapter 12). Thus, reduced inotropism and cardiac output, rather than reduced systemic vascular resistance, are responsible for hypotension seen with administration of midthoracic epidural local anesthetics.

Myocardial Oxygen Demand

Thoracic epidural anesthesia with local anesthetics is not contraindicated in ischemic cardiovascular disease. In fact, the negative inotropism, coupled with preservation of systemic vascular resistance, may have beneficial effects on myocardial oxygen demand.[29–33]

Blomberg et al[29] studied the effects of high thoracic epidural anesthesia on nine patients with unstable angina. The administration of thoracic epidural anesthesia during ischemic episodes decreased angina, mean arterial pressure, heart rate, pulmonary artery pressure, and pulmonary capillary wedge pressure without decreasing cardiac output or coronary perfusion pressure. They concluded that thoracic epidural anesthesia may favorably alter the oxygen supply/demand ratio in ischemic myocardium.

Davis et al[31] temporarily occluded the left anterior descending coronary artery (LAD) in dogs concomitantly receiving thoracic epidural anesthesia. Thoracic epidural anesthesia decreased heart rate, cardiac output, ST segment changes, and left ventricular stroke work compared with an ischemic period in the absence of neural blockade. Endocardial regional blood flow was greater with thoracic epidural anesthesia. In dogs that underwent permanent LAD occlusion, the infarct size was smaller in the thoracic anesthesia group.

Blomberg and Ricksten[32] also studied the effect of coronary artery ligation in the rat in the presence and absence of thoracic epidural anesthesia. Mortality was 10 percent in both groups. However, the incidence of ventricular fibrillation and tachycardia was much less in the presence of thoracic epidural anesthesia (20 percent) than in its absence (53 percent). In a separate study[33] using conscious rats after left coronary artery ligation, the same researchers were able to demonstrate that thoracic epidural anesthesia with local anesthetics had similar hemodynamic effects as compared with a single injection of metoprolol. They concluded that thoracic epidural analgesia had favorable effects on hemodynamics in the infarcted heart.

These data, along with the knowledge that high thoracic epidural blockade causes negative inotropism, would imply that thoracic epidural blockade may offer myocardial protection. This conclusion is supported by the work of Kock et al.[34] High-thoracic epidural blockade was achieved in 10 β-blocked patients with angiographically demonstrated symptomatic coronary artery disease. Thoracic epidural blockade resulted in a more normal exercise stress test, as measured by enhanced radionuclide angiographic ejection fraction, improved regional wall motion, and less ST segment depression. Exercise during thoracic epidural blockade resulted in lower arterial pressures but not heart rate, as compared with exercise without thoracic epidural blockade. Thus, thoracic epidural analgesia is not contraindicated in patients with ischemic heart disease. Moreover, it may have a salutary effect on myocardial oxygen supply/demand relationships, provided due care is paid to systemic hemodynamics. The predictability of the hemodynamic response does not obligate the insertion of pulmonary artery catheters into every patient with ischemic heart disease and thoracic epidural blockade.

CLINICAL APPLICATIONS

Thoracic epidural analgesia provides profound and consistent postoperative pain relief for surgery of the thorax and abdomen. Thoracic epidural analgesia has also been used in a number of acutely painful medical conditions including angina pectoris,[29-35] acute pancreatitis,[36,37] ureteric colic,[38] and acute and post-herpetic neuralgia.[39] The quality and consistency of the analgesia attendant to this technique make it the "gold standard" to which other regional anesthetic/analgesic techniques of the thorax and abdomen aspire.

COMPLICATIONS

Dural Puncture

Dural puncture from attempted midthoracic epidural analgesia is *not* a disaster. Dural puncture in the midthoracic spine is *not* synonymous with nerve injury. The patient should be questioned closely about paresthesiae (see below). In their absence, the epidural should be repeated at a more rostral interspace, preferably at least two spaces higher.

If subsequent attempts are successful, choice of analgesic becomes problematic. There is now a tear in the dura mater, and forceful pressure from intermittent injections or infusion devices can cause subarachnoid movement of epidurally administered agents. The test dose should be omitted because of the risk of "total" spinal block. The use of local anesthetics in subsequent postoperative epidural infusions is debatable. If the patient is able to be nursed in an intermediate or intensive care unit, the use of local anesthetics is probably justified, provided frequent assessment of the sensory level is made. In the absence of those nursing provisions, the use of epidural local anesthetics or hydrophilic opioids is probably not indicated. Epidural infusions of lipophilic opioids are probably best in this circumstance unless intensive nursing is available.

"Blood patching" of a persistent cerebrospinal fluid leak may be indicated. However, headache after midthoracic dural puncture is unusual because of the reduced hydrostatic pressure gradient between the cranial vault and the midthoracic region.

Venous Puncture

The presence of blood on aspiration of the epidural catheter is unusual in the midthoracic epidural space. This is especially true if the catheter has been inserted after injection of saline or local anesthetic into the epidural space. The management is no different from management of blood return in the lumbar epidural space. The catheter should be cleared of blood by injection of saline, and aspiration repeated. If blood is again obtained on aspiration, progressive withdrawal of the catheter with repeated aspiration or reinsertion of the catheter at another interspace is necessary.

Paresthesiae

Paresthesiae during performance of thoracic epidural technique are very unusual and are *not* a normal consequence of insertion of the needle or catheter. If a paresthesia is encountered, it must first be assumed that dural puncture has occurred. Safety therefore dictates that the needle or catheter must be withdrawn and the etiology of the paresthesia sought. If dural puncture has not occurred, the procedure can be reattempted at the same or another interspace. If dural puncture has resulted in a paresthesia, the technique should probably be abandoned. The patient should be examined by a neurologist both before and after surgery, and alternative means of postoperative analgesia should be used.

Urinary Retention

The incidence of urinary retention after thoracic epidural analgesia (i.e., opioids, local anesthetics, combinations) is approximately 40 percent.[7,40] It is our practice to remove the urinary catheter after 2 days if not needed for patient management. For men older than 70 years of age and those with prostatic symptomatology or prior prostatic surgery, the urinary catheter is left in until the epidural catheter is removed. It is important to appreciate that certain surgeons will fluid-restrict post-thoracotomy patients because of the fear of post-thoracotomy pulmonary edema. Such patients may not urinate for up to 12 hours after their catheter has been removed. It is our practice to remove the catheter on the morning of the second postoperative day so that possible urinary retention will occur during the day and not at night.

Nausea

Nausea is an occasional occurrence of thoracic epidural analgesia with opioids and is best managed by conventional antiemetics. (For a discussion of nausea and epidural opioids, see Ch. 11.)

Sedation

Sedation associated with overdose of epidural opioids is an occasional occurrence of thoracic epidural analgesia. It is usually mild and is best managed by decreasing the rate of the epidural infusion or the concentration of opioid in the infusion. Sedation will rarely need to be treated with opioid antagonists or agonist-antagonists if management of thoracic epidural analgesia has been appropriate.

After thoracotomy or extensive upper abdominal surgery, a mildly increased arterial PCO_2 is often found with adequate thoracic epidural analgesia. The PCO_2 will commonly be in the mid-40s (mm/Hg) and occasionally rise into the low 50s (mm/Hg). Provided the patient is appropriately alert, cooperative, and can perform coughing and other maneuvers on command, such elevation of PCO_2 is not a cause for concern and should not be treated. Administration of opioid antagonists, reduction of the infusion rate, or reduction of the concentration of opioid in the epidural infusion may result in inadequate analgesia and cause patient detriment, solely as a result of attempting to "make the numbers look good."

Hypotension

As previously described, hypotension with thoracic epidural anesthesia (signifying conduction blockade with local anesthetics) results from decreased inotropism from blockade of T1–T5. As segmental blockade of T10–L2 is not achieved, splanchnic bed vasoconstrictor capabilities are maintained. Decreased sympathetic vascular resistance plays little or a modest role in the genesis of hypotension.

With this in mind, what is the appropriate agent to treat hypotension, providing the volume status is adequate? The data would imply that an agent with predominantly β-activity (to restore inotropism) and some α-activity (to supply some vasoconstriction) would be the best choice.

Reiz et al[26] used midthoracic epidural anesthesia for aortic surgery and demonstrated that prenalterol (β1-agonism with very little β2-activity) caused positive inotropism without vasodilation. There was little increase in heart rate as a reflex response to the vasodilation, yet blood pressure was restored to normal. Kajimoto and Nishimyra[25] infused dobutamine (β1) or metaraminol (α1) into elderly patients with low-thoracic epidurals. Normalization of mean arterial pressure to preblockade levels occurred with both agents. For dobutamine, normalization of venous filling pressures and stroke volume occurred without change in systemic vascular resistance. Metaraminol resulted in a rise in filling pressures, a fall in heart rate, and a rise in systemic vascular resistance. Yet, stroke volume did not return to normal despite the increased filling pressures. Lundberg et al[28] used midthoracic epidural anesthesia for aortic aneurysm surgery in elderly patients. Dopamine was infused at rates of 0–8 μg/kg/min. An infusion rate of approximately 4 μg/kg/min restored mean arterial pressure and cardiac output to normal without a large change in heart rate or filling pressures. At infusion rates greater than 4 μg/kg/min, the increases in mean arterial pressure, cardiac output, and filling pressures were excessive. The combined β- and α-agonist activity of dopamine reversed the hemodynamic changes of midthoracic epidural blockade.

On balance, these data show that an agent with predominant β-activity and some α-activity provides restoration of mean arterial pressure without perturbations in other hemodynamic parameters. It is for this reason that intermittent injections of ephedrine or infusions of dopamine are the agents of choice for hypotension resulting from thoracic epidural anesthesia. Pure α-agonists should be avoided.

CONTRAINDICATIONS

Infection

Systemic bacterial or fungal infection or local infection at the epidural site is an absolute contraindication to epidural catheter placement. Absence of fever for 48 hours and a normal or decreasing white blood cell count is clear evidence of the safety of insertion. If the patient becomes febrile during continuous thoracic epidural analgesia, the low risk of a persisting foreign body combined with adequate analgesia must be weighed against the low risk of epidural abscess. If no specific site of sepsis can be identified and the fever is being ascribed to line sepsis by an infectious disease specialist, the epidural catheter should be removed after all other lines have been removed or replaced.

Reduced Cardiac Reserve

It is inadvisable to use local anesthetics with midthoracic epidural analgesia in patients with significantly reduced cardiac reserve (e.g., congestive heart failure). Sympathectomy and blockade of cardioaccelerator nerves may further reduce cardiac output. Ischemic heart disease is not, however, a contraindication to thoracic epidural analgesia and may actually be beneficial, as previously discussed.[29-35]

CONCLUSION

The careful management of thoracic epidural analgesia for thoracic and upper abdominal surgery is well within the capabilities of any comprehensive acute pain service. There is little to deter the careful practitioner with extensive lumbar epidural experience from performing thoracic epidural analgesia. In particular, the fear of spinal cord injury should be deemphasized, as the risk is very low, especially in the hands of the experienced practitioner. (In fact, there is no report of spinal cord trauma from thoracic epidural analgesia in the literature.) Thoracic epidural analgesia supplies consistently superb postoperative analgesia. In view of the profound analgesia, low risk of nerve or spinal cord damage, known physiologic sequelae, and easily treated side effects, fear of use of thoracic epidural analgesia is unwarranted and unwise.

References
1. Covino BG, Scott DB: Handbook of Epidural Anaesthesia and Analgesia. Grune & Stratton, Orlando, Fl, 1985
2. Katz J, Renck H: Handbook of Thoraco-Abdominal Nerve Block. Grune & Stratton, Orlando, Fl, 1987
3. Blomberg RG, Jaanivald A, Walther S: Advantages of the paramedian approach for lumbar epidural analgesia with catheter technique. A clinical comparison between midline and paramedian approaches. Anaesthesia 44:742, 1989
4. Cousins MJ, Bridenbaugh PO: Neural Blockade in Clinical Anesthesia and Management of Pain. 2nd Ed. JB Lippincott, Philadelphia, 1988
5. Sicard JA, Forestier J: Méthode radiographique d'exploration de la cavité epidurale par le lipiodol. Rev Neurol (Paris) 28:1264, 1921
6. Dogliotti AM: Segmental peridural anaesthesia. Am J Surg 20:107, 1933
7. Bromage PR: Epidural Analgesia. WB Saunders, Philadelphia, 1978
8. Sarna MC, Smith I, James JM: Paresthesia with lumbar epidural catheters. A comparison of air and saline in a loss-of-resistance technique. Anesthesia 45:1077, 1990

9. Gutierrez A: Valor de la aspiracion liquida en el especio peridural en la anestesia peridural. Rev Cir Buenos Aires 12:225, 1933

10. Janzen E: Der negativ vorschlag bei lumbalpunktion. Dtsch Z Nervenheilk 94:280, 1926

11. Macintosh RR, Mushin WW: Observations on the epidural space. Anaesthesia 2: 100, 1947

12. Durrans SF: High extradural segmental block. Anaesthesia 2:106, 1947

13. Usubiaga JE, Moya F, Usubiaga LE: Effect of thoracic and abdominal pressure changes on the epidural space pressure. Br J Anaesth 39:612, 1967

14. Bonniot M: Note sur la pression épidurale nègative. Bull Soc Nat Chir 60:124, 1934

15. James EC, Kolberg HL, Iwen GW, Gellatley TA: Epidural analgesia for post-thoracotomy patients. J Thorac Cardiovasc Surg 82:898, 1981

16. Gustafsson LL, Schildt B, Jacobsen KJ: Adverse effects of extradural and intrathecal opiates: report of a nationwide survey in Sweden. Br J Anaesth 54:479, 1982

17. Cousins MJ, Mather LE: Intrathecal and epidural administration of opioids. Anesthesiology 61:276, 1984

18. Conacher ID, Paes ML, Jacobson L et al: Epidural analgesia following thoracic surgery. A review of two years' experience. Anaesthesia 39:546, 1983

19. Zeldin RA, Normandin D, Landtwing D, Peters RM: Postpneumonectomy pulmonary edema. J Thorac Cardiovasc Surg 87:359, 1984

20. Verheijen-Breemhaar L, Bogaard JM, van den Berg B, Hilvering C: Postpneumonectomy pulmonary oedema. Thorax 43:323, 1988

21. Griffiths DPG, Diamond AW, Cameron JD: Postoperative extradural analgesia following thoracic surgery: a feasibility study. Br J Anaesth 47:48, 1975

22. Birnbach DJ, Johnson MD, Arcario T et al: Effect of diluent volume on analgesia produced by epidural fentanyl. Anesth Analg 68:808, 1989

23. Sundberg A, Wattwil M: Circulatory effects of short-term hypercapnia during high thoracic epidural anesthesia in elderly patients. Acta Anaesthesiol Scand 31:81, 1987

24. Otton PE, Wilson EJ: The cardiocirculatory effects of upper thoracic epidural analgesia. Can Anaesth Soc J 13:541, 1966

25. Kajimoto Y, Nishimura N: Metaraminol and dobutamine for the treatment of hypotension associated with epidural block. Resuscitation 12:47, 1984

26. Reiz S, Nath S, Ponten E: Hemodynamic effects of prenalterol, a β1-adrenoreceptor agonist, in hypotension induced by high thoracic epidural block in man. Acta Anaesthesiol Scand 23:93, 1979

27. McLean APH, Mulligan GW, Otton P, MacLean LD: Hemodynamic alterations associated with epidural anesthesia. Surgery 62:79, 1967

28. Lundberg J, Norgren L, Thomson D, Werner O: Hemodynamic effects of dopamine during thoracic epidural analgesia in man. Anesthesiology 66:641, 1987

29. Blomberg S, Emanuelsson H, Ricksten SE: Thoracic epidural anesthesia and central hemodynamics in patients with unstable angina pectoris. Anesth Analg 69:558, 1989

30. Blomberg S, Curelaru I, Emanuelsson H et al: Thoracic epidural anesthesia in patients with unstable angina pectoris. Eur Heart J 10:437, 1989

31. Davis RF, DeBoer LWV, Maroko PR: Thoracic epidural anesthesia reduces myocardial infarct size after coronary artery occlusion in dogs. Anesth Analg 65:711, 1986

32. Blomberg S, Ricksten S-E: Thoracic epidural anaesthesia decreases the incidence of ventricular arrhythmias during acute myocardial infarction in the anaesthetized rat. Acta Anesthesiol Scand 32:173, 1988

33. Blomberg S, Ricksten SE: Effects of thoracic epidural anaesthesia on central haemo-

dynamics compared to cardiac beta adrenoceptor blockade in conscious rats with acute myocardial infarction. Acta Anaesthesiol Scand 34:1, 1990

34. Kock M, Blomberg S, Emanuelsson H et al: Thoracic epidural anesthesia improves global and regional ventricular function during stress-induced myocardial ischemia in patients with coronary artery disease. Anesth Analg 71:625, 1990

35. Klassen GA, Bramwell RS, Bromage PR, Zborowska-Sluis DT: Effect of acute sympathectomy by epidural anesthesia on the canine coronary circulation. Anesthesiology 52:8, 1980

36. Kellum JM Jr, DeMeester TR, Elkins RC, Zuidema GD: Respiratory insufficiency secondary to acute pancreatitis. Ann Surg 175:657, 1972

37. Ranson JHC, Roses DF, Fink SD: Early respiratory insufficiency in acute pancreatitis. Ann Surg 178:75, 1973

38. Romagnoli A, Batra MS: Continuous epidural block in the treatment of impacted ureteric stones. Can Anaesth Soc J 109:968, 1973

39. Dan K, Kazuo H, Tanaka K, Mori R: Herpetic pain and cellular immunity. p. 293. In Yokodu T, Dubner R (eds): Current Topics in Pain Research and Therapy. Int. Cong. Ser. 613. Excerpta Medica, Amsterdam, 1983

40. Holmdahl MH, Sjögren S, Ström G, Wright B: Clinical aspects of continuous epidural blockade for postoperative pain relief. Ups J Med Sci 77:47, 1972

19

Regional Anesthesia/ Analgesia and Anticoagulation: Implications for Management of Postoperative Pain

John A. Fox
F. Michael Ferrante

During the past decade, regional anesthesia has enjoyed increasing popularity. Although the reasons for this are multifactorial, several studies (some controversial) have implied that regional anesthesia (either alone or in combination with general anesthesia) may decrease blood loss,[1] lower the incidence of thromboembolic events,[2] and eliminate the stress response to surgery.[3,4] Thus, these and other beneficial effects of regional anesthesia may effectively reduce the morbidity and mortality attendant on major surgical procedures.[5,6] In most studies, the benefits of regional anesthesia have occurred through continuation of the regional anesthetic as an analgesic after the surgical procedure (regional anesthesia/analgesia).

Thus, regional anesthesia/analgesia is often the anesthetic and analgesic of choice for the sickest patients because of the aforementioned effects on postoperative morbidity and mortality. Quite often, such patients are placed on an anticoagulant regimen, either preoperatively or postoperatively. At such times, a determination must be made as to whether regional anesthesia/analgesia poses any additional risks to the anticoagulated patient and whether those risks are worth the purported benefits of regional anesthesia/analgesia. This chapter is designed as an aid and guide to such critical decision analysis.

THE CLOTTING SYSTEM AND ITS PHYSIOLOGIC ASSESSMENT

The function of the clotting system is to form a stable clot and to lyse that clot once hemostasis has occurred. The physiologic phenomenon of clotting can be divided into four component processes: (1) disruption of vascular integrity (i.e., injury), (2) platelet recruitment, (3) activation of the clotting cascade, and (4) fibrinolysis.[7]

Once vascular integrity is violated, tissue thromboplastin (factor III) is released from the vascular endothelium (Fig. 19-1). Platelets in the area of the injury undergo membrane changes, making them adherent to the disrupted vas-

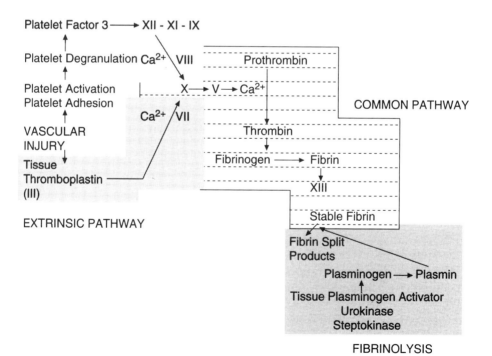

Fig. 19-1. The coagulation and fibrinolytic systems.

cular wall and other platelets. A number of chemical mediators are then released from intracellular granules within the platelets to recruit other platelets (platelet factor 3). Tissue thromboplastin and platelet factor 3 activate the extrinsic and intrinsic pathways of the coagulation cascade, respectively (Fig. 19-1).

Platelet function is clinically evaluated by determination of actual platelet numbers and the bleeding time. The Ivy bleeding time[8] is performed by placing a tourniquet around the biceps at 40 mmHg pressure. A lance is used to produce a small cut, and blood is gently blotted away using filter paper every 30 seconds until a clot appears. Normal bleeding times range between 2 and 10 minutes. Bleeding times increase linearly with sequential decreases in platelet numbers less than $100,000/mm^3$.[9] Additionally, studies of trauma victims show that most clinical bleeding occurs with platelet counts less than $100,000/mm^3$.

The coagulation cascade consists of a number of proteins whose function is to produce a stable fibrin clot (Fig. 19-1). The cascade consists of an extrinsic, intrinsic, and final common pathway. Calcium is a required cofactor for the activation of several of the coagulant proteins (II, VII, IX, and X).

The physiologic function of the extrinsic and intrinsic pathways is assessed by the activated partial thromboplastin time (aPTT) and prothrombin time (PT), respectively. Both tests measure the time required to form a stable fibrin clot in the presence of commercial reagents. Commercial reagents vary from laboratory to laboratory, necessitating the obligatory use of controls to assess normal clotting time. A 20 percent prolongation of clotting time above that of the controls is deemed to be abnormal.

Prolongation of aPTT can be clinically produced by administration of subcutaneous or intravenous heparin. Heparin[10] is a strongly anionic heterogeneous mucopolysaccharide with a molecular weight between 6,000 to 30,000. Heparin binds to antithrombin III (AT III), as well as many other coagulation factors.[11,12] The heparin/AT III complex binds thrombin, effectively removing it from use within the coagulation cascade. The positively charged histone protein protamine can reverse the physiologic effects of heparin.[13]

Prolongation of the PT is accomplished by administration of warfarin derivatives (coumadin). Coumadin inhibits vitamin K-dependent synthesis of factors II, VII, IX, and X within the liver.[14] Prolongation of the PT typically occurs within 1–3 days of oral administration of coumadin, but is subject to wide variability. The effects of coumadin can be reversed within 48 hours by administration of vitamin K_{15} or more immediately by administration of fresh-frozen plasma. Ostensibly, only 25 percent of the normal plasma levels of factors II, VII, IX, and X are required to form clots. Such replenishment can be accomplished with administration of two units of fresh-frozen plasma.[16]

Lysis of the fibrin clot is accomplished by activation of the fibrinolytic system. The enzyme plasmin, which actually lyses the fibrin clot, is formed from the proenzyme plasminogen. The lysosomal enzyme urokinase and tissue plasminogen activator (tPA) are responsible for the production of plasmin. Plasmin activity itself is difficult to measure. However, the presence of fibrinolysis is assessed by measurement of the breakdown products of fibrin, the so-called "fibrin split products" (FSPs) or D-dimers.[17]

EPIDURAL HEMATOMA

The controversies underlying administration of regional anesthesia/analgesia to patients with potential bleeding problems can best be understood in terms of the four component processes of coagulation (see Fig. 19-1). Few people would advocate use of spinal or epidural anesthesia in patients with a major violation of their "vascular integrity." Regional anesthesia is certainly contraindicated in the hypovolemic patient bleeding from a major vessel. Similarly, patients with disseminated intravascular coagulation (overactivity of the fibrinolytic system associated with consumption of coagulation factors) would not be candidates for regional anesthesia. However, absolute exclusion of the use of regional anesthesia/analgesia in patients with certain abnormalities of platelet function or the coagulation cascade is less clear-cut.

Regional anesthesia/analgesia can be broadly defined as involving two types of techniques: (1) neural blockade of the neuraxis, and (2) neural blockade of peripheral nerves. Neural blockade and pharmacologic manipulation of the neuraxis are most commonly used for postoperative pain management. Thus, discussion of the complications of regional anesthesia/analgesia will be restricted to the production of the epidural hematoma.

Clinical Course and Pathophysiology

In evaluating case reports of epidural hematoma after regional anesthesia/analgesia, it is important to recognize that the development of this condition is sudden and catastrophic. Epidural hematoma is usually manifested as excruciating pain localized to the site of needle insertion. This is rapidly followed by paraplegia caused by compression of the spinal cord by the extrinsic mass. Once suspected and diagnosed, early emergency decompression can restore function if performed within 12 hours of the onset of symptoms.[18] Fortunately, epidural hematomas are uncommon events.

Epidural Hematoma After Subarachnoid Puncture

As of August 1991, there are 37 reported cases of epidural hematoma complicating subarachnoid puncture. Thirty-four of these cases appeared in a review by Owens et al[19] in 1986. Three more reports have been published since 1986.[20-22] The risk factors, or lack thereof, for production of epidural hematoma in these 37 patients are listed in Table 19-1. Table 19-2 lists data from eight patients without identifiable risk factors. However, most of the patients in Table 19-2 had debilitating diseases that could have adversely affected the clotting mechanism.[23-29]

Reports of epidural hematoma occurring after attempted spinal anesthesia are listed in Table 19-3.[30-32] In all reports except that of Wille-Jørgensen and

TABLE 19-1. Risk Factors for Development of Epidural Hematoma After Subarachnoid Puncture
($N = 37$)

Risk Factor	Prevalence (N)
No known risk factor	8
Defined risk factor	29
Central neurologic event[a]	14
Leukemia[b]	9
Miscellaneous	6
Platelet abnormality	3
Systemic disease	2
Heparin therapy	1

[a] Lumbar puncture was diagnostically indicated. Each patient received an anticoagulant temporally related to performance of the lumbar puncture. Two patients received intravenous heparin before lumbar puncture.

[b] Diagnostic lumbar puncture was performed because of sepsis. Platelet count in all patients $<44,000/mm^3$.

co-workers,[22] performance of lumbar puncture was technically difficult and/or the cerebrospinal fluid was bloody. In the five cases in which information is available, large-gauge spinal needles were used (23-gauge or greater). Furthermore, seven of the nine patients listed had severe preexisting diseases that could have affected the clotting mechanism.

TABLE 19-2. Reports of Epidural Hematoma After Subarachnoid Puncture Without Identifiable Risk Factors

Author	Year	Disease/Surgery	Comments
Cooke[23]	1911	Tuberculous meningitis	Hematoma at autopsy
Hammes[24]	1920	Meningitis	Repetitive lumbar puncture ($N = 6$)
Courtin[25]	1952	Tertiary syphilis	
Kirkpatrick and Goodman[26]	1975	Sciatica	Chronic coumadin for 6 months before lumbar puncture
King and Glass[27a]	1959	Cystoscopy	Portal cirrhosis; no coagulation studies
Lerner et al[28a]	1973	Total knee replacement	No known risk factors
Rengachary and Murphy[29a]	1974	Femur fracture	General anesthesia after failed lumbar puncture; coagulation studies normal
Barker[20a]	1988	Total hip replacement	Asthmatic on prednisolone; no coagulation studies

[a] Anesthetic-related.

TABLE 19-3. Epidural Hematoma After Attempted Spinal Anesthesia (N = 9)

Author	Year	Difficult LP?	Bloody?	Needle Size (gauge)	Age (years)	Surgery	Comments
Bonica[30]	1953	?	Yes	?	?	?	Prolonged bleeding time
King and Glass[27]	1960	No	Yes	?	62	Cystoscopy	No anticoagulation
Lerner et al[28]	1973	Yes	Yes	22	70	Total knee replacement	Traumatic tap; no preexisting systemic disease
Rengachary and Murphy[29]	1974	Yes	No	?	64	Femur fracture	No preexisting systemic disease
Greensite and Katz[31]	1980	Yes	Yes	16	68	Total knee replacement	Subarachnoid catheter; received aspirin postoperatively
Mayumi and Dohi[32]	1983	Yes	No	23	70	Toe amputation	Antiplatelet drug (ticlopidine)
Barker[20a]	1988	No	?	22	87	Total hip replacement	Asthmatic on prednisolone
Grejda et al[21]	1989	Yes	Yes	22	58	Cystoscopy	Chronic renal failure; normal coagulation studies
Wille-Jørgensen et al[22]	1991	No	No	?	83	Femur fracture	Postoperative heparinization (36 h later)

[a] Subdural hematoma.

Epidural Hematoma After Epidural Anesthesia

There are at least 20 reported cases of epidural hematoma after epidural anesthesia. Before 1970, Usubiaga[33] described eight cases in a review of 75,000 epidural anesthetics (Table 19-4). Seven of the eight cases had either a traumatic epidural puncture or received intravenous heparin after performance of the epidural. In the 12 reports since 1969[34-42] (Table 19-4), 10 patients received an anticoagulant after placement of the epidural catheter. One patient had acute myelogenous leukemia and was thrombocytopenic.

Ballin[39] described the only reported instance of a possible epidural hematoma in a parturient. The patient was a 22-year-old woman without significant prior medical history or anticoagulant therapy. An epidural catheter was inserted twice. The first catheter was removed because of ineffective analgesia and was found to have blood in it. The second epidural anesthetic was inadequate for cesarean delivery, and a general anesthetic was subsequently administered. Bilateral lower extremity weakness and diffuse diminished pinprick sensation were noted postoperatively. The neurologic findings completely resolved within 6 weeks. Roentgenography of the lumbosacral spine revealed a "narrow spinal canal." No other diagnostic studies were performed. As blood was noted within the first epidural catheter, the resultant neurologic findings were attributed to a spontaneously resolving epidural hematoma. Based on the limited diagnostic studies, however, the neurologic findings cannot be conclusively attributed to an epidural hematoma.

Clinical Reports Demonstrating the Safety of Regional Anesthesia in Anticoagulated Patients

There are 50 reports of epidural hematoma after subarachnoid puncture or epidural anesthesia in patients with a defined abnormality of coagulation. However, several excellent studies demonstrate the safety of these same techniques in this same group of patients.

Rao and El-Etr[43] prospectively studied 4,015 patients undergoing peripheral vascular surgery with intraoperative heparinization. Either continuous spinal anesthesia ($N = 847$) or continuous epidural anesthesia ($N = 3,164$) was performed. All anesthetics were performed with a 17-gauge Tuohy needle, and catheters were threaded 1–2 cm. Patients with leukemia, a blood dyscrasia, thrombocytopenia, or preoperative anticoagulation (coumadin or heparin) were denied regional anesthesia. Preoperative PT and aPTT were obtained. Ivy bleeding time was not obtained. Four patients were canceled because of a significant amount of bleeding on initial puncture, and surgery was performed the next day under general anesthesia. Intraoperative heparinization was closely monitored by use of the activated clotting time (ACT). Incremental doses of 500 units of intravenous heparin were given every 3 minutes until the ACT was

TABLE 19-4. Epidural Hematoma After Epidural Anesthesia (N = 20)

Author	Year	Age (years)/Gender	Catheter?	Blood in Catheter?	Anticoagulation after Epidural?	Surgery
Usubiaga[33]	1975	80 M	No	Yes	Heparin	Laparotomy
Usubiaga[33]	1975	47 F	No	No	No	Myomectomy
Usubiaga[33]	1975	28 F	No	Yes	No	Nephropexy
Usubiaga[33]	1975	72 M	Yes	No	Heparin	Femoral embolectomy
Usubiaga[33]	1975	Neonate M	Yes	Yes	No	Omphalocele
Usubiaga[33]	1975	Middle-aged F	Yes	No	Heparin	Femoral embolectomy
Usubiaga[33]	1975	73 M	Yes	No	Heparin	Below-knee amputation
Usubiaga[33]	1975	48 F	Yes	Yes	Heparin	Incisional hernia
Massey Dawkins[34]	1969	?	?	?	Yes	?
Massey Dawkins[34]	1969	?	?	?	Yes	?
Butler and Green[35]	1970	70 M	Yes	No	Heparin	Femoral embolectomy
Helperin and Cohen[36]	1971	76 M	Yes	No	Heparin	Femoral-popliteal bypass
Janis[37]	1972	76 M	Yes	No	Heparin	Hip reduction
Varkey and Brindle[38]	1974	70 M	Yes	No	Heparin	Pain therapy for above-knee amputation
Ballin[39]	1981	22 F	Yes (twice)	Yes	No	Cesarean delivery
Wulf et al[40]	1988	21 M	Yes	No	No (AML)	Thoracotomy
Dickman et al[41]	1990	67 M	Yes	No	Urokinase	Catheter insertion
Dickman et al[41]	1990	74 M	Yes	No	Heparin	Femoral embolectomy
Tekkok et al[42]	1991	42 M	Yes	No	Heparin	Femoral-popliteal bypass
Wille-Jørgensen et al[22]	1991	68 M	Yes	No	Coumadin	Tibial fracture

twice baseline. Catheters were removed on the first postoperative day, but always 1 hour before initiation of the maintenance dose of intravenous heparin. Using these conservative measures, not a single patient demonstrated any signs or symptoms of epidural hematoma.[43]

Barron et al[44] retrospectively reviewed 912 patients undergoing vascular surgery with epidural anesthesia. All patients had normal preoperative PTs, aPTTs, and platelet counts. Intraoperative heparinization was performed with an initial injection of 75 U heparin/kg, with institution of an infusion at a rate of 1,000 U heparin/kg. This resulted in aPTTs greater than 100 seconds. Epidural catheters were removed at completion of the surgical procedure while the patients were still fully anticoagulated. In this retrospective analysis of nearly 1,000 patients, no major catastrophic neurologic event was noted.[44]

Odoom and Sih[45] reported the use of 1,000 lumbar epidural anesthetics in 950 patients undergoing vascular procedures. Epidural anesthetics were administered after induction of general endotracheal anesthesia. All patients had received preoperative anticoagulant therapy (medications and doses not specified), such that the preoperative aPTT was 20 percent above control. The Kaolin clotting test (similar to the ACT) was normal, however. Catheters were removed on the second postoperative day. No catastrophic neurologic events were noted.[45]

Waldman et al[46] reported on the use of 336 caudal anesthetics/analgesics in 37 patients referred to the authors' pain management service. All procedures were performed during full anticoagulation (PT or aPTT 1.5 times control). Twelve patients were receiving intravenous heparinization at the time of procedure, and 19 patients were severely thrombocytopenic (platelet counts less than 50,000/mm^3). Two patients developed hematomas at the puncture site, but no catastrophic permanent neurologic sequelae were noted.[46]

Finally, several studies[47–52] documented the safe administration of subarachnoid and epidural opioids before heparinization in patients undergoing coronary artery bypass grafting (Table 19-5). In all these studies, the authors attempted to administer the spinal opioids far in advance of heparinization for cardiopulmonary bypass. The actual times of administration ranged from the night before surgery (Joachimsson et al[52]) to shortly after induction of general anesthesia (Aun et al[48]). No epidural hematomas were noted in any of the studies.

TABLE 19-5. Administration of Spinal Opioids Before Cardiopulmonary Bypass

Author	Year	N	Analgesic	Needle (gauge)	Site	Morphine Dose
Mathews and Abrams[47]	1980	40	Subarachnoid	20–25	Lumbar	2 mg
Aun et al[48]	1985	40	Subarachnoid	25	Lumbar	2 and 4 mg
El Baz and Goldin[49]	1987	30	Epidural	17	High-thoracic	0.1 mg/h
Casey et al[50]	1987	40	Subarachnoid	25	Lumbar	0.02 mg/kg
Vanstrum et al[51]	1988	30	Subarachnoid	22 and 25	Lumbar	0.5 mg
Joachimsson et al[52]	1989	16	Epidural	16	High-thoracic	0.5% Bupivacaine

REGIONAL ANESTHESIA/ANALGESIA IN THE ANTICOAGULATED PATIENT: A GUIDE TO CRITICAL DECISION ANALYSIS

The aforementioned data unequivocally demonstrate that epidural hematomas, although rare, *do* occur in anticoagulated patients receiving regional anesthesia/analgesia. However, these same data also unequivocally demonstrate that regional anesthesia/analgesia *can* be safely performed in anticoagulated patients. The decision to administer a regional anesthetic/analgesic to an anticoagulated patient must be made on an individual basis. Always, the *benefits* of regional anesthesia/analgesia must be deemed to outweigh the *risks* attendant on production of an epidural hematoma. Only then should the practitioner proceed.

The following sections present guidelines for a rational approach to the administration of regional anesthesia/analgesia in anticoagulated patients.

Preoperative Evaluation

As previously outlined, the performance of neural blockade is contraindicated in the face of a major vascular injury or consumptive coagulopathy. Furthermore, regional anesthesia/analgesia is probably also unwarranted in fully anticoagulated patients receiving coumadin or intravenous heparin. However, consideration can be given to patients with (usually iatrogenically induced and pharmacologically mediated) abnormalities of the coagulation cascade and platelet function.

Subcutaneous ("Minidose") Heparin

As previously outlined, heparin acts directly in the bloodstream by complexing with a number of coagulation factors. At full anticoagulant dose, heparin inhibits the action of thrombin on fibrinogen. In low concentrations, ("minidose") heparin inhibits interactions between factors IXa and VIII and platelet factor 3.[53] At these low concentrations, heparin will not prevent the progression of preformed thrombi but can prophylax against the formation of new thrombi.[54] This is the rationale for its use in the prophylaxis of deep vein thrombosis and pulmonary embolism.

The question arises as to whether the degree of anticoagulation with "minidose" heparin is sufficient to warrant exclusion from regional anesthesia/analgesia. Subcutaneous administration of heparin in doses of 5,000 U two or three times daily is quite effective in prevention of venous thrombosis and pulmonary embolism.[54] Such dosage is not associated with abnormal aPTTs.[55]

As the first dose of subcutaneous heparin is given 2 hours before surgery, a single preoperative dose should not be deemed a contraindication to regional anesthesia in the operating room. For patients receiving a regimen of subcutaneous heparin for several days, a conservative approach would be to determine the aPTT before instrumentation.

Nonsteroidal Anti-inflammatory Drugs

For a complete discussion of the role of nonsteroidal anti-inflammatory drugs (NSAIDs) in the production of abnormal hemostasis, see Chapter 7. For the present discussion, suffice it to say that NSAIDs affect platelet function by inhibition of the enzyme cyclooxygenase. Aspirin will irreversibly inhibit cyclooxygenase, making platelets dysfunctional for their entire life span (6–10 days).[56] In comparison, all other NSAIDs reversibly inhibit platelet cyclooxygenase. Normal hemostasis will be restored in the time required to clear the NSAID from the body (five half-lives).[57]

Horlocker and co-workers[58] retrospectively examined 391 regional anesthetics that were administered while patients received NSAIDs. Aspirin was the most common medication (209 of 391). Unfortunately, only six patients had their bleeding times determined before surgery (all normal). No patient receiving NSAIDs developed an epidural hematoma.

The current practice of the Acute Pain Service at Brigham and Women's Hospital is to perform regional anesthesia/analgesia without discontinuation of NSAIDs or determination of a bleeding time.

Intraoperative and Postoperative Management

It is best to perform a regional technique as far in advance of any subsequent anticoagulation as possible. For vascular procedures, this usually means that the regional technique will be performed 1–3 hours before intravenous heparinization. If blood is obtained during performance of the anesthetic/analgesic, sufficient time will have elapsed for successful formation of a clot. Full anticoagulation with intravenous heparin will prevent progression of the clot but will not assist in its resolution.[54] Thus, if blood is obtained through inadvertent puncture of an epidural vein, the procedure may be repeated at another interspace without cancellation of surgery.

Unfortunately, recommendations regarding the most optimal time for removal of epidural catheters in anticoagulated patients are unclear. It would seem wise to remove epidural catheters at times of "maximal" coagulation. Some patients may receive intravenous heparin until their coumadin dose elevates PT. In such patients, the epidural catheter could be removed 4 hours after discontinuation of heparin. Unfortunately, no recommendations can be made regarding an "acceptable" PT for catheter removal. Such choices are purely arbitrary.

Some practitioners would state that as long as *either* the extrinsic pathway (clotting ability measured by PT) *or* the intrinsic pathway (clotting ability measured by aPTT) remained functionally intact, epidural catheters can be safely

**TABLE 19-6. Life Span of Plasma
Coagulation Factors**

Factor	$t^{1/2}$
Fibrinogen (I)	1.5–6.3 days
Prothrombin (II)	2–5 days
Factor V	12–35 hours
Factor VII	1–6 hours
Factor VIII	3 days
Factor IX	8 days
Factor X	32–48 hours
Factor XI	40–84 hours
Factor XII	48–52 hours
Factor XIII	4.5–7 days

(Data from Williams.[59])

removed. For instance, oral anticoagulation with coumadin is mediated by inhibition of vitamin K-dependent synthesis of factors II, VII, IX, and X. Once synthesis has been inhibited so that no new factors are released from the liver, clinical anticoagulation will not occur until factors within the plasma are exhausted. As factor VII has the shortest plasma half-life,[59] it will be the first to disappear from the blood (Table 19-6). This will cause prolongation of PT and dysfunction of the extrinsic pathway. However, coagulation should still be possible through the intrinsic and common pathways until factor X becomes exhausted (second shortest half-life)[59] (Table 19-6). Thus, after prolongation of PT with coumadin, coagulation should still be possible for 32–48 hours through the intrinsic and common pathways. Application of such logic to the removal of epidural catheters in patients receiving coumadin removes the need for arbitrarily determined ("acceptable") PTs.

Postoperative Monitoring

Neurologic status must be carefully monitored in anticoagulated patients receiving regional anesthesia/analgesia. Early surgical intervention with decompression will preserve neurologic function in patients sustaining an epidural hematoma.[18] In patients receiving postoperative epidural infusions, it is paramount that the evaluation of the neurologic examination should not be obscured by the administered agent. Thus, any residual motor deficit arising from the intraoperative regional anesthetic must resolve before institution of postoperative regional analgesic therapy. Epidural opioids are the agents of choice, as their administration will preserve motor function.

CONCLUSION

In summary, a review of the literature demonstrates that epidural hematomas have occurred in anticoagulated patients receiving regional anesthesia/analgesia. At the same time, the literature also shows that regional anesthesia/analgesia can be safely administered to anticoagulated patients. The benefits and risks must be weighed on an individual basis. An informed patient, consultation with the surgeon, and, most importantly, discretion are all necessary for safe administration of regional anesthesia/analgesia to anticoagulated patients.

References
1. Scott NB, Kehlet H: Regional anesthesia and surgical morbidity. Br J Surg 75:299, 1988
2. Modig J, Borg T, Karlström G et al: Thromboembolism after total hip replacement: role of epidural and general anesthesia. Anesth Analg 62:174, 1983
3. Kehlet H: The stress response to anaesthesia and surgery: release mechanisms and modifying factors. Clin Anaesthesiol 2:315, 1984
4. Kehlet H: Modification of responses to surgery by neural blockade: clinical implications. p. 145. In Cousins MJ, Bridenbaugh PO (eds): Neural Blockade in Clinical Anesthesia and Management of Pain. 2nd Ed. JB Lippincott, Philadelphia, 1987
5. Kehlet H: Surgical stress: the role of pain and analgesia. Br J Anaesth 63:189, 1989
6. Yeager MP, Glass DD, Neff RK, Brinck-Johnsen T: Epidural anesthesia and analgesia in high-risk surgical patients. Anesthesiology 66:729, 1987
7. Fischbach D, Fogdall R: Coagulation: The Essentials. Williams & Wilkins, Baltimore, 1981
8. Mielke CH Jr, Kaneshiro MM, Maher IA et al: The standardized normal Ivy bleeding time and its prolongation by aspirin. Blood 34:204, 1969
9. Freirich E: Effectiveness of platelet transfusions in leukemia and aplastic anemia. Transfusion 6:50, 1966
10. Wessler S, Gitel SN: Heparin: new concepts relevant to clinical use. Blood 53:525, 1979
11. Biggs R, Denson KW, Akman N et al: Antithrombin III, antifactor Xa and heparin. Br J Haematol 19:283, 1970
12. Yin ET, Nessler S, Stoll PJ: Identity of plasma-activated factor X inhibition with antithrombin III and heparin cofactor. J Biol Chem 246:3712, 1971
13. Parkin TW, Kvale WF: Neutralization of the anticoagulant effects of heparin with protamine (sulfate). Am Heart J 37:332, 1949
14. Deykin D: Warfarin therapy. N Engl J Med 283:691, 1970
15. Rehbein A, Jaretzki III A, Habif DV: The response of Dicumarol-induced hypoprothrombinemia to vitamin K. Ann Surg 135:454, 1962
16. Johnson AJ, Aronson DL, Williams WJ: Preparation and clinical use of plasma and plasma fractions. p. 1561. In Williams WJ, Beutler E, Erslev AJ, Rundles RW (eds): Hematology. 2nd Ed: McGraw-Hill, New York, 1977
17. Chesterman CN: The fibrinolytic system and haemostasis. Thromb Diathes Haemorrh (Stuttg) 34:368, 1975
18. Markham JW, Lynge HN, Stahlman GEB: The syndrome of spontaneous epidural hematoma: report of three cases. J Neurosurg 26:334, 1967
19. Owens EL, Kasten GW, Hessel II EA: Spinal subarachnoid hematoma after lumbar puncture and heparinization: a case report, review of the literature, and discussion of anesthetic implications. Anesth Analg 65:1201, 1986
20. Barker GL: Spinal subdural haematoma following spinal anaesthesia. Anaesthesia 43:663, 1988
21. Grejda S, Ellis K, Arino P: Paraplegia following spinal anesthesia in a patient with chronic renal failure. Reg Anesth 14:155, 1989
22. Wille-Jørgensen P, Jørgensen LN, Rasmussen LS: Lumbar regional anesthesia and

prophylactic anticoagulant therapy. Is the combination safe? Anaesthesia 46:623, 1991

23. Cooke JV: Hemorrhage into the cauda equina following lumbar puncture. Proc Path Soc Phila 14:104, 1911

24. Hammes EM: Hemorrhage into the cauda equina secondary to lumbar puncture. Arch Neurol Psychiatr (Chicago) 3:595, 1920

25. Courtin RF: Some practical aspects of lumbar puncture. Postgrad Med 12:157, 1952

26. Kirkpatrick D, Goodman SJ: Combined subarachnoid and subdural hematoma following spinal puncture. Surg Neurol 3:109, 1975

27. King OJ, Glass WW: Spinal subarachnoid hemorrhage following lumbar puncture. Arch Surg 80:574, 1960

28. Lerner SM, Gutterman P, Jenkins F: Epidural hematoma and paraplegia after numerous lumbar punctures. Anesthesiology 39:550, 1973

29. Rengachary SS, Murphy D: Subarachnoid hematoma following lumbar puncture causing compression of the cauda equina. Case report. J Neurosurg 41:252, 1974

30. Bonica JJ: Subarachnoid block. p. 457. The Management of Pain. Lea & Febiger, Philadelphia, 1953

31. Greensite FS, Katz J: Spinal subdural hematoma associated with attempted epidural anesthesia and subsequent continuous spinal anesthesia. Anesth Analg 59:72, 1980

32. Mayumi T, Dohi S: Spinal subarachnoid hematoma after lumbar puncture in a patient receiving antiplatelet therapy. Anesth Analg 62:777, 1983

33. Usubiaga JE: Neurological complications following epidural anesthesia. Int Anesthesiol Clin 13:1, 1975

34. Massey Dawkins CJ: An analysis of complications of extradural and caudal block. Anaesthesia 24:554, 1969

35. Butler AB, Green CD: Haematoma following epidural anaesthesia. Can Anaesth Soc J 6:635, 1970

36. Helperin SW, Cohen DD: Hematoma following epidural anaesthesia: report of a case. Anesthesiology 6:641, 1971

37. Janis KM: Epidural hematoma following epidural analgesia: a case report. Anesth Analg 51:689, 1972

38. Varkey GP, Brindle GF: Peridural anesthesia and anticoagulant therapy. Can Anaesth Soc J 21:106, 1974

39. Ballin NC: Paraplegia following epidural analgesia. Anaesthesia 36:952, 1981

40. Wulf H, Maier C, Striepling E: Epidural hematoma following epidural analgesia in a patient suffering from thrombocytopenia. Reg Anaesth 11:26, 1988

41. Dickman CA, Shedd SA, Spetzler RF et al: Spinal epidural hematoma associated with epidural anesthesia: complications of systemic heparinization in patients receiving peripheral vascular therapy. Anesthesiology 72:947, 1990

42. Tekkok IH, Cataltepe O, Tahta K, Bertan V: Extradural haematoma after continuous extradural anaesthesia. Br J Anaesth 67:112, 1991

43. Rao TL, El-Etr AA: Anticoagulation following placement of epidural and subarachnoid catheters: an evaluation of neurologic sequelae. Anesthesiology 55:618, 1981

44. Barron HC, LaRaja RD, Rossi G, Atkinson D: Continuous epidural analgesia in the heparinized vascular surgical patient: a retrospective review of 912 patients. J Vasc Surg 6:144, 1987

45. Odoom JA, Sih IL: Epidural anesthesia and anticoagulant therapy. Experience with one thousand cases of continuous epidurals. Anaesthesia 38:254, 1983

46. Waldman SD, Feldstein GS, Waldman HJ et al: Caudal administration of morphine sulfate in anticoagulated and thrombocytopenic patients. Anesth Analg 66:267, 1987

47. Mathews ET, Abrams LD: Intrathecal morphine in open heart surgery (letter). Lancet ii:543, 1980

48. Aun C, Thomas D, St. John-Jones L et al: Intrathecal morphine in cardiac surgery. Eur J Anaesthesiol 2:419, 1985

49. El-Baz N, Goldin M: Continuous epidural infusion of morphine for pain relief after cardiac operations. J Thorac Cardiovasc Surg 93:878, 1987

50. Casey WF, Wynands JE, Ralley FE et al: The role of intrathecal morphine in the anesthetic management of patients undergoing coronary artery bypass surgery. J Cardiothorac Anesth 1:510, 1987

51. Vanstrum GS, Bjornson KM, Ilko R: Postoperative effect of intrathecal morphine in coronary artery bypass surgery. Anesth Analg 67:261, 1988

52. Joachimsson PO, Nystrom SO, Tynden H: Early extubation after coronary artery surgery in effectively rewarmed patients: a postoperative comparison of opioid anesthesia versus inhalational anesthesia and thoracic epidural analgesia. J Cardiothorac Anesth 3:444, 1989

53. Wintrobe MM, Lee RG, Boggs DR et al: Thrombosis and antithrombotic therapy. p. 1233. In Clinical Hematology. 7th Ed. Lea & Febiger, Philadelphia, 1975

54. Salzman EW, Hirsch J: Prevention of venous thromboembolism. p. 1252. In Hemostasis and Thrombosis. 2nd Ed. JB Lippincott, Philadelphia, 1987

55. Turpie AG, Robinson JG, Doyle DJ et al: Comparison of high-dose with low-dose subcutaneous heparin to prevent left ventricular mural thrombosis in patients with acute transmural anterior myocardial infarction. N Engl J Med 320:352, 1989

56. Burch JW, Stanford N, Majerus PW: Inhibition of platelet prostaglandin synthetase by oral aspirin. J Clin Invest 61:314, 1978

57. Ali M, McDonald JWD: Reversible and irreversible inhibition of platelet cyclooxygenase and serotonin release by nonsteroidal anti-inflammatory drugs. Thromb Res 13:1057, 1978

58. Horlocker TT, Wedel DJ, Offord KP: Does preoperative antiplatelet therapy increase the risk of hemorrhagic complication associated with regional anesthesia? Anesth Analg 70:631, 1990

59. Williams WJ: Life-span of plasma coagulation factors. p. 1230. In Hematology. 3rd Ed. McGraw-Hill, New York, 1983

20

Transcutaneous Electrical Nerve Stimulation

Nathaniel Katz

The use of electric stimulation to treat pain and other ills dates back to antiquity. In the modern era, transcutaneous electrical nerve stimulation (TENS) has become a simple noninvasive method of delivering electric current to the underlying tissues. Despite methodologic flaws, studies suggest that TENS can be a useful adjunct in the treatment of postoperative pain. The mechanism of action of TENS is uncertain but is often explained in terms of the gate control theory of pain. Guidelines for the use of TENS for postoperative pain management are presented here.

HISTORY

Electricity has been used to treat pain and other disorders since ancient times. In 46 AD Scribonius Largin, a Roman physician, used the electric eel to treat gout, headache, and other disorders.[1,2] The patient's affected part was placed in a bucket of water with the fish. Although the patient often lost consciousness, pain relief was purportedly achieved.

In the 17th and 18th centuries, interest in electricity and its relationship to biology increased.[3] With the preliminary experiments by Gilbert, von Guericke, Gray, Galvani, and Volta, it was found that electricity could be generated, stored, and transmitted.[3] Many physicians and charlatans began to use electricity to treat a number of ailments. A book called *Electrical Medicine* was even published by Johann Schneffer in 1752.

By the mid-19th century, a hand-cranked electric stimulating unit was available in the United States.[4] These became popular in 1900–1940 and were marketed by large department stores. Attachments were available to treat acne, asthma, anemia, and numerous other disorders. Due to technologic limitations and advances in pharmacotherapy, interest in electrical stimulation waned.

In 1965, Melzack and Wall[5] proposed the *gate theory of pain*. They suggested that afferent activity from large myelinated fibers (A fibers) blocked central transmission of nociceptive impulses from small myelinated Aδ and unmyelinated C fibers, thus "closing the gate" to transmission of pain impulses. This theory gave new impetus to the study of nerve stimulation for analgesia.

In 1967, Wall and Sweet[6] delivered electric stimulation to the infraorbital nerve of normal subjects and noted diminished appreciation of pinprick on the face. Soon patients with a variety of chronic pain problems were being treated with implanted stimulators of peripheral nerves or the dorsal columns of the spinal cord.[7] In 1970 and 1971, Long[8] and Shealy,[9] among others, were looking for a way to screen patients for dorsal column stimulation and began using TENS for this purpose. Many patients noted diminution of their pain with TENS alone and would not proceed to implantation. Both Long and Shealy went on to establish pain clinics using TENS for chronic pain.

Hymes et al[10] were first to report the use of TENS for the management of acute postoperative pain. Within 20 minutes of application of a TENS unit to a thoracotomy incision, the patient reported dramatic pain relief and improvement in mobility. Hymes went on to study TENS in hundreds of patients, with encouraging results. Since the work of Hymes, TENS has been studied in many centers throughout the world and is gradually gaining acceptance as a useful (although unproven) adjunct for postoperative pain management.

MECHANISM OF ACTION

As previously stated, the gate control theory of Melzack and Wall[5] proposed that small fiber activity within the substantia gelatinosa "opened the gate" for rostral nociceptive transmission of nerve impulses. Large fiber input "closed the gate." The gate control theory has been cited as the explanation for the effectiveness of TENS.

The ability of large fiber stimulation to inhibit small fiber activity in the spinal cord has been amply documented, at least in animals.[11-13] The exact mechanism of this central inhibitory action is uncertain.[14] Presynaptic inhibition at the level of the dorsal horn has been suggested by the finding that A-fiber stimulation causes primary afferent depolarization of C-fiber terminals (as predicted by the gate control theory).[15,16] Segmental and suprasegmental inhibitory pathways have also been discovered.[17]

The concept of a central control trigger (promoted with the gate control theory) proposes that large fiber input ascends in the dorsal columns and activates descending inhibitory pathways. These descending pathways modulate nociceptive transmission at the level of the dorsal horn of the spinal cord. Such descending inhibition has been demonstrated in animals[13,18] and may be opioid-mediated.[13,19,20]

Peripheral mechanisms have also been proposed to explain the effectiveness of TENS. These have included peripheral blockade of $A\delta$ fibers,[21,22] diminished small fiber activation caused by antidromic overstimulation,[23] and diminished peripheral nerve fiber excitability with chronic stimulation.[24] These mechanisms have subsequently been shown to be untenable.[25]

A possible mechanism of action of TENS in certain clinical situations is the alteration of peripheral autonomic activity. Decreased sympathetic tone has been demonstrated in humans with use of TENS.[26]

Thus at the present time, TENS-induced analgesia is believed to be centrally mediated by large myelinated fiber activation. Peripheral mechanisms have been discounted, although the role of the sympathetic nervous system in TENS-induced analgesia requires further study.

TECHNICAL CONSIDERATIONS

The TENS unit (Fig. 20-1) consists of an electric pulse generator (usually battery-operated) with dials to adjust various electric stimulation parameters. The pulse generator is connected by wires to two or more electrodes, (Fig. 20-

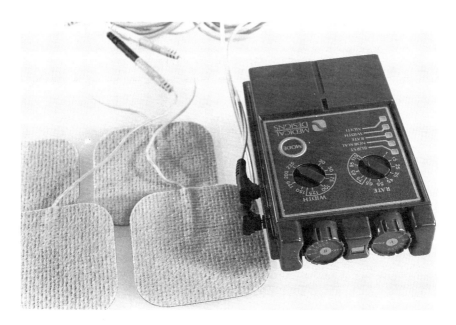

Fig. 20-1. A TENS unit and two electrode pairs.

1) which are placed on the skin. No studies have compared TENS parameters or electrode placements, and thus no firm statements can be made regarding ideal or optimal settings. The following discussion is therefore based largely on empiric observations.

Pulse Duration

The strength-duration curve[27] describes the relation between the durations of various applied electric stimuli and the amplitude of current needed to activate nerve or muscle fibers at those particular stimulus durations (Fig. 20-2). For impulses of short duration, strong currents are needed to activate the fiber. Eventually, a minimum pulse duration is reached, below which no current strength will activate the fiber. Similarly, there is a minimum threshold for current strength, below which the fiber cannot be activated irrespective of impulse duration. Both thresholds are higher for muscle than for nerve. Thus, there is a "window" of pulse duration and of current strength in which nerve will be selectively activated. Since activation of (myelinated) nerve fibers is the goal of (conventional) TENS, current strength and pulse duration values within this window are used. Empirically, the optimal range to achieve activation of myelinated nerve fibers without activation of muscle fibers is 60–150 μsec with respect to pulse duration. Below a pulse duration of 60 μsec, the high amplitudes required to activate a nerve fiber will deplete battery supplies. Above a pulse duration of 150 μsec, muscle contraction occurs even at low-frequency stimulation.

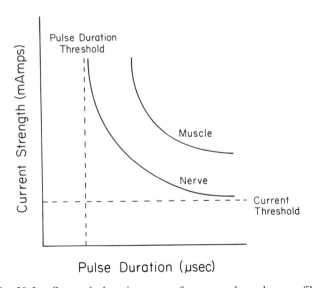

Fig. 20-2. Strength-duration curve for a muscle and nerve fiber.

Constant Current Versus Constant Voltage

TENS units deliver energy in two different forms, depending on the unit. In constant current units, the delivered current is set by the operator using a dial. In constant voltage machines, the voltage is set and the actual delivered current depends on the impedance of the electrode and underlying tissues. Skin impedance varies between 500 and 2,000 Ω depending on a number of factors.[28] In order to avoid variability in current delivery to the nerve, constant current stimulators are preferred.

Waveform

Originally, most stimulators delivered monophasic rectangular pulses, as these gave reliable current transmission to tissue (Fig. 20-3). At present, many stimulators give a balanced, biphasic potential to avoid iontophoresis (transfer of ions from electrode to skin or vice versa). Iontophoresis can change electrode impedance and interfere with current delivery.[27] Current may be symmetric or asymmetric, as long as the current remains equal in both phases. Asymmetric waveforms are purported to be more comfortable for the patient, causing less muscle contraction during low-frequency stimulation.[27,29] Patients may inexplicably respond to one waveform and not another, and therefore, units should have the availability of different waveform settings (Fig. 20-3).

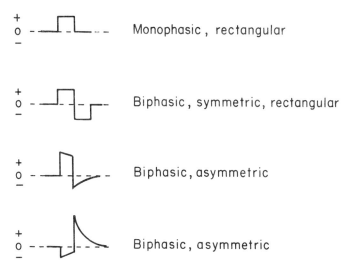

Fig. 20-3. Waveforms of electric pulses delivered by TENS units. Biphasic, symmetric, and asymmetric waveforms are most commonly used.

Frequency

In general, TENS may be administered by two variations in technique, dependent on the frequency of stimulation. *Conventional* TENS uses continuous stimulation at a constant high frequency (usually 50–100 Hz). The ideal frequency for conventional TENS is unknown, with most investigators using 80–100 Hz. *Acupuncture-like* TENS uses bursts of 100-Hz pulses delivered at a low frequency of 1–4 Hz. The goal of conventional TENS is to produce a strong but comfortable paresthesia in the area of application. Acupuncture-like TENS attempts to evoke local muscle contraction; onset of analgesia with this method may be slow, and the muscle contractions may be uncomfortable. Each method is purported to be more effective for certain indications. (Reliable comparative data are lacking.) Most of the experience in postoperative pain management has been with conventional TENS.

Amplitude

After the waveform and frequency have been selected, the operator gradually increases the amplitude to obtain a strong but comfortable paresthesia in the affected area. This amplitude tends to be two to three times the threshold current (i.e., the minimum current needed to evoke a paresthesia). The usual range is 10–20 mA. The amplitude can be set preoperatively during a patient education session so that stimulation can begin immediately after surgery at the predetermined amplitude. Some authors, however, have suggested that preoperative determination of amplitude will necessarily result in inadequate current for postoperative analgesia.[30]

Electrode Placement and Multiple Stimulation Channels

Most investigators have used a pair of electrodes aligned parallel to the incision for postoperative pain management. Some authors claim better results when a second pair is added. Such additional electrodes are usually placed (1) in series with the first pair to "cover" a long incision (Fig. 20-4), (2) parallel to a separate painful site, (3) on either side of the spine at the segmental level corresponding to the painful area (Fig. 20-5), or (4) straddling the major nerve trunk proximal to the painful area (Fig. 20-6). To achieve successful stimulation with each electrode pair, multiple independently adjustable channels are required.

Despite claims of superior analgesia, the effect of additional electrode pairs has not been directly studied in a single patient cohort. The only available data come from an inguinal herniorrhaphy model. Addition of a second paraspinal electrode pair[31] did not improve on the results obtained in a previous study (i.e., historic controls) using only a single paraincisional electrode pair.[32]

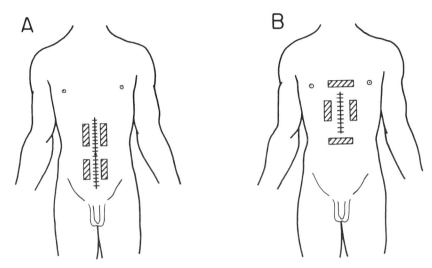

Fig. 20-4. Electrode placement. (**A**) Two pairs of electrodes are used to "cover" a long incision. (**B**) A second pair of electrodes is placed perpendicular to the first to "cover" an incision.

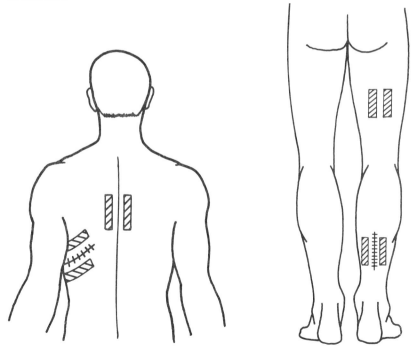

Fig. 20-5. Electrode placement. A second pair of electrodes is placed paraspinally at the appropriate segmental level after thoracotomy.

Fig. 20-6. Electrode placement. A second pair of electrodes is placed alongside the sciatic nerve in a patient with a leg incision.

Electrodes

Proper electrode size is important in order to obtain sufficient current intensity within tissue to stimulate nerves without damaging the skin. Too small an electrode may result in a high current density and skin damage; too large an electrode will dissipate the current, resulting in insufficient current density. A minimum electrode area of 10–15 cm^2 is generally used. For postoperative analgesia, a 2 × 15-cm electrode is commonly applied. Sterile, rectangular, self-adhesive electrodes are available and can be placed alongside the incision before dressings are applied.

Early electrodes suffered from a high incidence of skin damage caused by inhomogeneous electric contact, with areas of greater electric conductivity causing high current flows. To avoid this, the skin should be clean and free of surgical preparation and soap. A smooth layer of conducting gel should be used on the electrode surface.

Timing of Stimulation

Most investigators place electrodes in the operating room or recovery room. Stimulation is begun as soon as the patient awakens from general anesthesia. Stimulation is usually continuous for 48–72 hours, although some clinicians have used stimulation on an intermittent or as-needed schedule. Again, no comparative data are available.

Adverse Effects

Serious side effects occur rarely, if at all. Skin hypersensitivity occurs with an incidence of 10 percent. Therapy may continue by switching to hypoallergenic tape, gel, etc. The minimum effective frequency should be used in all patients to minimize delivery of electric energy to the skin. Electric burns to the skin can occur but are largely obviated by proper skin cleansing and electrode design. Patients with hypesthetic skin are at greatest risk. Other reported adverse effects include increased edema after mastectomy and transient increases in pain (usually in patients with crampy pain or psychological disturbances).

Contraindications

Contraindications to TENS (Table 20-1) are based on theoretic considerations rather than on reported adverse outcomes. Theoretic contraindications to use of TENS include patients with cardiac pacemakers, placement of electrodes on the neck (to avoid vagal stimulation), placement on the head in epileptics, pregnancy (possible uterine contractions in third trimester), and placement on

TABLE 20-1. Theoretic Contraindications to TENS

Patients with cardiac pacemakers
Placement on the head in epileptics
Placement on the chest in patients with cardiac arrhythmias
Pregnancy
Psychological instability, anxiety, narcissism
Inability to learn to use the device
Chronic opioid use

the chest in patients with cardiac dysrhythmias. These contraindications are not necessarily universally accepted. Of course, incompetent patients are not eligible for TENS.

EFFICACY OF POSTOPERATIVE TENS: REVIEW OF THE LITERATURE

Methodologic Issues

Studying the effectiveness of TENS for postoperative pain is a formidable task. Patient variables must be rigidly controlled, and basic guidelines for use of the device must be stated explicitly and rigorously followed. Valid outcome measures must be used, and a sufficient number of patients must be studied to obtain statistical power and derive meaningful conclusions. Despite a plethora of studies, *very few if any* of TENS trials meet even these most rudimentary of criteria for meaningful analgesic studies. Therefore, very few firm conclusions regarding the efficacy of TENS for postoperative pain relief can be drawn from the published literature.

As TENS is associated with a specific physical sensation, it is extremely difficult (and almost impossible) to design a placebo that would be subjectively similar to actual TENS. Some investigators have used TENS applied to the contralateral body site as a control ("remote TENS"—see below).[15] However, even this maneuver would not obviate experimenter bias or provide a disguise sufficiently adequate to double-blind a protocol.[33]

Although the best type of placebo for analgesic studies with TENS is controversial, the most popular placebo is "sham TENS." With sham TENS, a stimulator appears to be functioning but is not delivering current. A third "no TENS" group is used as a control to measure the degree of placebo effect. As described above, studies have also used "remote TENS", wherein a functioning stimulator is placed on a body site remote from the wound.[34] An active TENS unit placed on the contralateral body part would appear most appropriate.

Unfortunately, studies examining the differential effects of the various electric stimulation parameters have not been performed. Furthermore, many studies of TENS do not even specify the settings used. With these methodologic limitations in mind, the available literature on postoperative TENS will be reviewed. Studies will be divided into "preliminary" (poorly designed) trials (Table 20-2) and more definitive study designs (Table 20-3).

TABLE 20-2. Preliminary Clinical Trials of TENS for Postoperative Analgesia

Author	Year	N	Design	TENS	Results
Abdominal Surgery					
Ali et al[35]	1981	40	Cholecystectomy TENS vs sham vs no TENS ? rand ? blind	Asymmetric 10–100 Hz, 128–200 μsec, continuous for 48 h then as-needed, set to preop "tingling"	↓ pain, ↑ pulmonary function in TENS vs other groups
Taylor et al[36]	1983	77	Various operations TENS vs sham Prosp, rand	180 μsec, 70 Hz, 0–70 mA, adjusted to "tingling"	↓ pain and opioid use in TENS + sham
Rosenberg et al.[37]	1978	12	Cholecystectomy Prosp, rand TENS vs no TENS Unblinded	0–80 mA, 50–100 Hz, 20–100 μsec, adjusted by patient	↓ opioid use, no ▲ in ileus, pulmonary function
Bussey and Jackson[38]	1981	210	Cholecystectomy Herniorrhaphy TENS vs no TENS Retrospective	100 Hz, 100 μsec, amplitude set by patient	↑ opioid use
Caterine et al.[39]	1988	50	Gastroplasty TENS vs no TENS	85 Hz, 50 μsec, amplitude set by patient	↓ opioid doses, ↑ pulmonary function in no TENS group
Schomburg and Carter-Baker[40]	1983	150	Laparotomies TENS vs historic controls	0–90 V, 10–100 Hz, 120–340 μsec, set to preop "tingling", continuous for 48 h	↓ opioid use
Reuss et al[41]	1988	64	Cholecystectomy TENS vs no TENS Prosp, rand by surgeon	50 Hz, 170 μsec, 0–50 mA	No ▲ in ileus, pulmonary function, opioid use
Sodipo et al[42]	1980	30	Upper abdominal surgery TENS vs no TENS Prosp, rand	NS	↓ opioid use, ↑ pulmonary function, no ▲ in ileus
Orthopaedic Surgery					
Carman and Roach[43]	1988	45	Spine surgery, children TENS vs sham vs no TENS Rand, prosp, double-blind	60 Hz variable width, set to preop setting	Trend to ↓ opioid use with TENS

(Continued)

TABLE 20-2. Preliminary Clinical Trials of TENS for Postoperative Analgesia
(*continued*)

Author	Year	N	Design	TENS	Results
McCallum et al[44]	1988	20	Laminectomy TENS *vs* sham (each with patient-controlled analgesia) Rand, prosp	Asymmetric biphasic 180 μsec, 70 Hz amplitude set by patient (no instruction about "tingling") as-needed for 24 h	No ▲ in opioid use
Alm et al[45]	1979	125	Various podiatric surgeries TENS *vs* sham *vs* historic controls Unblinded, rand	Adjusted to "tingling"	↓ pain and opioid use in TENS and sham; more so in TENS
Harvie[46]	1979	34	Knee surgery	NS	↓ opioid use, ↑ tolerance of physiotherapy, ↓ hospital stay
Stabile and Mallory[47]	1978	107	Hip or knee replacement TENS *vs* sham *vs* no TENS Prosp, rand	10–100 Hz, 120–200 μsec, 0–100 V, set to preop "tingling"	↓ opioid use in sham, more so in TENS
Pike[48]	1978	40	Hip replacement TENS *vs* no TENS Prosp, rand	Modified rectangular 2 electrode pairs around hip, parameters set according to initial patient preference	↓ opioid use, pain, nausea, vomiting
Finley and Steward[49]	1983	22	Spine surgery TENS *vs* no TENS Rand, prosp	NS	↓ opioid use, pain
Richardson and Siqueira[50]	1980	38	Laminectomy, cervical and lumbar TENS *vs* no TENS	72–440 μsec, 9–240 Hz, 0.2–39 mA, patient adjusted, electrodes paraspinal	↓ pain, and opioid use
Cardiothoracic Surgery					
Stubbing and Jellicoe[51]	1988	40	Thoracotomy TENS *vs* no TENS Rand, prosp	70 Hz, modified rectangular, 180 μsec, set to preop "tingling", continuous for 48 h	No ▲ in opioid use, pulmonary function, ↓ nausea, vomiting Pain not assessed
Stratton and Smith[52]	1980	21	Thoracotomy Rand postoperatively, pulmonary function tested once with or without TENS	NS	↑ pulmonary function

(Continued)

TABLE 20-2. Preliminary Clinical Trials of TENS for Postoperative Analgesia
(*continued*)

Author	Year	N	Design	TENS	Results
Miscellaneous					
VanderArk and McGrath[53]	1975	100	Various abdominal + thoracic surgeries Prosp, rand TENS *vs* sham	100–150 Hz, 20–35 mA, 250–400 μsec, 20 min 3 times daily	↓ pain, no ▲ in ileus or atelectasis
Hymes et al.[10]	1973	130	Various operations, historic controls	20–35 mA, 250–400 μsec, 100–150 Hz, continuous for 24 h	↓ pain, ileus, respiratory complications, ICU stay
Hymes et al[54]	1974	115	Various operations, historic controls		↓ pain, ileus, respiratory complications, ICU stay
Solomon et al[55]	1980	196	Various operations Patients selected "randomly" by reviewing operative schedule, compared with "similar controls" Psychometric testing	Continuous for 48 h	↑ opioid use in "drug-naive" patients, ↑ opioid use in females with certain psychological traits

Abbreviations: 2-blind, double-blind; ▲, change; ↓, decrease(d); ↑, increase(d); NS, settings not specified; preop, preoperative; prosp, prospective; rand, randomized.

Abdominal Surgery

Initial studies of TENS did not typically stratify patients according to type of operation. Hymes et al[10,54] compared patients after various operations to historic controls and found 60–80 percent of patients reported "enhanced" pain relief with TENS. Patients receiving TENS had substantially less ileus, atelectasis, and shorter convalescence within intensive care units than historic controls. VanderArk and McGrath[53] in 1975 compared TENS versus sham TENS in 100 patients after a variety of abdominal and thoracic operations. In contrast to the findings of Hymes, use of TENS was associated with better analgesia without salutary changes in bowel or pulmonary function.[53]

Cooperman et al[56] were the first to study the use of TENS in a single cohort undergoing only abdominal surgery. Patients were prospectively divided into TENS and sham TENS groups. "Excellent" or "good" analgesia was found in 77 percent of patients receiving TENS in comparison with 33 percent of the sham-treatment patients. Patients with malignancy did not respond as well.

Solomon et al[55] studied 196 patients after various operations in an uncontrolled fashion and found TENS to benefit only opioid-naive patients. This study was responsible for generating the widely held notion that TENS is ineffective in patients with a history of opioid use. Several other studies (with various design flaws) have also found improved analgesia after abdominal surgery with

TABLE 20-3. "Well-Designed" Clinical Trials of TENS for Postoperative Analgesia

Author	Year	N	Design	TENS	Results
Abdominal Surgery					
Cooperman et al[56]	1977	50	Upper abd surgery Sham *vs* TENS Prosp, rand	NS	77% TENS *vs* 33% sham patients had excellent or good results
Smedley et al[31]	1988	62	Inguinal herniorrhaphy TENS *vs* sham Prosp, rand, 1-blind	Electrodes at incision + paralumbar 70 Hz rectangular amplitude adjusted to "tingling"	No difference in VAS, opioid use, pulmonary function
Lim et al[57]	1983	30	Upper abd surgery TENS *vs* sham Prosp, rand, 2-blind Psychometric testing	NS	Trend toward ↓ opioid and ↓ pain in TENS group; ↑ opioid use in patients with ↑ anxiety, neuroticism
Galloway et al[34]	1984	40	Cholecystectomy No TENS *vs* wound TENS *vs* remote TENS Prosp, rand	Rectangular, continuous for 48 h, otherwise NS	↓ pain, no change in opioid use or pulmonary function
Cuschieri et al[58]	1985	106	Various abd surgery TENS *vs* sham Prosp, rand	Rectangular, 170 μsec, 80 Hz, up to 15 mA	No ▲ in pain, opioid use, or pulmonary function
Gilbert et al[32]	1986	40	Herniorrhaphy TENS *vs* sham Prosp, rand	180 μsec, 70 Hz, 0–70 mA, adjusted to "tingling"	No ▲ in pain, opioid use, or pulmonary function
Conn et al[59]	1986	42	Appendectomy TENS *vs* sham *vs* no TENS Random, prosp, 1-blind	Continuous for 48 h, set to preop "tingling"	Trend to ↓ opioid use, no ▲ in VAS at 48 h
Orthopedic Surgery					
Arvidsson and Eriksson[60]	1986	15	Knee operations Recorded VAS, quad EMG at: time 0, after 15 min sham, after 15 min TENS, after epidural lidocaine	Electrodes on back and knee 100 Hz, 160 μsec, 30–40 mA, rectangular	Sham—modest ↓ pain TENS—substantial ↓ pain, ↑ EMG activity Epidural lidocaine—much better than TENS
Obstetric Surgery					
Smith et al[61]	1986	18	Cesarean delivery TENS *vs* sham Prosp, rand, 1-blind	80 μsec, 85 Hz, 0–75 mA, continuous for 3 days, set to preop "tingling"	↓ incisional pain, no ▲ in other pain types; no ▲ in opioid use

(Continued)

TABLE 20-3. "Well-Designed" Clinical Trials of TENS for Postoperative Analgesia (*continued*)

Author	Year	N	Design	TENS	Results
Davies[62]	1982	35	Cesarean delivery TENS *vs* sham Rand, prosp, 1-blind	Square, 200 μsec, 25 Hz, 0–40 V	↓ pain, opioid use in general anesthesia but not in epidural anesthesia patients
Cardiothoracic Surgery					
Rooney et al[63]	1983	44	Thoracotomy TENS *vs* sham Prosp, rand, 2-blind	120 Hz, 200 μsec, 14–20 mA, continuous for 24 h	22% of TENS *vs* 0% of sham required no opioids in 1st 24 h
Navaratham et al[64]	1984	31	Sternotomy TENS *vs* sham Prosp, rand, 2-blind	Rectangular 170 μsec, 80 Hz, 0–15 mA, set to preop "tingling"	↓ opioid use, ↑ pulmonary function, no ▲ in pain (nurses' assessment)
Warfield et al[65]	1985	24	Thoracotomy TENS *vs* sham Prosp, rand, 2-blind	Continuous for 48 h	↓ pain, ↓ ICU stay, ↑ tolerance of physiotherapy in TENS, no ▲ in opioid use
Miscellaneous					
Finsen et al[66]	1988	52	Amputations TENS *vs* sham *vs* sham + chlorpromazine	Electrode pairs over femoral + sciatic nerves, 100 Hz, 90 μsec, 7-pulse bursts at 2 Hz twice daily for 2 wk	No ▲ in phantom pain at 1 yr, ↓ reamputation, better stump healing

Abbreviations: abd, abdominal; 1-blind, single-blind; 2-blind, double-blind; ▲, change; ↓, decrease(d); EMG, electromyography; ↑, increase(d); NS, settings not specified; preop, preoperative; prosp, prospective; quad, quadriceps; rand, randomized; VAS, visual analogue pain score.

TENS.[35–40,42] However, two studies have found no benefit to be associated with the use of TENS after abdominal surgery.[41,58]

Two well-designed studies have focused on upper abdominal surgery. Lim et al[57] found a trend toward decreased postoperative analgesic use and decreased pain in patients using TENS. Greater analgesic consumption was associated with elevated "neuroticism" and "anxiety" scores on psychometric testing. Galloway et al[34] found the use of TENS to be associated with enhanced analgesia without change in pulmonary or bowel function, although the location of the remote TENS used for comparison was not specified.

Several fairly well-designed studies[5] investigated TENS after lower abdominal surgery (i.e., herniorrhaphy, appendectomy) and found no definite benefit compared with sham TENS.[31,32]

In summary, TENS seems to improve pain control and decrease opioid use after upper abdominal surgery, given the uniformly poor quality of the studies. Improvement in bowel and pulmonary function, although suggested by preliminary studies, has yet to be confirmed in well-designed trials. Some studies suggest that patients with previous opioid use, malignancy, or high anxiety or neuroticism scores on psychometric testing do not respond as well. TENS seems to offer no advantage over placebo for lower abdominal surgery.

Orthopaedic Surgery

A number of preliminary studies have shown decreased pain or opioid use to be associated with the use of TENS after orthopaedic surgery.[43,45-50] An elegant study[60] performed after knee surgery assessed pain and ability to extend the knee (as measured by quadriceps EMG) after one-time administration of sham TENS, TENS, and epidural lidocaine. Patients served as their own controls. TENS was substantially more effective than placebo, but not as effective as epidural lidocaine.[60]

In summary, TENS has been shown to significantly improve pain and motion after knee surgery in a single-dose study. Its utility in improving the postoperative course after orthopaedic surgery has been suggested by preliminary studies and remains to be confirmed.

Obstetric Surgery

Two well-designed studies evaluated the analgesic efficacy of TENS after cesarean delivery.[61,62] Smith et al[61] demonstrated that TENS reduced incisional (somatic) pain, but not other types of pain (e.g., uterine [visceral]). TENS did not influence postoperative analgesic use. This is not surprising, as patients do not discriminate among types of pain and will request opioids irrespective of the source of pain. Thus, the differential effectiveness of TENS for certain types of pain will not be reflected by decreased analgesic consumption.

Cardiothoracic Surgery

A "double-blind" (see previous comments), prospective, randomized, sham-controlled study demonstrated decreased opioid use in post-thoracotomy patients using TENS.[63] A similarly well-designed study demonstrated decreased pain, shorter duration of convalescence, and improved physiotherapy, but no change in postoperative opioid use.[65] A well-designed study of sternotomy pain after cardiac surgery demonstrated decreased opioid use and improved pulmonary function. There was no significant change in pain (assessed by nursing observations) with use of TENS as compared with controls. Two further studies of limited adequacy have been performed in post-thoracotomy patients, and show variable results.[51,52]

In summary, well-designed studies have demonstrated decreased pain and improved clinical parameters in patients with TENS compared with sham TENS after cardiothoracic surgery.

Postamputation

A prospective, randomized, sham-controlled, unblinded study of the efficacy of acupuncture-like TENS for prevention of phantom limb pain after lower extremity amputation demonstrated no effect on its prevalence at 1 year.[66] However, improved stump healing and a decreased rate of reamputation was found in the TENS group.[66]

Thus, TENS appears to improve postoperative pain control and decrease opioid use after upper abdominal surgery, cesarean delivery, thoracotomy, and median sternotomy; benefit has not been shown after lower abdominal surgery. Improved pain control after orthopaedic surgery has been suggested by many preliminary studies, but remains to be confirmed by well-designed studies. Improvement in clinical parameters such as bowel function, pulmonary function, and tolerance of physiotherapy has been suggested by many studies, but only confirmed in well-designed studies after thoracotomy.

GUIDELINES FOR USE OF POSTOPERATIVE TENS

Many decisions great and small must be made in establishing a postoperative TENS program, and detailed discussions of these issues are available.[67,68] In general, physical therapy departments usually administer TENS programs for chronic pain. Nursing or pain management departments may be better suited to manage postoperative TENS.[68]

Because the degree of clinical benefit and its cost-effectiveness remain controversial, the decision to offer TENS routinely to certain categories of patients or to reserve TENS for special cases must be made by the physician. Furthermore, since no data exist comparing different TENS parameters, only suggestions can be made. Rough guidelines appear in Tables 20-4 and 20-5.

TABLE 20-4. Patients Who May Benefit From TENS

After thoracotomy, upper abdominal surgery, cesarean delivery, or orthopaedic surgery
Patients with significant anticipated postoperative bowel or respiratory dysfunction
Clinical situations in which minimal opioid use is desirable (e.g., elderly, prior unfavorable reaction to opioids)
No other adjunctive analgesic therapy is available
Patients desiring participation or control in their management

TABLE 20-5. Suggested Electrode Placement and Stimulating Parameters for TENS

Electrode Placement
  One pair alongside wound
  A second pair placed paravertebrally at the appropriate segmental level, if desired
  In extremity surgery, a pair alongside the nerve innervating painful area
Stimulating Parameters
  Frequency: 80–100 Hz
  Waveform: biphasic
  Pulse width: 150–250 μsec
  Amplitude: set by patient to a comfortable "tingling"
  Timing: beginning as soon as possible after surgery, continuous for 24–48 h, then as-needed

CONCLUSION

In summary, TENS is an analgesic modality that has a convincing theoretic basis, is noninvasive, and exceptionally safe. Although its analgesic efficacy is supported by both clinical and laboratory investigations, a direct causal relationship between analgesia and stimulation has not been proven. Nevertheless, TENS is worth consideration in certain postoperative clinical scenarios, especially if use of opioids or regional anesthesia/analgesia is problematic.

References

1. Kellaway P: The part played by electrical fish in the early history of bioelectricity and electrotherapy. Bull Hist Med 20:112, 1946
2. Kane K, Taub A: A history of local electrical analgesia. Pain 1:125, 1975
3. Becker RO, Marino AA: Electromagnetism and Life. State University of New York Press, Albany, 1982
4. Sheon RP: Transcutaneous electrical nerve stimulation: from electric eels to electrodes. Postgrad Med 75:71, 1984
5. Melzack R, Wall PD: Pain mechanisms: a new theory. Science 150:971, 1965
6. Wall PD, Sweet WH: Temporary abolition of pain in man. Science 155:108, 1967
7. Burton CN: Neurosurgical treatment of intractable pain. Penn Med J 75:53, 1972
8. Long DM: Recent advances in the management of pain. Minn Med 57:705, 1974
9. Shealy CN: Transcutaneous electroanalgesia. Surg Forum 23:419, 1972
10. Hymes AG, Raab DE, Yonehiro EG et al: Electrical surface stimulation for control of acute postoperative pain and prevention of ileus. Surg Forum 24:447, 1973
11. Handwerker HO, Iggo A, Zimmermann M: Segmental and supraspinal actions on dorsal horn neurons responding to noxious and non-noxious skin stimuli. Pain 1:147, 1975
12. Wagman IH, Price DD: Responses of dorsal horn cells of *M. mulatta* to cutaneous and sural nerve A and C fiber stimuli. J Neurophysiol 32:803, 1969
13. Woolf CJ, Mitchell D, Barrett GD: Antinociceptive effect of peripheral segmental electrical stimulation in the rat. Pain 8:237, 1980
14. Howson DC: Peripheral neural excitability. Implications for transcutaneous electrical nerve stimulation. Phys Ther 58:1467, 1978
15. Woolf CJ: Segmental afferent fibre-induced analgesia: transcutaneous electrical nerve stimulation (TENS) and vibration. p. 884. In Melzack R, Wall PD (eds): Textbook of Pain. 2nd Ed. Churchill Livingstone, Edinburgh, 1989

16. Fitzgerald M, Woolf CJ: Effects of cutaneous nerve and intraspinal conditioning on C-fibre afferent terminal excitability in decerebrate spinal rats. J Physiol (Lond) 318: 25, 1981

17. Le Bars D, Dickenson AH, Besson JM: Diffuse noxious inhibitory controls (DNIC). I. Effects on dorsal horn convergent neurones in the rat. Pain 6:283, 1979

18. Shimizu T, Koja T, Fujusaki T, Fukuda T: Effects of methysergide and naloxone on analgesia induced by the peripheral electric stimulation in mice. Brain Res 208: 463, 1981

19. Sjölund BH, Eriksson MB: The influence of naloxone on analgesia produced by peripheral conditioning stimulation. Brain Res 173:295, 1979

20. Sjölund B, Eriksson M: Electroacupuncture and endogenous morphines (letter). Lancet ii:1085, 1976

21. Campbell JN, Taub A: Local analgesia from percutaneous electrical stimulation. A peripheral mechanism. Arch Neurol 28:347, 1973

22. Ignelzi RJ, Nyquist JK: Direct effect of electrical stimulation on peripheral nerve evoked activity: implications in pain relief. J Neurosurg 45:159, 1976

23. Wall PD, Gutnick M: Ongoing activity in peripheral nerves: the physiology and pharmacology of impulses originating from a neuroma. Exp Neurol 43:580, 1974

24. Ignelzi RJ, Nyquist JK: Excitability changes in peripheral nerve fivers after repetitive electrical stimulation. Implications in pain modulation. J Neurosurg 51:824, 1979

25. Swett JE, Law JD: Analgesia with peripheral nerve stimulation: absence of a peripheral nerve mechanism. Pain 15:55, 1983

26. Owens S, Atkinson ER, Lees DE: Thermographic evidence of reduced sympathetic tone with transcutaneous nerve stimulation. Anesthesiology 50:62, 1979

27. Tyler E, Caldwell C, Ghia JN: Transcutaneous electrical nerve stimulation: an alternative approach to the management of postoperative pain. Anesth Analg 61:449, 1982

28. Sjölund B, Eriksson M: Relief of Pain by TENS. John Wiley & Sons, 1985

29. Mannheimer JS, Lampe GN: Clinical Transcutaneous Electrical Nerve Stimulation. FA Davis, Philadelphia, 1984

30. Hardy PAJ: Transcutaneous electrical nerve stimulation following appendectomy: the placebo effect (letter). Ann R Coll Surg Eng 69:42, 1987

31. Smedley F, Taube M, Wastell C: Transcutaneous electrical nerve stimulation for pain relief following inguinal hernia repair: a controlled trial. Eur Surg Res 20:233, 1988

32. Gilbert JM, Gledhill T, Law N, George C: Controlled trial of transcutaneous electrical nerve stimulation (TENS) for postoperative pain relief following inguinal herniorrhaphy. Br J Surg 73:749, 1986

33. Fields HL: Nondrug methods for pain control. p. 307. In: Pain. McGraw-Hill, New York, 1987

34. Galloway DJ, Boyle P, Burns HJ et al: A clinical assessment of electroanalgesia following abdominal operations. Surg Gynecol Obstet 159:453, 1984

35. Ali J, Yaffe CS, Serrette C: The effect of transcutaneous electric nerve stimulation on postoperative pain and pulmonary function. Surgery 89:507, 1981

36. Taylor AG, West BA, Simon B et al: How effective is TENS for acute pain? Am J Nurs 83:1171, 1983

37. Rosenberg M, Curtis L, Bourke DL: Transcutaneous electrical nerve stimulation for the relief of postoperative pain. Pain 5:129, 1978

38. Bussey JG, Jackson A: TENS for postsurgical analgesia. Contemp Surg 18:35, 1981

39. Caterine JM, Smith DC, Olivencia J: TENS for postsurgical analgesia following gastroplasty. Iowa Med 78:369, 1988

40. Schomburg FL, Carter-Baker SA: Transcutaneous electrical nerve stimulation for postlaparotomy pain. Phys Ther 63:188, 1983

41. Reuss R, Cronen P, Abplanalp L: Transcutaneous electrical nerve stimulation for pain control after cholecystectomy: lack of expected benefits. South Med J 81:1361, 1988

42. Sodipo JO, Adedeji SA, Olumide O: Postoperative pain relief by transcutaneous electrical nerve stimulation (TENS). Am J Chin Med 8:190, 1980

43. Carman D, Roach JW: Transcutaneous electrical nerve stimulation for the relief of postoperative pain in children. Spine 13:109, 1988

44. McCallum MI, Glynn CJ, Moore RA et al: Transcutaneous electrical nerve stimulation in the management of acute postoperative pain. Br J Anaesth 61:308, 1988

45. Alm WA, Gold ML, Weil LS: Evaluation of transcutaneous electrical nerve stimulation (TENS) in pediatric surgery. J Am Podiatry Med Assoc 69:537, 1979

46. Harvie KW: A major advance in the control of postoperative knee pain. Orthopedics 2:26, 1979

47. Stabile M, Mallory T: The management of postoperative pain in total joint replacement: transcutaneous electrical nerve stimulation is evaluated in total hip and knee patients. Orthop Rev 7:121, 1978

48. Pike PMH: Transcutaneous electrical stimulation. Its use in the management of postoperative pain. Anaesthesia 33:165, 1978

49. Finley A, Steward DJ: Transcutaneous electric nerve stimulation for control of postoperative pain following spinal fusion in adolescents, abstracted. Can Anaesth Soc J 30:S67, 1983

50. Richardson RR, Siqueira EB: Transcutaneous electrical neurostimulation in postlaminectomy pain. Spine 5:361, 1980

51. Stubbing JF, Jellicoe JA: Transcutaneous electrical nerve stimulation after thoracotomy. Pain relief and peak expiratory flow rate — a trial of transcutaneous electrical nerve stimulation. Anaesthesia 43:296, 1988

52. Stratton SA, Smith MM: Postoperative thoracotomy. Effect of transcutaneous electrical nerve stimulation on forced vital capacity. Phys Ther 60:45, 1980

53. VanderArk GD, McGrath KA: Transcutaneous electrical nerve stimulation for the relief of postoperative pain. Am J Surg 130:338, 1975

54. Hymes AC, Yonehiro EG, Raab DE et al: Acute pain control by electrostimulation: a preliminary report. Adv Neurol 4:761, 1974

55. Solomon RA, Viernstein MC, Long DM: Reduction of postoperative pain and narcotic use by transcutaneous electrical nerve stimulation. Surgery 87:142, 1980

56. Cooperman AM, Hall B, Mikalacki K et al: Use of transcutaneous electrical stimulation in the control of postoperative pain. Am J Surg 133:185, 1977

57. Lim AT, Edis G, Kranz H et al: Postoperative pain control: contribution of psychological factors and transcutaneous electrical stimulation. Pain 17:179, 1983

58. Cuschieri RJ, Morran CG, McArdle CS: Transcutaneous electrical stimulation for postoperative pain. Ann R Coll Surg Engl 67:127, 1985

59. Conn IG, Marshall AH, Yadav SN et al: Transcutaneous electrical nerve stimulation following appendicectomy: the placebo effect. Ann R Coll Surg Engl 68:191, 1986

60. Arvidsson I, Eriksson E: Postoperative TENS pain relief after knee surgery: objective evaluation. Orthopedics 9:1346, 1986

61. Smith CM, Guralnick MS, Gelfand MM, Jeans ME: The effects of transcutaneous electrical nerve stimulation on postcaesarian pain. Pain 27:181, 1986

62. Davies JR: Ineffective transcutaneous nerve stimulation following epidural anaesthesia. Anaesthesia 37:453, 1982
63. Rooney SM, Jain S, Goldiner PL: Effect of transcutaneous nerve stimulation on postoperative pain after thoracotomy. Anesth Analg 62:1010, 1983
64. Navaratham RG, Wang IY, Thomas D, Klineberg PL: Evaluation of the transcutaneous nerve stimulator for postoperative analgesia following cardiac surgery. Anaesth Intensive Care 12:345, 1984
65. Warfield CA, Stein JM, Frank HA: The effect of transcutaneous electrical nerve stimulation on pain after thoracotomy. Ann Thorac Surg 39:462, 1985
66. Finsen V, Persen L, Lovlien M et al: Transcutaneous electrical nerve stimulation after major amputation. J Bone Joint Surg [Br] 70:109, 1988
67. Mannheimer JS, Lampe GN: Clinical Transcutaneous Electrical Nerve Stimulation. FA Davis, Philadelphia, 1984
68. Smith CM, LaFlamme CA: Managing a TENS program in the OR. AORN J 32:411, 1980

21

Hypnosis and the Relaxation Response

Elisabeth Kay

Twenty-nine million people underwent surgical procedures in 1986 according to data from the National Center of Health Statistics.[1] Of those, 40 percent experienced little or no pain, 35 percent had moderate pain, and the final 25 percent had severe pain that lasted 1–7 days.[2] Although the physical "injury" of surgery causes postoperative pain, psychosocial, cultural, and contextual factors also define the experience. Unfortunately, interventions to reduce pain have been largely chemoanalgesic in nature, ignoring the psychosocial context in which nociception occurs. This chapter looks at the role of nonchemoanalgesic adjunctive interventions, specifically hypnosis and the use of the relaxation response.[3,4]

THE PSYCHOSOCIAL CONTEXT OF POSTOPERATIVE PAIN

With respect to surgical patients, psychological stressors include the fear of loss of control, anxiety, and uncertainty about the degree of physical pain attendant on surgery. In addition, the inevitable dependency on staff contributes to the generalized feeling of vulnerability. Personality styles, as well as personal experiences, may impact on patients' perceptions as they wonder whether they can trust staff at a time when they will be totally dependent. If patients have been deprived of an emotionally supportive family or health care system in the past, it is likely that they will be more frightened when they come to the surgical experience. In other words, the capacity to develop trusting relationships with health care providers will impact on the underlying fears of being vulnerable. Because "pain is closely related to threat and stress,"[5] interventions need to deal with specific fears and anxieties.

Cultural attitudes are also important. In some cultures, the ability to scream represents a healthy adaptation to painful frightening stimuli. The affectivity does not equilibrate to "excruciating pain." This can often be readily misinterpreted by health care professionals. Similarly, noncomplaining joviality does not necessarily imply little or no pain. When highly stressed, patients often exacerbate their culturally accepted roles. To truly know the level of pain being experienced, staff will need to ask directly.

The context under which surgery occurs is in and of itself multifaceted. Surgery may be elective, thereby allowing the patient time to anticipate its meaning and to plan for time away from family, work, or school. Emergency surgery resulting from accident or acute disease will not allow time for planning or contemplation of significance. The severity of the underlying disorder, the extent of surgery and postoperative debilitation, and the possibility or impossibility of "cure" can alter a patient's sense of self-cohesiveness. Clearly, if the surgery can be anticipated, if it can "cure" the disease or the diseased organ within a reasonably short time, and if the procedure has little emotional meaning, patients will have less fear. Knowing the context under which surgery occurs helps the health care professional to begin to understand an individual patient's postoperative psychological stressors.

NONCHEMOTHERAPEUTIC ANALGESIC INTERVENTIONS

Development of a therapeutic relationship, education, hypnosis, and the relaxation response[3,4] are interventions designed to build on the patient's sense of control and self-esteem. Many studies have measured their analgesic efficacy when combined with traditional forms of analgesia.[6–11] Outcome measures have included decreased opioid used, early ambulation, early discharge, and positive long-term adjustments. According to Rogers and Reich,[6] "Psychological and behavioral preparation prior to surgery can affect postoperative recovery. The effect of interventions have been most consistently positive in reducing length of hospitalization and postoperative pain." However, it is difficult to precisely determine which interventions are at work—education, attention, relationship, relaxation, or hypnosis. Rogers and Reich[6] hypothesized that each might have a singular or "synergistic effect."

Education

Anesthesiologists have been using nonchemotherapeutic pain reduction strategies during preoperative education at the initial preanesthetic interview for quite some time. A classic study at the Massachusetts General Hospital correlated the preoperative visit (only 5 minutes on the eve of surgery) with a significant decrease in preoperative anxiety.[7] In fact, the level of anxiety was much reduced compared with a control group that received pentobarbital sedation without preoperative education.[7] Thus, educating patients about their potential postoperative pain empowers them with a sense of control and normality.[8] Insightful preoperative education gives patients the sense that the procedure and recovery is or will proceed uneventfully.[8]

Hypnosis

Hypnosis was initially described by Franz Anton Mesmer, an Austrian physician in the late 18th century. With the arrival of chemoanalgesia, hypnosis lost creditability and use. It has, during the past several decades, once again gained acceptability.

Hypnosis has been defined as an altered state of consciousness. It is "any mental state(s), induced by various physiologic, psychologic, or pharmacologic maneuvers or agents, which can be recognized subjectively by the individual himself (or by an objective observer of the individual) as representing sufficient deviation in subjective experience or psychologic functioning from certain general norms for that individual during alert, waking consciousness."[11] Brown and Fromm[12] pointed out that certain subjects have "special talents" with respect to hypnosis, in which they are more or less skilled. Understanding and using such talents as ideomotor skills, cognitive effects (such as perceived alterations of reality, hallucinatory capability, imagery, and memory), as well as post-trance suggestions, will help the clinician maximize the patient's benefit from hypnosis.[12]

The three schools of hypnosis are the directive, the permissive, and the Ericksonian. Of the three, the permissive philosophy engages the subject and hypnotist most equally, relying on the patient's inner resources and expansion of their coping capacities. It is less authoritarian than the directive school and more structured than the Ericksonian methods, which rely a great deal on metaphors and suggestion.

With the permissive method, the hypnotic experience consists of four parts: *induction of the trance, deepening the trance, hypnosis work* (or exploration of hypnosis), and *termination* (back to a normal state of awakening).

Induction of the Trance

There are a variety of inductions methods: eye closure, progressive muscle relaxation, coin drop, and the Chevreul pendulum. If patients are taught hypnosis preoperatively, using the same technique after surgery may be reassuring.

It is paramount that the patient assumes a comfortable position for induction. Thus, for the postsurgical patient, the practitioner will need to assess what positions are most comfortable. For example, sitting may be painful and an *eye closure technique* may therefore be the most efficacious. Other induction methods include *progressive muscle relaxation,* in which major muscle groups are repetitively tensed and released; the *coin drop technique,* wherein a coin drops to the floor as the palm of the hand turns over; and the *Chevreul pendulum.* When using this last modality, the patient holds a pendulum between his thumb and index finger. Using his attentional skills to focus on the tip of the pendulum, the suggestion is made that the pendulum will move in a particular direction. Next, the hypnotist suggests that the direction will change in some way. As it does, the linking of suggestion of a trance can be made. For example, one might say, "As the pendulum changes direction, you will find your arm getting heavier and heavier. As the pendulum hits the table, you will find yourself in a comfortable state of trance."

Deepening the Trance

Once the patient is in a trance, deepening of the trance is suggested to the patient. Levels of trance are regulated by the patient; they choose how deep they wish to go. Progressive muscle relaxation can be used as a deepening technique as well as an induction method. Other deepening techniques include staircase, elevator, boat, beach, or cloud imagery and fantasies. With all the deepening techniques, the hypnotist is helping the patient "to regress in the service of the ego."[13] Through the imagination of the hypnotist, patients enter a comfortable, warm, and rhythmically peaceful setting.

Hypnosis Work

With the deepening accomplished, the work of hypnosis for pain reduction can proceed in several ways. The hypnotist can directly suggest that the sensation causing discomfort will become less and less. Secondly, the hypnotist can suggest that the experience of the pain will decrease despite the fact that the patient will be aware of pain. In other words, the sensory experience will be the same, but the affective experience will be altered. Thirdly, the hypnotist can direct the patient's attention away from the pain and its source. For example, pain may be redirected to a hand, giving relief to the sensory experience of abdominal pain.[14] Fourth, the hypnotist can suggest an hallucination of anesthesia. Using the technique of "glove anesthesia," the patient initially imagines his hand is "gloved" with numbness as if receiving a local anesthetic. He then rubs the parts of the body with the anesthetized hand, "spreading" the numbness to painful places. A final method of pain reduction involves dissociation. This is especially useful in immobile patients. The patient is told that while the body will stay in the bed, the mind can wander to a place that is peaceful and comfortable. The more imaginative the patient and the hypnotist are, the better this experience will be. Remembering that hypnosis is a powerful and concrete experience, it is important that the hypnotist bring the mind and body back together before the termination phase of the session.

Termination

The termination phase of hypnosis is simple and direct, counting back from "five to one." At "one," the patient is told that he or she will be fully alert and awake and will remember only those parts of the experience that he or she is able to manage.

Certainly during the trance state itself, patients clinically report relaxation and analgesia. Posthypnotic suggestion and self-hypnosis are two methods that extend the benefits of the trance. Patients vary in their capacity for posthypnotic suggestions and self-hypnosis, however. According to Barber,[15] patients using self-hypnotic techniques achieve longer-lasting pain relief, as well as a sense of independence.

Used as an adjunct to chemoanalgesia, hypnosis can be an efficacious aid to pain reduction. Kolouch[10] studied 254 patients using hypnosis as adjunctive treatment for pain reduction. Based on objective criteria, hypnotized patients needed less analgesic medication and were discharged earlier than nonhypnotized patients.[10]

As it produces potent alterations in cognition and behavior, hypnosis must be performed with skill and sensitivity to patients' needs and experiences. The Society for Clinical and Experimental Hypnosis, the American Society of Clinical Hypnosis, and Division 30 of the American Psychological Association provide workshops for practitioners. Physicians, social workers, psychologists, dentists, and psychiatric nurses are eligible for training through one or more of these organizations.

The Relaxation Response

Systematic muscle relaxation was first used in the 1930s as a treatment for anxiety. Later, autogenic training was added to the repertoire. Patients learn to tense and release muscle groups in a systematic manner, which in turn results in deep relaxation and the ability to deal with fearful situations. Using systematic muscle relaxation, patients learn to feel their bodies and limbs as "warm and heavy." The warmth and heaviness expand into feelings of peace and serenity. Now a variety of techniques are used to reach this psychophysiologic state of low arousal known as the *relaxation response*.[3,4,16,17] In addition to progressive muscle relaxation and autogenic training, diaphragmatic breathing, the focused repetition of a word, phrase, or prayer, guided imagery, and meditation are examples of induction methods for the relaxation response.

The relaxation response is useful in any condition in which tension, fear, or anxiety may be augmenting the perception of pain.[17] Most patients are quite able to understand the relationship between tension and the increased perceptions of pain. These patients are easily taught relaxation techniques, become at least pleasantly if not deeply relaxed, develop a sense of mastery and inner peace, and can be provided with useful distraction from noxious stimuli when using the exercise. As with hypnosis, patients will be more comfortable using the relaxation response as a coping mechanism if preoperative rather than postoperative instruction is given.

Physiologic responses to relaxation techniques include reductions in respiratory rate, oxygen consumption, blood pressure, serum lactic acid, and heart rate. Benson[3] suggested that the relaxation response suppresses sympathetic hyperactivity by opposing the flight-or-fight response.

Physiologic changes may not fully explain why patients experience a decrease in pain perception. Syrjala[17] speculated that there may be changes in catecholamine or endogenous opioid levels. It must be kept in mind that patients using the relaxation response are also deriving benefit from "doing for themselves" in the totally dependent social situation of postoperative hospitalization. In addition, the concentration required to focus "mindful" meditation necessarily distracts from physical discomfort.

Achieving the Relaxation Response

As with hypnosis, patients are asked to get into a comfortable position. Permission is given for them to move in any way that feels comfortable during the exercise. Preparation includes turning off the telephone and requesting no interruptions from staff.

Breathing is used as the focal point of concentration. Patients seem adept at learning to "tune out" tension as they begin to notice the differences in temperature of inhalations and exhalations (cool on inhaling, warm on exhaling). Exhalation is done through the mouth. Patients are instructed to notice their shoulders rising a bit on inhalation and relaxing on exhalation.

Diaphragmatic breathing can be taught to patients who have not had abdominal surgery. Patients are taught to inhale from their diaphragm, filling their lungs from the lower to middle and finally upper parts. Patients are instructed to place their hands so that they just touch each other on their abdomen, and to notice that they separate as the abdomen extends on inhalation. Patients can be taught to notice tension or areas of physical discomfort on inhalation and to try as best as they can to dispel the discomfort on exhalation. Breathing training is at the core of the relaxation response.

Once patients are relaxed, they can repeat a word, phrase, or short prayer on inhalation. Exhalation provides the means to "focus away" all other thoughts, tension, anxiety, and pain. When thoughts intrude, as they will, patients are taught to notice them without judgment and to return to the chosen phrase of the meditation.

Guided imagery is a technique akin to hypnosis, without the induction of a formalized trance. In this technique, patients are asked to imagine a peaceful time in their lives and to recall that time in detail. Usually, patients choose times of solitude in which they have experienced some inner peace, or focus attention on intense feelings of connection with another person. The connection with others gives way to feelings of safety, warmth, and comfort. The practitioner can be more or less active at this time. The practitioners guide the patients, encouraging more and more detail; others leave the images for the patients to discover.

With postoperative patients worried about the results of biopsies, the success of the surgery, or present incisional pain, it can seem a daunting task to suggest that they release those concerns and relax. Nevertheless, the relaxation response provides an opportunity for patients who are worried, tense, and hurting to get relief. The duration of the exercise should be 15–20 minutes per session (up to 45 minutes), once or twice a day. Benson and others have also encouraged patients to use mini-relaxations. Patients take a few "mindful" short breaths when hurting or frightened. Concentration on breathing seems to temporarily break the pain cycle and can help patients to get back in control.[18]

Relaxation can induce changes in blood glucose levels in diabetic patients and blood pressure in hypertensive patients. It has also been suggested that psychotic or severely depressed patients, as well as patients with seizure disorders, may be adversely affected by the relaxation response.[18]

There are no extensive training requirements for therapists to teach meditation techniques. Nevertheless, practitioners need to be aware that patients may become in touch with profound, unanticipated feelings. They may also have hypersensitive or hyposensitive body experiences. An explanation that such experiences are normal is usually enough to reassure patients. If these remain troublesome, an exploration of the content of these experiences with a mental health professional will be necessary.

CONCLUSION

Instruction in the adjunctive interventions of hypnosis and the relaxation response is best administered preoperatively for postoperative pain management. Patients are told that such adjunctive strategies can be effective analgesic modalities and will be used in conjunction with typical analgesic regimens (e.g., epidural analgesia, patient-controlled analgesia). Both techniques can be augmented with tapes so patients can practice on their own. The creativity of either process, the willingness of the health care provider to better understand the meaning of the experience for the individual patient, and realistic hopefulness by the provider that the individual patient can cope with pain all contribute to successful management.

References
1. NCHS: Current Estimates from the National Health Interview Survey. United States. (DHHS publication no. (PHS) 87-1592). National Center for Health Statistics, Hyattsville, MD, 1987
2. Bonica JJ, Procacci P: General considerations of acute pain. p. 159. In Bonica JJ (ed): The Management of Pain. 2nd Ed. Lea & Febiger, Philadelphia, 1990
3. Benson H: The Relaxation Response. Avon, New York, 1976
4. Benson H: Beyond the Relaxation Response. Berkley Books, New York, 1985
5. Chapman RC, Turner JA: Psychologic and psychosocial aspects of acute pain. p.

122. In Bonica JJ (ed): The Management of Pain. 2nd Ed. Lea & Febiger, Philadelphia, 1990

6. Rogers M, Reich P: Psychological intervention with surgical patients: evaluation outcome. Adv Psychosom Med 15:23, 1986

7. Egbert LD, Battit GE, Turndof H, Beecher HK: The value of the preoperative visit by the anesthetist. JAMA 185:553, 1963

8. Egbert LD, Battit GE, Welch CE, Barlett MK: Reduction in postoperative pain by encouragement and instruction of patients. N Engl J Med 270:825, 1964

9. Flaherty GG, Fitzpatrick JJ: Relaxation technique to increase comfort level of postoperative patients: a preliminary study. Nurs Res 27:352, 1978

10. Kolouch FT: Hypnosis and surgical convalescence: a study of subjective factors in postoperative recovery. Am J Clin Hypn 7:1209, 1964

11. Ludwig AM: Altered states of consciousness. Arch Gen Psychiatry 15:225, 1966

12. Brown DP, Fromm E: Hypnotherapy and Hypnoanalysis. Lawrence Erlbaum, London, 1986

13. Kris E: Psychoanalytic Explorations in Art. International Universities Press, New York, 1952

14. Hilgard ER, and Hilgard JR: Hypnosis in the Relief of Pain. Wm Kaufman, Los Altos, California, 1983

15. Barber J: Hypnosis. p. 1733. In Bonica JJ (ed): The Management of Pain. 2nd Ed. Lea & Febiger, Philadelphia, 1990

16. Turk DC, Meichenbaum D, Genest M: Pain and Behavioral Medicine: A Cognitive Behavioral Perspective. Guilford Press, New York, 1983

17. Syrjala K: Relaxation techniques. p. 1742. In Bonica JJ (ed): The Management of Pain. 2nd Ed. Lea & Febiger, Philadelphia, 1990

18. Borysenko J: Minding the Body, Mending the Mind. Bantam Books, New York, 1988

22

Pediatric Postoperative Pain Management

Navil F. Sethna

For years, acute pediatric pain management has been practiced without clear rational use of analgesic therapy. Little, if any, useful information was readily available regarding opioid pharmacology in children. The recent improved understanding of opioid and local anesthetic pharmacology in infants and children has led to the development of formal analgesic regimens for the management of pain, particularly postoperative pain. Ongoing research will elucidate better dosing strategies and better methods of drug delivery in children of different ages.

Despite the advances in analgesic therapy, numerous studies show that postoperative pain is still inadequately treated in children, adolescents, and almost ignored in infants. Unwarranted concerns regarding opioid-induced respiratory depression and the potential for addiction are in part responsible for its undertreatment. Certainly, the inherent difficulty of assessing pain (particularly in the nonverbal child) is also contributory. Thus, opioids are customarily prescribed in subtherapeutic doses at unduly lengthy time intervals and administered only when a child requests them or the nurse perceives that the child is in pain.[1-4]

PREOPERATIVE CONSIDERATIONS AND PREPARATION

Hospitalization and surgery have long been recognized as sources of stress to most children and adults and may have a profound and long-lasting psychological impact.[5] A child's psychological constitution and cognitive function at different stages of development make the child unique in his or her individual distress and anxiety and also in his or her responses to pain and hospitalization. Thus, the child's reaction to the alien hospital environment and personnel is determined by how well the child and parents are prepared to deal with this unfamiliar and new experience. If unprepared, the child's ability to function is impaired and his or her secure state of everyday life is disturbed. The child's sense of security, control, and predictability of everyday events is threatened. The child may respond with maladaptive distress behavior brought on by feelings of defenselessness, anxiety, vulnerability, and the inability to cope.[6] Pain is a major contributor to stress and distress in hospitalized children and adolescents.[7] Conceivably, children exhibiting a higher degree of distress behavior are usually experiencing more intense pain.[8] Signs of stress and fear may include crying, restlessness, sleeplessness, or withdrawal from the environment. Emotional reactions to acute pain in children may be displayed as extreme anger, tantrums, demanding behavior, regression, and/or withdrawal.[9] Untreated pain could interfere with adaptation to hospitalization, recovery from surgery, and possibly, readjustment after discharge.

Parental preparation for their child's surgery and subsequent postoperative course can facilitate realistic expectations of the severity and duration of pain, optimize use of analgesic modalities, and promote greater coping skills for themselves and their child. Parental preparation is important because parental anxieties and fears may be projected onto and accentuate the child's distress and maladaptation. Omission of a realistic explanation, conveyance of misconception, or intentional deluding of the child about pain by the parents can unfavorably enhance the child's apprehensions and uncertainties.

The anesthesiologist can best serve both the child and the parents by planning the preoperative visit to aid in the adjustment to the hospital environment. This includes parental preparation and involvement and early preoperative bonding with the child. The child should be informed to expect pain in a truthful manner at his or her level of understanding. More importantly, the child should be instructed to report pain.

Intramuscular (IM) injections are at the center of anxiety and fear for almost all children. Children can certainly benefit from the reassurance that administration of analgesics via other routes is possible. With this in mind, it is important to familiarize children with the chosen alternative analgesic modality (e.g., epidural analgesia, intravenous [IV] opioids, patient-controlled analgesia [PCA],). Thus, the anesthesiologist is best suited to prepare both child and parents psychologically for the surgical experience by allaying anticipatory anxieties related to hospitalization, surgery, and postoperative pain.

PAIN ASSESSMENT

Pain in Nonverbal Children

As pain is a subjective experience, it is difficult to evaluate in neonates and in nonverbal children. Traditionally, such children were not viewed to experience pain as we know it.[10] Review of the available data indicates that the neurophysiologic and neurochemical components necessary for the transduction, transmission, modulation, and perception of nociception are present in term and preterm infants.[10] The hormonal-metabolic responses to noxious surgical stimuli (the surgical stress response—see Ch. 4) are also intact. Similarly, undesirable physiologic responses can be provoked by pain. Term and preterm infants can undergo substantial changes in hemodynamics, oxygen saturation, and intracranial pressure in response to noxious surgical stimuli. Both the surgical stress response and undesirable physiologic responses provoked by pain can be blunted or abolished by effective analgesia.[8,11-14] Thus, in contrast to previously held beliefs, the weight of evidence suggests that neonates experience pain and should be treated for it.

Pain Measurement

The difficulties of pain assessment in children can be explained by their constantly changing state of perception, interpretation and expression of pain related to age, developmental stage, previous pain experiences, and other modifying environmental factors.[15] Despite the shortcomings of our understanding of childhood pain experiences and our inability to assess pain accurately, the available instruments of pain assessment can be implemented in an age-appropriate manner in daily clinical practice. Such application can facilitate both the diagnosis of pain and the evaluation of the effectiveness of analgesic modalities. Selection of the appropriate assessment tool should emphasize ease of applicability and permit effective interventions at the bedside.

In general, infants and preverbal children younger than the age of 2 years are unable to communicate their pain and distress. Their physiologic and behavioral responses to painful stimuli are acceptable correlates of pain perception and distress. Their pain is best evaluated by observing their behavioral responses (i.e., body movements, facial expressions, cries) and physiologic responses (i.e., tachycardia, hypertension, tachypnea, palmar sweating, hypoxemia).

So far, simple and practical pain and distress measures in infants and preverbal children are lacking. In the clinical setting, the assessment of postoperative pain can be performed with a postoperative pain/comfort scale or objective pain scale, which incorporates both standardized behavioral and physiologic parameters.[16,17] Recently, the Children's Hospital of Eastern Ontario Pain Scale (CHEOPS) was developed to evaluate pain after surgery. It includes six behaviors that are repeatedly observed every 30 seconds by a trained observer. Preliminary results indicate that the scale is a sensitive, valid, and reliable behavioral measure of postoperative pain in children aged 1–5 years.[18]

Children between the ages of 2 and 7 years lack abstract thinking and the verbal skills necessary to express their feelings of pain. Thus, nonverbal techniques are used to assess their pain intensity. A number of projective methods have been evaluated to ascertain the presence of pain (and to a lesser degree the intensity of pain) as inferred from the child's selection of color, drawing, or facial emotional expressions.[19] A practical, reliable, and easy-to-apply bedside guide is a faces scale, such as the Oucher Scale. The Oucher Scale consists of a poster with six photographs of a child's face in various expressions of pain, matched alongside of a visual analogue scale (VAS) (see below).[20,21]

Older children (older than 7 years) often have the ability to understand, rationalize, and form relationships between cause and effect. They can often express their feelings and describe their pain experience. Therefore, they can self-report the quality *and* intensity of pain. Within their age group, a child's verbal description of his or her pain can be assessed by simple numerical-verbal rating scales (see Ch. 6).[22]

Children aged 12 years and older have the sophisticated vocabulary necessary to respond to a questionnaire similar to those used for pain assessment in adults.[23] (Please see Ch. 6 for a thorough discussion of pain assessment in adults.) The VAS is the most extensively used scale because of its simplicity.[24] This technique consists of a 10-cm line with two anchors. At one end are the words "no pain" and on the other end, "pain as severe as possible."

Pain ratings can be reliably assessed using an analogue chromatic continuous scale (ACCS),[25] which allows grading of a child's pain into a numeric value. The ACCS consists of a slide rule with graduated shades of red. The brightness of the color represents the intensity of the pain. The back of the ruler has a 100-mm scale corresponding to the color brightness (Fig. 22-1). The child is asked to rate his or her pain by moving a sliding line indicator onto the appropriate color. Thus, the choice of color brightness directly quantifies pain intensity into a numeric value.[25]

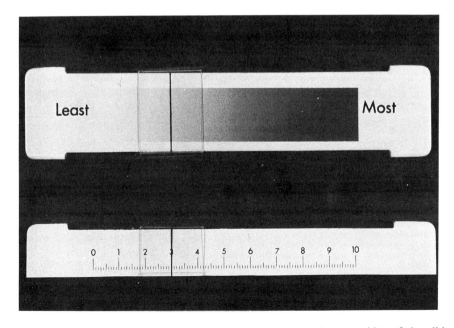

Fig. 22-1. Analogue chromatic continuous scale (ACCS). The two sides of the slide rule scale are shown.

THERAPEUTIC MODALITIES FOR PEDIATRIC POSTOPERATIVE PAIN MANAGEMENT

Effective systemic analgesics as well as routes of administration already exist for pediatric pain management. Unfortunately, these adequate analgesics and delivery systems are underused because of prevalent and persistent misconceptions regarding the propensity for respiratory depression and addiction in children and the actual presence of pain in certain age groups. Similarly, potent and safe regional anesthetic/analgesic techniques are well known but underused.

The remaining sections of this chapter discuss the appropriate use of systemic analgesics and regional anesthesia/analgesia for pain management in children. A tabular summary of dosing regimens for systemic analgesia maybe found in Tables 22-1 and 22-2. Pediatric dosages for regional anesthetic/analgesic techniques are found in Table 22-3.

TABLE 22-1. Systemic Analgesic Dosages for Pediatric Use

Name	Dose
Nonopioid	
Oral	
Acetaminophen	10–15 mg/kg po q 4 h prn
	15–20 mg/kg pr q 4 h prn
Acetylsalicylic acid	65–100 mg/kg 24 h in 4–6 doses
Opioids	
Oral	
Codeine	0.5–1 mg/kg po q 4 h prn
Morphine[a]	0.05–0.2 mg/kg po q 4 h
Meperidine[b]	1 mg/kg po q 4 h
Methadone	0.1 mg/kg po q 6–8 h[d]
Intramuscular[c]	
Morphine	0.1–0.15 mg/kg IM q 3–4 h prn
Intermittent IV injection	
Morphine	0.05–0.1 mg/kg IV q 2 h prn
Methadone	Loading dose: 0.2 mg/kg IV
	Supplemental loading after surgery: 0.05 mg/kg IV q 10 min prn
	Initial loading without prior opioid exposure: 0.1 mg/kg IV q 2–3 h to a maximum of 0.2 mg/kg
	Maintenance:
	0.07–0.08 mg/kg IV q 4 h for severe pain
	0.05–0.06 mg/kg IV q 4 h for moderate pain
	0.03 mg/kg IV q 4 h for mild or no pain
Continuous IV infusions	
Morphine	Less than 3 months old:
	Initially: 0.05 mg/kg IV q 15–20 min prn
	Maintenance: 10–15 μg/kg/h
	Older than 3 months of age:
	Initially: 0.1 mg/kg IV q 15–20 min prn
	Maintenance: 10–50 μg/kg h

[a] As there is wide clinical experience with use of morphine in children, there is little advantage to the use of other μ-agonists for *initial* management of pain.

[b] Meperidine is not routinely used in infants and children because of the prolonged elimination half-life in neonates.

[c] IM dosing should be avoided in children.

[d] Methadone requires careful titration because it accumulates with repetitive dosing, causing excessive somnalence. Adjustment of dosage or the dosing interval is required if sedation occurs.

TABLE 22-2. Postoperative PCA Morphine Regimens

Mode	Incremental Dose (mg/kg)	Continuous (mg/kg/h)	Lockout Interval (min)	4-Hour Limit (mg/kg)
Demand dose	0.025		10	0.24
Continuous + demand dose	0.018	0.015	10	0.24

(Data from Berde et al[70])

Systemic Analgesics

Nonopioid Analgesics

These agents provide relief of mild to moderate pain when used alone and provide additive analgesia when combined with opioids.

Acetaminophen is widely used as an analgesic in children of all ages as it is not associated with Reye syndrome like aspirin.[26] Acetaminophen has no anti-inflammatory properties.[27] Its analgesic and antipyretic effects are similar to aspirin, and the side effects are relatively infrequent when used in recommended doses.[27] Other advantages over aspirin include lack of gastric irritation, platelet dysfunction, and cross-sensitivity to aspirin. Hypersensitivity is rare.[27] The recommended dose is 10–15 mg/kg every 4 hours as needed.[28] Over-the-counter formulations include chewable tablets, elixirs, and suppositories. A higher dose is recommended for rectal use (15–20 mg/kg), but its absorption is incomplete and unreliable.[29]

Acetylsalicylic acid (aspirin) is the standard drug with which other nonopioid analgesics are compared. It is particularly useful in the presence of pain of inflammatory or rheumatic origin. Its use has been limited because of its association with Reye's syndrome in children with viral illnesses.[26,30]

Besides acetylsalicylic acid, relatively few nonsteroidal anti-inflammatory drugs are used in children, and only tolmetin is approved for use in juvenile rheumatoid arthritis. As a group, these drugs share common anti-inflammatory, antipyretic, and analgesic properties and produce varying degrees of gastropathy and platelet dysfunction. (See Ch. 7.) Their use in children is extrapolated from adult experience.[31]

Opioids

Morphine-like (μ) agonists differ in their potencies, but when given in equianalgesic dosages, the attendant degree of analgesia and the incidence of side effects are similar.[32–34] For this reason and because of the wide clinical experience with use of morphine in children, there is no advantage to the use of μ-agonists other than morphine for the *initial* management of postoperative pain.

Meperidine is not routinely used in infants and children because of the prolonged elimination half-life in neonates (6–39 h). Repeated administration of meperidine may lead to an accumulation of the normeperidine metabolite, which may produce central nervous system (CNS) excitation and seizures.[35,36]

TABLE 22-3. Pediatric Dosing Regimens for Regional Anesthesia/Analgesia

Block	Regimens
Caudal	Takasaki's formula for analgesia below T10 Total ml of 0.25% bupivacaine ± 1:200,000 epinephrine = 0.7 ml × body weight (kg) Armitage's rule Sacral analgesia = 0.5 ml/kg of 0.25% bupivacaine ± 1:200,000 epinephrine Lumbar and lower thoracic analgesia = 1 ml/kg of 0.25% bupivacaine ± 1:200,000 epinephrine Midthoracic analgesia = 1.25 ml/kg of 0.25% bupivacaine ± 1:200,000 epinephrine Morphine 0.033 mg/kg as initial injection
Epidural (lumbar or thoracic)	Initial dose 3–36 months of age: 0.75 ml/kg of 0.5% bupivacaine + 1:200,000 epinephrine Older children: 0.5 ml/kg of 0.5% bupivacaine + 1:200,000 epinephrine Top-up 0.5 ml/kg of 0.25% bupivacine + 1:200,000 epinephrine q 4 h prn Infusion 0.08 ml/kg/h of 0.25% bupivacaine
Ilioinguinal and iliohypogastric nerve blocks	0.4 ml/kg of 0.5% bupivacaine + 1:200,000 epinephrine
Penile blocks	Dorsal penile nerve block 2 injections of 1 ml of 1% lidocaine, 0.25% or 0.5% bupivacaine per injection Dorsal penile nerve block (subpubic space) 0.2 ml/kg of 1% lidocaine or 0.5% bupivacaine Topicalization of postcircumcision wound 10–20 mg of 10% lidocaine spray 0.5 ml of 5% lidocaine ointment 0.5–1.0 ml of 2% lidocaine jelly
Femoral nerve block	0.2 ml/kg of 0.5% bupivacaine (10 ml maximum) 0.3 ml/kg of 1% lidocaine
Fascia iliaca compartment block	0.5–0.75 ml/kg of equal volumes of 1% lidocaine and 0.5– bupivacaine, both with 1:200,000 epinephrine
Interpleural regional analgesic	For thoracotomy 0.5–1.0 ml/kg/h of 0.25% bupivacaine + 1:200,000 epinephrine For subcostal incision Initial dose: 0.5 ml/kg of 0.5% bupivacaine Infusion: 0.1–0.5 ml/kg/h of 0.25% bupivacaine + 1:200,000 epinephrine
Infiltration	0.5–1 ml/kg of 0.25% bupivacaine

Mixed agonist-antagonists are effective for mild to moderate pain, but no data are available on their use in children. Partial agonists, such as buprenorphine, have been evaluated in children.[37,38] Preliminary studies indicate that IV or sublingual buprenorphine produces analgesia comparable morphine. Buprenorphine has been safely used for the management of pain after thoracotomy and orthopedic procedures without distinct advantages over morphine.[37,38] At the time of this writing, the use of buprenorphine is not approved by the Food and Drug Administration for use in children.

SIDE EFFECTS

Respiratory depression is the most feared and potentially the most serious side effect of opioids. The incidence of respiratory depression with μ-agonists is directly related to dose.[32–34] In general, all μ-agonists administered in equianalgesic doses will depress the respiratory center to a similar degree.[32–34]

Minor opioid side effects such as nausea, vomiting, urinary retention, drowsiness, hallucinations, nightmares, light-headedness, and ileus occur no more frequently in children than in adults. Although these side effects are common to all opioids, their occurrence is related to dose, route of administration, and considerable interpatient pharmacodynamic variability.

Tolerance is an uncommon clinical problem in children when opioids are used in appropriate doses for short periods of time. Tolerance and physical dependence can occur when high doses are used for extended periods of time.[39] Withdrawal can be precipitated when an opioid is abruptly discontinued after prolonged use and can be averted by gradually discontinuing the opioid. The development of addiction (psychologic dependence) is rare in hospitalized children and adolescents, even when opioids are used in large doses for prolonged periods of time.[40]

Route of Administration

Oral Analgesia

Parenteral administration of opioids is necessary to achieve rapid relief of moderate to severe pain after surgery. The presence of nausea, vomiting, and delayed gastric emptying due to the effects of surgery and anesthesia preclude the use of oral analgesics in the early postoperative period. Subsequently, the oral route can maintain adequate analgesia when gastrointestinal tract function has recovered. When given the choice, most children prefer the oral route to painful IM injections. The present formulations of pediatric oral analgesics are acceptable to most children. These include oral elixirs (e.g., acetaminophen, codeine, hydromorphone, morphine, methadone, meperidine), chewable tablets (acetylsalicylic acid and acetaminophen), and flavored tablets. Analgesics commonly used in children by oral administration are acetaminophen, codeine, methadone, hydromorphone, morphine, meperidine, and less frequently, the nonsteroidal anti-inflammatory drugs.

Codeine is the most commonly used oral opioid in children for relief of mild to moderate postoperative pain.[41] It is well absorbed from the gastrointestinal tract. Its bioavailability is approximately 70 percent, and peak plasma concentrations are attained in 1–1.15 hours after ingestion. The plasma elimination half-life is 3–4 hours. It is recommended at doses of 0.5–1 mg/kg every 4 hours. The analgesic effect of codeine can be further enhanced by combining it with acetaminophen.[41]

Morphine can be used effectively for relief of moderate to severe pain after surgery in doses of 0.05–0.2 mg/kg every 4 hours. After orthopedic surgery, the use of oral morphine every 4 hours around the clock has been shown to be significantly more effective than equianalgesic doses of IM meperidine administered on a prn schedule.[42]

Other opioids are also used orally in older children, and the dosing schedule is extrapolated from adult clinical dosing regimens. The available data do not allow firm recommendations for their use as oral postoperative analgesics.

Intramuscular Administration

The IM route is undesirable and should be avoided because most children and adolescents fear and dislike injections. Moreover, the onset of analgesia is slow; absorption is unpredictable; the period of analgesia may be short; and the resultant blood levels may widely vary between subtherapeutic and toxic levels.[43,44] In adults, repeated IM injections of meperidine have a fivefold variation in the attendant maximum plasma concentrations and as much as sevenfold variation in the time to peak plasma concentrations.[43]

Intermittent Intravenous Opioids

Some of the difficulties inherent with IM injections can be circumvented by the IV route of administration. A steady therapeutic blood level of an opioid can be rapidly achieved and predictably maintained. Subsequent opioid doses can be easily and rapidly adjusted with a minimum of side effects.

Intermittent IV injections of morphine are suitable for short-term pain control.[45] The use of intermittent IV injections of morphine is associated with a rapid rise in the plasma concentration of opioid and, potentially, oversedation and respiratory depression. Injections must be administered slowly with careful monitoring of the patient. A rapid rise and decline in the plasma concentration of opioid produces a short duration of analgesia and requires redosing at frequent intervals (every 2–3 hours).

Opioid injections should be slowly delivered via burette over not less than 20 minutes under close monitoring. Recommended intermittent IV morphine doses are 0.05–0.1 mg/kg every 2 hours.

Methadone is a synthetic opioid of equal potency to morphine but with a slower systemic elimination and longer duration of analgesia. The mean elimination half-life is approximately 19 hours in children between the ages 1 and 18 years.[46] The duration of analgesia, however, is much shorter than the elimination half-life (see Ch. 8).

The recommended dosing strategy for methadone in children over one year of age is similar to adults.[47] An initial fixed loading dose of 0.2 mg/kg can be given intraoperatively. Supplemental doses may be necessary postoperatively when the child is awake and the intensity of pain can be assessed. In such instances, incremental loading doses of 0.05 mg/kg are administered every 10 minutes until the pain is alleviated. In an awake child with no prior anesthetic exposure, a loading dose of 0.1 mg/kg can be administered slowly over 20 minutes every 2–3 hours to a maximum of 0.2 mg/kg.

A steady-state concentration of methadone is maintained by the periodic assessment of pain and administration of incremental doses of methadone infused over 20 minutes, around the clock every 4 hours. Maintenance doses should match the child's pain on a sliding scale as follows: 0.07–0.08 mg/kg for severe pain; 0.05–0.06 mg/kg for moderate pain; 0.03 mg/kg for mild or no pain. Each maintenance dose should be administered only after assessment of the child's level of consciousness, pupillary size, and respiratory status. The maintenance dose should be withheld if the child appears to be drowsy. Methadone is a long-acting opioid, so repeated doses may accumulate and side effects will be of prolonged duration.[47]

Continuous Intravenous Opioids

Although most opioids with moderate to rapid clearance can be effectively used in continuous IV infusions, morphine and fentanyl are most commonly used for postoperative pain control via this modality in children. Various studies have demonstrated the efficacy and safety of continuous infusions of morphine sulfate for relief of moderate to severe pain from surgical procedures in newborns, children, and adolescents.[48–53]

The success of continuous IV infusions of opioids depends on attaining and maintaining an effective analgesic plasma concentration without exceeding the threshold concentration for ventilatory depression. Remember that the natural history of postoperative pain is dynamic with temporary exacerbations superimposed on generally decreasing intensity of pain. The threshold concentration for ventilatory depression therefore changes with time. Administration of a "fixed-rate" continuous infusion will not flexibly adapt to changing analgesic requirements, leading to respiratory depression. Furthermore, the therapeutic index of an opioid becomes smaller with decreasing age because of age-related changes in pharmacodynamics and pharmacokinetics. (The therapeutic index is traditionally defined in the pharmacologic literature as the ratio of ED_{50}/LD_{50}. The therapeutic index measures the drug doses producing the desired effect in 50 percent of a test population compared with doses producing death in 50 percent of the population. In contemporary terms, however, therapeutic index has come to be defined in terms of the plasma drug concentrations producing desired versus adverse effects, i.e., the "therapeutic window.") Thus, close patient monitoring and constant adjustment of the infusion rate are *mandatory* when using continuous IV opioid infusions in order to detect early signs of CNS depression.[54]

The therapeutic index of an opioid is further reduced in the presence of altered ventilatory control (preterm infants and term infants younger than 3 months), reduced pulmonary gas-exchange reserve (advanced cystic fibrosis, broncho-pulmonary dysplasia), restrictive lung mechanics (neuromuscular disorders, thoracotomy, upper abdominal operation), or clinical scenarios with increased risk for potential airway collapse (tracheomalacia, cleft palate surgery, forma-tion of a pharyngeal flap, excision of extensive cystic hygromas, hemangiomas and oromaxillary reconstructions). High-risk children receiving continuous IV infusions of opioids should be nursed in hospital locations where monitoring and proper equipment are available for immediate respiratory support and tracheal intubation.

The biotransformation of opioids occurs mainly in the liver. All hepatic en-zyme systems have reduced activity in the preterm infant and in term infants during the first 2–3 months of life. Reduced biotransformation may explain the prolonged elimination of opioids in early postnatal life.[55–57] The immaturity of the hepatic enzyme systems and the possible presence of enhanced CNS sensitivity to opioids may predispose infants to respiratory depression.[58]

With respect to morphine pharmacokinetic behavior, the elimination half-life is prolonged and body clearance is slow in infants younger than the age of 2 months. These parameters approximate those of adults by age 2–3 months. The mean elimination half-life of morphine in term newborn infants younger than the age of 4 days is significantly greater than that observed in older term infants at age 29–65 days (6.8 hours versus 3.9 hours). Morphine clearance in newborn infants is significantly lower than that in older infants (6.2 versus 23.8 ml/kg/min).[55,59]

Similar prolongation of clearance and elimination half-life has been observed with fentanyl in newborn infants (elimination half-life = 1–16 hours; mean = 5.3 hours) and in preterm infants (elimination half-life = 6–32 hours; mean = 17.7 hours).[60,61] Again, the immaturity of the hepatic enzyme systems and changes in hepatic blood flow are responsible.

Hertzka et al[62] showed that infants older than 3 months are more tolerant to fentanyl-induced ventilatory depression as compared with adults. Data on the effects of fentanyl on ventilation in infants younger than 3 months is not avail-able. No studies have investigated the pharmacokinetics of fentanyl infusions in neonates and children, although fentanyl is commonly used for postoperative pain management in the neonatal and pediatric intensive care units.

CONTINUOUS INTRAVENOUS INFUSIONS OF MORPHINE

Based on the aforementioned pharmacokinetic and pharmacodynamic con-siderations, continuous infusions of morphine can be administered at adjustable rates after achievement of analgesia in spontaneously breathing children older than 3 months of age. Maintenance infusion rates will range from 10 to 50 µ/kg/h. If a child has not received intraoperative opioids or a sufficient loading dose or is in moderate to severe pain, incremental doses of 0.1 mg/kg of IV morphine can be administered slowly every 15–20 minutes until adequate analgesia is achieved. (The peak period for respiratory depression usually occurs 7–10 minutes after an IV dose of morphine.) Using such an approach, a number of studies have demonstrated the effectiveness of continuous IV morphine infusions for postoperative pain management in large numbers of infants older than the age of 3 months and in older children.[47,4,51] In spontaneously breathing infants younger than the age of 3 months, the recommended infusion rate is 10–15 µg/kg/h. If a loading dose is required, it should be given in the smaller dose of 0.05 mg/kg of IV morphine every 15–20 minutes as needed. Larger infusion doses may be required after major surgical procedures in mechanically ventilated infants and older children.[52]

The aforementioned infusion rates are intended as a guideline. Because of the dynamic natural history of postoperative pain, the rate of morphine administration must be "titrated" in an age-appropriate manner for each individual child in order to obtain adequate analgesia without clinical signs of respiratory or CNS depression. Fixed-rate infusions are to be totally avoided. Careful monitoring of the patient is essential.

In general, administration of opioids for postoperative pain control to spontaneously breathing neonates (younger than 1 month of age) requires even greater clinical vigilance and closer monitoring. Given the increased susceptibility of newborn infants to hypoventilate, opioids should be administered judiciously and in smaller doses.[52] Term infants younger than 3 months of age should be routinely monitored for 24 hours after administration of the last dose of opioid. Premature infants receiving opioids demand even greater monitoring and continuous nursing attentiveness as they are at increased risk for apnea after inhalational general anesthesia[63,64] and administration of sedative drugs.[65] These infants should be nursed in a hospital setting where appropriate resuscitative measures and medical personnel skilled in airway management are immediately available.

Patient-Controlled Analgesia

Intravenous-PCA is a novel method whereby a microprocessor-operated infusion pump is programmed to deliver predetermined safe amounts of IV opioid at specified intervals on patient demand (see Ch. 10). PCA is a "flexible" modality, as patients use PCA to "titrate" their plasma concentration of opioid to achieve analgesia without respiratory depression. The mandatory requirement for frequent rate adjustments with continuous IV infusions of opioids is obviated by the patient's control of the delivery of an IV injection via the PCA infuser. A discussion of the factors underlying and modifying patients' individual analgesic requirements with PCA (i.e., how the individual patient uses the device) is found in Chapter 10.

Although the total experience with IV-PCA in children is small, a number of preliminary clinical trials have described favorable results.[66–70] (Recommended dosage regimens for IV-PCA in children are found in Table 22-3.) IV-PCA

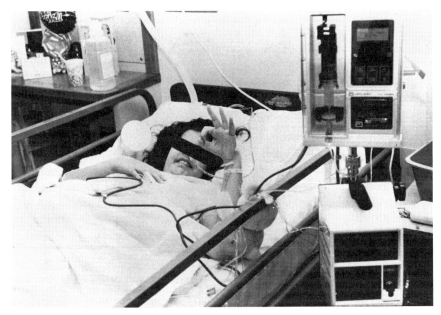

Fig. 22-2. Intravenous patient-controlled analgesia allows the postsurgical child to self-medicate and achieve satisfactory analgesia.

appears to be safe and effective in children and is frequently preferred by nursing staff, parents, and particularly adolescent patients[66,70] (Fig. 22-2). Despite its general appeal, however, there are a small number of older children and adolescents who may not wish to be bothered with self-medication, feel indifferent and even dissatisfied with PCA, and would rather receive analgesics by traditional methods.[66,68] Therefore, PCA is not a universal therapy for postoperative pain control, and alternative modalities should be offered if IV-PCA fails to satisfy the patient.

IV-PCA can be used in children as young as 7 years of age. Ultimately, the use of PCA is restricted by age, developmental understanding of the purpose of PCA, and inability to activate the pump in the presence of muscular weakness or immobilization. To circumvent these problems, some have proposed reliance on trustworthy parents for operation of the infuser (parent-controlled analgesia).[68] The safety and efficacy of parent-controlled analgesia remains to be determined.[68]

Further studies are needed to compare the efficacy and safety of PCA with other postoperative analgesic modalities commonly used in children, such as continuous infusions of opioids and regional anesthetic/analgesic techniques.

Regional Anesthesia/Analgesia

Although opioids are simple to administer, convenient, and an inexpensive means of managing postoperative pain, the judicious use of specific regional anesthetic techniques offers better pain relief for particular surgical procedures.

Neural blockade produces reliable and effective analgesia without the risk of sedation and respiratory depression. When combined with general anesthesia, adequate depth of surgical anesthesia can be provided with use of lower concentrations of potent inhalational anesthetics. Such techniques are associated with rapid recovery of airway reflexes and consciousness. Early child-parent bonding can be facilitated. Such features make most neural blockade techniques suitable for outpatient surgery.[71]

The most frequent indication for neural blockade is the provision of prolonged postoperative pain relief. In addition to negating the need for opioids, the child's cooperation can be more easily enlisted in order to facilitate activities such as effective deep breathing, dressing changes, and mobility. Regional anesthesia/analgesia also offers greater comfort than systemic opioids after reconstructive plastic procedures, complex congenital lower gastrointestinal/urogenital reconstructive procedure (e.g., cloacal reconstruction, bladder augmentation), and situations where postsurgical immobilization is necessary owing to limb traction.

All the regional techniques used in adults have been used safely and effectively in children. In the following section we review only those most commonly used in children. For a more detailed description of the regional anatomy, physiology, and technical considerations associated with pediatric neural blockade, the reader is referred to several recent publications.[72,73]

Caudal Block

Caudal anesthesia/analgesia is the most widely used neural blockade technique in children for the management of postoperative pain. It has been used following a vast range of surgical procedures on the lower abdomen, perineum, and lower extremity. Accumulating clinical experience suggests that caudal anesthesia/analgesia is simple to perform, reliable, and safe.[74–78]

ANATOMY

The sacrum is formed by fusion of the five sacral vertebrae (Fig. 22-3). This fusion is incomplete, however, and the sacral hiatus is formed by the failure of the laminae of S5 and usually part of S4 to fuse in the midline. This defect is of considerable variability in dimension[79,80] but is often described as an inverted U or V in shape. The remnants of the S5 inferior articular processes (the sacral cornua) are free, prominent and flank the hiatus. The sacral cornua are important landmarks for the identification of the hiatus and successful performance of the technique. The sacral hiatus is covered by the thick sacrococcygeal ligament. Penetration of the ligament with a needle gives direct access to the caudal aspect of the epidural space, as the sacral hiatus is the caudal termination of the spinal canal. Thus, caudal anesthesia/analgesia is in essence an epidural technique. The dura mater ends at S2, and insertion of a needle high into the caudal epidural space may cause accidental dural puncture.

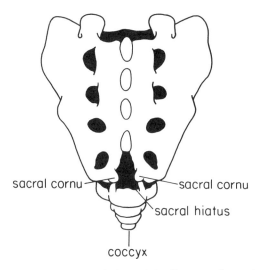

sacral cornu — sacral cornu

sacral hiatus

coccyx

Fig. 22-3. The sacrum is formed by fusion of the five sacral vertebrae. Failure of the laminae of S5 and part of S4 to fuse in the midline results in a bony defect called the sacral hiatus. Remnants of the S5 inferior articular processes (the sacral cornua) flank the hiatus on either side.

POSITIONING AND LANDMARKS

Caudal anesthesia/analgesia is quite easy to perform in children. It is customary to give the younger patient a light general anesthetic to aid positioning and performance of the technique. Depending on maturation, older adolescents may only need sedation.

The patient can be positioned in the lateral Sim's position (preferred), prone, or in the knee-chest position. In the lateral Sim's position, the lower leg is only slightly flexed at the hip. The upper leg is flexed to a greater extent so that it lies over and above the lower leg. Advantages of the lateral Sim's position include comfort for the patient, a comfortable and familiar work station for the anesthesiologist, and easy access to the airway.

In the prone position, a pillow is placed underneath the pelvis, and both legs are rotated so that the toes of both feet are facing medially. This relaxes the gluteal muscles and separates the buttocks. The disadvantage of this technique is the difficulty of airway access.

The knee-chest position is less popular in a pediatric population but is particularly useful for pregnant women.

PROCEDURE

The skin is cleaned and prepared over a large area to facilitate easy palpation of bony landmarks. The patient is draped as in preparation for lumbar epidural block.

Confirmation of the bony landmarks is the key to successful performance of this technique. In most children, the protrusions of the sacral cornua can be seen without palpation. The shallow depression of the sacral hiatus can be seen between the cornua. If landmarks are not easily visible, the coccyx may be palpated and the finger moved cephalad until the fingertip overlies the sacral hiatus with the cornua to either side.

For a single injection, a 2- to 3-cm-long, 23- or 25-gauge disposable needle may be used. In later adolescence, the greater rigidity of a 22-gauge needle may be preferable. Some practitioners prefer to insert over-the-needle catheters of small caliber, similar to those used for IV cannulation.[81] If of sufficient caliber, epidural catheters may be inserted through the properly positioned over-the-needle catheter. Similarly, pediatric epidural needles may be used to place epidural catheters for continuous analgesia.

An intradermal skin wheal of local anesthetic is raised over the sacral hiatus. The chosen needle is then inserted at a 45° angle to the sacrococcygeal ligament (Fig. 22-4). Penetration of the sacrococcygeal ligament has a characteristic "feel" or "pop." The anterior wall of the sacral canal is contacted, and the needle is redirected so that it is more in line with the long axis of spinal canal (Fig. 22-5). The needle is then advanced another 2–5 mm.

Confirmation of correct needle placement should be made before injection of analgesics. The location of bony landmarks should be checked again. Cerebrospinal fluid, air, or blood should not be obtained on aspiration. Light blood staining is not uncommon, as the area is fairly vascular and indicates entry into

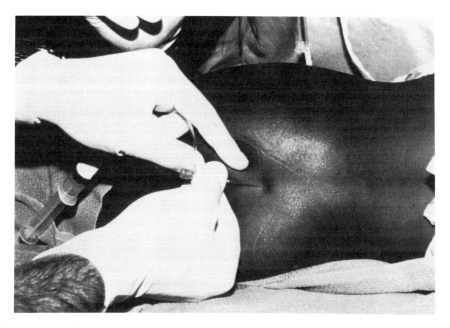

Fig. 22-4. A 23- or 25-gauge needle is inserted through the sacral hiatus at a 45° angle. Penetration of the sacrococcygeal ligament is appreciated as a characteristic "feel" or "pop."

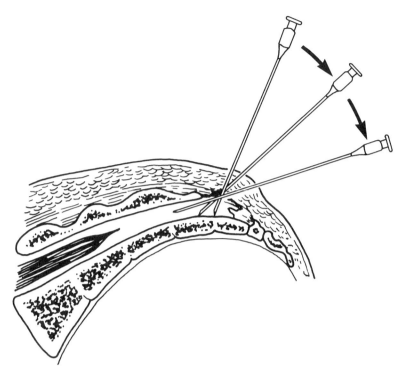

Fig. 22-5. After passage through the sacracoccygeal ligament, the anterior wall of the sacral canal is contacted. The needle is progressively reoriented to lie in the long axis of the spinal canal.

the sacral canal. Several cubic centimeters of normal saline should be rapidly injected through the needle while the skin over the needle tip is palpated for swelling. Swelling will be readily appreciated if the needle has been misplaced dorsally to the sacrum into the subcutaneous tissue. Should this occur, the needle is withdrawn and the technique attempted again.

CHOICE AND DOSING OF LOCAL ANESTHETIC

Bupivacaine is the most commonly used agent for postoperative pain management because of its differential blockade of sensory fibers at low concentrations and its long duration of action. A total dose of 2.5 mg/kg has resulted in safe peak plasma concentrations well below toxic thresholds.[82] Further prolongation of analgesia is obtained by adding epinephrine in a concentration of 1:200,000. Bupivacaine in a concentration of 0.25 percent is most suitable for a single caudal injection when used as an adjunct to general anesthesia.[77] Lower concentrations of bupivacaine (0.125 percent) have been shown to be equally effective when administered at the conclusion of surgery and to produce significantly less motor weakness.[83] Increasing the concentration to 0.30 percent or 0.375 percent does not offer any additional advantages.[84]

Many dosing regimens have been recommended for local anesthetics based on age, body weight, the distance from the sacral hiatus to the C7 vertebra, and the number of segments to be anesthetized.[85-91] A practical and effective method of calculation is Takasaki's formula for children younger than the age of 7 years.[88] The total dose of bupivacaine calculated from this formula is well below the maximum permissible dose. The total volume of 0.25 percent bupivacaine required for analgesia below the T10 dermatomal level is calculated as follows:

$$
\begin{aligned}
\text{Total volume (ml)} &= 0.056 \text{ ml} \times \text{number of segments} \times \text{body weight (kg)} \\
&= 0.056 \text{ ml} \times 12 \times \text{body weight (kg)} \\
&= 0.672 \times \text{body weight (kg)} \\
&= \text{approximately } 0.7 \text{ ml} \times \text{body weight (kg)}
\end{aligned}
$$

Armitage reported a 98 percent success rate with a simple and easily remembered method of calculating effective analgesic volumes of 0.25 percent bupivacaine.[76] A volume of 0.5 ml/kg is used for sacral analgesia, 1 ml/kg for lower thoracic analgesia, and 1.25 ml/kg for midthoracic analgesia.[91a]

DURATION OF ANALGESIA

The median duration of caudal analgesia after administration of a single dose of 1 ml/kg of 0.25 percent bupivacaine with 1:200,000 epinephrine at the beginning of surgery is about 5 hours.[92] Motor weakness is significant at such a dose.[92]

Using Takasaki's formula, the duration of analgesia with a single caudal injection at the beginning of surgery is 4–6 hours. Postoperative pain control was reported to be satisfactory in 85 percent of patients.[88]

Continuous analgesia can be provided by caudal infusions of local anesthetic, opioid, or a combination of both.

CAUDAL MORPHINE

A single injection of caudal morphine at a dose of 0.1 mg/kg in children older than the age of 1 year has been shown to produce prolonged postoperative analgesia.[92] This dose was reported to have a median duration of 12 hours when used for urologic and lower-extremity orthopedic procedures. Such a dose of caudal morphine has been reported to produce delayed life-threatening hypoventilation in a 1½-year-old child after penile surgery.[93] A lower dose of caudal morphine (0.033 mg/kg) administered to children older than 1 year of age has been shown to be equally effective and probably safer. However, duration of analgesia was slightly shorter with 0.033 mg/kg as compared with 0.1 mg/kg dosing (10.0 ± 3.3 hours versus 13.3 ± 4.7 hours, respectively).[94] The authors recommended that 0.033 mg/kg of caudal morphine be administered as the initial dose. The dose could be incrementally increased if longer durations of analgesia were required.[94] Close monitoring for respiratory depression is recommended for a minimum of 24 hours after each dose.[94]

SIDE EFFECTS AND COMPLICATIONS

The true incidence of side effects associated with caudal anesthesia/analgesia is difficult to ascertain as different studies have used varying methods for calculation of total dose and different study designs. Most reports agree that the incidence of postoperative vomiting after caudal anesthesia/analgesia with local anesthetics is less than 30 percent[95–97] and is comparable with the incidence after caudal administration of morphine.[92] Some degree of motor weakness has been reported in all children receiving 1 ml/kg of 0.25 percent bupivacaine with 1:200,000 epinephrine.[92] Urinary retention or delayed micturition has not been reported to be a problem after a single injection of 0.25 percent bupivacaine. Other potential but rare problems associated with caudal anesthesia/analgesia include accidental intravascular or intramarrow injection, dural puncture, neuralgia, and infection.

Lumbar and Thoracic Epidural Analgesia

Since the preliminary report by Meignier et al[98] of the feasibility and potential benefits of thoracic epidural analgesia in children, the interest and experience in lumbar and thoracic epidural analgesia has increased. Numerous reports have documented the safety, efficacy, and reliability of epidural analgesia in *experienced* hands.[99–105] Intermittent injection and continuous infusion regimens have been described for postoperative pain management.[99–105]

Ecoffey et al[99] demonstrated adequate postoperative segmental analgesia using lumbar and thoracic catheters in infants and children. They used an initial anesthetic dose of 0.75 ml/kg of 0.5 percent bupivacaine with 1:200,000 epinephrine (3.75 mg/kg) in infants younger than the age of 18 months. A lower dose of 0.5 ml/kg of the same solution (2.5 mg/kg) was used in older children. Intermittent "top-up" doses of 0.5 ml/kg of 0.25 percent bupivacaine with 1:200,000 epinephrine (1.5 mg/kg) were administered when the child appeared to be agitated and in pain. One to two doses were reported to be adequate over a period of 24 hours.[99]

Desparmet et al[101] showed the efficacy and safety of continuous epidural analgesia in children older than the age of 11 months for procedures requiring analgesia below the T10 spinal segment. Initial loading dose was 0.5 ml/kg of 0.25 percent bupivacaine (1.25 mg/kg) followed by a 0.08 ml/kg/h (0.2 mg/kg/h) infusion for up to 48 hours postoperatively. Pain was reported to be minimal in older children as assessed by VAS. Other children too young to evaluate their pain gave no outward sign of agitation or discomfort during the study period. There was no accumulation of bupivacaine in the plasma during the infusion period, and plasma levels remained well below the concentration considered toxic in adults.[101]

As in adults, the decision regarding placement of the catheter at lumbar, thoracic, or caudal locations is dependent on the site of the surgery, the choice of the analgesic, and the experience of the anesthesiologist. The caudal approach is the simplest in infants and younger children, as catheters can safely

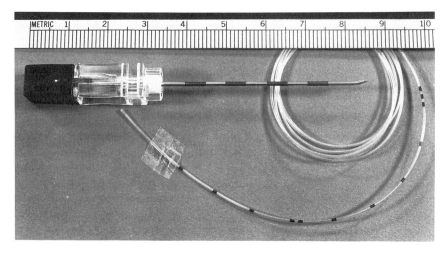

Fig. 22-6. A 19-gauge pediatric epidural needle with accompanying 21-gauge catheter (Portex System 1 Epidural Minipack).

be threaded to the thoracic region. Performance of lumbar or thoracic epidural anesthesia/analgesia should only be undertaken by experienced practitioners. Use of a 19-gauge epidural needle and 21-gauge catheter is suggested (Fig. 22-6), as—in our experience—smaller gauge catheters are associated with a higher incidence of failure to thread, kinking, and inability to infuse via mechanical pump.

Ilioinguinal and Iliohypogastric Nerve Blocks

Of the many peripheral nerve blocks performed in children, the ilioinguinal and iliohypogastric nerve blocks are the easiest to perform. These blocks are widely used for postoperative pain relief after inguinal herniotomy, varicocele ligation, and orchiopexy. Used as the sole anesthetic, these blocks will not provide surgical anesthesia of sufficient depth to allow exploration and manipulation of the spermatic cord during surgery. When used in conjunction with "light" general anesthesia, emergence is rapid; the requirement for postoperative analgesia is significantly reduced, and earlier ambulation is promoted as compared with use of caudal or opioid analgesia.[106,107] These nerve blocks are easily performed by means of percutaneous infiltration.[106–112]

ANATOMY

The peripheral extensions of the ilioinguinal and iliohypogastric nerves pass near the readily palpable anterior superior iliac spine (ASIS) (Fig. 22-7). The

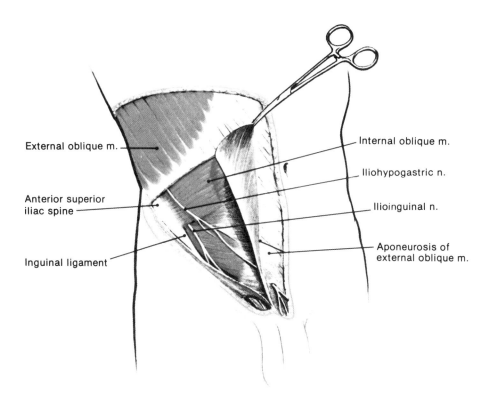

Fig. 22-7. Ilioinguinal and iliohypogastric nerve blocks. From Katz,[109] with permission.)

iliohypogastric nerve lies between the internal and external oblique muscles at the level of the ASIS. The ilioinguinal nerve initially lies between the transversus abdominis and internal oblique muscles and penetrates the internal oblique muscle at a variable distance medial to the ASIS. Neural blockade of these nerves can be achieved by using the ASIS as the point of orientation and spreading a large volume of local anesthetic between the abdominal muscle layers.

PROCEDURE

A 23-gauge needle is inserted perpendicular to the skin at a point 0.5–2 cm medial and inferior to the anterior superior iliac spine. The distance varies with the size of the child. The needle is advanced through the skin, subcutaneous tissue, and until a loss of resistance is felt as the needle pierces the aponeurosis of the external oblique. The local anesthetic solution is injected after negative aspiration for blood and in the absence of resistance to injection (Fig. 22–7).

The aforementioned pattern of injection is insufficient to provide surgical anesthesia, as structures that enter the internal inguinal ring (i.e., genitofemoral nerve, sympathetic fibers, spermatic cord) will not be anesthetized. A spermatic cord block will anesthetize these structures and is best performed by the surgeon under direct vision.

CHOICE AND DOSING OF LOCAL ANESTHETIC

Various doses and concentrations of bupivacaine have been successfully used without untoward effects. Shandling and Steward[107] recommended 0.4 ml/kg of 0.5 percent bupivacaine (2 mg/kg) with 1:200,000 epinephrine for infants and children. This dose was used effectively and without any clinical evidence of toxicity. Epstein et al[110] used a similar dose of bupivacaine in children older than the age of 13 months and reported a mean maximum plasma concentration of 1.35 ($\pm$ 0.4) μg/ml (well below the concentration for CNS toxicity in adults).

SIDE EFFECTS AND COMPLICATIONS

A rare complication of ilioinguinal and iliohypogastric nerve block is unintentional femoral nerve block, resulting in transient paresis of the quadriceps muscle group and/or numbness over the cutaneous distribution of the femoral nerve.[111] Such blockade may result from local anesthetic diffusing and tracking between fascial planes to reach the femoral nerve. No special treatment other than observation is required until femoral neural blockade dissipates.

Postoperative vomiting after pediatric herniorraphy is a common and distressing problem. The incidence of vomiting after ilioinguinal and iliohypogastric nerve blocks is not significantly different from the incidence associated with systemic opioid analgesia.[112]

Penile Nerve Block

Dorsal penile nerve block (DPNB) is a reliable means of managing pain and distress in infants and children undergoing circumcision or correction of distal hypospadias.[113,114] It is often used as the sole anesthetic during neonatal circumcision, and has been shown to modify the neuroendocrine stress response.[12,115,116] DPNB is also used in conjunction with general anesthesia for circumcision and hypospadias repair in older children. Advantages of such a combined technique include a reduced requirement for inhalational anesthetics, quick emergence, considerably less agitation during emergence, and a shorter recovery time and earlier discharge from the hospital. Postoperative analgesic requirements are also diminished for a considerable period of time when long-acting local anesthetics are used.[117,118]

Caudal anesthesia/analgesia has also been used to alleviate postcircumcision pain and is more effective than parenteral opioid or DPNB in the early postoperative period.[119,120] DPNB with bupivacaine affords longer pain relief than single injection caudal anesthesia/analgesia. DPNB is also free of undesirable effects that may be associated with caudal analgesia such as delayed mobilization and micturition, vomiting, and lower extremity numbness. However, analgesic requirements after the first 6 hours are considerably reduced with use of DPNB as compared with caudal analgesia.[120]

ANATOMY

The dorsal nerves of the penis are bilateral structures that emerge from under the pubis and pass forward on the surface of the crura of the penis (Fig. 22-8). The dorsal nerves of the penis lie in the deep aspect of a triangle bounded superiorly by Buck's fascia, posteriorly by the symphysis pubis and inferiorly by the crura, and subsequently, the corpora cavernosa. The suspensory ligament of the penis vertically divides this triangular space. The dorsal nerves of the penis lie on the crura deep to the suspensory ligament.

PROCEDURE

The dorsal nerves of the penis may be blocked by two separate injections using a 26- or 27-gauge needle as shown in Figure 22-8. The needle should pierce the deep fascia. Aspiration is necessary to ensure that a blood vessel has not been entered.

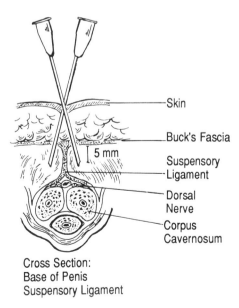

Fig. 22-8. Dorsal penile nerve block.

CHOICE AND DOSING OF LOCAL ANESTHETIC

Two separate injections of 1 ml of 1 percent lidocaine are sufficient for surgical anesthesia. Postoperative analgesia may be obtained with use of the same volumes of 0.25 percent or 0.5 percent bupivacaine.

Maxwell et al[121] measured the serum lidocaine concentrations in 30 healthy term newborns after penile block with 0.8 ml of 1 percent lidocaine. Serum concentrations were considerably lower than toxic threshold in adults.

COMPLICATIONS

Although penile block is an easy procedure to perform, serious complications can result. Inadvertent puncture of the dorsal penile artery or the corpus cavernosum can produce a localized hematoma. Accidental injection of the anesthetic solution into these structures can lead to systemic toxicity.[122] The use of large volumes of local anesthetic is not recommended because such volumes may cause pressure-induced compression of the penile blood vessels.

OTHER TECHNIQUES FOR ANESTHESIA/ANALGESIA OF THE PENIS

In contrast to an anesthetic block of the dorsal penile nerves, penile cutaneous analgesia can be achieved merely by infiltrating local anesthetic subcutaneously around the base of the penile shaft. Such a block produces effective and prolonged postcircumcision analgesia when a long-acting local anesthetic is used. An infiltration technique does not require specialized training, and it avoids injection of local anesthetic in the vicinity of major penile neurovascular structures.[123]

Recently, Dalens et al[124] described a simple two puncture technique for penile nerve block via the subpubic fat. The needle is inserted in the two compartments of the subpubic space on either side of the midline. This technique does not require special skills, and there is no risk of damaging neurovascular or other penile structures. An effective block can be achieved within 15 minutes of injection of a small volume of local anesthetic (0.2 mg/kg). Either 1 percent lidocaine or 0.5 percent bupivacaine can be used with excellent reliability.[124] Prolonged analgesia of up to 24 hours can be achieved with the latter solution.[124]

Topical analgesia of the postcircumcision wound can be achieved with lidocaine in the form of a spray (10–20 mg of a 10 percent solution), an ointment (0.5 ml of a 5 percent preparation), or a jelly (0.5–1.0 ml of a 2 percent preparation).[125] The surface analgesia achieved with these topical preparations is similar in intensity to that achieved with DPNB.[125]

Systemic lidocaine toxicity has not been reported with use of these topical preparations. However, as the plasma concentrations of lidocaine associated with use of the preparations have not been measured, their absorption and safety for neonatal circumcision has not as yet been determined. Despite the similarity in effectiveness of all the topical preparations of lidocaine, the spray appears to be the most acceptable to children because it can be applied repeatedly without wound contact.

Femoral and Lateral Femoral Cutaneous
Nerve Blocks

The femoral nerve (Fig. 22-9) supplies motor innervation to the quadriceps muscle, sensation to the skin overlying the anterior aspect of the thigh, and sensory innervation to the periosteum of the femoral shaft. Femoral nerve block can be used to relieve quadriceps muscle spasm, to permit pain-free manipulation of femoral shaft fractures, and to provide operative analgesia during muscle biopsy in children.[126–129] The technique of femoral nerve block is similar to that in adults, and the reader is referred to Chapter 13 for details.

Of note, a simple single-needle technique with a high success rate in children has recently been described by Khoo and Brown.[130]

Selection of the anesthetic solution depends on the desired length of neural blockade. The actual volumes required to block the femoral nerve as a function of age have not been determined. Grossbard and Love[127] reported effective analgesia in children with femoral shaft fractures using 0.2 ml/kg of 0.5 percent bupivacaine (1 mg/kg) up to a maximum of 10 ml. Analgesia lasted 4 hours.[127]

Ronchi et al[131] performed a pharmacokinetic study using 0.4 ml/kg of 0.5 percent bupivacaine (2 mg/kg) for femoral nerve block in seven children aged 2–7 years. Mean peak plasma concentration (0.87 µg/ml) was well below toxic level. Duration of analgesia was only 3 hours.[131]

At Children's Hospital in Boston, 0.3 ml/kg of 1 percent lidocaine (3 mg/kg)

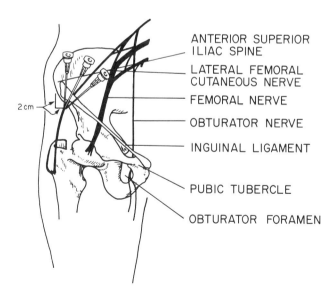

ANTERIOR SUPERIOR ILIAC SPINE

LATERAL FEMORAL CUTANEOUS NERVE

FEMORAL NERVE

OBTURATOR NERVE

INGUINAL LIGAMENT

PUBIC TUBERCLE

OBTURATOR FORAMEN

2 cm

Fig. 22-9. Infiltration technique for lateral femoral cutaneous nerve block. Note formation of both the femoral and lateral femoral cutaneous nerves from the lumbar plexus with subsequent passage into the thigh. The lateral femoral cutaneous nerve is easily blocked by infiltration of local anesthetic 1–2 cm below and 1–2 cm medial to the anterior superior iliac spine.

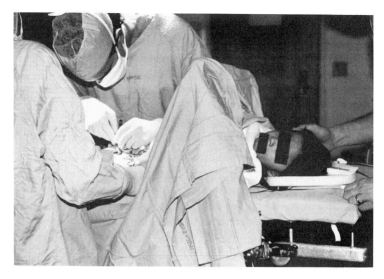

Fig. 22-10. A 6-year-old child having a diagnostic muscle biopsy under femoral and lateral femoral cutaneous nerve block.

without epinephrine is used for short procedures such as muscle biopsy. Onset of anesthesia occurs within 10 minutes. The duration of analgesia is short.

When used in combination with lateral femoral cutaneous nerve block, anesthesia is provided for the quadriceps muscle, overlying skin, and the skin on the lateral aspect of the thigh. (Lateral femoral cutaneous nerve block can be simply performed by infiltration of local anesthetic 1–2 cm below and 1–2 cm medial to the anterior superior iliac spine. See Fig. 22-9.) This combination can be used to obtain diagnostic open muscle biopsy specimens from children with suspected malignant hyperthermia, muscular dystrophy, and other neuromuscular disorders. With use of this combined neural blockade technique, unnecessary parental anxiety regarding general anesthesia is avoided, some analgesia is provided during the postoperative period, and muscle biopsy can be performed on a day-surgery basis (Fig. 22-10).

Fascia Iliaca Compartment Block

This is a new technique whereby femoral, lateral femoral cutaneous, and obturator neural blockade can be accomplished with a single injection. These nerves lie on the anterior surface of the iliacus muscle and are enclosed by iliacus fascia (Fig. 22-11). The iliacus compartment is safely approached at the junction of the lateral one-third and medial two-thirds of the inguinal ligament. The needle is directed inward at right angles to the skin, approximately 0.5–1 cm below the inguinal ligament. The needle is advanced until two losses of resistance are felt as the needle pierces the fascia lata and iliacus to enter the iliacus compartment. Prolonged postoperative analgesia can be provided via an indwelling catheter.

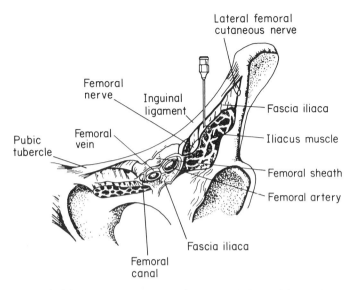

Fig. 22-11. Fascia iliaca compartment block. Femoral, lateral femoral cutaneous, and obturator nerves lie on the anterior surface of the iliacus muscle and are invested by the iliacus fascia to form the iliacus compartment. (The iliacus compartment is outlined in *bold lines*.) Thus, all three nerves may be blocked by injection of local anesthetic into the compartment.

A prospective comparison of the fascia iliacus block with the 3-in-1 block demonstrated that the fascia iliaca compartment block is easy to perform, free of complications, and effective in more than 90 percent of children. The mean duration of postoperative analgesia is 5 hours. Recommended dose ranges are 0.5–0.75 ml/kg of a combination of equal volumes of 1 percent lidocaine and 0.5 percent bupivacaine, both with 1:200,000 epinephrine.[132]

Interpleural Regional Analgesia

In contradistinction to the findings in adults, use of continuous interpleural regional analgesia after thoracotomy in children provides consistent analgesia[133] (see Ch. 16). Infusion rates of 0.5–1.0 ml/kg/h of 0.25 percent bupivacaine with 1:200,000 epinephrine are recommended.[133] At this rate of infusion, however, peak plasma concentrations of bupivacaine have been reported to be greater than 7 μg/ml in some patients after 24 hour of infusion. Although none of the children exhibited CNS toxicity, many children in this study also received benzodiazepines and hypnotics during the infusion period.[133] Interpleural regional analgesia has also been used in the management of subcostal incisional pain in children. The recommended initial dose is 0.5 ml/kg of 0.5 percent bupivacaine (2.5 mg/kg) with 1:200,000 epinephrine, followed by 0.1–0.5 ml/kg/h of 0.25 percent bupivacaine with 1:200,000 epinephrine by infusion.[134]

Infiltration Analgesia of the Surgical Wound

Incisional pain in adults has been effectively alleviated by the simple technique of local anesthetic infiltration, topicalization, or perfusion into the surgical wound.[135,136] In children, injection of local anesthetic into the incision at the end of inguinal herniotomy produces analgesia comparable to that rendered by caudal analgesia. Doses of 0.5 ml/kg of 0.25 percent bupivacaine are effective for wound infiltration and are half the dose required for caudal blockade (1 ml/kg).[137] The absorption of bupivacaine from subcutaneous infiltration is considerably slower in children than adults, and the resultant plasma concentrations of local anesthetic are far below toxic levels.[138]

Unfortunately, this technically simple and safe means of managing incisional pain has not received the attention it deserves. Furthermore, infiltration analgesia is widely underused or not used at all in neonates undergoing surgery.

CONCLUSION

The past decade has witnessed a growing realization that children of all ages do experience pain similar to adults. It is essential that medical personnel caring for postsurgical children routinely assess pain, taking into consideration the child's developmental level. Most children can be made comfortable if a suitable analgesic is selected to match the intensity of the child's pain, and it is prescribed in adequate doses at pharmacokinetically appropriate time intervals. With the proper use of systemic opioids and the use of various regional anesthetic/analgesic techniques, traditional IM injections and all the fear they engender in children can become a thing of the past.

References
1. Beyer JE, DeGood DE, Ashley LC, Russell GA: Patterns of postoperative analgesic use with adults and children following cardiac surgery. Pain 17:71, 1983
2. Mather L, Mackie J: The incidence of postoperative pain in children. Pain 15:271, 1983
3. Purcell-Jones G, Dorman F, Sumner D: Paediatric anaesthetists' perceptions of neonatal and infant pain. Pain 33:181, 1988
4. Schechter NL, Allen DA, Hanson K: Status of pediatric pain control: a comparison of hospital analgesic usage in children and adults. Pediatrics 77:11, 1986
5. Chapman AH, Loeb DG, Gibbons MJ: Psychiatric aspects of hospitalized children. Arch Pediatr 73:77, 1956
6. Lamontagene LL: Children's locus of control beliefs as predictors of preoperative coping behavior. Nurs Res 33:76, 1984
7. Stevens M: Adolescents' perception of stressful events during hospitalization. J Pediatr Nurs 1:303, 1986
8. Anand KJ, Sippell WG, Aynsley-Green A: Randomized trial of fentanyl anaesthesia in preterm neonates undergoing surgery: effects on the stress response. Lancet i:62, 1987
9. Kavanagh C: A new approach to dressing change in the severely burned child and its effect on burn-related psychopathology. Heart Lung 12:612, 1983

10. Anand KJ, Hickey PR: Pain and its effects in the human neonate and fetus. N Engl J Med 317:1321, 1987

11. Anand KJS, Hickey PR: Randomized trial of high-dose sufentanil anesthesia in neonates undergoing cardiac surgery: hormonal and hemodynamic stress response, abstracted. Anesthesiology 67:A501, 1987

12. Kirya C, Werthmann MW Jr: Neonatal circumcision and penile dorsal nerve block—a painless procedure. J Pediatr 92:998, 1978

13. Holve RL, Bromberger PJ, Groveman HD et al: Regional anesthesia during new-born circumcision. Effect on infant pain response. Clin Pediatr 22:813, 1983

14. Anand KJ, Aynsley-Green A: Metabolic and endocrine effects of surgical ligation of patent ductus arteriosus in the human preterm neonate: are there implications for further improvement of postoperative outcome? Mod Probl Paediatr 23:143, 1985

15. Beyer JE, Wells N: The assessment of pain in children. Pediatr Clin North Am 36: 837, 1989

16. Barrier G, Attia J, Mayer MN et al: Measurement of post-operative pain and nar-cotic administration in infants using a new clinical scoring system. Intensive Care Med, suppl 15:S37, 1989

17. Broadman LM, Rice LJ, Hannallah RS: Testing the validity of an objective pain scale for infants and children, abstracted. Anesthesiology 69:A747, 1988

18. McGrath PJ, Johnson G, Goodman JT et al: The CHEOPS: a behavioral scale to measure postoperative pain in children. p. 395. In Fields HL, Dubnar R, Ververo F (eds): Advances in Pain Research and Therapy. Raven Press, New York, 1985

19. McGrath PJ, Unruh AM: The measurement and assessment of pain. p. 72. In Pain in Children and Adolescents. Elsevier, Amsterdam, 1987

20. Beyer J: The Oucher: a user's manual and technical report. Judson Press, Evans-ton, IL, 1984

21. Beyer JE, Aradine CR: Content validity of an instrument to measure young chil-dren's perceptions of the intensity of their pain. J Pediatr Nurs 1:386, 1985

22. Richardson GM, McGrath PJ, Cunningham SJ, Humphreys P: Validity of the head-ache diary for children. Headache 23:184, 1983

23. Wilkie J, Holzema WL, Tester MD et al: Measuring pain quality: validity and reliability of children's and adolescents' pain language. Pain 44:151, 1990

24. Abu-Saad H: Assessing children's responses to pain. Pain 19:163, 1984

25. Grossi E, Borghi C, Cerchiari EL et al: Analogue chromatic continuous scale (ACCS): a new method for pain assessment. Clin Exp Rheumatol 1:337, 1983

26. Porter JD, Robinson PH, Glasgow JF et al: Trends in the incidence of Reye's syndrome and the use of aspirin. Arch Dis Child 65:826, 1990

27. Ameer B, Greenblatt DJ: Acetaminophen. Ann Intern Med 87:202, 1977

28. Temple AR: Pediatric dosing of acetaminophen. Pediatr Pharmacol 3:321, 1983

29. Gaudreault P, Guay J, Nicol O, Dupuis C: Pharmacokinetics and clinica! efficacy of intrarectal solution of acetaminophen. Can J Anaesth 35:149, 1988

30. Rahwan GL, Rahwan RG: Aspirin and Reye's syndrome: the change in prescribing habits of health professionals. Drug Intell Clin Pharm 20:143, 1986

31. Shannon M, Berde CB: Pharmacologic management of pain in children and adoles-cents. Pediatr Clin North Am 36:855, 1989

32. Mather LE, Owen H: The pharmacology of patient-administered opioids. p.27. In Ferrante FM, Ostheimer GW, Covino BG (eds): Patient-Controlled Analgesia. Blackwell Scientific, Boston, 1990

33. Bellville JW, Seed JC: The effects of drugs on the respiratory response to carbon dioxide. Anesthesiology 21:727, 1960

34. Foley KM, Inturrisi CE: Analgesic drug therapy in cancer pain: principles and practice. Med Clin North Am 71:207, 1987

35. Morselli PL, Rovei V: Plancental transfer of pethidine and norpethidine and their pharmacokinetics in the newborn. Eur J Clin Pharmacol 18:25, 1980

36. Kaiko RF, Foley KM, Grabinski PY et al: Central nervous system excitatory effects of meperidine in cancer patients. Ann Neurol 13:180, 1983

37. Maunuksela EL, Korpela R, Olkkola KT: Double-blind, multiple-dose comparison of buprenorphine and morphine in postoperative pain of children. Br J Anaesth 60: 48, 1988

38. Maunuksela EL, Korpela R, Olkkola KT: Comparison of buprenorphine with morphine in the treatment of postoperative pain in children. Anesth Analg 67:233, 1988

39. Arnold JH, Truog RD, Orav JE et al: Tolerance and dependence in neonates sedated with fentanyl during extracorporeal membrane oxygenation. Anesthesiology 73:1136, 1990

40. Miser AW, Miser JS: The treatment of cancer pain in children. Pediatr Clin North Am 36:979, 1989

41. Koren G, Maurice L: Pediatric uses of opioids. Pediatr Clin North Am 36:1141, 1989

42. O'hara M, McGrath PJ, D'Astous J, Vair CA: Oral morphine versus injected meperidine (Demerol) for pain relief in children after orthopedic surgery. J Pediatr Orthop 7:78, 1987

43. Austin KL, Stapleton JV, Mather LE: Multiple intramuscular injections: a major source of variability in analgesic response to meperidine. Pain 8:47, 1980

44. Austin KL, Stapleton JV, Mather LE: Relationship between blood meperidine concentrations and analgesic response: a preliminary report. Anesthesiology 53: 460, 1980

45. Purcell-Jones G, Dormon F, Sumner E: The use of opioids in neonates. A retrospective study of 933 cases. Anaesthesia 42:1316, 1987

46. Berde CB, Beyer JE, Bournaki MC et al: Comparison of morphine and methadone for prevention of postoperative pain in 3- to 7-year old children. J Pediatr 119:136, 1991

47. Gourlay GK, Willis RJ, Wilson PR: Postoperative pain control with methadone: influence of supplementary methadone doses and blood concentration-response relationships. Anesthesiology 61:19, 1984

48. Hendrickson M, Myre L, Johnson DG et al: Postoperative anaglesia in children: a prospective study of intermittent intramuscular injection versus continuous intravenous infusion of morphine. J Pediatr Surg 25:185, 1990

49. Millar AJ, Rode H, Cywes S: Continuous morphine infusion for postoperative pain in children. S Afr Med J 72:396, 1987

50. Bray RJ: Postoperative analgesia provided by morphine infusion in children. Anaesthesia 38:1075, 1983

51. Lynn AM, Opheim KE, Tyler DC: Morphine infusion after pediatric cardiac surgery. Crit Care Med 12:863, 1984

52. Koren G, Butt W, Chinyanga H et al: Postoperative morphine infusion in newborn infants: assessment of disposition characteristics and safety. J Pediatr 107:963, 1985

53. Beasley SW, Tibballs J: Efficacy and safety of continuous morphine infusion for postoperative analgesia in the paediatric surgical ward. Aust N Z J Surg 57:233, 1987

54. Berde CB: Pediatric postoperative pain management. Pediatr Clin North Am 36: 921, 1989

55. Lynn AM, Slattery JT: Morphine pharmacokinetics in early infancy. Anesthesiology 66:136, 1987

56. Koehntop DE, Rodman JH, Brundage DM et al: Pharmacokinetics of fentanyl in neonates. Anesth Analg 65:227, 1986

57. Hudson RJ: Variability of fentanyl pharmacokinetics in neonates (letter). Anesth Analg 65:1369, 1986

58. Way WL, Costley EC, Way EL: Respiratory sensitivity of the newborn infant to meperidine and morphine. Clin Pharmacol Ther 6:454, 1965

59. Lynn AM, Slattery JT: Morphine pharmacokinetics in early infancy. Anesthesiology 66:136, 1987

60. Collins C, Koren G, Crean P et al: Fentanyl pharmacokinetics and hemodynamic effects in preterm infants during ligation of patent ductus arteriosus. Anesth Analg 64:1078, 1985

61. Hug CC Jr: Pharmacokinetics and dynamics of narcotic analgesics. p. 187. In Prys-Roberts C, Hug CC Jr (eds): Pharmacokinetics of Anaesthesia. Blackwell Scientific, London, 1984

62. Hertzka RE, Gauntlett IS, Fisher MD, Spellman MJ: Fentanyl-induced ventilatory depression: effects of age. Anesthesiology 70:213, 1989

63. Liu LMP, Cote CJ, Coudsouzian NG et al: Life-threatening apnea in infants recovering from anesthesia. Anesthesiology 59:506, 1983

64. Welborn LG, Ramirez N, Oh TH et al: Postanesthetic apnea and periodic breathing in infants. Anesthesiology 65:658, 1986

65. Welborn LG, Rice L, Hannallah RS et al: Postoperative apnea in former preterm infants: prospective comparison of spinal and general anesthesia. Anesthesiology 72:838, 1990

66. Brown RE, Broadman LM: Patient-controlled analgesia (PCA) for postoperative pain in adolescents, abstracted. Anesth Analg 66:S22, 1987

67. Means LJ, Allen HM, Lookabill SJ, Krishna G: Recovery room initiation of patient-controlled analgesia in pediatric patients, abstracted. Anesthesiology 69:A772, 1988

68. Rodgers BM, Webb CJ, Stergios D, Newman BM: Patient-controlled analgesia in pediatric surgery. J Pediatr Surg 23:259, 1988

69. Tyler DC: Patient-controlled analgesia in adolescents. J Adolesc Health Care 11:154, 1990

70. Berde CB, Lehn BM, Yee JD et al: Patient-controlled analgesia in children and adolescents: a randomized, prospective comparison with intramuscular morphine for postoperative analgesia. J Pediatr 118:460, 1991

71. Steward DJ: Outpatient pediatric anesthesia. Anesthesiology 43:268, 1975

72. Sethna NF, Berde CB: Pediatric regional anesthesia. p. 647. In Gregory GA (ed): Pediatric Anesthesia. 2nd Ed. Churchill Livingstone, New York, 1990

73. Dalens B: Regional anesthesia in children. Anesth Analg 68:654, 1989

74. Yaster M, Maxwell LG: Pediatric regional anesthesia. Anesthesiology 70:324, 1989

75. Broadman LM, Hannallah RS, Norden JM, McGill WA: "Kiddie caudals": experience with 1154 consecutive cases without complications, abstracted. Anesth Analg 66:S18, 1987

76. Gunter JB, Dunn CM, Bennie JB: Optimum concentration of bupivacaine for combined caudal-general anesthesia in children. Anesthesiology 75:57, 1991

77. Dalens B, Hasnaoui A: Caudal anesthesia in pediatric surgery: success rate and adverse effects in 750 consecutive patients. Anesth Analg 68:83, 1989

78. Desparmet J, Desmazes N, Mazoit X, Ecoffey C: Evolution of regional anesthesia

in a pediatric surgical practice. p.201. In Tyler DC, Krane EJ (ed): Advances in Pain Research Therapy. Raven Press, New York, 1990

79. Thompson JE: An anatomical and experimental study of sacral anaesthesia. Ann Surg 66:718, 1917

80. Black MG: Anatomic reasons for caudal anesthesia failure. Anesth Analg 28:33, 1949

81. Owens WD, Slater EM, Battit GE: A new technique of caudal anesthesia. Anesthesiology 50:549, 1979

82. Ecoffey C, Desparmet J, Maury M et al: Bupivacaine in children: pharmacokinetics following caudal anesthesia. Anesthesiology 63:447, 1985

83. Wolf AR, Valley RD, Fear DW et al: Bupivacaine for caudal analgesia in infants and children: the optimal effective concentration. Anesthesiology 69:102, 1988

84. Broadman LM, Hannallah RS, Norrie WC et al: Caudal analgesia in pediatric outpatient surgery: a comparison of three different bupivacaine concentrations, abstracted. Anesth Analg 66:S19, 1987

85. Spiegel P: Caudal anesthesia in pediatric surgery: a preliminary report. Anesth Analg 41:218, 1962

86. Satoyoshi M, Kamiyama Y: Caudal anaesthesia for upper abdominal surgery in infants and children: a simple calculation for the volume of local anaesthetic. Acta Anaesthesiol Scand 28:57, 1984

87. Lourey CJ, McDonald IH: Caudal anaesthesia in infants and children. Anaesth Intensive Care 1:547, 1973

88. Takasaki M, Dohi S, Kawabata Y, Takahashi T: Dosage of lidocaine for caudal anesthesia in infants and children. Anesthesiology 47:527, 1977

89. Schulte-Steinberg O, Rahlfs VW: Caudal anaesthesia in children and spread of 1 percent lignocaine. A statistical study. Br J Anaesth 42:1093, 1970

90. Melman E, Arenas JA, Tandazo WE: Caudal anesthesia for pediatric surgery. An easy and safe method for calculating dose requirements, abstracted. Anesthesiology 63:A463, 1985

91. Fortuna A: Caudal Analgesia: a simple and safe technique in paediatric surgery. Br J Anaesth 39:165, 1967

91a. Armitage EN: Caudal block in children, abstracted. Anaesthesia 34:396, 1979

92. Krane EJ, Jacobson LE, Lynn AM et al: Caudal morphine for postoperative analgesia in children: a comparison with caudal bupivacaine and intravenous morphine. Anesth Analg 66:647, 1987

93. Krane EJ: Delayed respiratory depression in a child after caudal epidural morphine. Anesth Analg 67:79, 1988

94. Krane EJ, Tyler DC, Jacobson LE: The dose response of caudal morphine in children. Anesthesiology 71:48, 1989

95. Lunn JN: Postoperative analgesia after circumcision. A randomized comparison between caudal analgesia and intramuscular morphine. Anaesthesia 34:552, 1979

96. Bramwell RG, Bullen C, Radford P: Caudal block for postoperative analgesia in children. Anaesthesia 37:1024, 1982

97. Martin LV: Postoperative analgesia after circumcision in children. Br J Anaesth 54:1263, 1982

98. Meignier M, Souron R, Le Neel JC: Postoperative dorsal epidural analgesia in the child with respiratory disabilities. Anesthesiology 59:473, 1983

99. Ecoffey C, Dubousset AM, Samii K: Lumbar and thoracic epidural anesthesia for urologic and upper abdominal surgery in infants and children. Anesthesiology 65:87, 1986

100. Desparmet J, Saint-Maurice C: Continuous epidural anesthesia in children under 10 years old. Reg Anesth 11:168, 1986
101. Desparmet J, Mesitelman C, Barre J, Saint-Maurice C: Continuous epidural infusion of bupivacaine for postoperative pain relief in children. Anesthesiology 67:108, 1987
102. Bosenberg AT, Bland BA, Schulte-Steinberg O, Downing JW: Thoracic epidural anesthesia via caudal route in infants. Anesthesiology 69:265, 1988
103. Rasch DK, Webster DE, Pollard TG, Gurkowski MA: Lumbar and thoracic epidural analgesia via the caudal approach for postoperative pain relief in infants and children. Can J Anaesth 37:359, 1990
104. Attia J, Ecoffey C, Sandouk P et al: Epidural morphine in children: pharmacokinetics and CO_2 sensitivity. Anesthesiology 65:590, 1986
105. Berde CB, Sethna NF, Yemen TA et al: Continuous epidural bupivacaine-fentanyl infusions in children following ureteral re-implantation, abstracted. Anesthesiology 73:A1128, 1990
106. Langer J, Shandling KB, Rosenberg M: Intraoperative bupivacaine during outpatient hernia repair in children: a randomized double-blind trial. J Pediatr Surg 22:267, 1987
107. Shandling B, Steward DJ: Regional analgesia for postoperative pain in pediatric outpatient surgery. J Pediatr Surg 15:477, 1980
108. Hinkle AJ: Percutaneous inguinal block for the outpatient management of post-herniorrhaphy pain in children. Anesthesiology 67:411, 1987
109. Katz J: Atlas of Regional Anesthesia. p. 115 Appleton-Century-Crofts, Norwalk, CT, 1985
110. Epstein RH, Larijani GE, Wolfson PJ et al: Plasma bupivacaine concentrations following ilioinguinal-iliohypogastric nerve blockade in children. Anesthesiology 69:773, 1988
111. Roy-Shapira A, Amoury RA, Ashcraft KW et al: Transient quadriceps paresis following local inquinal block for postoperative pain control. J Pediatr Surg 20:554, 1985
112. Hannallah RS, Broadman LM, Belman AB et al: Comparison of caudal and ilioinguinal/iliohypogastric nerve blocks for control of post-orchiopexy pain in pediatric ambulatory surgery. Anesthesiology 66:832, 1987
113. Soliman MG, Tremblay NA: Nerve block of the penis for postoperative pain relief in children. Anesth Analg 57:495, 1978
114. Blaise G, Roy WL: Postoperative pain relief after hypospadias repair in pediatric patients: regional analgesia versus systemic anaglesics. Anesthesiology 65:84, 1986
115. Williamson PS, Williamson ML: Physiologic stress reduction by a local anesthetic during newborn circumcision. Pediatrics 71:36, 1983
116. Stang HJ, Gunnar RM, Snellman L et al: Local anesthesia for neonatal circumcision. Effects on distress and cortisol response. JAMA 259:1507, 1988
117. Carlsson P, Svensson J: The duration of pain relief after penile block to boys undergoing circumcision. Acta Anaesthesiol Scand 28:432, 1984
118. Lau JTK: Penile block for pain relief after circumcision in children. A randomized, prospective trial. Am J Surg 147:797, 1984
119. May AE, Wandless J, James RH: Analgesia for circumcision in children. A comparison of caudal bupivacaine and intramuscular buprenorphine. Acta Anaesthesiol Scand 26:331, 1982
120. Yeoman PM, Cooke R, Hain WR: Penile block for circumcision? A comparison with caudal blockade. Anaesthesia 38:862, 1983

121. Maxwell LG, Yaster M, Wetzel RC, Niebyl JR: Penile nerve block for newborn circumcision. Obstet Gynecol 70:415, 1987

122. Sara CA, Lowry CJ: A complication of circumcision and dorsal nerve block of the penis. Anaesth Intensive Care 13:79, 1984

123. Broadman LM, Hannallah RS, Belman B et al: Postcircumcision analgesia—a prospective evaluation of subcutaneous ring block of the penis. Anesthesiology 67: 399, 1987

124. Dalens B, Vanneuville G, Dechelotte P: Penile block via the subpubic space in 100 children. Anesth Analg 69:41, 1989

125. Tree-Trakarn T, Pirayavaraporn S: Postoperative pain relief for circumcision in children: comparison among morphine, nerve block, and topical analgesia. Anesthesiology 62:519, 1985

126. Berry FR: Analgesia in patients with fracture shaft of femur. Anaesthesia 32:576, 1977

127. Grossbard GD, Love BR: Femoral nerve block: a simple and safe method of instant analgesia for femoral shaft fractures in children. Aust N Z J Surg 49:592, 1979

128. Tondare AS, Nadkarni AV: Femoral nerve block for fractured shaft of femur. Can Anaesth Soc J 29:270, 1982

129. Berkowitz A, Rosenberg H: Femoral block with mepivacaine for muscle biopsy in malignant hyperthermia patients. Anesthesiology 62:651, 1985

130. Khoo ST, Brown TCK: Femoral nerve block—the anatomical basis for a single injection technique. Anaesth Intensive Care 11:40, 1983

131. Ronchi L, Rosenbaum D, Athouel A et al: Femoral nerve block with bupivacaine in children. Anesthesiology 70:622, 1989

132. Dalens B, Vanneuville G, Tanguy A: Comparison of the facia iliaca compartment block with the 3-in-1 block in children. Anesth Analg 69:705, 1989

133. McIlvaine WB, Knox RF, Fennessey PV, Goldstein M: Continuous infusion of bupivacaine via intrapleural catheter for analgesia after thoracotomy in children. Anesthesiology 69:261, 1988

134. McIlvaine WB, Chang JH, Jones M: The effective use of intrapleural bupivacaine for analgesia after thoracic and subcostal incisions in children. J Pediatr Surg 23: 1184, 1988

135. Hashemi K, Middleton MD: Subcutaneous bupivacaine for postoperative analgesia after herniorrhaphy. Ann R Coll Surg Engl 65:38, 1983

136. Tree-Trakarn T, Pirayavaraporn S, Lertakyamanee J: Topical analgesia for relief of post-circumcision pain. Anesthesiology 67:395, 1987

137. Fell D, Derrington MC, Taylor E, Wandless JG: Paediatric postoperative analgesia. A comparison between caudal block and wound infiltration of local anaesthetic. Anaesthesia 43:107, 1988

138. Eyres RL, Kidd J, Oppenheim R, Brown TC: Local anaesthetic plasma levels in children. Anaesth Intensive Care 6:243, 1978

23

Analgesia After Cesarean Delivery

Beth Minzter

Provision of effective pain control after cesarean delivery can be exceedingly demanding. Not only is superior analgesia important to the patient, but minimal sedation and the ability to ambulate are essential in order to allow the new mother to interact with her newborn. Moreover, it is desirable to maximize pain control rapidly while keeping maternal drug concentrations low, thereby minimizing the opportunity for drug transfer to the infant during breast-feeding. Mindful of these goals, this chapter reviews analgesic modalities of potential use after cesarean delivery.

PUERPERAL RESOLUTION OF THE PHYSIOLOGIC ADAPTATIONS OF PREGNANCY

Although this chapter is not meant to be a review of the physiologic adaptations of pregnancy (Table 23-1), it would be incorrect to ignore completely a discussion of the resolution of those changes. In particular, the question should be raised as to how these physiologic adaptations affect subsequent analgesic management after cesarean delivery. For a thorough discussion of the physiologic adaptations of pregnancy and their impact on anesthetic management during labor and delivery, a number of excellent reviews are available.[1]

Cardiac output rises sharply after birth and returns to nonpregnant levels by 2–4 weeks postpartum.[2] Patients with stenotic valvular lesions or pulmonary hypertension are at high risk for decompensation during the immediate postpar-

TABLE 23-1. Maternal Physiologic Adaptations at Term

Variable	Direction	Average Change (%)
Cardiovascular alterations		
Cardiac output	+	40
Stroke volume	+/−	0–30
Heart rate	+	15
Respiratory alterations		
Minute ventilation	+	50
Alveolar ventilation	+	70
Tidal volume	+	40
Respiratory rate	+	15
Closing volume	+/−	0
Residual volume	−	20
Vital capacity	+/−	0
Functional residual capacity	−	20
Airway resistance	−	36
Oxygen consumption	+	20
Hematologic alterations		
Plasma volume	+	45
Erythrocyte volume	+	20
Blood urea nitrogen	−	33

tum period. Otherwise, the return to nonpregnant levels of cardiac output has little physiologic impact on the vast majority of women.

Uterine involution causes rapid resolution of the pulmonary changes induced by mechanical compression of the diaphragm and lungs (Table 23-1). Functional residual capacity and residual volume quickly return to normal. Alveolar ventilation mirrors the gradual fall in blood progesterone levels with a return to nonpregnant values within 2–3 weeks postpartum.[3]

The edematous changes of the upper airway begin to resolve with the onset of postpartum diuresis. Plasma volume gradually declines, and airway edema resolves over a 2- to 4-week period.[4]

Elevated levels of circulating progesterone may still cause decreased gastrointestinal motility, reduced food absorption, and lowered esophageal sphincter pressure.[5] Although mechanical effects on the gastrointestinal tract from uterine enlargement will resolve in 2–3 days, elevated progesterone levels will persist for several weeks.

Thus, with the quick return of functional residual capacity and residual volume to normal, and despite the lingering effects of progesterone levels and expanded plasma volume, the resolving physiologic adaptations of pregnancy should have little impact on analgesic management after cesarean delivery. Certainly airway edema and lowered esophageal sphincter pressure could be of clinical significance in an obtunded patient. However, with proper analgesic management such situations should not occur.

As the resolving physiologic adaptations of pregnancy have little impact on analgesic management and subsequent outcome after cesarean delivery, it must follow that "improved" analgesia will be unlikely to affect the low morbidity and mortality inherent in this healthy group of patients.[6] Therefore, reversal of aberrant postsurgical physiology cannot be used as an outcome measure for the postcesarean delivery patient. Thus, the primary goal of analgesic management should be to promote maternal-newborn bonding. Ultimately, patient satisfaction (rather than improved outcome) becomes the final arbiter for success of an analgesic modality after cesarean delivery.

ANALGESIC MODALITIES

Intramuscular Opioids

Conventional treatment of postoperative pain has consisted of intramuscular (IM) injections of opioids, usually meperidine or morphine. Traditional doses include 50–100 mg of meperidine every 3–4 hours prn (*pro re nata,* or "as needed"), 5–15 mg of morphine every 3–4 hours prn, or 1–2 mg of hydromorphone (dilaudid) every 3–4 hours prn. Variable absorption from IM injection sites results in fluctuating and unpredictable plasma concentrations.[7] This uneven absorption accounts for the wide variations in peak plasma concentrations and the time to reach peak plasma concentrations. (For a full discussion of the vagaries of the IM route of administration, please see Ch. 10.)

Although IM dosing of opioids can produce effective analgesia (particularly when administered around the clock), these drugs are often prescribed in insufficient dosages (e.g., less than 75–100 mg of meperidine in a single injection).[8] Furthermore, opioids have been traditionally prescribed in fixed doses administered prn without evaluating the efficacy of the first dose. There is almost always a delay in administration of subsequent doses despite the prescribed frequency of administration.[9,10] Fixed dose around-the-clock or prn administration more often than not results in inadequate analgesia. Administration is routine rather than varied by actual dosage and/or interval between doses. (For a complete discussion of the inadequacies of prn administration, please see Ch. 1.)

Intravenous Opioids

Given the variable absorption and unpredictable plasma concentration of opioids after IM administration, intravenous (IV) administration is a more desirable route of delivery. IV administration of opioids (especially in small, on-demand, repetitive doses) can eliminate variability in peak plasma concentration as well as decrease the time required to reach peak concentration. Generally, IV dosing is best accomplished with patient-controlled analgesia (PCA). With IV-PCA, opioid is delivered directly into the central venous compartment, and the wide variations in plasma concentration seen with IM dosing are avoided. Highly variable analgesic requirements can be accommodated, and PCA allows patients to "titrate" medication to their specific needs. The immediate accessibility of opioid on patient demand also decreases the anxiety associated with the normal delay in receiving conventional IM medication.[11] (For a complete discussion of PCA, see Ch. 10.)

In general, the suggested PCA or demand doses are 0.5–2 mg morphine every 5–12 minutes (the lockout interval) or 10–20 mg meperidine every 5–12 minutes. Opioids other than morphine and meperidine can be administered by PCA (see Ch. 10 for suggested prescriptions), but most patients will achieve adequate pain control with these two agents. PCA also affords the physician the option of treating the patient with a continuous infusion of opioid in addition to the typical intermittent dose. Common infusion rates are 0.2–0.5 mg/h of morphine or 4–6 mg/h of meperidine.

Quite often after cesarean delivery, patients have not been premedicated and therefore require large loading doses of opioids in order to achieve a comfortable state. Furthermore, these women may have been laboring for extended periods of time (unless scheduled for an elective cesarean delivery). The high circulating levels of endogenous opioids associated with term pregnancy and labor[12,13] may now decrease precipitously, thereby augmenting the need for analgesics. It is important to initially administer sufficient amounts of opioid so that a state of comfort is achieved before commencement of PCA. PCA is much better in maintaining a comfortable level of analgesia than at attaining it. The amount of drug needed to produce acute pain relief cannot be given rapidly enough within usual PCA dosing parameters.

If patients experience nausea or pruritus, it is often helpful to decrease the demand dose or modify the lockout interval. Changing from one opioid to another may also be helpful in some cases, as is the use of antihistamines (e.g., diphenhydramine) or antiemetics. In the event of intractable nausea or pruritus, opioid antagonists may be necessary.

Epidural Opioids

Opioids commonly used to provide epidural analgesia after cesarean delivery are morphine, meperidine, fentanyl, and sufentanil (Table 23-2). For an extensive review of the pharmacology of epidural opioids, please see Chapter 11. Only their use after cesarean delivery will be reviewed here.

Morphine

Epidural morphine provides prolonged analgesia and has been extensively studied in the postcesarean patient.[14,15] Usually 5 mg (or less) of preservative-free morphine is administered before the epidural catheter is removed, providing analgesia of up to 26 hours for the parturient.[15] Alternatively, the epidural catheter can be left in place and additional doses can be administered on the return of pain. Side effects include moderate pruritus in 20 to 30 percent of patients, nausea or vomiting in 20 percent, and rare delayed respiratory depression (0.1 to 0.9 percent).[14] As the onset of analgesia with morphine is slow, a small amount of fentanyl (50–100 µg) can be administered concomitantly with epidural morphine.

TABLE 23-2. Dosing Regimens for Epidural and
Subarachnoid Opioids for Analgesia after Cesarean Delivery

Epidural	
Morphine	2–5 mg[a]
Meperidine	30–100 mg[b]
Fentanyl	50–100 μg[b]
Sufentanil	20–30 μg[b]
Butorphanol	2 mg[b]
Buprenorphine	0.3 mg[b]
Subarachnoid	
Morphine	0.2–0.3 mg
Fentanyl	6.25 μg
Sufentanil	10–20 μg

[a] As morphine has a slow onset of action, more rapid analgesia may be achieved with coadministration of 50–100 μg fentanyl.

[b] Diluent volume affects time of onset and duration of analgesia with a single injection of epidural fentanyl. Administration of fentanyl in a volume of 10 ml will optimize time of onset and duration of analgesia. Although such an effect has not been definitively proven for sufentanil, butorphanol, meperidine, or buprenorphone, most studies have administered these opioids in a diluent volume of 10 or 15 ml.

Meperidine

Epidural meperidine has a rapid onset of action with little risk of delayed respiratory depression; 30–100 mg affords good pain relief for 6–8 hours. Side effects include pruritus and mild sedation. The advantage of meperidine over morphine is a much reduced risk of late respiratory depression, but the duration of analgesia is concomitantly decreased by as much as two-thirds.

Fentanyl

The minimum reliable epidural dose of fentanyl is 50 μg.[16] Fentanyl should be injected in a volume of at least 10 ml of preservative-free normal saline for maximum effectiveness.[17] Onset of analgesia is rapid (about 7 minutes with 50 μg injection).[16] Larger doses result in a slightly more rapid onset of analgesia (3–6 minutes). The duration of analgesia is short, usually 4 hours or less (range = 3–7 hours).[16] To provide more continuous analgesia, a single injection of 50–100 μg can be administered, followed by a continuous infusion of 50–100 μg of fentanyl per hour. Because of the high lipid solubility of fentanyl and the resultant systemic absorption of the opioid, epidural infusions of fentanyl may provide analgesia largely through a supraspinal mechanism.[18,19]

Sufentanil

Epidural sufentanil has been administered in doses of 30–60 μg (diluted in 10 ml of preservative-free normal saline) in order to provide postoperative analgesia after cesarean delivery.[20–23] Twenty μg of epidural sufentanil is equipotent to 100 μg of epidural fentanyl.[20] At least in preliminary studies, there appears to be a rapid onset of analgesia and possibly a greater incidence of side effects than would be predicted by its partition coefficient (see Ch. 11). Rosen et al[22] found the onset of analgesia to be rapid (about 15 minutes). In that particular study, duration of analgesia was about 4 hours (range = 2.8–5.2 hours) after a 30-μg injection. Fifty μg of sufentanil has been reported to produce an unacceptably high incidence of somnolence, pruritus, and emesis.[20,23] Epidural infusions of sufentanil have been studied, but infusion rates of up to 10 μg/h have failed to produce sustained patient comfort.[22]

The disadvantage of both fentanyl and sufentanil for use as a single injection is their markedly short durations of analgesia as compared with morphine.[21] This is consistent with the high lipid solubility of these agents. Like fentanyl, the analgesia attendant on sufentanil may have a substantial supraspinal component because of its lipid solubility and extensive systemic absorption from the epidural space.

Butorphanol

Butorphanol (a mixed agonist-antagonist) has been shown to provide good analgesia after cesarean delivery.[24–26] Doses of up to 66 mg of butorphanol produced substantial somnolence but no nausea or pruritus.[24] Two milligrams in 10 ml of preservative-free normal saline is recommended as the optimal dose for single injection.

Buprenorphine

Epidural buprenorphine (a partial agonist) has been administered to patients either as a single dose or as an infusion.[27] A dose of 0.3 mg in 15 ml normal saline produced analgesia for 12 hours.[27] Cohen et al[28,29] evaluated buprenorphine (0.3 mg/ml) and bupivacaine coadministered by infusion and found an unacceptable incidence of vomiting associated with use of these infusions. At the present time, buprenorphine has been insufficiently studied to suggest a recommended dose, although a single dose of 0.3 mg has been used in most studies.

Combinations

Concomitant epidural administration of two opioids has been studied in order to take advantage of (1) the differing lipophilicities, or (2) the differing intrinsic activities of the two agents. Concomitant use of hydrophilic and lipophilic agents (morphine/fentanyl or sufentanil) would provide the rapid onset of analgesia inherent in use of lipophilic agents with the prolonged analgesia of hydrophilic opioids (see Ch. 11). Combinations of 50–100 μg fentanyl with 4 mg morphine or 20 μg sufentanil with 2.5 mg morphine have been studied.[30] Such combinations could potentially reduce the incidence of side effects while effectively using the most desirable characteristics of each class of agent.

Concomitant epidural administration of agonist/antagonists with μ-agonists could potentially reduce the incidence of side effects attendant on the use of epidural opioids without adversely affecting the quality of analgesia.[31,32] Coadministration of 3 mg butorphanol with 50 μg epidural fentanyl or 4 mg epidural morphine has been shown to reduce the incidence of pruritus and nausea.[31,32] The duration of analgesia and the incidence of respiratory depression and sedation were unaffected.[31,32] Certainly, further work is necessary in order to clarify the utility of coadministration of epidural opioids of differing liphophilicities or intrinsic activities.

Subarachnoid Opioids

Subarachnoid opioids are very useful after cesarean delivery and are injected with local anesthetic at the time of induction of spinal anesthesia. Fentanyl, sufentanil, and morphine have been studied (Table 23-2).

Morphine

Subarachnoid morphine achieves the longest duration of analgesia because of its hydrophilic properties. The usual dose of subarachnoid morphine for analgesia after delivery is 0.2–0.3 mg. Abouleish et al[33] combined 0.2 mg with hyperbaric bupivacaine and achieved an average duration of analgesia of 27 hours.

Side effects limit the maximum dose of subarachnoid morphine that can be used. Abboud et al[34] found that doses as small as 0.1 mg and 0.25 mg of morphine produced 18 and 28 hours of analgesia, respectively, when administered with hyperbaric bupivacaine. However, these low doses were associated with a significant incidence of pruritus. Respiratory depression has been reported with subarachnoid doses as low as 0.3 mg of morphine.[35]

It has been reported that the risk of delayed respiratory depression is four times as frequent for subarachnoid as compared with epidural administration of morphine.[35] In large surveys, the reported incidence of ventilatory depression after epidural morphine is 0.1–0.9 percent, as compared with 4–7 percent after subarachnoid administration.[14,36,37] There is only one study, however, comparing equianalgesic doses of epidural and subarachnoid morphine. Chadwick and Ready[38] compared the effects of administration of 0.3–0.5 mg of subarachnoid morphine with 3–5 mg of epidural morphine for analgesia after cesarean delivery. A significantly greater proportion of patients receiving subarachnoid morphine experienced more than 20 hours of analgesia. There was no difference in the incidence of side effects. The results of this single study using equianalgesic dosages suggest that the analgesia attendant on administration of subarachnoid morphine after cesarean delivery may be of greater duration than that of epidural administration. This occurred despite a similar incidence of side effects.[38] Certainly, more investigations are necessary to corroborate these findings.

Fentanyl

Fentanyl in doses of 6.25–50 μg has been shown to intensify the degree of spinal anesthesia when coadministered with hyperbaric bupivacaine.[39] Doses greater than or equal to 6.25 μg of fentanyl resulted in approximately 3 hours of effective analgesia. There was no influence on the incidence of side effects or 24-hour postoperative opioid requirements, irrespective of dose.

Sufentanil

Subarachnoid administration of 10 μg of sufentanil has resulted in approximately 2.5 hours of analgesia in women undergoing elective cesarean delivery.[40] Although larger doses resulted in longer durations of analgesia, the incidence of side effects was also increased. No respiratory depression was seen with up to 20 μg of sufentanil.[40]

Epidural Clonidine

Clonidine, an α_2-agonist (see Ch. 31), has been used experimentally for analgesia after cesarean delivery. In a study by Mendez et al,[41] epidural injections of 400 and 800 μg of clonidine followed by 10 μg/h and 20 μg/h epidural infusions, respectively, were compared with epidural injections and infusions of saline. Supplemental analgesia was provided by IV-PCA morphine. Analgesia and time to first use of supplemental morphine were similar between the two clonidine dosage groups but significantly greater than in patients receiving saline during the first 6 hours after injection. However, only the 20 μg/h clonidine infusion resulted in decreased morphine use over 24 hours. Thus, continuous infusions of epidural clonidine are required for analgesia of more than 6 hours duration. Epidural use of clonidine decreased blood pressure and heart rate and produced transient sedation.

In a second study, use of epidural 2-chloroprocaine for anesthesia was found to profoundly inhibit subsequent use of clonidine for postoperative analgesia.[42] It was suggested that epidural clonidine in a dose of 400 μg followed by a 40-μg/h infusion was an appropriate regimen for postoperative analgesia. Side effects included decreases in blood pressure, heart rate, and sedation.

The ultimate applicability of epidural clonidine for postcesarean analgesia requires further study. Despite the apparently excellent analgesia, the tendency to cause sedation would be dissatisfactory to new mothers.

OPIOID ANALGESIA AND THE NURSING MOTHER

A consideration unique to pain control in the parturient after cesarean delivery is the uptake of opioids in breast milk and their effects on nursing neonates. The more routine side effects of parenteral and neuraxial opioids and their treatment have been previously discussed in Chapters 8 and 11.

Recently Wittels et al[43] reported on the evaluation of neonatal neurobehavior in the nursing infants of postcesarean delivery patients receiving morphine and meperidine by IV-PCA, both of which provided equivalent maternal analgesia and overall satisfaction. Neonates of mothers receiving morphine were significantly more alert and better oriented than those receiving meperidine as measured by the Brazelton Neonatal Behavioral Assessment Scale on the third day of life. Such neurobehavioral findings were attributed to accumulation of normeperidine, which has a prolonged elimination half-life in neonates (as do morphine and meperidine). At the time of neonatal examination (72 hours postpartum), the ratio of normeperidine/meperidine in breast milk was approximately 3:1. This is in contrast to the observed ratio of approximately 1:1 for morphine and its inactive metabolite morphine-3-glucuronide. (Morphine-6-glucuronide was not measured; see Ch. 8.)[43]

Other studies have contrasted the amount of opioid in breast milk and maternal plasma after epidural or parenteral administration. In a study by Feilberg et al,[44] lactating women undergoing surgery during the nursing period (at least 1 month after having given birth) were treated with epidural or parenteral (IV/IM) morphine. In all cases the concentration of morphine was higher in breast milk than in plasma, irrespective of route of administration. After parenteral administration of 15 mg morphine, maximal concentration in milk was approximately 500 ng/ml (within about 30 minutes). This was followed by a rapid decline to 100 ng/ml at 2 hours. This maximum concentration in milk after 4 mg epidural morphine was 82 ng/ml. The milk/plasma (M:P) ratio in all patients varied between 3.6 and 1.1, in accordance with previous work that found an M:P ratio for morphine of 2.46.[45] The authors concluded that the amount of morphine transferred during nursing is small, even at a peak concentration of 500 ng/ml in the milk, and will hardly cause respiratory depression or drowsiness.[46]

Bernstein et al.[47] measured colostrum morphine concentrations after administration of 5 mg epidural morphine immediately after delivery. The colostrum samples were collected as soon as patients began lactation (24–100 hours after morphine administration). Conjugated morphine concentrations of 1.2–8.6 ng/ml and free morphine concentrations of 0.6 and 4.5 ng/ml were demonstrated. No free morphine was detectable in four of the six samples. Given the low concentrations of free morphine, it is unlikely that the neonate will be appreciably affected by epidural morphine administration.[47]

In summary, available data suggest that morphine administered in conventional dosages by epidural or parenteral routes has little effect on the nursing neonate. Although a single study suggests significant normeperidine accumulation in the neonate from meperidine administered via IV-PCA, only a small number of patients were studied. Much valuable research remains to be done on the neonatal neurobehavioral effects of analgesics administered to postpartum nursing mothers.

CHOOSING AN ANALGESIC MODALITY FOR POSTCESAREAN MOTHERS

As is evident from perusal of this chapter, a large number of modalities provide effective and potent analgesia after cesarean delivery. As previously stated, the resolving physiologic adaptations of pregnancy have little impact on outcome after cesarean delivery. Thus, "better" analgesia will be unlikely to affect the low morbidity inherent in this group of patients.[6] The primary goal of analgesic management for the postcesarean mother should therefore be promotion of maternal-newborn bonding. Maternal satisfaction with the chosen analgesic technique will facilitate such bonding. Maternal satisfaction thus becomes a valid and legitimate outcome measure of the success of postoperative care.

Several studies compare and contrast the analgesia, side effects, and maternal satisfaction associated with use of IM, IV-PCA, and epidural opioids in postcesarean delivery patients.[46,48,49] All studies report improved satisfaction with IV-PCA as compared with IM or epidural opioids.[49,50] The difference between IM and PCA administration with respect to drug usage, quality of analgesia, and sedation were variable, except for the superior satisfaction associated with PCA.[46,48,49] Single injections of epidural morphine provided the best pain relief with the least amount of opioid.[46,49] However, the bothersome side effects of epidural morphine probably contributed to the superior satisfaction associated with use of PCA.

Certainly these preliminary studies should *not* be used as an indictment of the use of epidural and subarachnoid opioids in the postcesarean mother. However, these studies do emphasize that mothers wish to have quality time with their new families. Return of a sensation of "control" after a surgical procedure may facilitate such an appreciation.[50] Untoward side effects may adversely affect maternal-newborn bonding and, thereby, eliminate the potential for a sensation of control and satisfaction. Perhaps the future lies in combining the superior analgesia associated with administration of epidural opioids with the satisfaction inherent in PCA (i.e., patient-controlled epidural analgesia).[51,52]

For the present, the ultimate aim of analgesic therapy in the postcesarean mother should be promotion of maternal-newborn bonding. The success of any analgesic modality in this patient population should be judged by its ability to foster such interaction and not simply by the results of pain scores.

References

1. Camann WR, Ostheimer GW: Physiologic adaptation during pregnancy. p. 1. In Ostheimer GW (ed): Manual of Obstetric Anesthesia. Churchill Livingstone, New York, 1992
2. Ueland K: Maternal cardiovascular hemodynamics. VII. Intrapartum blood volume changes. Am J Obstet Gynecol 126:671, 1976
3. Gugell DW: Pulmonary function in pregnancy. I. Serial observations in normal women. Am Rev Tuberc 67:568, 1953
4. Davison JM: Kidney function in pregnant women. Am J Kidney Dis 9:248, 1987
5. Lind LJ, Smith AM, McIver DK et al: Lower esophageal sphincter pressures in pregnancy. Can J Anaesth 98:571, 1968
6. Eisenach JC: Patient-controlled analgesia for the treatment of obstetric pain: postcesarean delivery. p. 122. In Ferrante FM, Ostheimer GW, Covino BG (eds): Patient-Controlled Analgesia. Blackwell Scientific, Boston, 1990
7. Austin KL, Stapleton JV, Mather LE: Multiple intramuscular injections: a major source of variability in analgesic response to meperidine. Pain 8:47, 1980
8. Marks RM, Sachar EJ: Undertreatment of medical inpatients with narcotic analgesics. Ann Intern Med 78:173, 1973

9. Ferrante FM, Orav EJ, Rocco AG, Gallo J: A statistical model for pain in patient-controlled analgesia and conventional intramusular opioid regimens. Anesth Analg 67:457, 1988

10. Graves DA, Foster TS, Batenhorst RL et al: Patient-controlled analgesia. Ann Intern Med 99:360, 1983

11. Ferrante FM: Patient characteristics influencing effective use of patient-controlled analgesia. p. 51. In Ferrante FM, Ostheimer GW, Covino BG (eds): Patient-Controlled Analgesia. Blackwell Scientific, Boston, 1990

12. Goland RS, Wardlaw SL, Stark RI, Frantz AG: Human plasma beta-endorphin during pregnancy, labor and delivery. J Clin Endocrinol Metab 52:74, 1981

13. Lyrenas S, Nyberg F, Lindberg B, Terenius L: Cerebrospinal fluid activity of dynorphin-converting enzyme at term pregnancy. Obstet Gynecol 72:54, 1988

14. Leicht CII, IIughcs SC, Dailey PA et al: Epidural morphine sulfate for analgesia after cesarean section: a prospective report of 1000 patients, abstracted. Anesthesiology 65:A366, 1986

15. Rosen MA, Hughes SC, Shnider SM et al: Epidural morphine for the relief of postoperative pain after cesarean delivery. Anesth Analg 62:666, 1983

16. Naulty JS, Datta S, Ostheimer GW et al: Epidural fentanyl for postcesarean delivery pain management. Anesthesiology 63:694, 1985

17. Birnbach DJ, Johnson MD, Arcario T et al: Effect of diluent volume on analgesia produced by epidural fentanyl. Anesth Analg 68:808, 1989

18. Loper KA, Ready LB, Downey M et al: Epidural and intravenous fentanyl infusions are clinically equivalent after knee surgery. Anesth Analg 70:72, 1990

19. Glass PSA, Estok P, Ginsberg B et al: Use of patient-controlled analgesia to compare the efficacy of epidural to intravenous fentanyl administration. Anesth Analg 74:345, 1992

20. Madej TH, Strunin L: Comparison of epidural fentanyl with sufentanil. Analgesia and side effects after a single bolus dose during elective cesarean section. Anaesthesia 42:1156, 1987

21. Rosen MA, Dailey PA, Hughes SC et al: Epidural sufentanil for postoperative analgesia after cesarean section. Anesthesiology 68:448, 1988

22. Rosen MA, Hughes SC, Shnider MD et al: Continuous infusion epidural sufentanil for postoperative analgesia, abstracted. Anesth Analg 70:S331, 1990

23. Cohen SE, Tan S, White PF: Sufentanil analgesia following cesarean section: epidural versus intravenous administration. Anesthesiology 68:129, 1988

24. Naulty JS, Weintraub S, McMahon J et al: Epidural butorphanol for post-cesarean delivery pain management, abstracted. Anesthesiology 61:A415, 1984

25. Abboud TK, Moore M, Zhu J: Epidural butorphanol for the relief of postoperative pain after cesarean section, abstracted. Anesthesiology 65:A397, 1986

26. Abboud TK, Moore M, Zhu J et al: Epidural butorphanol or morphine for relief of post-cesarean section pain: ventilatory responses to carbon dioxide. Anesth Analg 66:887, 1987

27. Lanz E, Simko G, Teiss D, Glocke MH: Epidural buprenorphine—a double-blind study of postoperative analgesia and side effects. Anesth Analg 63:593, 1984

28. Cohen S, Amar D, Pantuck CB et al: Continuous epidural-PCA post-cesarean section: buprenorphine-bupivacaine 0.03% vs fentanyl-bupivacaine 0.03%, abstracted. Anesthesiology 73:A975, 1990

29. Cohen S, Amar D, Pantuck CB et al: Epidural patient-controlled analgesia after cesarean section: buprenorphine-0.15% bupivacaine with epinephrine vs fentanyl-0.015% bupivacaine with and without epinephrine. Anesth Analg 74:226, 1992

30. Naulty JS, Parmet J, Pate A et al: Epidural sufentanil and morphine for post-cesarean delivery analgesia, abstracted. Anesthesiology 73:A965, 1990

31. Lawhorn CD, McNitt JD, Fibuch EE et al: Epidural morphine with butorphanol for postoperative analgesia after cesarean delivery. Anesth Analg 72:53, 1991

32. Hunt CO, Naulty JS, Malinow AM et al: Epidural butorphanol-bupivacaine for analgesia during labor and delivery. Anesth Analg 68:323, 1989

33. Abouleish E, Rawal N, Fallon K, Hernandez D: Combined intrathecal morphine and bupivacaine for cesarean section. Anesth Analg 67:370, 1988

34. Abboud TK, Dror A, Mosaad P et al: Mini-dose intrathecal morphine for the relief of post-cesarean section pain: safety, efficacy, and ventilatory responses to carbon dioxide. Anesth Analg 67:137, 1988

35. Rawal N, Arner S, Gustafsson LL, Allvin R: Present state of extradural and intrathecal opioid analgesia in Sweden. Br J Anaesth 59:791, 1987

36. Cousins MJ, Mather LE: Intrathecal and epidural administration of opioids. Anesthesiology 61:276, 1984

37. Gustafsson LL, Schildt B, Jacobsen K: Adverse effects of extradural and intrathecal opiates: report of a nationwide survey in Sweden. Br. J Anaesth 54:479, 1982

38. Chadwick HS, Ready LB: Intrathecal and epidural morphine sulfate for postcesarean analgesia—a clinical comparison. Anesthesiology 68:925, 1988

39. Hunt CO, Naulty JS, Bader AM et al: Perioperative analgesia with subarachnoid fentanyl-bupivacaine for cesarean delivery. Anesthesiology 71:535, 1989

40. Courtney M, Bader AM, Hartwell BL et al: Perioperative analgesia with subarachnoid sufentanil-bupivacaine, abstracted. Anesthesiology 73:A994, 1990

41. Mendez R, Eisenach JC, Kashtan K: Epidural clonidine analgesia after cesarean section. Anesthesiology 73:848, 1990

42. Huntoon M, Eisenach JC, Boese P: Epidural clonidine after cesarean section. Appropriate dose and effect of prior local anesthetic. Anesthesiology 76:187, 1992

43. Wittels B, Scott DT, Sinatra RS: Exogenous opioids in human breast milk and acute neonatal behavior: a preliminary study. Anesth Analg 73:864, 1990

44. Feilberg VL, Rosenborg D, Christensen CB, Mogensen JW: Excretion of morphine in human breast milk. Acta Anaesthesiol Scand 33:426, 1989

45. Findlay JWA, DeAngelis RL, Kearney MF et al: Analgesic drugs in breast milk and plasma. Clin Pharmacol Ther 29:625, 1981

46. Harrison DM, Sinatra R, Morgese L, Chung JH: Epidural narcotic and patient-controlled analgesia for post-cesarean section pain relief. Anesthesiology 68:454, 1988

47. Bernstein J, Patel N, Moszczynski Z et al: Colostrum morphine concentrations following epidural administration, abstracted. Anesth Analg 68:S23, 1989

48. Rayburn WF, Geranis BJ, Ramadei CA et al: Patient-controlled analgesia for post-cesarean pain. Obstet Gynecol 72:136, 1988

49. Eisenach JC, Grice SC, Dewan DM: Patient-controlled analgesia following cesarean section: a comparison with epidural and intramuscular narcotics. Anesthesiology 68:444, 1988

50. Egan KJ: What does it mean to a patient to be "in control"? p. 17. In Ferrante FM, Ostheimer GW, Covino BG (eds): Patient-Controlled Analgesia. Blackwell Scientific, Boston, 1990

51. Ferrante FM, Lu L, Jamison SB, Datta S: Patient-controlled epidural analgesia: demand dosing. Anesth Analg 73:547, 1991

52. Parker RK, White PF: Epidural patient-controlled analgesia: an alternative to intravenous patient-controlled analgesia for pain relief after cesarean delivery. Anesth Analg 75:245, 1992

24

Analgesia After Orthopaedic Surgery

Gilbert J. Fanciullo
F. Michael Ferrante

Pain after major orthopaedic surgery is among the most severe encountered by the clinician. This fact, together with the amenability of these operations to regional anesthesia/analgesia and a desire for early painless physical therapy, make this surgical population among the most frequently cared-for by an acute pain service. This chapter focuses on the postoperative analgesic management of several common orthopaedic procedures.

ANALGESIA FOR SPECIFIC ORTHOPAEDIC OPERATIONS

Hip Arthroplasty and Replacement

Patients undergoing hip arthroplasty or total replacement are generally elderly patients. Arthroplasty is most commonly performed for hip fractures sustained from minor falls. Hip replacement is performed because of pain and disabling immobility caused by a number of chronic conditions such as osteoarthritis, rheumatoid arthritis, or avascular necrosis of the femoral head. Patients undergoing either procedure usually have a number of comorbid conditions requiring preoperative evaluation and, possibly, treatment.[1-3] In a series of more than 200 patients with fractured hips, Haljamae et al[1] found significant nonorthopaedic findings in 92 percent of patients. The average patient had correctable abnormalities in two major organ systems.[1] Thus, besides the attendant surgical risks of hypotension from cementing,[4–7] fat embolization,[8] and deep vein thrombosis and subsequent embolism caused by postsurgical immobility,[9] the comorbid conditions associated with this group of patients increase the chances for substantial morbidity and mortality.

A number of series study the relation between choice of anesthetic and subsequent mortality and morbidity associated with hip arthroplasty and joint replacement. Unfortunately, few if any of the studies examine the impact of extension of neural blockade into the postoperative period. Thus, these studies really only look at the effects of choice of intraoperative anesthetic. The influence of postoperative analgesic techniques on morbidity and mortality can therefore only be extrapolated from the existing data.

A fair amount of data[10–17] exist regarding the effect of anesthetic technique on mortality after hip arthroplasty (Table 24-1). The cumulative data show an almost 50 percent reduction in mortality associated with use of regional anesthesia (6.6 percent versus 12.3 percent for general anesthesia). Review of these series, however, demonstrates only a short-term initial reduction in mortality with regional anesthesia. Identical survival rates are found with long-term follow-up. Analysis of the cause of death is incompletely defined, but most fatalities resulted from pulmonary complications. Thus, data exist that suggest that intraoperative regional anesthesia may impact on early postoperative mortality after hip surgery. It is intriguing to speculate as to whether aggressive, prolonged regional analgesia (instead of anesthesia) coupled with aggressive inpatient and outpatient physical therapy would have impacted on long-term mortality rates.

The influence of regional anesthesia/analgesia on postoperative thromboembolic complications after hip surgery has been examined in several controlled studies[13,18,19,20] (Table 24-2). As verified by phlebography or ^{125}I-fibrinogen scanning, regional anesthesia reduced the incidence of thromboembolic complications in the lower extremities by about 50 percent after hip surgery. Continuous postoperative epidural analgesia for 24 hours after hip replacement reduced the incidence of pulmonary embolism from 33 percent to 10 percent, as assessed

TABLE 24-1. Effect of Regional Anesthesia on Mortality after Hip Arthroplasty

Study	Regional Technique	Mortality: Regional Anesthesia	Mortality: General Anesthesia	Follow-up (months)
Couderc et al[10]	Epidural	7/50	12/50	3
McKenzie et al[11]	Spinal	5/49	8/51	1
White and Chapell[12]	Spinal	0/20	0/20	1
Davis and Laurenson[13]	Spinal	3/64	9/68	1
McLaren[14]	Spinal	4/56	17/60	1
Wickström et al[15]	Epidural	2/32	6/97	1
McKenzie et al[16]	Spinal	3/73	12/75	2
Valentin et al[17]	Spinal	17/281	24/297	24
Cumulative mortality		41/625 (6.6%)	88/718 (12.3%)	

TABLE 24-2. **Effect of Regional Anesthesia/Analgesia on Thromboembolic Complications after Hip and Knee Surgery**

Reference	Regional	Complications (% of Group)	
		Regional	General
Hip			
Davie et al[3]	Spinal	19	77
Modig et al[18]	Epidural	20	73
Modig et al[19]	Epidural[a] (1)	40	77
Wille-Jorgensen et al[20]	Both	9	31
Knee			
Nielsen et al[29]	Epidural	16	63
Sharrock et al[30]	Epidural	48	64
Jorgensen et al[31]	Epidural[a] (3)	18	59
Mitchell et al[32]	Epidural[b]	46	64

[a] Epidural anesthesia/analgesia was continued into the postoperative period. Numbers in parentheses represent number of days of postoperative epidural analgesia.

[b] There was no difference in the overall incidence of thromboembolism between regional and general anesthesia in this study. However, the incidence of proximal vein thrombosis was significantly decreased in the epidural group. The incidence of proximal vein thrombosis is listed.

by perfusion lung scanning.[19] Similar to the discussion regarding mortality after hip surgery, the extant studies do not allow determination as to whether continuous postoperative epidural analgesia is superior to intraoperative regional anesthesia alone for the prevention of thromboembolism.

Patient-Controlled Analgesia

Despite the considerations of decreased morbidity and mortality attendant to intraoperative use of regional anesthesia, with respect to postoperative pain, patients can be managed equally well with either continuous epidural analgesia or patient-controlled analgesia (PCA). As there is insufficient data to determine whether *postoperative* epidural analgesia impacts on outcome after hip surgery, PCA is a reasonable first choice because of the decreased intensity of labor, risk, and cost. Elderly or debilitated patients (common features in an orthopaedic population) or opioid-naive patients should be prescribed smaller demand doses and longer lockout intervals than robust, healthy, young people (e.g., traumatic hip fractures) or those tolerant to opioids[21] (Table 24-3). Certainly, advanced age may be a consideration for choosing an alternate analgesic modality, as inability to access the demand button, "sundowning," and dementia would affect patients' ability to effectively use PCA.

Subarachnoid Opioids

Many patients receive spinal anesthesia for hip surgery. Single dose subarachnoid opioids can provide satisfactory (and perhaps protracted) analgesia. A dosage range cannot be precisely recommended, as most of the original stud-

TABLE 24-3. Analgesic Dosage Regimens for Open Hip and Knee Surgery

Analgesic Modality	Hip Surgery	Knee Surgery
PCA[a]	Morphine: 1–2-mg demand dose; 5–10 min lockout interval Meperidine: 10–20-mg demand dose; 5–10 min lockout interval	Same
Subarachnoid opioids (see Table 24-4)	0.2–0.5 mg morphine	0.5 mg morphine
Epidural morphine (single injection)	2–4 mg intraoperatively; "titrate" to effect with repetitive dose of 1–2 mg	4 mg intraoperative; "titrate" to effect with repetitive dose of 1–3 mg
Epidural fentanyl (single injection)	50–100 μg in 10 ml diluent	Not recommended[b]
Combined epidural opioid (single injection)	Morphine 4 mg with 50–100 μg fentanyl[c]	Not recommended[b]
Epidural local anesthetic (infusion)	Not recommended[d]	0.25% bupivacaine at 5–7 ml/h; "titrate" appropriately
Epidural local anesthetic and opioid (infusion)	Not recommended[d]	0.125% or 0.25% bupivacaine with 1–2.5 mg meperidine or 5 μg fentanyl, or 0.05–0.1 mg morphine at 5–7 ml/h; titrate appropriately
Continuous lumbar plexus neural blockade	Not recommended[e]	20 ml of 0.25% bupivacaine as a single injection followed by 7–10 ml/h as an infusion; "titrate" appropriately

[a] Elderly patients should be prescribed smaller doses and longer lockout intervals.

[b] Single dose epidural fentanyl is not efficacious for analgesia after open knee surgery.[39]

[c] In a single dose combination, epidural fentanyl provides short-term analgesia while awaiting the onset of analgesia attendant to morphine.

[d] Epidural administration of local anesthetics may mask hip dislocation. However, patients should receive some kind of anticoagulant therapy (if they do not receive epidural local anesthetics) to provide prophylaxis against thromboembolism.

[e] Continuous administration of local anesthetics to the lumbar plexus may mask hip dislocation.

ies of subarachnoid opioids for hip surgery were performed early in the history of the use of neuraxial opioids[22–25] (Table 24-4). Thus, very large doses of morphine were used.[22–25] Later studies used much less opioid.[26,27] A dose-response study is needed to compare the side effects and analgesic intensity and duration attendant to "minidose" (0.2–0.5 mg morphine) versus larger doses of opioids (0.5–2 mg morphine). Given this degree of imprecision, 0.2–0.5 mg administered as a single subarachnoid dose is safe and effective in the experience of the Acute Pain Service at the Brigham and Women's Hospital.

Epidural Opioids and Local Anesthetics

Similar to the situation with subarachnoid opioids, there has been little organized or comparative study of the epidural administration of local anesthetics and/or opioids for postoperative analgesia after hip surgery. Modig and Paalzow[28] demonstrated an average duration of analgesia of 28 hours after 5 mg of epidural morphine. No comparisons have been made of epidural opioids and

TABLE 24-4. Use of Subarachnoid Opioids for Hip and Knee Arthroplasty and Replacement

Reference	Dose	Comments
Hip		
Barron and Strong[22]	Morphine 2 mg; diamorphine[a] 0.5mg	Unacceptably high incidence of vomiting: one patient required resuscitation
Gjessing and Tomlin[23]	Morphine 0.8–2 mg	Two patients developed late respiratory depression
Moore et al[24]	Morphine 2.5 mg	Hypercarbia; median time to request of additional analgesic was 22 hours
Paterson et al[25]	Morphine 0.625 mg, 1.25 mg, and 2.5 mg	Increasing duration of analgesia with increased dose; greater incidence of side effects at doses >0.625 mg of morphine; no difference in incidence of side effects and quality of analgesia between morphine and diamorphine at corresponding doses
Hedenstierna and Lofstrom[26]	Morphine 0.3 mg	Hypercarbia; decreased functional residual capacity and closing capacity
Knee		
Jacobson et al[37]	Diamorphine 0.25 mg, 0.75 mg, 1.5 mg, and 2.5 mg	Inconsistent and incomplete analgesia at all doses
Both		
Drakeford et al[27]	Morphine 0.5 mg; hydromorphone 0.002 mg/kg	Minimal side effects and good analgesia with both doses

[a] Heroin.

local anesthetics for pain after hip surgery. Thus, much of the information regarding dosing schedules for epidural analgesia after hip surgery has been empirically derived from the experience of the individual practitioner or extrapolated from studies of other procedures.

Recommendations derived from the experience at Brigham and Women's Hospital are found in Table 24-3. As practically no data correlate the relation between the dose of epidural morphine and side effects (e.g., pruritus, nausea, respiratory depression), initial doses of 2–4 mg are recommended if the epidural catheter is not removed after surgery. (A single dose of 5 mg can be given if the catheter is to be removed.) Repetitive doses of 1–2 mg of epidural morphine can then be administered and adjusted according to patient response. Ignoring concerns regarding thromboembolism, as patients often receive oral anticoagulants, continuous use of local anesthetics (either by epidural administration or continuous lumbar plexus neural blockade) is best avoided after hip fracture. In our experience, several postoperative hip dislocations have been masked by use of local anesthetic.

Open Knee Surgery

Patients who have undergone knee arthroplasty or joint replacement or anterior or posterior cruciate ligament repair (all examples of open knee surgery) are managed much differently from the patient after hip surgery. The knee has a major role in proprioception for the lower extremity. It is extensively innervated, and any surgery tends to be excruciatingly painful. The postoperative course usually includes both vigorous physical therapy and the use of continuous passive motion of the joint. These two therapeutic modalities generate intensive pain in the freshly operated knee.

As in hip surgery, a number of studies have looked at the impact of anesthesia on the incidence of thromboembolism after knee surgery[29–32] (Table 24-2). Once again, provision of regional anesthesia (with possible continuation as regional analgesia after surgery[31]) is shown to beneficially affect the incidence of deep vein thrombosis.

Systemic Opioids

Conventionally administered (intramuscular [IM]) systemic opioids[33] as well as intravenous-PCA (IV-PCA)[34,35] are often inadequate for the relief of postoperative pain after knee surgery. When compared, the degree of analgesia attendant to administration of IM opioids and IV-PCA is equivalent after total knee replacement.[36] Epidural analgesia with morphine[34,35] and bupivacaine alone[33] have been shown to provide analgesia superior to the administration of systemic opioids after open knee surgery.

Subarachnoid Opioids

Like its use after hip surgery, all too little research has been done on the use of subarachnoid opioids after knee arthroplasty and replacement.[27,37] Unlike the experience with hip surgery, however, a dose-response study for the use of subarachnoid opioids (diamorphine [heroin] in this case) does exist.[37] Inconsistent and incomplete analgesia was found at all doses (0.25 mg, 0.75 mg, 1.5 mg, and 2.5 mg of diamorphine). There was no difference in the quality of analgesia as a function of dose. Subarachnoid diamorphine was unable to provide profound and consistent analgesia after knee surgery and cannot be recommended for use. However, 0.5 mg of morphine or 0.002 mg/kg of hydromorphone produced good analgesia after both knee and hip surgery.[27]

Epidural Opioids

When comparing the use of epidural opioids for open knee surgery, it is important to note whether ligamentous repair or actual bone surgery had been performed.

Both epidural morphine[34] and fentanyl[38] have been shown to provide excellent analgesia after anterior cruciate ligament repair. (It is impossible to determine from the pertinent studies, however, whether continuous passive motion of the knee joint was used. This certainly would have dramatically increased the level of pain.)

With respect to knee joint arthroplasty or replacement and use of continuous passive motion, the complete adequacy of epidural opioids is more controversial. Pierrot et al[39] were unable to use epidural fentanyl effectively in 50 percent of their patients undergoing continuous passive motion after knee surgery, despite single doses ranging from 245 to 450 μg of fentanyl. (In actuality, it was *impossible* to use continuous passive motion in 30 percent of their patients.) Nielsen et al[40] were able to demonstrate good pain relief with epidural morphine but no attendant increase in range of motion. However, Baker et al[41] found inconsistent analgesia associated with use of epidural morphine after total knee replacement. Epidural morphine was associated with an increased range of knee motion and decreased hospital stay. However, the attendant side effects and inconsistent analgesia forced the authors to conclude that epidural morphine was untenable as a single analgesic agent after total knee replacement.[41]

Our experience at Brigham and Women's Hospital corroborates the findings of Pierrot et al.[39] Epidural fentanyl is ineffective as an analgesic in a large percentage of patients undergoing continuous passive motion of the knee. However, in our experience, epidural fentanyl appears to be more effective for soft tissue than for bone surgery. Similar to the results of Baker et al,[41] we find inconsistent analgesia associated with the use of epidural morphine. Such experiences have lead the Acute Pain Service at Brigham and Women's Hospital to rely on epidural infusions of local anesthetic and opioid or regional analgesic techniques (lumbar plexus analgesia).

Epidural Local Anesthetics

Continuous infusions of local anesthetic have been uniformly found to provide consistent, excellent, and protracted analgesia in patients undergoing continuous passive knee motion after knee replacement[33,42] and arthrolysis.[43] Although not reported in relation to knee surgery, tachyphylaxis can occur with prolonged epidural infusion of local anesthetic alone.[44-46] Furthermore, the incidence of tachyphylaxis has been shown to be reduced or ablated by coadministration of an opioid.[47,48] Thus, infusions of local anesthetics and opioids would seem the most optimal method for provision of analgesia after open knee surgery.

Combinations

Unfortunately, only two studies look at the combined use of local anesthetics and opioids for postoperative analgesia after total knee replacement, and their results are contradictory. Mahoney et al[49] demonstrated that concomitant epidural infusion of morphine and bupivacaine produced less moderate-to-severe pain and greater joint mobility than epidural morphine alone. However, Badner et al[50] were unable to demonstrate any benefit from addition of 0.1 percent bupivacaine to continuous epidural infusions of fentanyl. (It is uncertain whether patients underwent continuous passive motion of the knee.)

Ligamentous repair of the knee joint or total knee arthroplasty are two of the most demanding postoperative pain management problems. Much time has been spent reviewing the literature regarding the use of subarachnoid opioids, epidural opioids, and local anesthetics so that the reader may appreciate the inconsistencies of the literature and the need for further research. Most studies have used pain or pain relief as an outcome measure. Ultimately, perhaps, a better outcome measure after knee surgery is enhanced mobilization. Little difference in pain scores would be expected at rest when comparing epidural administration of local anesthetics and/or opioids. However, much improved mobility of a knee joint would be expected with combination therapy. Indeed, this has been demonstrated in knee patients by Mahoney et al[49] and in abdominal surgery patients by Dahl et al.[51] Our experience in the management of knee arthroplasty and total joint replacement corroborates these findings, and combinational infusions have been adopted as the standard of care at Brigham and Women's Hospital.

Lumbar Plexus Neural Blockade

Another very effective analgesic option for patients undergoing open knee surgery is lumbar plexus neural blockade. (Lumbar plexus blockade is extensively discussed in Ch. 13.) Few studies compare the efficacy of lumbar plexus blockade to epidural opioids and/or local anesthetics. Schultz et al[52] were unable to demonstrate any difference in pain relief after open knee surgery when comparing epidural morphine and continuous lumbar plexus blockade with bupivacaine. (Once again, it is impossible to determine whether continuous passive knee motion was used postoperatively, and improved facility with this modality may be a better outcome measure after knee surgery.) However, use of lumbar plexus analgesia was associated with a lower incidence of nausea, vomiting, pruritus, and urinary retention.[52]

Given the paucity of comparative data, lumbar plexus blockade, in our experience, is best used in patients without epidural catheters who have inadequate analgesia or intolerable opioid side effects.

Clinical Practice at Brigham and Women's Hospital

If epidural morphine is to be used for knee arthroplasty or joint replacement, 4 mg should be administered in the operating room 1 hour before termination of surgery. (As explained in Ch. 11, epidural morphine has a prolonged onset of action.) Alternatively for ligamentous repair, 50–100 μg of fentanyl can be coadministered with 3–4 mg of epidural morphine at the very end of surgery. Concomitant administration of fentanyl allows for short-term analgesia while awaiting the onset of analgesia attendant to morphine. If we believe the work of Pierrot et al,[39] such a technique of coadministration should not be efficacious for knee arthroplasty or joint replacement, although no study directly addresses this question.

When using a local anesthetic-opioid combination, the local anesthetic of choice is bupivacaine. Bupivacaine is selected because of its long duration of action, differential blockade of sensory rather than motor fibers, and low incidence of tachyphylaxis. The remarkable differential block reported with the new local anesthetic ropivacaine, as well as its long duration of action and lower cardiac toxicity, may make ropivacaine appealing as the local anesthetic of choice for continuous epidural analgesia in the future.[53-56]

A concentration of 0.25 percent bupivacaine combined with an opioid provides good analgesia for most patients undergoing open knee surgery.[33] A small percentage of patients will develop motor block with this concentration,[33] which can then be reduced to 0.125 percent bupivacaine. If there is inadequate analgesia with use of 0.125 percent bupivacaine, the concentration can then be increased to 0.1875 percent, at which point good analgesia is usually achieved. A dense motor block is undesirable because of the possible development of pressure ulcers.[57]

Meperidine[58,59] is a good choice of opioid for continuous epidural infusions of local anesthetic and opioid when used for analgesia after open knee surgery. Concentrations of 1-2.5 mg/ml provide excellent analgesia when combined with bupivacaine, and there is less of a risk of respiratory depression when compared with morphine, particularly in elderly or debilitated patients. The lipophilicity of meperidine, intermediate between fentanyl and morphine, may provide better spread (covering more dermatomes) than fentanyl and may account for a lower incidence of respiratory depression than morphine (see Ch. 11). Despite the local anesthetic properties of meperidine,[60-62] there does not seem to be an increased incidence of motor block when used at the recommended dosages.[63]

Morphine or fentanyl can also be used. The standard concentration of fentanyl for epidural infusion is 5 μg/ml. If the patient is young and otherwise healthy, a concentration of fentanyl of 10 μg/ml may be necessary at times. The customary concentration of morphine is 0.05-0.1 mg/ml. As suggested by Pierrot et al,[39] we have found epidural fentanyl to be inconsistent in the effective management of pain after knee arthroplasty or joint replacement, particularly in patients undergoing continuous passive motion of the knee. In our experience, fentanyl works quite well for analgesia after ligamentous repair. Morphine provides adequate analgesia after both soft tissue and bony knee surgery.

Initial infusion rates are 5-7 mg/h. It may be prudent to select a maximum rate of continuous infusion that should not be exceeded, because higher rates of administration may be associated with a greater risk of respiratory embarrassment. When using the aforementioned concentrations of opioid with bupivacaine, excellent analgesia can be obtained at a rate of 10 ml/h or less. The maximum rate can be exceeded, but it should rarely be necessary. Whenever it is necessary to exceed an infusion rate of 10 ml/h, one should be suspicious of a malpositioned catheter (not in the epidural space).

A summary of the recommendations for neuraxial administration of opioids and/or local anesthetics for open knee surgery is found in Table 24-3.

Knee Arthroscopy

Intra-articular Bupivacaine

Lidocaine,[64] prilocaine,[65,66] and bupivacaine[64,65,67–72] have been administered intra-articularly to provide intra-operative local anesthesia[64,67] and postoperative analgesia for knee arthroscopy. Usual bupivacaine doses have ranged from 20 to 30 ml of 0.25 or 0.5 percent bupivacaine and provide several hours of analgesia. Addition of epinephrine has no analgesic effect but does decrease plasma concentrations.[64,70]

Intra-articular Morphine

Intra-articular morphine has recently been proposed as an effective modality for pain management after arthroscopy.[73,74] According to Stein et al,[74] 0.5–1.0 mg of intra-articular morphine provided 3–6 hours of analgesia and reduced supplemental opioid use. Analgesia was reversible by intra-articular injection of naloxone. The authors proposed that analgesia was produced by the binding of morphine to opioid receptors in inflamed tissue within the knee.[74] Further research is necessary before the exact role of intra-articular opioids for postoperative pain relief after joint surgery can be determined.

Shoulder Arthroplasty

Patient-Controlled Analgesia

Most patients can be effectively managed with IV-PCA alone or in combination with ketorolac for pain after shoulder surgery. Certainly, analgesia is not as complete as that achieved by continuous brachial plexus blockade. However, because of the simplicity and ease of applicability of PCA, it is a reasonable first choice as an analgesic modality for many practitioners.

Brachial Plexus Blockade

Consideration should be given to the use of regional anesthesia/analgesia if the practitioner is facile with brachial plexus regional anesthesia and continuous brachial plexus catheter techniques (see Ch. 14). Brachial plexus blockade should also be considered if inadequate analgesia and/or intolerable side effects are associated with the use of systemic analgesics.

A single injection interscalene approach to the brachial plexus has been shown to provide excellent analgesia in several studies.[75,76] In the study of Brandl et al,[76] superior analgesia was demonstrated for up to 24 hours in many patients after using 40 ml of 0.375 percent bupivacaine. Thirty-five percent of patients required no further analgesic supplementation over 24 hours.[76] Of course, cervical plexus block should be combined with brachial plexus blockade to achieve analgesia over the skin of the shoulder and neck.[75,77]

Continuous brachial plexus catheter technique using the interscalene approach has been described for intraoperative anesthesia and postoperative analgesia after shoulder surgery.[78] Because of the perpendicular angle of approach of the needle to the brachial plexus, advancement of a catheter may prove problematic when using the interscalene technique (see Ch. 14). A 20 percent failure rate was reported by Haasio et al.[78]

Cervical Epidural Anesthesia/Analgesia

There is one study in the literature examining the use of cervical epidural anesthesia for shoulder surgery.[79] All epidural catheters were inserted at C7-T1 and advanced 2–3 cm into the epidural space. Incremental doses of 3–4 ml of 0.5 percent bupivacaine with 1:200,000 epinephrine were administered every 5 minutes to a maximum of 12–15 ml. The authors advocated use of the cervical epidural catheter for postoperative analgesia, although none of their small series of seven patients received analgesia in this manner. Because of the paucity of data and the obvious potential for physiologic trespass, the regular use of cervical epidural anesthesia/analgesia cannot be advocated at this time.

Amputation

Amputation is a procedure that is performed less frequently than hip or knee arthroplasty or replacement. Although amputations do not usually present as major postoperative pain management problems, subsequent development of phantom limb pain is a very serious problem indeed.[80] The success rate for treating established phantom pain is dismal. One large study of American war veterans showed an 85 percent incidence of phantom limb or stump pain of such severity that it interfered with social and work responsibilities every year.[81] As the success in treating established phantom limb pain is poor, it would seem optimal to prophylax against its occurrence, if possible.

A great deal of excitement was therefore engendered by the study of Bach et al,[82] suggesting that preamputation epidural analgesia could prophylax against the occurrence of phantom limb pain and sensations. Unfortunately, there are a number of methodologic problems with this study (small numbers of patients, dropouts caused by death, and lack of uniformity in treatment: patients received lumbar epidural morphine *or* bupivacaine *or* both). According to the authors, a larger, more rigorous study is underway.

On a theoretic basis, preoperative neural blockade may only be seen to be efficacious if a peripheral[80,83] or spinal cord[84] mechanism is believed to be involved in the genesis of phantom pain. However, if phantom pain is believed to be the reaction of a nociceptive ''imprint'' on cerebral structures,[85,86] preoperative neural blockade should not be efficacious.

At present, the use of preoperative neural blockade for prophylaxis of phantom limb pain is unproven. The decision to submit an individual for such preoperative therapy must be made with the consensus of the surgeon and the informed consent of the patient when viewed in this light.

Open Reduction and Interval Fixation of Ankle Fractures

Open reduction and internal fixation of ankle fractures can be very painful postoperatively and difficult to manage. IV-PCA alone or IV-PCA plus ketorolac is only modestly effective. Epidural analgesia with local anesthetic is efficacious but may be less than satisfactory in some patients because of the difficulty in affecting sacral roots with lumbar catheters.[87] Epidural analgesia with opioid is effective for postoperative analgesia after ankle surgery, but no specific study addresses its use. Another effective option is to perform a popliteal space sciatic nerve block.[88,89]

Popliteal Space Sciatic Nerve Block

ANATOMY

The anatomy of the popliteal fossa is shown in Figure 24-1. Note that two branches of the sciatic nerve (the tibial and common peroneal nerves) lie within the popliteal fossa in easy access.

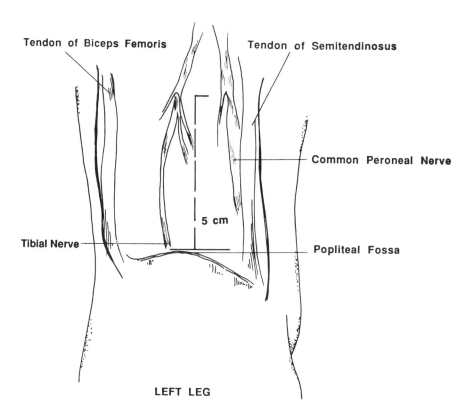

Fig. 24-1. Anatomy of the posterior compartment of the knee.

POSITIONING AND LANDMARKS

Neural blockade is performed with the patient in the prone or lateral position. A peripheral nerve stimulator (PNS) with a variable amperage output is used. An 18- or 20-gauge insulated 1½- or 2-inch needle is selected. The PNS is then arranged with one lead grounded to the patient and the other lead attached to the block needle. A line is then drawn in the popliteal crease between the ligaments of insertion of the semimembranosis muscle and the biceps femoris muscle. (These two large ligaments lie perpendicular to and on either side of the crease and are easily appreciated.) A perpendicular line bisecting the crease is drawn upward and extended for 10 cm. A point 5 cm cephalad from the crease is located along this line. The insertion point for the block needle is 1 cm lateral to this point (Fig. 24-1).

PROCEDURE

The area is prepared with betadine. Using sterile technique, the needle is gently inserted with the PNS current set at 2 mA. Either dorsiflexion or plantar flexion of the foot implies needle proximity to the peroneal component or the tibial component of the sciatic nerve, respectively. If the current can be decreased to about 0.5 mA and dorsiflexion or plantar flexion maintained, the needle is likely abutting against a nerve. Thirty milliliters of 0.25 percent bupivacaine with epinephrine is then injected in increments, providing 12–24 hours of analgesia.

COMPLICATIONS

Popliteal hematomas are extremely rare but can occur. They may be difficult to detect because of the loose and roomy anatomic compartment of the popliteal space. A compartment syndrome may be masked by successful technique because of the lack of increasing pain as a symptom. If the surgeon is not worried about a compartment syndrome or if another method to monitor for its occurrence is standard practice at your facility (e.g., compartment pressures), this block can be most rewarding.

CONCLUSION

Many modalities are available for the management of postoperative pain after orthopaedic surgery. This chapter is an attempt to present a current state-of-the-art review. As more data are available about the sequelae of orthopaedic surgery and as more comparisons of techniques become available, management of postoperative pain will continue to be refined and improved.

References
1. Haljamae H, Stefansson T, Wickström I: Preanesthetic evaluation of the female geriatric patient with hip fracture. Acta Anaesth Scand 26:393, 1982
2. Allen HL, Metcalf DW: Fractured hip: a study of anesthesia in the aged. Anesth Analg 44:408, 1965

3. Davie IT, MacRae WR, Malcom-Smith NA: Anesthesia for the fractured hip: a survey of 200 cases. Anesth Analg 49:165, 1970
4. Ellis RH, Mulvein J: The cardiovascular effects of methylmethacrylate. J Bone Joint Surg 56B:59, 1974
5. Anderson KH: Air aspirated from the venous system during total hip replacement. Anaesthesia 38:1175, 1983
6. Bengtson A, Larsson M, Gammer W, Heideman M et al: Anaphylatoxin release in association with methylmethacrylate fixation of hip prostheses. J Bone Joint Surg 69A:46, 1987
7. Crout DHG, Corkill JH, James ML, Ling RS: Methylmethacrylate metabolism in man. The hydrolysis of methylmethacrylate to methacrylate acid during total hip replacement. Clin Orthop 141:90, 1979
8. Orsini EC, Byrick RJ, Muller JBM et al: Cardiopulmonary function and pulmonary microemboli during arthroplasty using cemented and noncemented components. The role of intramedullary pressure. J Bone Joint Surg 69A:822, 1987
9. Kakkar VV, Fok PJ, Murray WJG et al: Heparin and dihydroergotamine prophylaxis against thrombo-embolism after hip arthroplasty. J Bone Joint Surg 67B:538, 1985
10. Couderc E, Mauge F, Duvaldestin P, Desmonts JM: Résultats comparatifs de l'anesthésia générale et peridurale chez le grand vieillard dans la chirurgie de la hanche. Anesth Analg Réan 34:987, 1977
11. McKenzie PJ, Wishart HY, Dewar KMS et al: Comparison of the effects of spinal anesthesia and general anaesthesia on postoperative oxygenation and perioperative mortality. Br J Anaesth 52:49, 1980
12. White IWC, Chapell WA: Anaesthesia for surgical correction of fractured femoral neck. A comparison of three techniques. Anaesthesia 35:1107, 1980
13. Davis FM, Laurenson VG: Spinal anaesthesia or general anaesthesia for emergency hip surgery in elderly patients. Anaesth Intensive Care 9:352, 1981
14. McLaren AD: Mortality studies. A review, abstracted. Reg Anaesth 7:S172, 1982
15. Wickström I, Holmberg I, Stefansson T: Survival of female geriatric patients after hip fracture surgery. A comparison of 5 anesthetic methods. Acta Anaesthesiol Scand 26:607, 1982
16. McKenzie PJ, Wishart HY, Smith G: Long-term outcome after repair of fractured neck of femur. Comparison of subarachnoid and general anaesthesia. Br J Anaesth 56:581, 1984
17. Valentin N, Lomholt B, Jensen JS et al: Spinal or general anaesthesia for surgery of the fractured hip? A prospective study of mortality in 578 patients. Br J Anaesth 58:284, 1986
18. Modig J, Hjelmstedt Å, Sahlstedt B, Maripuu E: Comparitive influences of epidural and general anaesthesia on deep vein thrombosis and pulmonary embolism after hip replacement. Acta Chir Scand 147:125, 1981
19. Modig J, Borg T, Karlström G et al: Thromboembolism after total hip replacement: role of epidural and general anesthesia. Anesth Analg 62:174, 1983
20. Wille-Jorgensen P, Christensen SW, Bjerg-Nielsen A et al: Prevention of thromboembolism following elective hip surgery. The value of regional anesthesia and graded comparison stockings. Clin Orthop 247:163, 1989
21. Ferrante FM: Patient-controlled analgesia. Anesthesiol Clin North Am 10:287, 1992
22. Barron DW, Strong JE: Postoperative analgesia in major orthopedic surgery. Epidural and intrathecal opiates. Anaesthesia 36:937, 1981
23. Gjessing J, Tomlin PJ: Postoperative pain control with intrathecal morphine. Anaesthesia 36:268, 1981

24. Moore RA, Paterson GM, Bullingham RE et al: Controlled comparison of intrathecal cinchocaine with intrathecal cinchocaine and morphine. Clinical effects and plasma morphine concentrations. Br J Anaesth 56:837, 1984

25. Paterson GM, McQuay HJ, Bullingham RE, Moore RA: Intradural morphine and diamorphone. Dose response studies. Anaesthesia 39:113, 1984

26. Hedenstierna G, Lofstrom J: Effect of anaesthesia on respiratory function after major lower extremity surgery. A comparison between bupivacaine spinal analgesia with low-dose morphine and general anesthesia. Acta Anaesthesiol Scand 29:55, 1985

27. Drakeford MK, Pettine KA, Brookshire L, Ebert F: Spinal narcotics for postoperative analgesia in total joint arthroplasty. A prospective study. J Bone Joint Surg 73A:424, 1991

28. Modig J, Paalzow L: A comparison of epidural morphine and epidural bupivacaine for postoperative pain relief. Acta Anaesthesiol Scand 25:437, 1981

29. Nielsen PT, Jorgensen LN, Albrecht-Beste E et al: Lower thrombosis risk with epidural blockade in knee arthroplasty. Acta Orthop Scand 61:29, 1990

30. Sharrock NE, Haas SB, Hargett MJ et al: Effects of epidural anesthesia on the incidence of deep-vein thrombosis after total knee arthroplasty. J Bone Joint Surg 73A:502, 1991

31. Jorgensen LN, Rasmussen LS, Nielsen PE et al: Antithrombitic efficacy of continuous extradural analgesia after knee replacement. Br J Anaesth 66:8, 1991

32. Mitchell D, Friedman RJ, Baker JD III et al: Prevention of thromboembolic disease following total knee arthroplasty. Epidural versus general anesthesia. Clin Orthop 269:109, 1991

33. Raj PP, Knarr DC, Vigdorth E et al: Comparison of continuous epidural infusion of a local anesthetic and administration of systemic narcotics in the management of pain after total knee replacement surgery. Anesth Analg 66:401, 1987

34. Loper KA, Ready LB: Epidural morphine after anterior cruciate ligament repair: a comparison with patient-controlled intravenous morphine. Anesth Analg 68:350, 1989

35. Weller R, Rosenblum M, Conard P, Gross JB: Comparison of epidural and patient-controlled intravenous morphine following joint replacement surgery. Can J Anaesth 38:582, 1991

36. Ferrante FM, Orav EJ, Rocco AG, Gallo J: A statistical model for pain in patient-controlled analgesia and conventional intramuscular opioid regimens. Anesth Analg 67:457, 1988

37. Jacobson L, Kokri MS, Pridie AK: Intrathecal diamorphone: a dose-response study. Ann R Coll Surg Engl 71:289, 1989

38. Loper KA, Ready LB, Downey M et al: Epidural and intravenous fentanyl infusions are clinically equivalent after knee surgery. Anesth Analg 70:72, 1990

39. Pierrot M, Blaise M, Dupuy A et al: Peridural analgesia with high doses of fentanyl: failure of the method for early postoperative kinesitherapy in knee surgery. Can Anaesth Soc J 29:587, 1982

40. Nielsen PT, Blom H, Nielsen SE: Less pain with epidural morphione after knee arthroplasty. Acta Orthop Scand 60:447, 1989

41. Baker MW, Tullos AS, Bryan WJ, Oxspring H: The use of epidural morphine in patients undergoing total knee arthroplasty. J Arthroplasty 4:157, 1989

42. Pettine KA, Wedel DJ, Cabanella ME, Weeks JL: The use of epidural bupivacaine following total knee arthroplasty. Orthop Rev 18:894, 1989

43. Ulrich C, Burri C, Worsdorfer O: Continuous passive motion after knee-joint arthrolysis under catheter peridural anesthesia. Arch Orthop Trauma Surg 104:346, 1986

44. Mogensen T, Hjortsø NC, Bigler D et al: Unpredictability of regression of analgesia during the continuous postoperative extradural infusion of bupivacaine. Br J Anaesth 60:515, 1988
45. Mogensen T, Scott NB, Hjortsø NC et al: The influence of volume and concentration of bupivacaine on regression of analgesia during continuous postoperative epidural infusion. Reg Anesth 13:122, 1988
46. Renck H, Edstrøm H, Kinnberger B, Brandt G: Thoracic epidural analgesia II. Prolongation in the early postoperative period by continuous injection of 1% bupivacaine. Acta Anaesthesiol Scand 20:47, 1976
47. Lund C, Mogensen T, Hjortsø NC, Kehlet H: Systemic morphine enhances spread of sensory analgesia during postoperative epidural bupivacaine infusion. Lancet ii: 1156, 1985
48. Hjortsø NC, Lund C, Mogensen T et al: Epidural morphine improves pain relief and maintains sensory analgesia during continuous bupivacaine after abdominal surgery. Anesth Analg 65:1033, 1986
49. Mahoney OM, Noble PC, Davidson J, Tullos HS: The effect of continuous epidural analgesia on postoperative pain, rehabilitation, and duration of hospitalization in total knee arthroplasty. Clin Orthop 260:30, 1990
50. Badner NH, Reimer EJ, Komar WE, Moote CA: Low-dose bupivacaine does not improve postoperative epidural fentanyl analgesia in orthopaedic patients. Anesth Analg 72:337, 1991
51. Dahl JB, Rosenberg J, Hansen BL et al: Differential analgesic effects of low-dose epidural morphine and morphine-bupivacaine at rest and during mobilization after major abdominal surgery. Anesth Analg 74:362, 1992
52. Schultz P, Anker-Møller E, Dahl JB et al: Postperative pain treatment after open knee surgery: continuous lumbar plexus block with bupivacaine versus epidural morphine. Reg Anesth 16:34, 1991
53. Bader AM, Datta S, Flanagan H, Covino BG: Comparison of bupivacaine- and ropivacaine-induced conduction blockade in the isolated rabbit vagus nerve. Anesth Analg 68:724, 1989
54. Feldman HS, Arthur GR, Covino BG: Comparative systemic toxicity of convulsant and supraconvulsant doses of intravenous ropivacaine, bupivacaine, and lidocaine in the conscious dog. Anesth Analg 69:794, 1989
55. Concepcion M. Arthur GR, Steele SM et al: A new local anesthetic, ropivacaine. Its epidural effects in humans. Anesth Analg 70:80, 1990
56. Scott DB, Lee A, Fagan D et al: Acute toxicity of ropivacaine compared with that of bupivacaine. Anesth Analg 69:563, 1989
57. Peduto VA, Boero G, Marchi A, Tani R: Bilateral extensive skin necrosis of the lower limbs following prolonged epidural blockade. Can J Anaesth 35:628, 1988
58. Glynn CJ, Mather LE, Cousins MJ et al: Peridural meperidine in humans: analgesic response, pharmacokinetics and transmission into CSF. Anesthesiology 55:520, 1981
59. Sjöström S, Hartvig D, Tamsen A: Patient-controlled analgesia with extradural morphine or pethidine. Br J Anaesth 60:358, 1988
60. Famewo CE, Naguib M: Spinal analgesia with meperidine as the sole agent. Can Anaesth Soc J 32:533, 1985
61. Acalovschi I, Ene V, Lorinczi E, Nicolaus F: Saddle block with pethidine for perineal operations. Br J Anaesth 58:1012, 1986
62. Sangarlangkarn S, Klaewtanong V, Jonglerttrakool P, Khankaew V: Meperidine as a spinal anesthetic agent: a comparison with lidocaine-glucose. Anesth Analg 66: 235, 1987

63. Power I, Brown DT, Wildsmith JAW: The effect of fentanyl, meperidine, and diamorphine on nerve conduction in vitro. Reg Anesth 16:204, 1991

64. Weiker GG, Kuivila TE, Pippinger CE: Serum lidocaine and bupivacaine levels in local technique knee arthroscopy. Am J Sports Med 19:499, 1991

65. Moulin M, Debruyne D, Thomassin C et al: Comparison of the course of blood levels of bupivacaine and prilocaine after intra-articular irrigation administration for arthroscopy of the knee. Therapie 40:217, 1985

66. White AP, Laurent S, Wilkinson DJ: Intra-articular and subcutaneous prilocaine with adrenaline for pain relief in day case arthroscopy of the knee joint. Ann R Coll Surg Engl 72:350, 1990

67. Debruyne D, Moulin M, Carnes C et al: Monitoring serum bupivacaine levels during arthroscopy. Eur J Clin Pharmacol 27:733, 1985

68. Katz JA, Kaeding CS, Hill JR, Henthorn TK: The pharmacokinetics of bupivacaine when injected intraarticularly after knee arthroscopy. Anesth Analg 67:872, 1988

69. Solanki DR, Enneking FK, Ivey FM et al: Serum bupivacaine concentrations after intraarticular injection for pain relief after knee arthroscopy. Arthroscopy 8:44, 1992

70. Butterworth JF IV, Carnes RS III, Samuel MP et al: Effects of adrenaline on plasma concentrations of bupivacaine following intra-articular injection of bupivacaine for knee arthroscopy. Br J Anaesth 65:537, 1990

71. Henderson RC, Campion ER, DeMasi RA, Taft TN: Postarthroscopy analgesia with bupivacaine. A prospective, randomized, blinded evaluation. Am J Sports Med 18:614, 1990

72. Milligan KA, Mowbray MJ, Mulrooney L, Standen PJ: Intra-articular bupivacaine for pain relief after arthroscopic surgery of the knee joint in day case patients. Anaesthesia 43:563, 1988

73. Khoury GF, Stein C, Garland DE: Intra-articular morphine for pain after knee arthroscopy (letter). Lancet ii:874, 1990

74. Stein C, Comisel K, Haimerl E et al: Analgesic effect of intraarticular morphine after arthroscopic knee surgery. N Engl J Med 325:1123, 1991

75. Conn RA, Cofield RH, Byer DE, Linstromberg JW: Interscalene block anesthesia for shoulder surgery. Clin Orthop 216:94, 1987

76. Brandl F, Taeger K: The combination of general anesthesia and interscalene block in shoulder surgery. Anaesthesist 40:537, 1991

77. Winnie AP, Ramamurthy S, Durrani Z, Radonjic R: Interscalene cervical plexus block: a single-injection technic. Anesth Analg 54:370, 1975

78. Haasio J, Tuominen M, Rosenberg PH: Continuous interscalene brachial plexus block during and after shoulder surgery. Ann Chir Gynaecol 79:103, 1990

79. Zablocki AD, Baysinger CL, Epps JL, Bucknell AL: Cervical epidural anesthesia for surgery of the shoulder. Orthop Rev 16:98, 1987

80. Melzack R: Phantom limb pain: implications for treatment of pathologic pain. Anesthesiology 35:409, 1971

81. Sherman RA, Sherman CJ, Parker L: Chronic phantom and stump pain among American veterans: results of a survey. Pain 18:83, 1984

82. Bach S, Noreng MF, Tjéllden NU: Phantom limb pain in amputees during the first 12 months following limb amputation, after preoperative lumbar epidural blockade. Pain 33:297, 1988

83. Wall PD, Gutnik M: Ongoing activity in peripheral nerves: the physiology and pharmacology of impulses generating from a neuroma. Exp Neurol 43:580, 1974

84. Omer GE Jr: Nerve, neuroma, and pain problems related to upper limb amputations. Orthop Clin North Am 12:751, 1981

85. Bromage PR, Melzack R: Phantom limbs and the body schema. Can Anesth Soc J 21:267, 1974

86. Fischer R: Out on a (phantom) limb. Variations on the theme: stability of body image and the golden section. Perspect Biol Med 12:259, 1969

87. Galindo A, Hernandez J, Benavides O et al: Quality of spinal and extradural anaesthesia: the influence of spinal nerve root diameter. Br J Anaesth 47:41, 1975

88. Singelyn FJ, Gouverneur JA, Gribomont BF: Popliteal sciatic nerve block aided by a nerve stimulator: a reliable technique for foot and ankle surgery. Reg Anaesth 16:278, 1991

89. Rorie DK, Byer DE, Nelson DO et al: Assessment of block of the sciatic nerve in the popliteal fossa. Anesth Analg 59:371, 1980

25

Postoperative Thoracic Analgesia

Simon C. Body
F. Michael Ferrante

The advent of rational protocols for the management of carcinoma of the lung in the 1980s has brought about a reversal in the declining incidence of thoracic surgery for that disease.[1] Advances in chemotherapy and radiotherapy have allowed preoperative improvement in disease status, permitting increasing numbers of patients to undergo thoracic surgery. Similar advances have also been made in the diagnosis, staging, and surgery of lymphoma and cancer of the esophagus. Thus, there has been an increasing requirement for thoracic surgery and, consequently, a renewed interest in thoracic anesthesia. In addition, enhanced knowledge of the physiology and pharmacology of the lung has placed the art of thoracic anesthesia on a more scientific footing. Despite the developments in intra-operative management, the greatest advances have been made in thoracic analgesia in the postoperative period.

Implicit in the development of the numerous modalities for provision of analgesia after thoracotomy has been the observation that earlier methods have been either inadequate, too labor-intensive, too complicated, or fraught with immediate or late side effects. This appreciation has led to the era of thoracic epidural analgesia with continuous infusions of local anesthetic and opioid in the late 1980s. This technique is not without its own risks and side effects, but has clearly become the optimal modality for postoperative pain management after thoracotomy in the 1990s.

PHYSIOLOGIC ALTERATIONS AFTER
THORACIC SURGERY

Pulmonary function is reduced to a greater extent after thoracotomy than after any other surgical procedure. The causes of respiratory dysfunction after thoracotomy are outlined in Table 25-1. Each of these factors plays a role (to a greater or lesser extent) in the genesis of postoperative respiratory depression and pulmonary failure. These processes cause decreased forced vital capacity (FVC), decreased forced expired volume in 1 second (FEV_1), and decreased functional residual capacity (FRC) (Fig. 25-1). The reductions in FEV_1 and FVC frequently reach 30 percent of preoperative values, especially in the presence of poor analgesia.[2] These changes allow the closing capacity (CC) of the lung to impinge on the FRC (Fig. 25-2). Individual alveoli and, eventually, focal lung areas develop atelectasis on both the operative and nonoperative sides, especially in the presence of high inspired oxygen concentrations.[3] The resultant atelectasis causes ventilation/perfusion (V/Q) mismatching with attendant hypoxemia and pneumonia.[4] Inadequate analgesia results in the inability to cooperate with physical therapy, poor pulmonary toilet, and poor ambulation and represents a tremendous impediment to patient recovery.

Although analgesia improves pulmonary function, most analgesic techniques carry the concomitant potential for decreasing pulmonary function. For instance, parenteral opioids can result in a blunting of the ventilatory response to

TABLE 25-1. Causes of Post-thoracotomy Respiratory Dysfunction

Factors resulting from the preoperative state of the patient
    Prior smoking, bronchospasm
    Preoperative decreased lung function

Factors resulting from residual anesthetic agents
    Decreased O_2 and CO_2 responsiveness
    Decreased cough
    Decreased sighing

Factors resulting from analgesic agents
    Decreased O_2 and CO_2 responsiveness
    Decreased cough
    Decreased sighing
    Increased sedation
    Increased risk of aspiration with vomiting

Factors resulting from surgery
    Pain
    Reduced alveolar numbers
    Decreased chest wall function
    Increased risk of pulmonary embolism
    Increased risk of vocal cord or neuronal injury

Factors with multiple etiologies
    Decreased FEV_1
    Decreased FVC
    Decreased FRC
    Increased CC/FRC ratio
    V/Q mismatch

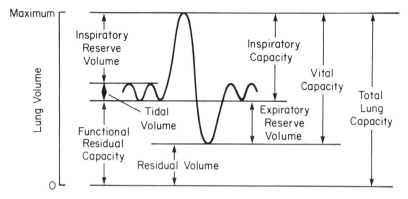

Fig. 25-1. Dynamic lung volumes as measured by simple spirometry.

hypercapnia and hypoxia.[5] In addition, the patient decreases the frequency of sighing and fails to cough. Parenteral use of opioids may cause significant sedation. Epidural and subarachnoid opioids carry similar risks. Techniques such as interpleural regional analgesia and intercostal cryotherapy have a low incidence of cardiac and pulmonary side effects. Unfortunately, these modalities are not as potent as the administration of opioids (both parenteral and spinal) for relief of pain after thoracotomy.

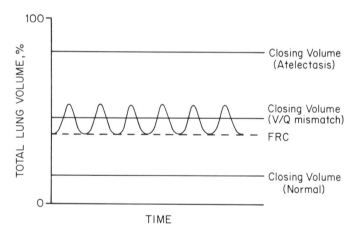

Fig. 25-2. Relationship between functional residual capacity (FRC) (*dashed line* at trough of tidal breathing curve) and the closing capacity (CC) in three physiologic states. As lung volume decreases during expiration, small airways have a tendency to close. In the presence of inadequate analgesia after thoracotomy, the volume at which some airways close may be greater than that achieved during tidal breathing (atelectasis). If the closing volume of some airways lies within tidal volume, these airways will alternately open and close during tidal breathing. Because these opening and closing airways have a shorter time than normal for fresh gas exchange, ventilation/perfusion mismatching occurs. (In the normal state, the closing volumes of all airways are always below the volumes attendant to tidal breathing, and no airways are closed at any time.)

ANALGESIC MODALITIES

Parenteral Opioids

Although the development of the hollow needle and syringe in 1853 was a huge advance in analgesia, it took more than a century to show that most patients receive inadequate dosages or insufficient frequency of administration (see Ch. 1). The literature (summarized by Ferrante and Covino[6]) clearly shows that at least 50 percent of patients do not obtain adequate analgesia. This problem is especially marked after thoracic and upper abdominal surgery when concerns over adequacy of respiration have mistakenly caused the withholding of analgesics. This perception, along with a misguided fear of addiction,[7] the highly variable individual requirements for opioids,[8] the unreliable absorption after intramuscular (IM) injection,[9] and the nursing effort required for scheduled around-the-clock administration[10] result in underadministration of opioids. Because of these factors, the incidence of inadequate analgesia probably exceeds 50 percent in post-thoracotomy patients receiving conventional opioid regimens.

Patient-controlled analgesia (PCA) has to some extent resolved several of these issues. Obese patients undergoing upper abdominal surgery have been shown to have better pulmonary function with intravenous-PCA (IV-PCA) than with conventional regimens of IM opioids.[11] In a study of post-thoracotomy patients receiving PCA-administered or IM buprenorphine, patients in the IV-PCA group were found to have fewer postoperative radiographic pulmonary abnormalities (atelectasis), use less drug, and have a lower incidence of postoperative fever.[12]

IV-PCA has significant advantages over intermittent IM opioids. However, compared with epidural analgesia, IV-PCA provides poorer analgesia with more sedation.[13–15]

Intercostal Neural Blockade

Conventional intercostal nerve blocks (the injection of 3–5 ml of local anesthetic into individual intercostal spaces at multiple levels) has been used for decades to provide analgesia after thoracotomy. It may be performed by the surgeon while the lung is collapsed[16] or percutaneously by the anesthesiologist after chest closure.[17]

The beneficial effects of intercostal neural blockade on pulmonary function are well known.[18–20] The major disadvantages of the technique include (1) a small risk of pneumothorax (although the incidence is further reduced in thoracotomy patients because of the presence of thoracostomy tubes), (2) the necessity for multiple injections, (3) the requirement for administration of a large dose of local anesthetic, and (4) the short duration of analgesia.

The technique of continuous intercostal neural blockade (see Ch. 15) can circumvent many of the shortcomings of conventional multilevel injection. Continuous intercostal neural blockade involves catheterization of an intercostal space and injection of a large volume of local anesthetic (10–20 ml) to provide analgesia over a large number of thoracic dermatomes.[21,22] A comparison of continuous intercostal neural blockade versus thoracic or lumbar epidural analgesia for the management of post-thoracotomy pain has not been performed.

Interpleural Regional Analgesia

The technique of interpleural regional analgesia[23] (see Ch. 16) is easy to perform, and originally it was hoped to be a simple answer to the problem of post-thoracotomy pain. Although there are sporadic reports of its efficacy,[24] the overwhelming majority of studies have documented inadequate analgesia.[25–27]

The reasons for the failure of interpleural regional analgesia to achieve satisfactory pain relief in the thoracotomy patient are multifactorial. At least one-third of any intrapleural injection is lost through thoracostomy tube drainage.[25,26] The tissue edema and extravasation of tissue fluid attendant on surgical incision and manipulation of the thorax form an actual physical barrier for diffusion of local anesthetic to nerve.[27] Intrathoracic collections of blood and exudate will dilute and bind local anesthetic (protein-binding).[25] The distribution of local anesthetic throughout the interpleural space by normal respiratory movement of the lung will be altered. Restricted motion of an operated lung (or lack thereof) may cause uneven spread, channeling of flow, and sequestration of local anesthetic.[27]

The advocates of interpleural regional analgesia for post-thoracotomy pain have attributed poor efficacy to improper technique.[28] Remaining supporters suggest administration of large volumes of local anesthetic at high concentrations (30–40 ml of 0.5 percent bupivacaine) with clamping of the thoracostomy tube for 15 minutes.[28] However, no published study to date has used such a regimen, and the potential for significant systemic toxicity may be significant. In the face of accumulating evidence, it is incumbent on the advocates of interpleural analgesia to demonstrate its safety and efficacy for post-thoracotomy pain. Until such data are available, it is wise for the individual practitioner to use other techniques for post-thoracotomy analgesia.

Paravertebral Neural Blockade

Unlike interpleural regional analgesia, continuous thoracic paravertebral neural blockade (see Ch. 17) can provide excellent and predictable analgesia.[29–31] Similar to continuous intercostal neural blockade, this technique is underused, probably because of the fear of potential pneumothorax.[32] In thoracotomy patients, however, the incidence of pneumothorax should be limited by the presence of thoracostomy tubes. Until more widespread experience is gained with this modality, the ultimate applicability of paravertebral neural blockade for the treatment of post-thoracotomy pain will remain undefined.

Cryoanalgesia

Cryoanalgesia involves application of low temperatures to nerves to produce anesthesia or analgesia[33] (Fig. 25-3). The most common type of cryoprobe causes freezing by expansion of high-pressure nitrous oxide (N_2O) through a

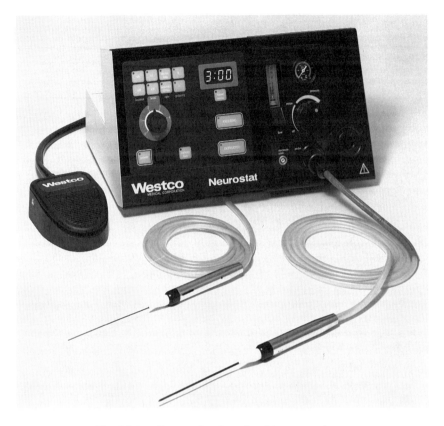

Fig. 25-3. Cryoanalgesia unit with cryoprobes.

small orifice at the tip of the probe (Fig. 25-4). Freezing of tissue occurs because of the latent heat of vaporization of N_2O (or carbon dioxide). Temperatures of $-75°C$ in the tip of the probe and $-20°C$ in the nerve are achieved.[33,34] Maiwand et al[35] have shown that optimal blockade is achieved when each nerve is cooled for at least 30 seconds. A single freeze cycle, instead of two 30-second freeze cycles, is associated with a 1-month period of analgesia and a reduced incidence of dysesthesia. Use of a single freeze cycle will still cause neuronal injury. However, the endoneurium is spared, thus allowing neuronal regrowth over time.[35]

A number of authors[35–37] have published their experiences with cryoanalgesia of the intercostal nerves. The largest series is that of Maiwand et al.[35] In more than 600 cases, analgesia persisted for 1–3 months, facilitating enhanced cooperation with physical therapy and decreased need for supplemental opioids.

The intensity of analgesia associated with cryoanalgesia is incomplete and inferior to that provided by epidural opioids.[38] Cryoanalgesia does not significantly improve pulmonary function[39] as compared with intercostal nerve blocks or opioids,[38] and supplemental opioid administration is required with cryoanal-

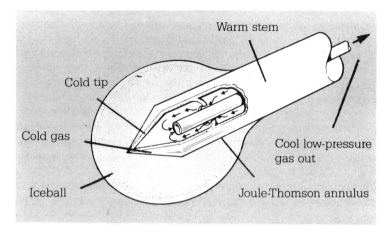

Fig. 25-4. Nerve freezing is accomplished by expanding high-pressure N_2O or CO_2 gas through a small orifice (Joule-Thomson annulus). This causes heat to be withdrawn from the cryoprobe tip.

gesia.[22,36] The risks of cryoanalgesia include neuronal destruction with subsequent neuralgia,[40] intercostal artery avulsion, spinal cord injury by direct cold, nipple anesthesia,[35] and intercostal motor blockade.[33]

Transcutaneous Electrical Nerve Stimulation

Some investigators have described good post-thoracotomy analgesia with transcutaneous electrical nerve stimulation (TENS).[41–43] However, as discussed in Chapter 20, a direct causal relationship between stimulation and analgesia has not been defined. TENS is noninvasive and safe. The use of TENS is worth consideration, especially in clinical situations where the use of opioids or regional anesthesia/analgesia is problematic.

Subarachnoid Opioids

The use of subarachnoid opioids for post-thoracotomy pain is greatly limited by the necessity for repetitive injections, owing to the potential dangers of continuous subarachnoid catheterization. Although single administrations of subarachnoid morphine have been used to provide 18–24 hours of pain relief after thoracotomy,[44,45] the problem of subsequent provision of analgesia remains. Because the epidural route of administration can provide continuous analgesia, it has generally replaced subarachnoid administration.

Epidural Local Anesthetics and Opioids

Local Anesthetics

There is a large amount of clinical experience with the use of local anesthetics as the sole analgesic for thoracic epidural analgesia.[2,29,46–49] Thoracic epidural analgesia with local anesthetics produces analgesia similar to intercostal neural blockade, with improved pulmonary function and decreased opioid requirements. However, provision of thoracic epidural analgesia with local anesthetics alone requires concentrations that produce a significant incidence of hypotension[29,46,47] and sedation.[46] Combinations of local anesthetic and opioid administered to the thoracic epidural space allow use of lower concentrations of local anesthetic while providing excellent analgesia (see below).

Opioids

Treatment of post-thoracotomy pain with epidural opioids has several advantages: (1) no sympathetic blockade is obtained; (2) there is no motor blockade or sensory anesthesia, and (3) analgesia is profound and predictable. Liphophilic (fentanyl,[38,50–52] sufentanil,[53–55] and methadone[56]) and hydrophilic (hydromorphone,[57] morphine[48,58–62]) opioids have been used successfully.

Thoracic or Lumbar Epidural Placement

At least with respect to the administration of epidural morphine alone, there appears to be a consensus regarding the question of optimal location for catheter placement.[62,63] Morphine is equally efficacious for treatment of upper abdominal or thoracic postoperative pain when administered to the thoracic or lumbar epidural space. This is to be expected in view of the partition coefficient of morphine and its hydrophilic properties (see Ch. 11). Because of its hydrophilic behavior, morphine will spread rostrally in cerebrospinal fluid (CSF)[64] and can effectively treat pain over a wide number of dermatomes. Morphine has been administered by intermittent injection[58–60,62] or continuous infusion[61] to treat post-thoracotomy pain. Administration of smaller doses of morphine is advisable in the thoracic as compared with the lumbar epidural space.[65] Use of thoracic morphine is associated with a higher incidence of delayed respiratory depression.[66]

However, there is considerable debate regarding the optimal catheter location for epidural administration of lipophilic opioids. Thoracic administration of analgesics has the theoretic advantage of delivering drug directly to the spinal cord segments immediately involved in nociceptive transmission. With respect to lipophilic opioids, direct thoracic administration may allow a greater spinal rather than supraspinal (systemic) effect. Thoracic catheter placement may decrease the dose requirement for opioid (and local anesthetic), thereby reducing the incidence of side effects from systemic absorption of opioids.

Evidence is accumulating to suggest that these suppositions are true. Chamberlain et al[51] compared lumbar versus thoracic epidural administration of fentanyl using epidural PCA. (Use of a patient-controlled modality allows patients to find their own dose ranges without the influence of experimenter bias.) Patients receiving thoracic fentanyl required less opioid and obtained better pain scores.[51] Panos et al[52] compared lumbar epidural and intravenous administration of fentanyl for post-thoracotomy pain. Although different infusion rates were used between sites, the quality of analgesia was dependent on the plasma fentanyl level. The data indicated that lumbar fentanyl achieved analgesia through systemic absorption of the opioid rather than a direct spinal effect. The supraspinal mechanism of action for lumbar administration of epidural fentanyl has also been corroborated in patients undergoing lower abdominal and lower extremity surgery.[67,68]

Combinations of Local Anesthetics and Opioids

There is much evidence to suggest that coadministration of local anesthetics and opioids may have a synergistic interaction, improving analgesic effect while at the same time reducing the dose requirement for each agent.[69–72] Coupled with the preceding arguments regarding the advisability of thoracic administration of lipophilic opioids, coadministration of local anesthetics and lipophilic opioids in the thoracic epidural space would seem optimal.

Great fear has been associated with the use of local anesthetics in the midthoracic space because of the potential for profound hypotension.[47] (See Ch. 18 for a discussion of the cardiovascular effects of thoracic epidural analgesia.) Maintenance of the patient in a relatively hypovolemic state because of the fear of post-thoracotomy pulmonary edema will accentuate the potential for hypotension.[73,74] As described earlier, the intermittent administration of local anesthetics has been associated with an appreciable incidence of hypotension.[29,47] Use of infusions rather than intermittent injections probably results in fewer episodes of hypotension, especially if dilute concentrations are used in the infusions.[46]

Quite interestingly, little data exist regarding combinational therapy for thoracic epidural analgesia. Logas et al[48] found no difference in analgesic efficacy between thoracic epidural morphine and thoracic epidural morphine and bupivacaine. However, George et al[75] found enhanced analgesia and pulmonary function in post-thoracotomy patients receiving continuous thoracic epidural fentanyl and 0.2 percent bupivacaine in comparison with thoracic epidural fentanyl alone. However, differences between groups were obscured by the second postoperative day. Of note, the incidence of side effects attributable to fentanyl was appreciable, but hypotension did not occur.[75]

As reviewed by Dahl et al,[70] the results of studies comparing epidural local anesthetic/opioid combinations with epidural opioids for other surgical procedures are contradictory.[48,72,76–80] No benefit has been documented from the addition of local anesthetic in most clinical studies.[48,78–80] However, in none of these studies was pain assessed during activity. As Dahl et al[70] so elegantly demonstrated, the combination of low-dose thoracic epidural bupivacaine and morphine enhanced mobilization and coughing after major abdominal surgery as compared with thoracic epidural morphine alone. The improved ability to clear secretions and the improved mobilization associated with combinational therapy has lead to its adoption as the standard for treatment of post-thoracotomy pain at Brigham and Women's Hospital.

Respiratory Effects

There is good evidence to show that the inevitable respiratory changes seen after thoracic surgery can be attenuated by thoracic epidural anesthesia/analgesia.[60,75,81,82] The beneficial effects on pulmonary function are denoted by improvement in FRC, FVC, FEV_1, the alveolar-to-arterial oxygen gradient (A-a DO_2), peak flow, and radiographic appearance. Diaphragmatic function is also improved.[2] Improvement in these parameters of pulmonary function can occur despite intercostal motor blockade attendant on the use of high concentrations of local anesthetic. The ventilatory response to hypercapnia, however, is blunted after thoracic epidural blockade with local anesthetics, probably as a result of intercostal motor blockade.[83] It is probable that the improved pulmonary function lowers the incidence of postoperative pulmonary complications.

Unfortunately, epidural opioids are associated with a moderate incidence of mild respiratory depression and a small incidence of severe respiratory depression from systemic absorption of lipophilic opioids or rostral spread of hydrophilic opioids. Shulman et al[60,84] have demonstrated that lumbar epidural morphine provides better analgesia and improves FVC and FEV_1, as compared to intravenous administration of morphine. However, an incidence of respiratory depression of 27 percent has been reported after thoracic epidural administration of morphine.[61]

There is a very low incidence of severe respiratory depression associated with thoracic epidural administration of fentanyl, although mild respiratory depression ($pCO_2 > 50$ mm Hg) can be quite frequent. Such repeated mild hypercarbia may, in actuality, be due to relative overdosage. Welchew[85] has reported that the optimal concentration for infusion of thoracic epidural fentanyl alone is between 5–10 µg/ml. Higher concentrations confer no advantages.[85] The analgesic synergy achieved with combined epidural infusion of local anesthetic and fentanyl allows administration of lower concentrations of fentanyl. A fentanyl concentration of 5 µg/ml is optimal when infused with a local anesthetic, and results in a lower incidence of respiratory depression and sedation.

There are several reports of severe respiratory depression associated with the thoracic epidural administration of sufentanil.[53–55]

PROTOCOL FOR THE MANAGEMENT OF POST-THORACOTOMY THORACIC EPIDURAL ANALGESIA

The previous discussion suggests that the optimal modality for treatment of post-thoracotomy pain is a continuous thoracic epidural infusion of local anesthetic and opioid. Of course, the epidural catheter must be placed within a few segments of the surgical incision in order to optimize delivery of analgesic to the area of the cord receiving afferent nociceptive transmission. Our practice at Brigham and Women's Hospital is listed below and in Table 25-2.

TABLE 25-2. Protocol for Thoracic Epidural Analgesia with Combinations of Local Anesthetic and Opioid

Midthoracic epidural catheterization (T5T6, T6T7, or T7T8) is performed before surgery

Test dosing is always performed to confirm placement (2-ml aliquots of 2 percent lidocaine with 1:200,000 epinephrine at 5-min intervals ×2)

Re-establish sensory anesthesia prior to the end of surgery (2-ml aliquots of 2 percent lidocaine with 1:200,000 epinephrine at 5-min intervals ×2)

Start initial postoperative infusion at 3–5 ml/h (0.125 percent bupivacaine with 5 μg/ml fentanyl or 0.125 percent bupivacaine with 1–2.5 mg/ml meperidine)

1. Midthoracic epidural catheterization is performed preoperatively in an awake, sedated patient.
2. Confirmation of correct placement is performed by preoperative test dosing of the catheter with 2 percent lidocaine with 1:200,000 epinephrine. Test dosing should be performed using 2-ml aliquots at 5-minute intervals. Loss of sensation over the midthoracic dermatomes is used as confirmation of correct placement.
3. The thoracic epidural can be used intraoperatively (if so desired, although not essential), provided significant blood loss is not anticipated. Repeated injections of 0.25 percent bupivacaine with 5 μg/ml of fentanyl[85] can be administered as blood pressure allows. Two milliliters should be administered no more frequently than every 20 minutes. More frequent administration or larger volumes of injection can result in undesired hypotension.
4. The epidural catheter should be injected before the end of surgery to ensure adequate analgesia on emergence. Alternatively, the postoperative epidural infusion (Table 25-3) can be commenced during the operative period.
5. Initial postoperative infusion rates are 3–5 ml/h. Infusion rates can be adjusted as blood pressure permits.
6. The patient is monitored with ECG, pulse oximetry, and periodic blood gases on a 1:1 or 1:2 nursing basis (at least until the first postoperative day). In-hospital 24-hour acute pain service coverage is recommended.

Dosage guidelines for use of opioids alone for thoracic epidural analgesia, as well as suggestions for the treatment of breakthrough pain, are found in Table 25-3.

SPECIFIC PROBLEMS IN POST-THORACOTOMY ANALGESIA

Shoulder pain on the operative side represents an occasional but annoying problem after thoracotomy. Shoulder pain can occur despite the presence of complete chest wall analgesia. The etiology is unclear but may be due to diaphragmatic irritation carried by phrenic afferents, by referred pain from intercostal innervation of the diaphragm, or by true pain in the area of the cupola of

TABLE 25-3. Dosage Guidelines for Thoracic Epidural Analgesia

Test dose
  2 ml of 2% lidocaine $\times$2 at 5-min intervals

Opioids
  Intermittent injection
    Fentanyl 50–100 µg in 10 ml preservative-free saline[a]
    Meperidine 30–100 mg
    Morphine 1–2 mg
  Infusion[b]
    Fentanyl 30–100 µg/h
    Meperidine 10–25 mg/h

Local anesthetic and opioid
  Infusion[b]
    0.125% bupivacaine with 3–5 µg/ml fentanyl at 3–7 ml/h
    0.125% bupivacaine with 1–2.5 mg/ml meperidine at 3–7 ml/h

"Rescue" for breakthrough pain
  Increase infusion rate after
    Fentanyl 50–100 µg in 10 ml preservative-free saline[a]
    Meperidine 30–50 mg
    2 ml of 2% lidocaine $\times$1 or $\times$2 at 5-min intervals
    Ketorolac 60 IM or IV then 30 mg IM or IV q6h

[a] Diluent volume affects time of onset and duration of analgesia with a single injection of epidural fentanyl. Administration of fentanyl in a volume of 10 ml will optimize time of onset and duration of analgesia. No such effect has been described for morphine or meperidine, though meperidine is customarily administered in a volume of 10 ml.

[b] The use of continuous infusions of morphine into the thoracic epidural space is not suggested. Excessive administration of morphine in the thoracic epidural space enhances the risk of late respiratory depression.

the lung caused by thoracostomy tube irritation.[86] Possible therapies include: (1) supplemental administration of epidural analgesics, (2) injection of 20–25 ml of 0.5 percent bupivacaine with 1:200,000 epinephrine through the chest tube with clamping of the tube for 10–15 minutes (interpleural regional analgesia)[87], (3) administration of IM or IV ketorolac, or (4) pulling the thoracostomy tube back 2–5 cm. Administration of ketorolac is the most successful of these modalities. In the presence of hypovolemia, however, there is an enhanced risk of nephrotoxicity associated with the liberal use of ketorolac and other nonsteroidal anti-inflammatory drugs (NSAIDs)[88,89] (see Ch. 7). As a result, the use of ketorolac and other NSAIDs should be judicious, and renal function should be carefully monitored.

CONCLUSION

The management of post-thoracotomy pain has always been a vexing problem. The problem of post-thoracotomy pain, however, is particularly amenable to regional analgesic techniques. Use of thoracic epidural analgesia and combinations of local anesthetics and opioids can greatly relieve pain and enhance mobilization. There are few clinical situations in which the results of regional analgesia are so dramatic or gratifying.

References

1. Naruke T, Goya T, Tsuchiya R, Suemasu K: Prognosis and survival in resected lung carcinoma based on the new international staging system. J Thorac Cardiovasc Surg 96:440, 1988

2. Mankikian B, Cantineau JP, Bertrand M et al: Improvement of diaphragmatic function by a thoracic extradural block after upper abdominal surgery. Anesthesiology 68:379, 1988

3. Dantzker DR, Wagner PD, West JB: Proceedings: Instability of poorly ventilated lung units during oxygen breathing. J Physiol (Lond) 242:72P, 1974

4. Lockwood P: Respiratory function and cardiopulmonary complications following thoracotomy for carcinoma of the lung. Respiration 29:468, 1972

5. Weil JV, McCullough RE, Kline JS, Sodal IE: Diminished ventilatory response to hypoxia and hypercapnia after morphine in normal man. N Engl J Med 292:1103, 1975

6. Ferrante FM, Covino BG: Patient controlled analgesia: an historical perspective. In: Ferrante FM, Ostheimer GW, Covino BG (eds): Patient-Controlled Analgesia. Blackwell Scientific, Boston, 1990

7. Marks RM, Sachar EJ: Undertreatment of medical inpatients with narcotic analgesics. Ann Intern Med 78:173, 1973

8. Austin KL, Stapleton JV, Mather LE: Relationship between blood meperidine concentrations and analgesic response: a preliminary report. Anesthesiology 53:460, 1980

9. Austin KL, Stapleton JV, Mather LE: Multiple intramuscular injections: a major source of variability in analgesic response to meperidine. Pain 8:47, 1980

10. Graves DA, Foster TS, Batenhorst RL et al: Patient-controlled analgesia. Ann Intern Med 99:360, 1983

11. Bennett RL, Batenhorst RL, Foster TS et al: Postoperative pulmonary function with patient-controlled analgesia, abstracted. Anesth Analg 61:171, 1982

12. Lange MP, Dahn MS, Jacobs LA: Patient-controlled analgesia versus intermittent analgesia dosing. Heart Lung 17:495, 1988

13. Eisenach JC, Grice SC, Dewan DM: Patient-controlled analgesia following cesarean section: a comparison with epidural and intramuscular narcotics. Anesthesiology 68:444, 1988

14. Harrison DM, Sinatra R, Morgese L, Chung JH: Epidural narcotic and patient-controlled analgesia for postcesarean section pain relief. Anesthesiology 68:454, 1988

15. Purves PG, Sperring SJ, Dykes V, Stanley TD: Improved post-operative analgesia: epidural vs patient controlled intravenous morphine, abstracted. Anesth Analg 66: S143, 1987

16. Skretting P: Hypotension after intercostal nerve block during thoracotomy under general anaesthesia. Br J Anaesth 53:527, 1981

17. Moore DC: Intercostal nerve block for postoperative somatic pain following surgery of the thorax and upper abdomen. Br J Anaesth, suppl. 47:289, 1975

18. Bergh NP, Dottori O, Lof BA et al: Effects of intercostal blockade or lung function after thoracotomy. Acta Anaesthesiol Scand, suppl. 24:85, 1966

19. Faust RJ, Nauss LA: Post-thoracotomy intercostal block: comparison of its effect on pulmonary function with those of intramuscular meperidine. Anesth Analg 55: 542, 1976

20. Toledo-Pereyra LH, DeMeester TR: Prospective randomized evaluation of intrathoracic intercostal nerve block with bupivacaine on postoperative ventilatory function. Ann Thorac Surg 27:203, 1979

21. Kaplan JA, Miller ED Jr, Gallagher EG Jr: Postoperative analgesia for thoracotomy patients. Anesth Analg 54:773, 1975
22. de la Roche AG, Chambers K: Pain amelioration after thoracotomy: a prospective, randomized study. Ann Thorac Surg 37:239, 1984
23. Reiestad F, Strømskag KE: Interpleural catheter in the management of postoperative pain. A preliminary report. Reg Anesth 11:89, 1986
24. Kambam JR, Hammon J, Parris WCV, Lupinetti FM: Intrapleural analgesia for post-thoracotomy pain and blood levels of bupivacaine following intrapleural injection. Can J Anaesth 36:106, 1989
25. Ferrante FM, Chan VWS, Arthur GR, Rocco AG: Interpleural analgesia after thoracotomy. Anesth Analg 72:105, 1991
26. Rosenberg PH, Scheinin BM-A, Lepäntalo MJA, Lindfors O: Continuous intrapleural infusion of bupivacaine for analgesia after thoracotomy. Anesthesiology 67: 811, 1987
27. El-Baz N: The experts opine. Interpleural analgesia: advantages and limitations in comparison to thoracic epidural analgesia (editorial). Survey Anesthesiol 23:193, 1989
28. Reiestad F, McIlvaine WB: The experts opine. Interpleural analgesia: advantages and limitations in comparison to thoracic epidural analgesia. Survey Anesthesiol 23: 188, 1989
29. Matthews PJ, Govenden V: Comparison of continuous paravertebral and extradural infusions of bupivacaine for pain relief after thoracotomy. Br J Anaesth 62:204, 1989
30. Purcell-Jones G, Pither CE, Justin DM: Paravertebral somatic block: a clinical, radiographic, and computed tomographic study in chronic pain patients. Anesth Analg 68:32, 1989
31. Eason MJ, Wyatt R: Paravertebral thoracic block—a reappraisal. Anaesthesia 34: 638, 1979
32. Conacher ID, Kokri M: Postoperative paravertebral blocks for thoracic surgery. A radiological appraisal. Br J Anaeth 59:155, 1987
33. Evans PJ: Cryoanalgesia. The application of low temperatures to nerves to produce anaesthesia or analgesia. Anaesthesia 36:1003, 1981
34. Nehme AE, Wardield CA: Cryoanalgesia: freezing of peripheral nerves. Hosp Pract 22:71, 1987
35. Maiwand MO, Makey AR, Rees A: Cryoanalgesia after thoracotomy. Improvement of technique and review of 600 cases. J Thorac Cardiovasc Surg 92:291, 1986
36. Nelson KM, Vincent RG, Bourke RS et al: Intraoperative intercostal nerve freezing to prevent post-thoracotomy pain. Ann Thorac Surg 18:280, 1974
37. Katz J, Nelson W, Forest R, Bruce DL: Cryoanalgesia for post-thoracotomy pain. Lancet 1:512, 1980
38. Gough JD, Williams AB, Vaugh RS et al: The control of post-thoracotomy pain. A comparative evaluation of thoracic epidural fentanyl infusions and cryo-analgesia. Anaesthesia 43:780, 1988
39. Rooney SM, Jain S, McCormack P et al: A comparison of pulmonary function tests for postthoracotomy pain using cryoanalgesia and transcutaneous nerve stimulation. Ann Thorac Surg 41:204, 1986
40. Conacher ID, Locke T, Hilton C: Neuralgia after cryoanalgesia for thoracotomy (letter). Lancet i:277, 1986
41. Rooney SM, Jain S, Goldiner PL: Effect of transcutaneous nerve stimulation on postoperative pain after thoracotomy. Anesth Analg 62:1010, 1983
42. Stratton SA, Smith MM: Postoperative thoracotomy. Effects of transcutaneous electrical nerve stimulation on forced vital capacity. Phys Ther 60:45, 1980

43. Warfield CA, Stein JM, Frank HA: The effect of transcutaneous electrical nerve stimulation on pain after thoracotomy. Ann Thorac Surg 39:462, 1985

44. Katz J, Nelson W: Intrathecal morphine for postoperative pain relief. Reg Anesth 6:1, 1981

45. Gray JR, Fromme GA, Nauss LA et al: Intrathecal morphine for post-thoracotomy pain. Anesth Analg 65:873, 1985

46. Griffiths DPG, Diamond AW, Cameron JD: Postoperative extradural analgesia following thoracic surgery. a feasibility study. Br J Anaesth 47:48, 1975

47. Conacher ID, Paes ML, Jacobson L et al: Epidural analgesia following thoracic surgery. A review of two years' experience. Anaesthesia 38:546, 1983

48. Logas WG, El-Baz N, El-Ganzouri A et al: Continuous thoracic epidural analgesia for postoperative pain relief following thoracotomy: a randomized prospective study. Anesthesiology 67:787, 1987

49. James EC, Kolberg HL, Iwen GW, Gellatly TA: Epidural analgesia for post-thoracotomy patients. J Thorac Cardiovasc Surg 82:898, 1981

50. Welchew EA, Thornton JA: Continuous thoracic epidural fentanyl. A comparison of epidural fentanyl with intramuscular papaveretum for postoperative pain. Anaesthesia 37:309, 1982

51. Chamberlain DP, Bodily MN, Olssen GL, Ramsey DH: Comparison of lumbar versus thoracic epidural fentanyl for post-thoracotomy analgesia using patient controlled dosage, abstracted. Reg Anesth 14:26S, 1989

52. Panos L, Sandler AN, Stringer DG et al: Continuous infusions of lumbar epidural fentanyl and intravenous fentanyl for post-thoracotomy pain relief. I. Analgesic and pharmacokinetic effects. Can J Anaesth, suppl. 37: 66, 1990

53. Rosseel PM, van den Broek WGM, Boer EC, Prakash O: Epidural sufentanil for intra- and post operative analgesia in thoracic surgery: a comparative study with intravenous sufentanil. Acta Anaesthesiol Scand 32:193, 1988

54. Whiting WC, Sandler AN, Lau LC et al: Analgesic and respiratory effects of epidural sufentanil in patients following thoracotomy. Anesthesiology 69:36, 1988

55. Hasenbos MA, Gielen MJM, Bos J et al: High thoracic epidural sufentanil for post-thoracotomy pain: influence of epinephrine as an adjuvant—a double blind study. Anesthesiology 69:1017, 1988

56. Welch DB, Hrynaszkiewicz A: Postoperative analgesia using epidural methadone. Administration by the lumbar route for thoracic pain relief. Anaesthesia 36:1051, 1981

57. Shulman MS, Wakerlin G, Yamaguchi LY, Brodsky JB: Experience with lumbar hydromorphone for post-thoracotomy pain relief. Anesth Analg 66:1331, 1987

58. Fromme GA, Steidl LJ, Danielson DR: Comparison of lumbar and thoracic epidural morphine for relief of post-thoracotomy pain. Anesth Analg 64:454, 1985

59. Baxter AD, Samson B, Penning J et al: Prevention of epidural morphine-induced respiratory depression with intravenous nalbupine infusion in post-thoracotomy patients. Can J Anaesth 36:503, 1989

60. Shulman M, Sandler AN, Bradley JW et al: Postthoracotomy pain and pulmonary function following epidural and systemic morphine. Anesthesiology 61:569, 1984

61. El-Baz NM, Faber LP, Jensik RJ: Continuous epidural infusion of morphine for treatment of pain after thoracic surgery: a new technique. Anesth Analg 63:757, 1984

62. Pelliccia E, Falchi C, Angelotti G, Lombardi M: Postoperative analgesia with peridural morphine. Comparative study in thoracic and abdominal surgery. Minerva Anestesiol 54:521, 1988

63. Larsen VH, Iversen P, Christensen P, Andersen PK: Postoperative pain treatment after upper abdominal surgery with epidural morphine at thoracic or lumbar level. Acta Anesthesiol Scand 29:566, 1985

64. Bromage PR, Camporesi EM, Durant PAC, Nielsen CH: Rostral spread of epidural morphine. Anesthesiology 56:431, 1982

65. Ready LB: Spinal opioids in the management of acute and postoperative pain. J Pain Symptom Manage 5:138, 1990

66. Cousins MJ, Mather LE: Intrathecal and epidural administration of opioids. Anesthesiology 61:276, 1984

67. Loper KA, Ready LB, Downey M et al: Epidural and intravenous fentanyl infusions are clinically equivalent after knee surgery. Anesth Analg 70:72, 1990

68. Glass PSA, Estok P, Ginsberg B et al: Use of patient-controlled analgesia to compare the efficacy of epidural to intravenous fentanyl administration. Anesth Analg 74:345, 1992

69. Åkerman B, Arwestrom E, Post C: Local anesthetics potentiate spinal morphine antinociception. Anesth Analg 67:943, 1988

70. Dahl JB, Rosenberg J, Hansen BL et al: Differential analgesic effects of low-dose epidural morphine and morphine-bupivacaine at rest and during mobilization after major abdominal surgery. Anesth Analg 74:362, 1992

71. Abouleish E, Rawal N, Fallon K, Hernandez D: Combined intrathecal morphine and bupivacaine for cesarean section. Anesth Analg 67:370, 1988

72. Bisgaard C, Mouridsen P, Dahl JB: Continuous lumbar epidural bupivacaine plus morphine versus epidural morphine after major abdominal surgery. Eur J Anaesthesiol 7:219, 1990

73. Zeldin RA, Normandin D, Landtwing D, Peters RM: Postpneumonectomy pulmonary edema. J Thorac Cardiovasc Surg 87:359, 1984

74. Verheijen-Breemhaar L, Bogaard JM, van den Berg B, Hilvering C: Postpneumonectomy pulmonary oedema. Thorax 43:323, 1988

75. George KA, Wright PMC, Chisakuta A: Continuous thoracic epidural fentanyl for post-thoracotomy pain relief: with or without bupivacaine? Anaesthesia 46:732, 1991

76. Lee A, Simpson D, Whitfield A, Scott DB: Postoperative analgesia by continuous extradural infusion of bupivacaine and diamorphine. Br J Anaesth 60:845, 1988

77. King MJ, Bowden MI, Cooper GM: Epidural fentanyl and 0.5% bupivacaine for elective caesarean section. Anaesthesia 45:285, 1990

78. Douglas MJ, McMorland GH, Janzen JA: Influence of bupivacaine as an adjuvant to epidural morphine for analgesia after cesarean section. Anesth Analg 67:1138, 1988

79. Badner NH, Reimer EJ, Komar WE, Moote CA: Low-dose bupivacaine does not improve postoperative epidural fentanyl analgesia in orthopedic patients. Anesth Analg 72:337, 1991

80. Cullen ML, Staren ED, El-Ganzouri A et al: Continuous epidural infusion for analgesia after major abdominal operations: a randomized, prospective, double-blind study. Surgery 98:718, 1985

81. Hakanson E, Bengtsson M, Rutberg H, Ulrick AM: Epidural morphine by the thoracic or lumbar routes in cholecystectomy. Effect on postoperative pain and respiratory variables. Anaesth Intensive Care 17:166, 1989

82. Hendolin H, Lahtinen J, Lansimies E et al: The effect of thoracic epidural analgesia on respiratory function after cholecystectomy. Acta Anaesthesiol Scand 31:645, 1987

83. Kochi T, Sako S, Nishino T, Mizuguchi T: Effect of high thoracic extradural anaes-

thesia on ventilatory response to hypercapnia in normal volunteers. Br J Anaesth 62:362, 1989

84. Shulman BS, Brebner J, Sandler AN: The effect of epidural morphine on postoperative pain relief and pulmonary function in thoracotomy patients, abstracted. Anesthesiology 59:A192, 1983

85. Welchew EA: The optimum concentration for epidural fentanyl. A randomized, double-blind comparison with and without 1:200,000 adrenaline. Anaesthesia 38: 1037, 1983

86. Bonica JJ: General considerations of pain in the chest. p. 959. In Bonica JJ (ed): The Management of Pain. 2nd Ed. Lea & Febiger, Philadelphia, 1990

87. Lee VC, Abram SE: Intrapleural administration of bupivacaine for post-thoracotomy analgesia (letter). Anesthesiology 66:586, 1987

88. Clive DM, Stoff JS: Renal syndromes associated with nonsteroidal antiinflammatory drugs. N Engl J Med 310:563, 1984

89. Patrono C, Dunn MJ: The clinical significance of inhibition of renal prostaglandin synthesis. Kidney Int 32:1, 1987

26

Analgesia After Abdominal Surgery

F. Michael Ferrante
Niall Hughes

The goal of aggressive postoperative analgesic care after surgery of the abdomen and its contents is to provide profound analgesia while hastening functional recovery. Unfortunately, the role of "balanced analgesia" (see Ch. 12) in bringing about hastened recovery after abdominal surgery has been incompletely studied. The problems attendant on shortening the time of convalescence are complex, due in part to the multiplicity of pathophysiologic mechanisms involved in production of postoperative abdominal pain. Moreover, the degree of physiologic trespass is appreciable, particularly after upper abdominal surgery. This chapter discusses (1) the pathophysiologic mechanisms underlying postoperative abdominal pain, (2) the physiologic alterations attendant to this surgery, (3) appropriate management techniques for specific surgical scenarios, and (4) the potential role of balanced analgesia in hastening postoperative recovery.

THE PATHOPHYSIOLOGY OF POSTOPERATIVE ABDOMINAL PAIN

Postoperative abdominal pain has seven distinct components. (The physiologic processes underlying nociception itself have already been extensively reviewed in Ch. 2.)

Cutaneous Somatic Pain

Cutaneous somatic pain is distinguished from deep somatic and deep visceral pain by its quality and localization. Superficial tissue injury caused by the surgical incision is described as "sharp, pricking, burning, throbbing, and/or stabbing." The neuroanatomy has been extensively reviewed in Chapter 2.

Sensitization of Nociceptors

After repeated stimulation, high-threshold mechanoreceptors, mechanothermal nociceptors, and C-polymodal nociceptors in the skin (see Ch. 2) will increase their frequency of discharge and achieve a lower stimulatory threshold. This process is referred to as *sensitization*.[1,2] Sensitization is responsible for the hyperalgesia and allodynia associated with abdominal (as well as other) incisions.

Deep Somatic Pain

Deep somatic pain is appreciated in muscles, ligaments, and fasciae and is characterized by a "dull, aching" quality. It is less localizable than cutaneous pain but is still fairly circumscribed. Prolonged[3] or intense[4] stimulation of deep somatic structures will lead to diffuse spread of pain, however. Like visceral and cutaneous pain, deep somatic pain is associated with cutaneous hyperalgesia, tenderness, reflex muscle spasm, and sympathetic hyperactivity.

Visceral Pain

Transduction

Clinical observation has revealed that viscera are relatively insensitive to cutting, heat, or pinching,[5-7] but twisting or distention are effective noxious stimuli.[8-10] Pain is perceived in or near the injured viscus or is referred to a remote location. Teleologically, the insensitivity of viscera to somatic stimuli such as cutting or pinching is not surprising, as viscera are not normally exposed to such stimuli.

As viscera do not respond to somatic stimuli, some early investigators were lead to believe that viscera do not possess nociceptors.[7,11] It is perhaps best to conceptualize visceral nociceptors as the "sensory" innervation of viscera.[12] These fibers will not be activated unless the "appropriate" or "adequate stimulus"[10] is applied.

Transmission

The viscera are innervated by two routes: (1) via the body wall through nerves primarily innervating somatic structures, or (2) through the splanchnic nerves, which are primarily involved with autonomic function (see Ch. 3). The splanchnic innervation has been most extensively studied because of the complete lack of somatic fibers. This has led to the erroneous conclusion among many practitioners that visceral afferent fibers are equivalent to sympathetic fibers.

The range of fiber sizes within visceral afferents is comparable with that of cutaneous fibers, although there is a considerably higher proportion of small fibers.[13] Moreover, the ratio of A to C fibers is only about 1:8 or 1:10 in visceral nerves, in comparison with a ratio of 1:2 in dorsal roots.[14]

Splanchnic afferents enter the spinal cord in the thoracic and upper lumbar regions. These visceral afferents synapse primarily in laminae I and V but also in deeper laminae (VII and VIII). All neurons excited by visceral afferents also receive somatic input. No spinal neurons respond specifically to visceral afferents alone (perhaps explaining the poor localization of visceral pain). Similar to somatic afferents, visceral input is transmitted to higher centers through the spinothalamic[15] and spinoreticular[16] tracts.

Referred Pain

The term *referred pain* is used for pain that is appreciated adjacent or at a distance from the site of its cause (Fig. 26-1). Although somewhat variable depending on the individual, the pattern of referral has a distribution that is characteristic for the particular structures being noxiously simulated. For instance, mechanical stimulation of the central region of the diaphragm produces pain in the shoulder on the ipsilateral side (Fig. 26-1). Referred pain is usually accompanied by cutaneous and deep hyperalgesia, reflex muscle spasm, deep tenderness, and autonomic hyperactivity.

Proposed Mechanisms for Referred Pain

BRANCHED PRIMARY AFFERENTS

A proportion of the afferent fibers approaching the dorsal root of a single spinal segment is bifurcated, with the collateral axons innervating both visceral somatic structures.[18–20] Such a somatotopic arrangement could produce referred pain in two ways[21] (Fig. 26-2): (1) sensory transmission is received from two sources (only one source is nociceptive). This causes confusion as to discrimination of the location of actual noxious stimulation. (2) Afferent nociceptive transmission in the branch of the nociceptor innervating the noxiously stimulated deep structure could be antidromically conducted to the collateral branch. Nociceptors in the unstimulated structure could become sensitized by antidromic release of algogenic substances.[21] Pain could be produced by response of these sensitized nociceptors to innocuous stimuli.[21]

The actual contribution of branched primary afferents to the phenomenon of referred pain is unknown as the proportion of bifurcate afferents within the dorsal roots is unknown. A recent study has demonstrated that only 1 percent of cervical dorsal root ganglion cells have bifurcate branches supplying the diaphragm and the shoulder.[18] Thus, the contribution of branched primary affer-

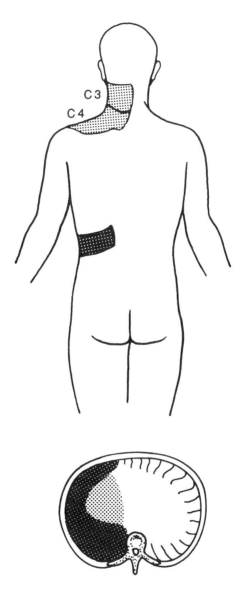

Fig. 26-1. Referral patterns of pain from diaphragm. Nociceptive stimulation of pleural or peritoneal surface of left side of diaphragm (**bottom**) produces pain at two sites. If central region of diaphragm is stimulated (*light stripping,* **bottom**), a sharp pain is appreciated in the shoulder. Central portion of diaphragm is innervated by the phrenic nerve, which originates from the third and fourth cervical spinal segment. Pain is thereby referred to approximately the C3 and C4 dermatomes (*light stippling,* **top**). When a nociceptive stimulus is applied to peripheral portion of diaphragm (*dark stippling,* **bottom**), pain is appreciated in the adjacent lower chest and upper abdominal wall (*dark stippling,* **top**). (Modified from Fields,[17] with permission.)

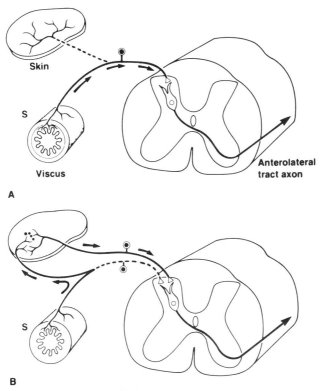

Fig. 26-2. Theories of referred pain. **(A)** Branched primary afferent. According to this theory, a single primary afferent branches to supply both the stimulated deep structure(**S**) and the structure to which pain is referred. **(B)** Referred pain caused by antidromic activation of receptors at a distant secondary site. According to this theory, misperception is due to antidromic conduction of impulses in a peripheral branch of stimulated structure(**S**). Algogenic substances are released from peripheral terminals of the branch at site of pain referral. Other nociceptors are activated and conduct nociceptive transmission orthodromically and rostrally. In this case, the brain correctly localizes site of origin of the nociceptive message but not the site of the original pathologic process (*Figure continues.*)

ents to referred diaphragmatic pain may be rather small. It is not known in what proportion such branched afferents are found elsewhere in other dorsal roots.

REFLEX ACTIVATION OF NOCICEPTORS: SEQUENTIAL
REFLEX RESPONSES

Segmental (spinal) reflexes occur in response to somatic and visceral afferent input to the dorsal horn of the spinal cord. Such reflexes may be viscerosomatic, viscerosympathetic, or viscerovisceral in origin (Fig. 26-3) and can produce referred pain as well as deleterious alterations in ventilatory, circulatory, gastrointestinal, and urinary function.[22,23] Reflexes are believed to be generated through interneuronal connections between the somatic and visceral afferent

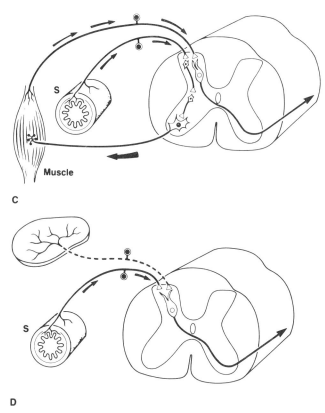

Fig. 26-2. (*Continued*) **(C)** Referred pain resulting from reflex muscle contraction that causes activation of a distant secondary site. In this situation, impulses originating in the stimulated structure(**S**) cause reflex activation of motor neurons, which produce muscle contraction and activation of muscle nociceptors. The brain correctly localizes active muscle nociception but not the site of original pathology. **(D)** Convergence projection theory. According to this hypothesis, visceral afferent nociceptors (**S**) converge on the same pain-projection neurons as afferents from somatic structures in which pain is perceived. The brain has no way of knowing the actual source and mistakenly "projects" sensation to the somatic structure. (From Fields,[17] with permission.)

inputs to the dorsal horn and sympathetic efferent and motor neurons in the intermediolateral gray column and ventral horn, respectively (Figs. 26-2 and 26-3). Reflex somatic motor activity results in muscle spasm. Reflex sympathetic efferent activity may cause visceral sphincteric spasm over a wide area. Sympathetic efferent activity may also produce visceral ischemia, resulting in further noxious stimulation. Besides generating, sustaining, and intensifying pain, such reflexes contribute to the phenomenon of referred pain.

VISCERAL-SOMATIC CONVERGENCE

The "convergence-projection" hypothesis[24] is the most widely accepted explanation for the mechanism underlying referred pain. Experimental evidence demonstrates the convergence of visceral and somatic input onto second-order

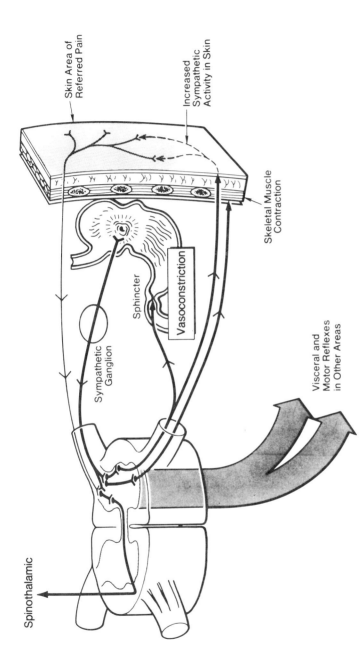

Fig. 26-3. Reflex activation of nociceptors and convergence of visceral and somatic nociceptive afferents. Visceral afferents converge on same dorsal horn neurons as somatic nociceptive afferents. Visceral nociceptive transmission is then conveyed along with somatic nociceptive transmission through spinothalamic tract to the brain. Note the following: (1) Referred pain is appreciated in cutaneous area corresponding to dorsal horn neurons on which visceral afferents converge. Increased sympathetic activity may influence cutaneous nociceptors, and this may be at least partially responsible for "referred" pain. (2) Reflex somatic motor activity results in muscle spasm, which may stimulate parietal peritoneum and initiate somatic nociceptive transmission to dorsal horn. (3) Reflex sympathetic efferent activity may result in spasm of sphincters of viscera over a wide area. (4) Reflex sympathetic efferent activity may result in visceral ischemia and further nociceptive stimulation. (From Cousins,[23] with permission.)

Labels in figure:
Skin Area of Referred Pain
Increased Sympathetic Activity in Skin
Skeletal Muscle Contraction
Vasoconstriction
Sphincter
Sympathetic Ganglion
Visceral and Motor Reflexes in Other Areas
Spinothalamic

neurons in laminae V–VII of the dorsal horn.[25,26] Visceral afferents enter the same spinal segments as nociceptive somatic afferents innervating the region of the body to which the pain is referred.[27] According to the theory, the two types of afferents converge onto the same spinothalamic tract (projection) neurons. Visceral nociceptive input is then conveyed together with somatic nociceptive input to the brain by the spinothalamic tract. Referred pain is then perceived in the somatic area corresponding to the dorsal horn neurons on which the visceral afferents converge (Figs. 26-2 and 26-3).[27]

For instance, diaphragmatic irritation is caused by blood from a ruptured viscus underneath the diaphragm. Such pain is referred to the shoulder. The central region of the diaphragm is innervated by visceral afferents that synapse in the dorsal horn at the third and fourth spinal segments. Thus, the site of referred pain and cutaneous hyperalgesia is the C3 and C4 dermatomes (i.e., the shoulder) (Fig. 26-1).

Sequential Reflex Responses

As already described in the discussion of referred pain, a number of viscero-somatic, viscerosympathetic, and viscerovisceral reflexes can occur after abdominal surgery (Fig. 26-3). It is important to appreciate the role of such reflexes in the activation of nociceptors over a wide area of the body and the contribution of such activation to the phenomenon of referred pain.

Cortical Responses

Acute pain is invariably associated with anxiety, fear, and, perhaps, feelings of helplessness. Such emotions can greatly enhance the neuroendocrine response to stress[28] (see Ch. 4).

The complexity of the pathophysiology of postoperative abdominal pain underscores the difficulty of improving functional recovery with single modality analgesic care. Use of single analgesic techniques (intravenous patient-controlled analgesia [IV-PCA] or epidural opioids) can only affect certain discreet aspects of the previously outlined pathophysiologic mechanisms. A more "balanced" multimodal approach to postoperative abdominal pain would seem more efficacious. Certainly, a more balanced approach would seem to be better able to reverse deleterious physiologic alterations after surgery.

PHYSIOLOGIC ALTERATIONS AFTER ABDOMINAL SURGERY

Pulmonary Dysfunction

Pulmonary dysfunction is particularly common after upper abdominal surgery. Decreased lung volumes are associated with hypoxemia and atelectasis. Functional residual capacity (FRC) is reduced about 30 percent at 24 hours after operation and remains reduced for several days.[29] Forced vital capacity (FVC) is reduced by approximately 60 percent in the immediate postoperative period. These changes in pulmonary function tests are even more striking in obese patients.

Diaphragmatic dysfunction may be the etiology of altered pulmonary function.[30,31] Diaphragmatic dysfunction may be due to an impairment of diaphragmatic mechanics related to an increase in abdominal wall tone (reflex muscle spasm) and/or a reflex decrease of phrenic nerve activity by inhibitory visceral afferent input.[29]

Clinically, pulmonary dysfunction is expressed as decreased deep inspiration, decreased clearance of secretions, and diminished cough. Such patients develop an "atelectatic" FRC: closing capacity relationship (Fig. 26-4). This predisposes to premature airway closure during tidal ventilation with resultant development of areas of ventilation/perfusion (V/Q) mismatch. Ventilation/perfusion mismatch is manifested as a reduction in arterial oxygen tension and widened alveolar-arterial O_2 difference.

In summary, patients undergoing upper abdominal surgery develop a severe restrictive breathing pattern with reductions in FRC, FVC, and diaphragmatic function lasting up to 1 week after surgery.[30] Such alterations will, of course, be most detrimental in patients with preexisting lung disease.

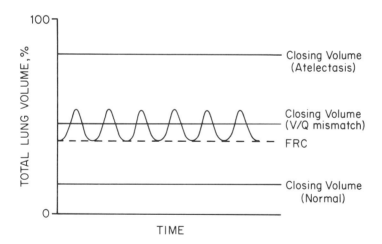

Fig. 26-4. Relationship between functional residual capacity (FRC) (*dashed line* at trough of tidal breathing curve) and closing capacity (*CC*) in three physiologic states. As lung volume decreases during expiration, small airways have a tendency to close. In presence of inadequate analgesia after thoracotomy, volume at which some airways close may be greater than that achieved during tidal breathing (atelectasis). If closing volume of some airways lies within tidal volume, these airways will alternately open and close during tidal breathing. Because these opening and closing airways have a shorter time than normal for fresh gas exchange, ventilation/perfusion mismatching occurs. (In normal state, closing volumes of all airways are always below volumes attendant to tidal breathing, and no airways are closed at any time.)

Gastrointestinal Complications

Segmental reflexes may result in paralytic ileus causing nausea, vomiting, and abdominal distension. Abdominal distention may further contribute to a restrictive breathing pattern and pulmonary dysfunction.

Thromboembolic Complications

Postoperative abdominal pain reduces physical activity because of fear of aggravating pain. Immobility causes venous stasis and pooling of blood in the lower limbs. In addition, pain-induced anxiety may produce cortically mediated increases in blood viscosity,[32] clotting time,[33] and platelet aggregation (neuroendocrine stress response). The combination of stasis and hypercoagulability places the patient at increased risk for development of deep venous thrombosis and pulmonary embolism.

ANALGESIA FOR SPECIFIC ABDOMINAL PROCEDURES

Despite the plethora of abdominal surgical procedures performed daily, there has been little to no systematic study of the role of aggressive analgesic care in the rehabilitation of these patients. There is a diverse literature, however, regarding postoperative analgesia after biliary tract surgery. Unfortunately, such a literature was perhaps generated more from the ease of procurement of patients rather than any innate interest in the natural history of the postoperative course of biliary tract surgery. Thus, the role of "balanced" analgesic techniques in the rehabilitation and functional recovery of patients after many types of abdominal surgery remains to be defined.

With the present level of sophistication, it is perhaps best to grossly divide the abdomen into upper and lower portions on the basis of the degree of physiologic trespass and neuroendocrine sequelae. As described previously, upper abdominal surgery is associated with a greater degree of pulmonary dysfunction. Furthermore, despite the ability of regional anesthesia/analgesia to restore vital capacity and functional residual capacity to normal,[34] resolve V/Q mismatch,[35] and reverse diaphragmatic dysfunction,[31] the neuroendocrine response to surgical stress remains unaltered[36–38] (see Ch. 4). This is in contradistinction to lower abdominal surgery where production of pulmonary dysfunction in not an issue, and the neuroendocrine response to surgery can be successfully interdicted.[36,39] Thus, division of the abdomen into upper and lower portions forms a convenient method to study the effect of various analgesic modalities on postoperative abdominal pain.

Upper Abdominal Surgery

Nonsteroidal Anti-inflammatory Drugs

Nonsteroidal anti-inflammatory drugs (NSAIDs) are best used as part of a "balanced" analgesic regimen.[40] Indomethacin rectal suppositories have been shown to provide good adjunctive analgesia after abdominal surgery and a morphine "sparing" effect.[41] With respect to injectable preparations, lysine acetyl salicylate[42,43] and diclofenac[44,45] have been available in Europe for some time. Ketorolac is now available as an injectable NSAID in the United States. The pharmacology of the NSAIDs has been reviewed in Chapter 7.

Patient-Controlled Analgesia

IV-PCA is now a mainstay of analgesic therapy after abdominal surgery.[46,47] There does not appear to be an increased incidence of nausea, vomiting, or ileus associated with use of PCA after abdominal surgery.[47,48] Production of side effects appears to be related to total dose of opioid rather than the use of a particular drug[46] or the modality per se.[48]

Of note, PCA has been shown to have little effect on the stress response after upper abdominal surgery despite improved patient satisfaction and analgesia.[49] (IV-PCA has been shown to possibly decrease cortisol levels after hysterectomy, however.[50])

Intercostal Neural Blockade

Most reports of the use of intercostal neural blockade after cholecystectomy have demonstrated improved analgesia and improved pulmonary function as compared with parenteral opioids.[51-55] However, a few studies have been unable to demonstrate any advantages over parenteral opioids.[56,57] Discrepancies in results may be due to differences in type of incision (midline versus subcostal),[55] type of surgery or surgical technique,[55] and the intermittent administration of local anesthetic used in conventional intercostal nerve blocks.[51-57] It is interesting to speculate whether the more uniform provision of analgesia through continuous intercostal catheterization[58,59] (see Ch. 15) would obviate "peak and trough" analgesic and pulmonary effects associated with intermittent administration. Overall, there is consensus that intercostal neural blockade results in superior analgesia with improved pulmonary function.

Interpleural Regional Analgesia

Interpleural regional analgesia (see Ch. 16) has been extensively studied after cholecystectomy. Unlike intercostal neural blockade, there is no consensus as to the superiority of this technique with respect to degree of analgesia or effect on pulmonary function (Table 26-1).[60-67] Furthermore, interpleural regional analgesia has been shown to have no effect on the neuroendocrine response to cholecystectomy.[68] Interpleural analgesia does not provide analgesia of sufficient intensity or duration to be used as a single analgesic modality after cholecystectomy. This has lead several authors to supplement interpleural regional analgesia with IV-PCA.[60-62]

TABLE 26-1. Effect of Interpleural Regional Analgesia (IRA) and Conventional Opioid Regimens on Analgesia and Pulmonary Function after Cholecystectomy

Reference	Analgesia with IRA	Pulmonary Function with IRA
VadeBoncouer et al[61]	Superior[a]	Improved
Lee et al[62]	Superior	No difference
Frank et al[63]	Superior[b]	No difference
Frenette et al[64]	Superior	Improved
Schroeder et al[65]	Superior	Improved
Kastrissios et al[66]	No difference	Improved[c]
Oxorn and Whatley[67]	No difference	Worse

[a] Analgesia was superior for 3 h after injection and then became comparable with that of the controls.

[b] Analgesia was superior for 4 h after injection and then became comparable with that of the controls.

[c] No difference between groups was found in pulmonary function tests. However, patients with interpleural regional analgesia had a significantly lower incidence of hypercarbia and hypoxemia.

Subarachnoid Opioids

Only a single study by Yamaguchi et al[69] examines the dose-response relations for administration of subarachnoid morphine after upper abdominal surgery (i.e., cholecystectomy). Preservative-free morphine was given to 139 patients undergoing cholecystectomy in a dose ranging from 0.0 to 0.2 mg at time of administration of the hyperbaric tetracaine spinal anesthetic. A dose of 0.06–0.12 mg appeared optimal, providing "effective analgesia" (no request for supplement opioids) without respiratory depression for 24 hours.

Epidural Local Anesthetics and Opioids

THORACIC VERSUS LUMBAR EPIDURAL PLACEMENT

The question of thoracic versus lumbar epidural catheterization for analgesia after upper abdominal surgery is somewhat controversial. The considerations for catheter placement along a specific part of the spine when using certain opioids or combinations of opioid and local anesthetic are the same as in Chapters 11 and 25. The reader is referred to these sources for a discussion of the benefits and disadvantages of thoracic or lumbar epidural catheterization.

LOCAL ANESTHETICS

As would be expected, thoracic epidural analgesia with local anesthetics uniformly improves postoperative pulmonary function after upper abdominal surgery.[70] Quite interestingly, such beneficial effects did not translate into decreased morbidity and mortality in a study by Hendolin et al.[71] In another study, however, the incidence of deep vein thrombosis as determined by [125I]fibrinogen uptake was reduced by thoracic epidural analgesia.[72]

BALANCED ANALGESIA

In laboratory studies, local anesthetics given in doses insufficient to produce an analgesic effect by themselves have been shown to potentiate the analgesic effects of spinal opioids.[73] When used in combination after upper and lower abdominal surgery, combinations of epidural local anesthetics and opioids have been shown to improve pain relief[74-77] and maintain sensory analgesia[76,77] as compared to epidural local anesthetics alone.

The concept of *balanced* analgesia implies provision of agents to selectively affect several of the physiologic processes involved in nociception: transduction (NSAIDs[78-80] or steroids[81]), transmission (local anesthetics, peripheral[82,83] and/or neuraxial,[74-77,82]), and modulation (epidural opioids).[74-77] Such combined therapy can almost completely eliminate postoperative pain after abdominal surgery (or any surgery for that matter) at both rest and during mobilization.[78-80]

Despite the provision of almost complete analgesia, the possibility of shortened convalescence is not assured after upper abdominal surgery. With upper abdominal surgery, afferent nociceptive transmission is not ablated at clinically used (and safe) concentrations of local anesthetic.[36-38] Thus, despite potent analgesia, the neuroendocrine response to upper abdominal surgery is not suppressed.[36,38] However, the neuroendocrine response to lower abdominal surgery is more easily ablated. Its suppression has been associated with decreased morbidity and shortened time of convalescence.[36,84] Obviously, the benefit of "balanced" combinations of analgesics on facilitation of patient mobilization and time of convalescence is an important and fruitful topic for future research.

Lower Abdominal Surgery

The literature regarding the use of individual analgesic modalities for lower abdominal surgery is less extensive than that for procedures of the upper abdomen. Thus we will confine our discussion to two common surgical procedures.

Appendectomy

Despite the frequency of performance of this operation, little organized attention has been given to amelioration of its attendant postoperative pain. As simple a technique as intercostal neural blockade has been shown to provide at least 12 hours of superior analgesia as compared with parenteral opioids.[85] It is interesting to speculate as to (1) the reason why this technique is not used more often after appendectomy, (2) the potential use of continuous intercostal neural blockade, and (3) the effect of the addition of NSAIDs (both oral and parenteral) on the analgesic efficacy of intercostal neural blockade.

Colonic Surgery

Balanced analgesia has been definitively shown to prevent the neuroendocrine response to colonic surgery.[79] Furthermore, besides providing almost complete pain relief, combinations of epidural opioids and local anesthetics and systemic NSAIDs have been shown to improve mobilization.[79,80] Thus, balanced analgesia may significantly shorten the time of convalescence, although no study directly addresses this question.

Despite the considerable benefits of epidural analgesia, several reports have implicated early anastamotic dehiscence to be associated with its use.[86-88] The mechanism for such dehiscence has been hypothesized to be increased colonic activity resulting from epidural analgesia.[87,88] A more recent experiment using a porcine model suggests that epidural local anesthetics and opioids will individually accelerate colonic transit time.[89] However, anastomotic complications did not occur in any animal, suggesting that epidural analgesia is a safe technique after colorectal resection and anastamosis.[89]

THE EFFECT OF EPIDURAL ANESTHESIA/ANALGESIA ON GASTROINTESTINAL MOTILITY

Abdominal nociceptive stimulation, such as that occurring after surgery, results in reflex inhibition of gastrointestinal motility.[90,91] This inhibition is believed to be due to spinal cord reflexes[92,93] whose efferent limb involves the sympathetic nervous system.[94] Retardation of gastrointestinal motility is most persistent in the stomach[95] and colon,[96,97] whereas activity in the small intestine returns rapidly to normal after surgery (within a few hours).[97] Inhibition of gastrointestinal motility may be further compounded by administration of parenteral opioids, which affect motility by binding to opioid receptors within the gut.[98]

This section examines the role of epidural anesthesia/analgesia in potentiating or retarding gastrointestinal motility. Two models have been used: (1) human volunteers with experimentally induced pain, and (2) actual postsurgical patients. One must remember that these two models may not be physiologically equivalent.

Gastric Emptying and Small Intestinal Motility

All studies of the effects of epidural morphine on gastric emptying and small intestinal transit have been performed in volunteers.[99,100] Epidural morphine has been shown to slow gastric emptying[99,100] and reduce orocecal and small intestinal transit.[99] The mechanism underlying these effects is believed to be centrally mediated and not produced through systemic concentrations of opioid.[100] Interestingly, however, systemic opioids resulted in a greater slowing of gastric emptying after abdominal surgery than subarachnoid opioids.[101] This occurred despite provision of equivalent analgesia by the two modalities. Route of administration has been implicated to be important in the genesis of opioid-mediated motility effects in other experimental models.[102]

Thoracic epidural anesthesia blocks efferent sympathetic innervation to the stomach (T6–T10). Administration of sufficient 0.5 percent bupivacaine to cause sensory blockade in corresponding dermatomes has been shown to have no effect on gastric emptying in volunteers.[100,103] Thoracic epidural anesthesia has likewise been shown to have no effect on orocecal or small intestinal transit.[103]

Colonic Motility

In comparison with both systemic[86,104] and epidural[89,105,106] administration of opioids, both thoracic and lumbar administration of bupivacaine have been shown to almost uniformly enhance colonic motility.

The effects of morphine on the colon were first described by Painter in 1963.[107] Segmental contraction of the colon was noted after intravenous or intramuscular administration. Wilson,[108] however, was unable to demonstrate an effect of postoperative parenteral opioids on colonic motility. Epidural opioids are believed to inhibit colonic motility through spinal cord reflexes.[102]

Increased colonic motility with epidural local anesthetics is believed to be mediated by the attendant sympathetic blockade, thereby inhibiting the efferent limb of potential spinal reflexes.[92] Sympathetic block results in an increase in the propulsive force of peristalsis and an increase in the muscular force of bowel wall.[89] To date, only one study has failed to show enhanced colonic motility associated with epidural administration of local anesthetics, despite efficient block of sympathetic efferents.[109] The authors of this study suggest that ileus may be due to mechanisms other than activation of spinal sympathetic reflexes.[109–111]

Only one study examines the use of combinations of epidural local anesthetics and opioids on colonic motility.[112] As the duration of postoperative ileus was not shortened, it can be hypothesized that the negative motile effects of opioids are predominant in combinational epidural regimens. However, this question is certainly open to further investigation.

CONCLUSION

Balanced analgesic techniques have the greatest potential for hastening patient rehabilitation and shortening convalescence after abdominal surgery. The role of such techniques has been incompletely studied, however. With a greater appreciation of the pathophysiologic mechanisms underlying postoperative abdominal pain and its sequelae (e.g., impaired gastrointestinal function), research in balanced analgesia may provide answers to basic concerns in the rehabilitation and convalescence of abdominal surgical patients.

References

1. Adriaensen H, Gybels J, Handwerker H, Van Hees J: Response properties of thin myelinated (Aδ) fibers in human skin nerves. J Neurophysiol 49:111, 1983
2. Besson P, Perl ER: Response of cutaneous sensory units with unmyelinated fibers to noxious stimuli. J Neurophysiol 32:1025, 1969

3. Wolff HG: Headache and Other Head Pain. Oxford University Press, New York, 1948

4. Kellgren JH: Observations on referred pain arising from muscle. Clin Sci 3:176, 1937

5. Capps JA, Coleman GH: An Experimental and Clinical Study of Pain in the Pleura, Pericardium and Peritoneum. Macmillan, New York, 1932

6. Lewis T: Pain. Macmillan, New York, 1942

7. Lennander KG: Über die sensibilitat der Bauchhoehle und über lokale und allegemeine Anasthesie bei Bruch und Bachoperationen. Zentralbl Physiol 28:209, 1901

8. Kast L, Meltzer SJ: Die sensibilitat der bauchorgane. Mitt, a.d. Grenzgebiet Med Chirurg 19:586, 1908

9. Hurst AF: On the sensibility of the alimentary canal in health and disease. Lancet i:105, 1911

10. Holmes G: Some clinical aspects of pain. Practitioner 158:165, 1947

11. Mackenzie J: Some points bearing on the association of sensory disorders and visceral disease. Brain 16:321, 1893

12. Cervero F: Mechanisms of visceral pain. p. 1. In Persistent Pain. Vol. 4. Grune and Stratton, New York, 1983

13. Bonica JJ: Anatomic and physiologic basis of nociception and pain. p. 28. In The Management of Pain. 2nd Ed. Lea & Febiger, Philadelphia, 1990

14. Janig W, Morrison JFB: Functional properties of spinal visceral afferents supplying abdominal and pelvic organs with special emphasis on visceral nociception. p. 87. In Cervero F, Morrison JF (eds): Visceral Sensation. Elsevier, Amsterdam, 1986

15. Milne RJ, Foreman RD, Giesler GJ Jr, Willis WD: Convergence of cutaneous and pelvic visceral nociceptive inputs onto primate spinothalamic neurons. Pain 11: 163, 1981

16. Cervero F: Supraspinal connections of neurones in the thoracic spinal cord of the cat: ascending projections and effects of descending impulses. Brain Res 275:251, 1983

17. Fields HL: Pain from deep tissues and referred pain. p. 79. In: Pain. McGraw Hill, New York, 1987

18. Laurberg S, Sorensen KE: Cervical dorsal root ganglion cells with collaterals to both shoulder skin and the diaphragm. A fluorescent double labelling study in the rat. A model for referred pain? Brain Res 331:160, 1985

19. Willis WD: The Pain Systems: The Neural Basis of Nociceptive Transmission in the Mammalian Nervous System. Karger, Basel, 1985

20. Perl ER: Pain and nociception. p. 915. In Darian-Smith I (ed): Handbook of Physiology. Section I, The Nervous System. Vol. 3. American Physiologic Society, Bethesda, MD, 1984

21. Sinclair DC, Weddell G, Feindel WH: Referred pain and associated phenomena. Brain 71:184, 1948

22. Bing HI: Viscerocutaneous and cutaneovisceral thoracic reflexes. Acta Med Scand 89:57, 1936

23. Cousins MJ: Introduction to acute and chronic pain: implications for neural blockade. p. 739. In Cousins MJ, Bridenbaugh PO (eds): Neural Blockade in Clinical Anesthesia and Management of Pain. 2nd Ed. JB Lippincott, Philadelphia, 1988

24. Ruch TC: Pathophysiology of pain. p. 345. In Ruch TC, Patton HD (eds): Physiology and Biophysics. WB Saunders, Philadelphia, 1965

25. Pomeranz B, Wall PD, Weber WV: Cord cells responding to fine myelinated afferents from viscera, muscle and skin. J Physiol (Lond) 199:511, 1968

26. Selzer M, Spencer WA: Convergence of visceral and cutaneous afferent pathways in the lumbar spinal cord. Brain Res 14:331, 1969

27. Fields HL, Meyer GA, Partridge LD Jr: Convergence of visceral and somatic input onto spinal neurons. Exp Neurol 26:36, 1970

28. Hume DH, Egdahl RH: The importance of the brain in the endocrine response to injury. Ann Surg 150:697, 1959

29. Craig DB: Postoperative recovery of pulmonary function. Anesth Analg 60:46, 1981

30. Ford GT, Whitelaw WA, Rosenal TW et al: Diaphragm function after upper abdominal surgery in humans. Am Rev Respir Dis 127:431, 1983

31. Mankikian B, Cantineau JP, Bertrand M et al: Improvement of diaphragmatic function by a thoracic extradural block after upper abdominal surgery. Anesthesiology 68:379, 1988

32. Schneider RA: The relation of stress to clotting time, relative viscosity and certain biophysical alterations of the blood in normotension and hypertensive subjects. p. 818. In Wolff HG, Wolff SG, Hare CC (eds): Life Stresses and Bodily Disease. Williams & Wilkins, Baltimore, 1950

33. Dreyfuss F: Coagulation time of the blood, level of blood eosinophiles and thrombocytes under emotional stress. J Psychosom Res 1:252, 1956

34. Bromage PR: Epidural Analgesia. WB Saunders, Philadelphia, 1978

35. Pflug AE, Murphy TM, Butler SH, Tucker GT: The effects of postoperative peridural analgesia on pulmonary therapy and pulmonary complications. Anesthesiology 41:8, 1974

36. Kehlet H: Surgical stress: the role of pain and analgesia. Br J Anaesth 63:189, 1989

37. Lund C, Hansen OB, Mogensen T, Kehlet H: Effect of thoracic epidural bupivacaine on somatosensory evoked potentials after dermatomal stimulation. Anesth Analg 66:731,1987

38. Rutberg H, Håkansson E, Anderberg B et al: Effects of extradural administration of morphine, or bupivacaine on the endocrine response to upper abdominal surgery. Br J Anaesth 56:233, 1984

39. Scott NB, Kehlet H: Regional anaesthesia and surgical morbidity. Br J Surg 75: 299, 1988

40. Dahl JB, Rosenberg J, Dirkes WE et al: Prevention of postoperative pain by balanced analgesia. Br J Anaesth 64:518, 1990

41. Reasbeck PG, Rice ML, Reasbeck JC: Double-blind controlled trial of indomethacin as an adjunct to narcotic analgesia after major abdominal surgery. Lancet ii: 115, 1982

42. Kweekel-de Vries WJ, Spierdijk J, Mattie H, Herman JM: A new soluble acetylsalicylic acid derivative in the treatment of postoperative pain. Br J Anaesth 46:133, 1974

43. Launo C, Molinino M, Bassi C et al: Postoperative analgesia with lysine salicylate and pentazocine. Minerva Anestesiol 47:237, 1981

44. Hodsman NBA, Burns J, Blyth A et al: The morphine sparing effects of diclofenac sodium following abdominal surgery. Anaesthesia 42:1005, 1987

45. Moffat AC, Kenny GNC, Prentice JW: Postoperative neofam and diclofenac. Evaluation of their morphine sparing effect after upper abdominal surgery. Anaesthesia 45:302, 1990

46. Bahar M, Rosen M, Vickers MD: Self-administered nalbuphine, morphine and pethidine. Comparison, by intravenous route, following cholecystectomy. Anaesthesia 40:529, 1985

47. Bollish SJ, Collins CL, Kirking DM, Bartlett RH: Efficacy of patient-controlled versus conventional analgesia for postoperative pain. Clin Pharm 4:48, 1985

48. Callan CM: An analysis of complaints and complications with patient-controlled analgesia. p. 139. In Ferrante FM, Ostheimer GW, Covino BG (eds): Patient-Controlled Analgesia. Blackwell Scientific, Boston, 1990

49. Moller IW, Dinesen K, Sondergard S et al: Effect of patient-controlled analgesia on plasma catecholamine, cortisol and glucose concentrations after cholecystectomy. Br J Anaesth 61:160, 1988

50. Wasylak TJ, Abbott FV, English MJ, Jeans ME: Reduction of post-operative morbidity following patient-controlled morphine. Can J Anaesth 37:726, 1990

51. Moore DC, Bridenbaugh LD: Intercostal nerve block in 4333 patients. Anesth Analg 41:1, 1962

52. Moore DC: Intercostal nerve block for postoperative somatic pain following surgery of thorax and upper abdomen. Br J Anaesth, suppl. 47:284, 1975

53. Bridenbaugh PO, DuPen SL, Moore DC et al: Postoperative intercostal nerve block analgesia versus narcotic analgesia. Anesth Analg 52:81, 1973

54. Bridenbaugh PO, Bridenbaugh LD, Moore DC, Thompson GE: The role of intercostal block and three general anesthetic agents as predisposing factors to postoperative pulmonary problems. Anesth Analg 51:638, 1972

55. Engberg G: Respiratory performance after upper abdominal surgery. A comparison of pain relief with intercostal blocks and centrally acting analgesics. Acta Anaesthesiol Scand 29:427, 1985

56. Ross WB, Tweedie JH, Leong YP et al: Intercostal blockade and pulmonary function after cholecystectomy. Surgery 105:166, 1989

57. Hollmén A, Saukkonen J: Postoperative elimination of pain following upper abdominal surgery. Anesthetics, intercostal block and epidural anesthesia and their effects on respiration. Anaesthesist 18:298, 1969

58. Murphy DF: Continuous intercostal nerve blockade for pain relief after cholecystectomy. Br J Anaesth 55:521, 1983

59. Hashimi H, Stewart AL, Ah-Fat G: Continuous intercostal nerve block for postoperative analgesia after surgical treatment of the upper part of the abdomen. Surg Gynecol Obstet 173:116, 1991

60. Laurito CE, Kirz LI, VadeBoncouer TR et al: Continuous infusion of interpleural bupivacaine maintains effective analgesia after cholecystectomy. Anesth Analg 72:516, 1991

61. VadeBoncouer TR, Riegler FX, Gautt RS, Weinberg GL: A randomized, double-blind comparison of the effects of interpleural bupivacaine and saline on morphine requirements and pulmonary function after cholecystectomy. Anesthesiology 71:339, 1989

62. Lee A, Boon D, Bagshaw P, Kempthorne P: A randomized double-blind study of interpleural analgesia after cholecystectomy. Anaesthesia 45:1028, 1990

63. Frank ED, McKay W, Rocco A, Gallo JP: Interpleural bupivacaine for postoperative analgesia following cholecystectomy: a randomized prospective study. Reg Anesth 15:26, 1990

64. Frenette L, Boudreault D, Guay J: Interpleural analgesia improves pulmonary function after cholecystectomy. Can J Anaesth 38:71, 1991

65. Schroeder D, Baker P: Interpleural catheter for analgesia after cholecystectomy: the surgical perspective. Aust N Z J Surg 60:689, 1990

66. Kastrissios H, Mogg GA, Triggs EJ, Higbie JW: Interpleural bupivacaine infusion compared with intravenous pethidine infusion after cholecystectomy. Anaesth Intensive Care 19:539, 1991

67. Oxorn DC, Whatley GS: Post-cholecystectomy pulmonary function following interpleural bupivacaine and intramuscular pethidine. Anaesth Intensive Care 17:440, 1989

68. Rademaker BM, Sih IL, Kalkman CJ et al: Effects of interpleurally administered bupivacaine 0.5% on opioid analgesic requirements and endocrine response during and after cholecystectomy: a randomized double-blind controlled study. Acta Anaesthesiol Scand 35:108, 1991

69. Yamaguchi H, Watanabe S, Motokawa K, Ishizawa Y: Intrathecal morphine dose-response data for pain relief after cholecystectomy. Anesth Analg 70:168, 1990

70. Hendolin H, Lahtinen J, Lansimies E et al: The effect of thoracic epidural analgesia on respiratory function after cholecystectomy. Acta Anaesthesiol Scand 31:645, 1987

71. Hendolin H, Lahtinen J, Lansimies E, Tuppurainen T: The effect of thoracic epidural analgesia on postoperative stress and morbidity. Ann Chir Gynaecol 76:234, 1987

72. Hendolin H, Tuppurainen T, Lahtinen J: Thoracic epidural analgesia and deep vein thrombosis in cholecystectomized patients. Acta Chir Scand 148:405, 1982

73. Åkerman B, Arwestroem E, Post C: Local anesthetics potentiate spinal morphine antinociception. Anesth Analg 67:943, 1988

74. Cullen ML, Staren ED, El-Ganzouri A et al: Continuous epidural infusion for analgesia after major abdominal operations: a randomized, prospective, double-blind study. Surgery 98:718, 1985

75. Lee A, Simpson D, Whitfield A, Scott DB: Postoperative analgesia by continuous extradural infusion of bupivacaine and diamorphine. Br J Anaesth 60:845, 1988

76. Hjortsø N-C, Lund C, Mogensen T et al: Epidural morphine improves pain relief and maintains sensory analgesia during continuous epidural bupivacaine after abdominal surgery. Anesth Analg 65:1033, 1986

77. Scott NB, Mogensen T, Bigler D et al: Continuous thoracic extradural 0.5% bupivacaine with or without morphine: effect on quality of blockade, lung function and the surgical stress response. Br J Anaesth 62:253, 1989

78. Schulze S, Roikjaer O, Hasselström L et al: Epidural bupivacaine and morphine plus systemic indomethacin eliminates pain but not systemic response and convalescence after cholecystectomy. Surgery 103:321, 1988

79. Dahl JB, Rosenberg J, Dirkes WE et al: Prevention of postoperative pain by balanced analgesia. Br J Anaesth 64:518, 1990

80. Dahl JB, Rosenberg J, Hansen BL et al: Differential analgesic effects of low-dose epidural morphine and morphine-bupivacaine at rest and during mobilization after major abdominal surgery. Anesth Analg 74:362, 1992

81. Schulze S, Møller IW, Bang V et al: Effect of combined prednisolone, epidural analgesia and indomethacin on pain, systemic response and convalescence after cholecystectomy. Acta Chir Scand 156:203, 1990

82. Tverskoy M, Cozacov C, Ayache M et al: Postoperative pain after inguinal herniorrhaphy with different types of anesthesia. Anesth Analg 70:29, 1990

83. Patel JM, Lanzafame RJ, Williams JS et al: The effect of incisional infiltration of bupivacaine hydrochloride upon pulmonary functions, atelectasis and narcotic need following elective cholecystectomy. Surg Gynecol Obstet 157:338, 1983

84. Scott NB, Kehlet H: Regional anaesthesia and surgical morbidity. Br J Surg 75:299, 1988

85. Bunting P, McGeachie JF: Intercostal nerve blockade producing analgesia after appendicectomy. Br J Anaesth 61:169, 1988

86. Bredtmann RD, Herden HN, Teichmann W et al: Epidural analgesia in colonic surgery: results of a randomized prospective study. Br J Surg 77:638, 1990

87. Treissman DA: Disruption of colonic anastomosis associated with epidural anesthesia. Reg Anesth 5:22, 1980

88. Bigler D, Hjortsø N-C, Kehlet H: Disruption of colonic anastomosis during continuous epidural analgesia. An early postoperative complication. Anaesthesia 40:278, 1985

89. Schnitzler M, Kilbride MJ, Senagore A: Effect of epidural analgesia on colorectal anastomotic healing and colonic motility. Reg Anesth 17:143, 1992

90. Glise H, Lindahl B-O, Abrahamsson H: Reflex adrenergic inhibition of gastric motility by nociceptive intestinal stimulation and peritoneal irritation in the cat. Scand J Gastroenterol 15:673, 1980

91. Dubois A, Henry DP, Kopin IJ: Plasma catecholamines and postoperative gastric emptying and small intestinal propulsion in the rat. Gastroenterology 68:466, 1975

92. Petri G, Szenohradszky J, Porszasz-Gibiszer K: Sympatholytic treatment of "paralytic" ileus. Surgery 70:359, 1971

93. Neely J, Catchpole B: Ileus: the restoration of alimentary tract motility by pharmacologic means. Br J Surg 58:21, 1971

94. Glise A, Abrahamsson H: Reflex inhibition of gastric motility—pathophysiological aspects. Scand J Gastroenterol, suppl. 19(89):77, 1984

95. Nachlas M, Younis MT, Roda CP, Wityk JJ: Gastrointestinal motility as a guide to postoperative management. Ann Surg 175:510, 1972

96. Woods JH, Erickson LW, Condon RE et al: Postoperative ileus: a colonic problem? Surgery 84:527, 1978

97. Graber JN, Schulte WJ, Condon RE, Cowles VE: Relationship of postoperative ileus to extent and site of operative dissection. Surgery 92:87, 1982

98. Mather LE, Owen H: The pharmacology of patient-administered opioids. p. 27. In Ferrante FM, Ostheimer GW, Covino BG (eds): Patient-Controlled Analgesia. Blackwell Scientific, Boston, 1990

99. Thorén T, Tanghöj H, Wattwil M, Järnerot G: Epidural morphine delays gastric emptying and small intestinal transit in volunteers. Acta Anaesthesiol Scand 33:174, 1989

100. Thorén T, Wattwil M: Effects on gastric emptying of thoracic epidural analgesia with morphine or bupivacaine. Anesth Analg 67:687, 1988

101. England DW, Davis IJ, Timmins AE et al: Gastric emptying: a study to compare the effects of intrathecal morphine and I.M. papaveretum analgesia. Br J Anaesth 59:1403, 1987

102. Bardon T, Ruckebusch Y: Comparative effects of opiate agonists on proximal and distal colonic motility in dogs. Eur J Pharmacol 110:329, 1985

103. Thorén T, Wattwil M, Järnerot G, Tanghöj H: Epidural and spinal anesthesia do not influence gastric emptying and small intestinal transit in volunteers. Reg Anesth 14:35, 1989

104. Ahn H, Bronge A, Johansson K et al: Effects of continuous postoperative epidural analgesia on intestinal motility. Br J Surg 75:1176, 1988

105. Wattwil M, Thorén T, Hennerdal S, Garvill J-E: Epidural analgesia with bupivacaine reduces postoperative paralytic ileus after hysterectomy. Anesth Analg 68:353, 1989

106. Scheinin B, Asantila R, Orko R: The effect of bupivacaine and morphine on pain and bowel function after colonic surgery. Acta Anaesthesiol Scand 31:161, 1987

107. Painter NS: The effect of morphine in diverticulosis of the colon. Proc R Soc Med 56:800, 1963

108. Wilson JP: Postoperative motility of the large intestine in man. Gut 16:689, 1975
109. Wallin G, Cassuto J, Högström S et al: Failure of epidural anesthesia to prevent postoperative paralytic ileus. Anesthesiology 65:292, 1986
110. Olivecrona H: An experimental study of postoperative, so called paralytic ileus. Acta Chir Scand 61:485, 1927
111. David VC, Loring M: Splanchnic anesthesia in the treatment of paralytic ileus. Ann Surg 92:721, 1930
112. Hjortsø NC, Neumann P, Frøsig F et al: A controlled study on the effect of epidural analgesia with local anaesthetics and morphine on morbidity after abdominal surgery. Acta Anesthesiol Scand 29:790, 1985

27

Analgesia for the Victim of Trauma

Phillip Kistler

The provision of comfort to the victim of trauma is one of the most challenging responsibilities a practitioner of acute pain management may encounter. The enormity of the problem is illustrated by the fact that accidental injury is the leading cause of death for individuals younger than 45 years of age in the United States.[1] It has been calculated that more productive years are lost as a result of trauma than any other disease source.[1] The trauma patient is typically a young, healthy adult with multiple injuries who must be delivered to the medical care system as rapidly as possible to minimize morbidity and mortality. Initial evaluation and therapeutic maneuvers are carried out with great intensity and rapidity. It is during this period that the sometimes dichotomous goals of comfort and diagnosis first come to be at odds with each other. The great fear in this period of rapid evaluation and intervention is that analgesic comfort measures may mask evolving or yet undiagnosed processes that may be potentially associated with severe morbidity or even death.

DICHOTOMOUS GOALS: ANALGESIA VERSUS DIAGNOSIS?

There are many advantages to be gained by the provision of analgesia. A calm, comfortable, cooperative patient is obviously desirable so that the necessary verbal questioning, physical examinations, and therapeutic maneuvers might be readily accomplished. The initial control of pain and anxiety may reduce the extent of hormonal alteration (the stress response, see Ch. 4) and immunosuppression encountered with traumatic injury.[2] Amelioration of the effects of noxious stimuli may improve conditions for examination and reduce systemic hypertension. The restoration of function associated with adequate analgesia may eliminate secondary morbidity (e.g., the patient with multiple rib fractures). The provision of comfort is desirable, may provide for optimal patient evaluation and care, and reduces physiologic trespass associated with a given injury.

The method of providing analgesia must be carefully tailored to the individual.[3] The injuries, therapeutic priorities, and requirements for continuing evaluation of the patient must be considered. Consensus as to the plan of care must be established before the initiation of analgesic therapy. Centrally acting analgesics and sedatives may interfere with patient evaluation by depression of consciousness, depression of respiration, and production of hypotension. Major conduction blockade of the neuraxis may result in profound hypotension (especially in the hypovolemic patient). Major conduction anesthesia may also potentially mask evolving injuries by preventing detection of alterations in serial physical examinations.[4] Peripheral neural blockade may be advantageous by production of a limited area of hyperemia with minimal incidence of hypotension (particularly useful in reimplantation of the extremities). Potential masking of associated compartment syndromes remains a consideration.

The selection of an analgesic regimen in a trauma patient is a complicated task that must encompass many disparate and often competing interests. The risks of masking evolving pathology must be weighed against the increased patient cooperation and potentially improved physiologic parameters that effective analgesia can provide. Although not *necessarily* dichotomous goals, the risks and benefits of analgesia versus diagnosis must be weighed on an individual basis.

PHYSIOLOGIC ALTERATIONS ASSOCIATED WITH TRAUMATIC INJURY

The trauma patient may be subjected to any of a great number of physiologic trespasses. The patient may have head injuries that result in depressed consciousness, coma, or shock. Blunt chest trauma may result in injury to the heart, great vessels, and lungs, with attendant difficulties in maintenance of circulation and respiration. Major organs and vessels of the abdomen may be injured, resulting in hemorrhage, disruption of visceral integrity, and predisposition to multisystem organ failure. Injury to the skeleton and extremities may result in concealed hemorrhage, compartment syndromes, release of embolic material, or nerve injury. Disruption of vital structures and the attendant physiologic alterations may create a tenuous situation in which effective intervention may be the difference between life and death.

The release of humoral (i.e., protaglandins, leukotrienes, and kinins) and hormonal (i.e., catacholamines, cortisol, glucagon) mediators of the stress response after injury results in many deleterious physiologic alterations (see Ch. 4). These mediators produce a state in which hypermetabolism[5] (i.e., increased oxygen consumption), catabolism[6] (i.e., increased lipolysis, gluconeogenesis, and protein breakdown), and impaired immune competence[2,7] conspire to retard patient recovery. Reduction of the magnitude of the stress response by regional anesthetic/analgesic techniques is a compelling argument for their early institution.[8-10] (see Ch. 4).

ANALGESIC MODALITIES

Parenteral Analgesics

The most commonly used method of supplying analgesia to the trauma victim is the administration of centrally and peripherally acting parenteral analgesics (i.e., acetaminophen, nonsteroidal anti-inflammatory drugs [NSAIDs], and opioids).

The use of enteral medications in the victim of severe injury is best avoided. The effects of pain on gastric emptying and subsequent absorption are well documented. The delay in onset of action of orally administered medications and their unpredictable absorption limit their use. The subcutaneous and intramuscular routes of administration are also affected by the varying degrees of peripheral vasoconstriction present in severely injured patients.

The intravenous route of administration of analgesics is preferred for the trauma patient. The intravenous route provides for the reliable uptake and distribution of medication and allows for titration of effect without the possibility of delayed absorption.

Besides opioids, NSAIDs are now available in the United States as injectable medications (i.e., ketorolac) (see Ch. 7). Ketorolac (and potentially other NSAIDs) offer advantages over opioids in providing analgesia of similar intensity but without the attendant respiratory depressive, psychomotor, and sedative effects.[11-13]

Regional Anesthesia/Analgesia

The use of regional anesthesia/analgesia can be particularly effective in the victim of traumatic injury (Fig. 27-1). Subcutaneous infiltration about a localized site of injury can be simply performed with excellent results. The more specialized techniques of field block (Fig. 27-2), peripheral neural blockade, plexus blockade, and central neuraxial anesthesia and/or analgesia may also be used in the victim of trauma during the initial diagnostic, operative, or recuperative phases of hospitalization.

Infiltration

Local infiltration of anesthetic is most useful for smaller areas of injury (e.g., lacerations and minor operative repairs), as local anesthetic toxicity limits the mass of drug that may be administered (Table 27-1). No extensive knowledge

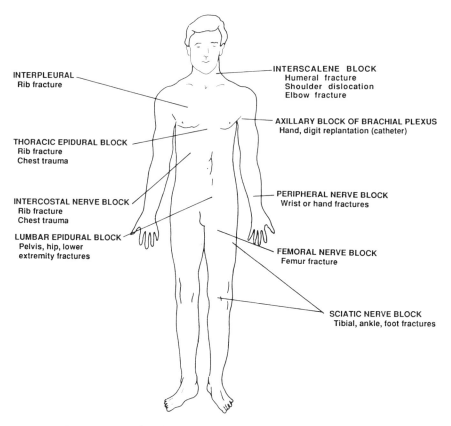

INTERPLEURAL
Rib fracture

INTERSCALENE BLOCK
Humeral fracture
Shoulder dislocation
Elbow fracture

AXILLARY BLOCK OF BRACHIAL PLEXUS
Hand, digit replantation (catheter)

THORACIC EPIDURAL BLOCK
Rib fracture
Chest trauma

INTERCOSTAL NERVE BLOCK
Rib fracture
Chest trauma

PERIPHERAL NERVE BLOCK
Wrist or hand fractures

LUMBAR EPIDURAL BLOCK
Pelvis, hip, lower
extremity fractures

FEMORAL NERVE BLOCK
Femur fracture

SCIATIC NERVE BLOCK
Tibial, ankle, foot fractures

Fig. 27-1. Regional analgesic techniques for traumatic injury.

of anatomy is required. An initial skin wheal of local anesthetic is made, and subsequent extensions of the wheal are initiated from previously anesthetized areas. Accidental intravascular injection and deposition of epinephrine along the distribution of end arteries must be avoided.

Field Blockade

Field blockade involves infiltration of local anesthetic along the divisions of nerves supplying a given area. Large areas of superficial structures may be made analgesic with acceptable doses of local anesthetic. This technique is commonly used for abdominal incisions, as somatic nerves radiating from the spine are easily blocked by infiltration of local anesthetic subcutaneously across their course. An excellent example of a field block used in conjunction with the ilioinguinal and iliohypogastric nerve blocks to provide inguinal anesthesia is found in Figure 27-2.

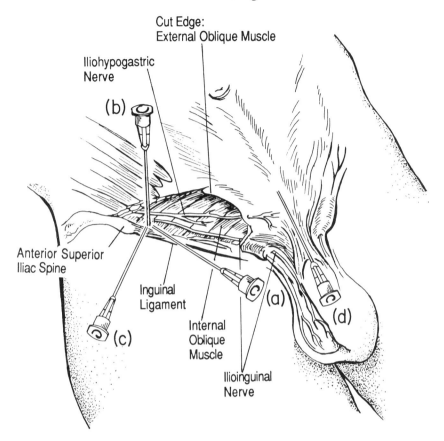

Cut Edge:
External Oblique Muscle

Iliohypogastric
Nerve

(b)

Anterior Superior
Iliac Spine

Inguinal
Ligament

(c)

Internal
Oblique
Muscle

(a)

(d)

Ilioinguinal
Nerve

Fig. 27-2. Ilioinguinal and iliohypogastric nerve blocks and accompanying field block for inguinal anesthesia/analgesia. (The external oblique muscle has been cut away to reveal the underlying neural structures.) (**a**) Local anesthetic is infiltrated in a superolateral direction until the ilium is contacted. (**b**) Infiltration is then performed at a steeper angle to ensure penetration of all abdominal wall muscles. (**c**) Subcutaneous infiltration is performed from the anterior superior iliac spine to the umbilicus. (**d**) Infiltration is performed from the pubis to the umbilicus. Of course, the site of surgical incision is also anesthetized.

Peripheral Neural Blockade

Peripheral neural blockade is more technically demanding. The instillation of local anesthetic sufficiently close to a nerve trunk or plexus in adequate volume and concentration to block impulse conduction without causing nerve injury is a refined skill. Particular knowledge of the anatomic location of nerves in relation to other structures is required. The danger of intravascular injection and local anesthetic toxicity must be respected. The advantage of the technique lies in the fact that injections can be made remote from the actual site of injury. Use of the longer-acting local anesthetic agents (e.g., bupivacaine with epinephrine) can make twice daily administration of medication a complete analgesic

TABLE 27-1. Infiltration Anesthesia

Local Anesthetic	Concentration (%)	Duration (min + range) Plain	Duration (min + range) Epinephrine (1:200,000)	Maximum Single Dose (mg) Plain	Maximum Single Dose (mg) Epinephrine (1:200,000)
Procaine	0.5	20 (15–30)	60 (15–120)	500	600
Lidocaine	0.5	75 (30–90)	200 (60–300)	300[a]	500
Lidocaine	1.0	120 (90–140)	400 (360–420)	Same	Same
Mepivacaine	0.5	108 (30–120)	240 (140–310)	300[a]	500
Prilocaine	1.0	100 (90–110)	280 (250–300)	400[a]	600[b]
Bupivacaine	0.25	190 (180–210)	430 (400–450)	175	250

[a] In the hands of specialists other than anesthesiologists, dosage of these agents without epinephrine should not exceed 200 mg.

[b] Single doses of prilocaine over 600 mg or repeated doses of lesser amounts will produce methemoglobinemia.

regimen for selected applications. The application of catheter techniques is possible, making repeated injections or continuous infusions feasible. The use of a nerve sheath catheter for prevention of phantom limb pain has been recently described.[14]

Plexus Blockade

Plexus blockade uses the existence of connective tissue planes and sheaths to make the blockade of an extensive area possible (brachial or lumbar plexuses, see Chs. 13 and 14, respectively) with a single injection. The use of continuous plexus anesthesia/analgesia via catheter techniques is illustrated by improved outcome after extremity reimplantation[15,16] (see Ch. 14). The technical expertise required for catheter techniques has limited the use of these methods. Also, maintenance of catheters in the proper anatomic compartment is difficult because of patient movement. However, the advantages of limited sympathectomy, prolonged use, and peripheral location may make this technique the treatment of choice in certain circumstances. The masking of compartment syndromes because of hemorrhage, edema, or compression is possible, and surgical team members must be prepared to use alternative measures to monitor for these complications.

Interpleural Regional Analgesia

Interpleural administration of local anesthetic has been described for the treatment of pain caused by multiple rib fractures.[17] The technique involves placement of a catheter between the visceral and parietal pleura with production of multiple intercostal nerve blocks (see Ch. 16). The administration of large volumes of local anesthetic is required, and toxicity is possible. Delayed splenic rupture has been masked by use of interpleural analgesia.[18]

Epidural Analgesia

Epidural anesthetic/analgesic techniques are widely used in both the postoperative and post-traumatic injury patient. Restoration of respiratory mechanics after multiple rib fractures can speed recovery and reduce morbidity associated with these conditions.[19,20] The use of regional anesthesia has been shown to decrease the incidence of deep venous thrombosis.[21] Reduction in the magnitude of the stress response to lower abdominal and hip procedures is also a known feature of epidural anesthesia.[22]

Ease of application of the technique and the ability to place catheters at the spinal cord level appropriate to the level of injury are distinct advantages. Disadvantages of epidural anesthesia/analgesia are the potential for extensive sympathectomy (with use of local anesthetics), the possibility of catheter migration or infection, the possibility of epidural hematoma formation (in the patient with abnormal coagulation), the masking of evolving injuries at many levels, and close proximity to the central nervous system.

Subarachnoid Analgesia

The use of subarachnoid (spinal) analgesia is commonly limited to one-time administration of opioids. The fear of postdural puncture headache has limited repetitive administration. The concern regarding potential infection of the subarachnoid space has led to a reluctance to use continuous catheters. The use of local anesthetics in very dilute solutions for continuous analgesia has been reported.[23] The extensive and rapid sympathectomy associated with local anesthetic administration may make the technique suitable only for stable patients with adequate monitoring. The adaptability of epidural anesthetic/analgesic techniques makes subarachnoid analgesia a second-line modality in most instances.

HEAD INJURY

The management of the patient with severe head injury allows little room for error. The patient has frequently consumed alcohol or drugs and is at great risk for aspiration caused by depression of protective airway reflexes. The presence of anxiety, pain, and combativeness may adversely affect intracranial pressure in patients with reduced intraventricular compliance. The use of opioids or anxiolytics in such patients may be risky because of the effects of respiratory depression (hypoxia and hypercarbia) on cerebral blood flow.[24] Once ventilation has been controlled, the use of opioids and barbiturates may be beneficial in reducing cerebral oxygen requirements. The use of local anesthetic techniques is quite attractive in those patients in whom consciousness is used as an indicator of the severity of head injury. Provision of analgesia without alteration in mental status is a very useful characteristic of regional anesthesia/analgesia. Central neuraxial anesthesia/analgesia is contraindicated in the presence of elevated intracranial pressure because of the fear of herniation or further increases in intracranial pressure. The provision of analgesia to the head-injured patient is a service of potentially great benefit, but extreme caution and planning must be used to avoid morbidity.

CHEST INJURY

Blunt chest trauma is a frequent sequela of automobile accidents. Lacerations of the aorta, myocardial and/or pulmonary contusions, multiple rib fractures, and hemopneumothorax may occur. It is incumbent on the practitioner to rule out the presence of immediately life-threatening conditions before applying therapy that might mask their detection.[25]

Treatment of multiple rib fractures is particularly effective in restoration of homeostasis. Inspiratory pain leads to atelectasis and hypoxia, which require additional ventilatory work. Increased ventilatory effort leads to more pain and more decrement in respiratory function. This cycle can be interrupted with adequate analgesia. Analgesia is most often provided by epidural,[26] intercostal,[27] or interpleural analgesia.[17] These modalities have been shown to be superior to conventional opioid administration. Avoidance of intubation with superior analgesia may be possible, and this may result in decreased morbidity.[28]

ORTHOPAEDIC INJURY

The orthopaedic surgeon is often already very familiar with the advantages of regional anesthesia/analgesia. A reduction in intraoperative blood loss and an associated decrease in postoperative opioid requirements is well documented with use of spinal and epidural anesthesia.[29] Continuous brachial plexus blockade for intraoperative anesthesia and postoperative sympathectomy and analgesia can increase the success of reimplantation procedures of the hand.[14] Epidural analgesia has become immensely popular in providing postoperative analgesia in lower extremity procedures. Early mobilization, painless physical therapy, and a possible reduction in the incidence of deep venous thrombosis[21,30] are advantages to the technique. Preoperative epidural anesthesia[31] and intraoperative placement of nerve sheath catheters with subsequent use of local anesthetic infusions[14] have been successful in preventing phantom limb pain.

Many orthopaedic injuries involve large amounts of tissue damage and hemorrhage, predisposing to hypovolemia and compartment syndromes. Neural blockade may obscure detection of the development of compartment syndrome. Use of neuraxial opioids will not obscure the diagnosis of compartment syndrome, however.[32]

CONCLUSION

The provision of analgesia to the victim of traumatic injury is a reasonable goal. In many instances, improved outcome may result from the timely application of analgesic techniques. The goals of the surgical trauma team remain paramount: preservation of life, limb, and function. Any maneuvers that can improve patient comfort, as well as outcome, should be provided as soon as is practical without endangering the aforementioned goals. The practitioner of acute pain management has many tools that can be used to great effect in the management of the trauma patient. The role of pain management must not be relegated to the level of a mere afterthought, and more active participation in the care of the trauma patient is to be encouraged.

References

1. Committee on Trauma Research, Commission of Life Sciences, National Research Council and Institute of Medicine: Injury in America. A Continuing Public Health Problem. National Academic Press, Washington, DC, 1985
2. Hole A, Unsgaard G, Brivick H: Monocyte functions are depressed during and after surgery under general anesthesia but not under epidural anesthesia. Acta Anaesthesiol Scand 26:301, 1982
3. Sharar SR, Cullen BF: Regional anesthesia and analgesia for the trauma and burn patient. Clin Anesth Updates 1:1, 1990
4. Strecker WB, Wood MB, Bieber EJ: Compartment syndrome masked by epidural anesthesia for postoperative pain. Report of a case. J Bone Joint Surg [Am] 68:1447, 1986
5. Jaattela A, Alho A, Avikainen V et al: Plasma catacholamines in severely injured patients: a prospective study on 45 patients with multiple injuries. Br J Surg 62:177, 1975
6. Brandt MR, Fernandes A, Mordhorst R et al: Epidural analgesia improves postoperative nitrogen balance. Br Med J 1:1106, 1978
7. Slade MS, Simmons RL, Yunis E, Greenberg LJ: Immunodepression after major surgery in normal patients. Surgery 78:363, 1974
8. Gann DS, Lilly MP: The neuroendocrine response to multiple trauma. World J Surg 7:101, 1983
9. Kehlet H: The modifying effect of general and regional anesthesia on the endocrine—metabolic response to surgery. Reg Anaesth 7:838, 1982
10. Kehlet H: The modifying effect of anesthetic technique on the metabolic and endocrine responses to anesthesia and surgery. Acta Anesthesiol Belg 39:143, 1988
11. Rubin P, Yee JP, Murthy VS, Seavey W: Ketorolac tromethamine (KT) analgesia: no post-operative respiratory depression and less constipation. Clin Pharmacol Ther 41:182, 1987
12. MacDonald FC, Gough KJ, Nicoll RAG, Dow RJ: Psychomotor effects of ketorolac in comparison with buprenorphine and diclofenac. Br J Clin Pharmacol 27:453, 1989
13. Kenny CNC: Ketorolac trometamol—a new non-opioid analgesic (editorial). Br J Anaesth 65:445, 1990
14. Fisher A, Meller Y: Continuous postoperative regional analgesia by nerve sheath block for amputation surgery—a pilot study. Anesth Analg 72:300, 1991
15. Rosenblatt R, Pepitone-Rockwell F, McKillop MJ: Continuous axillary analgesia for traumatic hand injury. Anesthesiology 51:565, 1979
16. Berger A, Tizian C, Zana M: Continuous plexus blockade for improved circulation in microvascular surgery. Ann Plast Surg 14:16, 1985
17. Rocco A, Reiestad F, Gudman J, McKay W: Interpleural administration of local anesthetics for pain relief in patients with multiple rib fractures. Reg Anesth 12:10, 1987

18. Pond WW, Somerville, GM, Thong SH et al: Pain of delayed splenic rupture masked by intrapleural lidocaine. Anesthesiology 70:154, 1989

19. Pederson VM, Schulze S, Hoier-Madsen K, Halkier E: Air flow meter assessment on the effect of intercostal nerve blockade on respiratory function in rib fractures. Acta Chir Scand 149:119, 1983

20. Mackersie RC, Shackford SR, Hoyt DB, Karagianes TG: Continuous epidural fentanyl analgesia: ventilatory function improvement with routine use in treatment of blunt chest injury. J Trauma 27:1207, 1987

21. Stewart GJ: Antithrombotic activity of local anesthetics in several canine models, abstracted. Reg Anaesth 7:S89, 1982

22. Kehlet H: The stress response to anesthesia and surgery: release mechanisms and modifying factors. Clin Anesth 2:315, 1984

23. Bevacqua BK, Slucky AV, Adusumilli SB: Postoperative analgesia with continuous intrathecal lidocaine infusion, abstracted. Anesthesiology 73:A833, 1990

24. Buchweitz E, Grandison C, Weiss HR: Effect of morphine on regional cerebral oxygen consumption and supply. Brain Res 291:301, 1984

25. Ward AJ, Gillat DA: Delayed diagnosis of traumatic rupture of the spleen: a warning of the use of thoracic epidural analgesia in chest trauma. Injury 20:178, 1989

26. Dittman M, Keller R, Wolff G: A rationale for epidural analgesia in the treatment of multiple rib fractures. Intensive Care Med 4:193, 1978

27. Bridenbaugh PO, DuPen SL, Moore DC et al: Postoperative intercostal nerve block analgesia versus narcotic analgesia. Anesth Analg 52:81, 1973

28. Trinkle JK, Richardson JD, Franz JL et al: Management of flail chest without mechanical ventilation. Ann Thorac Surg 19:355, 1975

29. Valentin H, Lomholt B, Jensen JS et al: Spinal or general anesthesia for surgery of the fractured hip? A prospective study of mortality in 578 patients. Br J Anaesth 58:284, 1986

30. McKenzie PJ, Wishart HY, Gray I, Smith G: Effects of anesthetic technique on deep vein thrombosis. A comparison of subarachnoid and general anesthesia. Br J Anaesth 57:853, 1985

31. Bach S, Noreng MF, Tjéllden NU: Phantom limb pain in amputees during the first 12 months following limb amputation, after preoperative lumbar epidural blockade. Pain 33:297, 1988

32. Montgomery CJ, Ready LB: Epidural opioid analgesia does not obscure diagnosis of compartment syndrome resulting from prolonged lithotomy position. Anesthesiology 75:541, 1991

28

Financial Aspects of Acute Pain Management

Edward M. Le Sage

It is important to recognize from the outset that all states differ with respect to policies and procedures for insurance claim submission and reimbursement, especially where Blue Cross, Medicare, and Welfare are concerned. Still, for each individual state, the data and formats for these three carriers alone create a maze of rules and regulations that is enough to discourage any potential provider. This is a pessimistic view, but a realistic one. Recognition of the realities of billing for an acute pain service (APS) is the first step toward fiscal responsibility and financial success.

COMMUNICATION

The essential first step or starting point for creation of an APS is *communication*. This would appear rudimentary, and yet it cannot be stressed enough. It is not easy to coordinate or to achieve communication and collaboration without great effort, but it is a necessary preliminary for the establishment of any APS billing office.

Professional representatives of the various insurance carriers should be contacted. Ideally, you should meet with them to become familiar with their specific concerns and priorities. Obviously, this ideal is not always possible. In lieu of meetings, most third-party carriers have manuals that should contain a plethora of useful and necessary information.

Billing data, the format of that data, rules, regulations, and laws vary tremendously. This is true within a state *and* from state to state. For example, the Department of Health and Human Services Health Care Financing Administration legislates nationally for Medicare. In general, however, this legislation is often interpreted and implemented differently from state to state and among major defined regions. Knowledge of regional specifications is necessary in order to submit a claim and be reimbursed for that claim. The oft-quoted phrase from the computer world "garbage in, garbage out" summarizes the scenario fairly well.

PHYSICIAN INPUT

Development of comfortable working relations with the physicians of the APS (especially the director or head of the pain service) cannot help but be beneficial. In fact, physician input, or lack of it, could make or break an APS billing operation. This is true for the actual billing process, as well as the office administration. More crucially, it is important for definition of the goals of the service, financial and otherwise.

THE CONCEPT OF THE GLOBAL FEE

With respect to definitions, a quick look at the etymology of the word *anesthesia* shows its derivation from the Greek "anaisthesia" (*an* = without; *aisthesis* = feeling). Thus, "*anesthesia*" means partial or total loss of the sense of pain, temperature, touch, etc., produced by disease or an anesthetic.[1] The definition of *anesthesiologist* flows from this. The anesthesiologist's pharmacologic and neuroanatomic knowledge of pain and the ability to administer effective treatment firmly places the expertise of the field squarely in his or her hands.

Ready et al[2] and Ramsey[3] have cogently argued that "organized" management of postoperative pain belongs to the discipline of anesthesiology. They note that "initial concerns from some surgical colleagues regarding loss of control of the management of their patients . . . have been replaced by enthusiasm for the quality of care being provided by the APS."[2] Insurance companies and the various agencies paying for the services rendered have yet to be convinced.

Traditionally, care rendered by anesthesiologists has been viewed as a sort of package deal, infamously labeled the *global fee*. The preoperative, intraoperative, and postoperative work of the anesthesiologist is viewed as a continuum by insurance carriers. Traditionally it has been billed as such to insurance carriers. They have come to see it as such, expect it to be so, and in turn, pay accordingly.

The concept of the global fee is a narrow view that is being increasingly challenged by the work and success of physicians and other health care professionals involved in postoperative pain management. Unfortunately, the concept of the global fee has a great negative impact on the financial viability of organized acute pain management. To paraphrase the most common reason given for the rejection of claims for APS care, "these services have already been covered by the global anesthesia charge. No further payment will be made." Such a "package-deal" mentality could eventually make provision of acute pain services economically untenable and destroy what are in essence *new* services.

The matter is further complicated because billing for APS services falls under the rubrics of internal medicine. An anesthesiologist providing postoperative pain management must charge for these services with the same procedure codes an internist would use for in-hospital patient care. At the present time, internal medicine billing codes are the only categories available to him or her. How accurately do internal medicine codes describe the work an anesthesiologist does in providing acute pain care? As you can imagine, this causes great confusion in the insurance world. The need then is to argue for, get the recognition of, and be paid for acute pain management that goes beyond the neatly accepted categories of pre-, intra-, and postanesthetic care generally equated with the concept of the global anesthesia fee.

In an address given on November 20, 1990, before the Agency for Health Care Policy and Research on the Management of Acute Postoperative Pain, Michel DuBois, M.D. (representing the American Society of Anesthesiologists) presented the case as follows:[4]

> *Relief of postoperative pain must no longer be considered ancillary to the surgical service. The days of standing surgical orders for p.r.n. oral and intramuscular pain relief, with no patient specificity and wide latitude as to dosage, are surely coming to an end. The pain results from the surgical procedure, but postoperative pain has its own diagnosis, its own treatments, its own side effects, its own specialists. The physiologic responses triggered by postsurgical pain include increases in cardiac functions, muscle tension, hormone imbalances and a host of other problems. Relief of pain is what the patient appreciates; avoidance of complications needs appreciation by the medical community.*
>
> *Anesthesiologists and other specialists now have the capability, working with nurses and pharmacists, to decrease morbidity and mortality, achieve earlier ambulation and discharge, and enhance patient satisfaction. In addition to these clinical improvements, one must consider the cost efficiency of earlier discharge and fewer complications—savings which more than offset the cost of a sophisticated pain service.*
>
> *However, the overwhelming amount of research, the skill required to deliver the service, and the obvious efficacy have not dispelled the opinion of some physicians, hospital administrators, and payors that pain management is no more than patient comfort. If this panel accomplishes nothing more, a valuable service will be done if this notion is put aside.*

In the end, the concept of global care and the global fee still remain the biggest stumbling blocks to the financial health of organized postoperative pain management. Until third-party payors view acute pain management as more than comfort measures and until there are concise and unambiguous billing and procedural codes specific for acute pain services, the financial viability of acute pain management must remain uncertain.

ADMINISTRATION

Departmental Administration

To state the obvious, an APS will not succeed without the support of both departmental and hospital administration. Departmental administration must fund salaries for attending staff, residents, fellows, physician's assistants or nurses, and office support staff, as well as select an appropriate vehicle for billing. The financial ramifications for an anesthesia department are obvious. Viewed in purely a financial sense, more revenue would be accrued from staffing operating rooms with personnel rather than an APS struggling to be self-sustaining. Monies have to be provided to initially support and bolster an APS during its fledgling years. Before institution of an APS, a department should scrutinize and assess its average payor mix, patient populations, and how the various group percentages work out in order to determine if an APS will ever be financially successful in the particular economic climate. It is wise and perhaps crucial to perform a cost analysis regarding patient payment from Blue Cross and Medicare Part A versus payment from Blue Shield and Medicare Part B.

More important than funding, departmental administration's role will be to facilitate communication and collaboration between all the different components of the anesthesia department. An APS will have absolutely no hope of becoming self-sustaining if operations between the operating room and APS are not streamlined and efficient.

Hospital Administration

Hospital administration's perspective of an APS is, naturally, seen in the context of the demands made on and the attention required by all the other services in the hospital. In supporting an APS, a hospital will have to assume responsibility for a number of basic necessities. Hospital administration must allot space, purchase needed equipment (infusion pumps), market the APS, and educate both the medical and nursing staff regarding the services of the APS.

Procurement of Equipment

Capital equipment for the APS is a major expense. A more educated choice of patient-controlled analgesia (PCA) or epidural infusion devices is always made through multidisciplinary input. Thus, particular devices can be chosen that best meet the particular needs of an institution's nursing staff and pharmacy department, as well as APS. With the fiscal power of a large institution, hospital administration is ideally suited to negotiate with vendors for procurement of infusion devices. Individuals, rather than institutions, are at a distinct disadvantage when purchasing or procuring capital equipment from vendors. After procurement of the devices, the role of administration is central in setting policies and procedures for the storage, maintenance, and dispensing of the chosen infusion pumps.

Infusion pumps can be (1) purchased and their use charged to the patient, (2) purchased and amortized through the budget, or (3) given to the hospital on signature of a contract for exclusive purchase and use of a particular vendor's analgesics. The wisest plan for procurement depends on individual state regulations. If the first option is chosen, hospital administration should set up the mechanism for charging third-party payors for daily use of the pumps. Charge codes must be in place before service begins. The budget department of the hospital will be aware of the various eccentricities of billing for individual carriers. Familiarity with Medicare and Welfare carriers is vital. Their mandated rules and regulations affect not only patient charges per se, but also the method used for procurement of infusion devices and disposables relative to purchase or amortization. Incorrect submission of claims, especially with Medicare, can result in the levying of substantial fines.

Marketing

Marketing of the APS is an integral part of administrative responsibility. The main target group should be the medical community, but the patient population should not be ignored. An informational brochure useful for both physician and patient should be designed and published. When available, the initial distribution should be to surgeons, obstetricians, and oncologists whose names may be obtained from hospital staff lists.

It is best to start slowly. Acute pain services are very popular. It is important to have sufficient staff and equipment so that the demand for services does not outstrip the ability to supply it.

There are two relatively uncomplicated ways of distributing APS literature to patients. Physicians can keep brochures on display in their waiting rooms. However, such an approach relies too heavily on individuals not intimately associated with the APS. A better approach is to distribute brochures in a preadmission testing center. Before the preoperative visit with an anesthesiologist, the patient can read about the availability of epidural analgesia and PCA. During the preoperative anesthesia interview, the patient can speak with an anesthesiologist about their postoperative analgesic care. Subsequently, they can express their interest in APS care to their surgeon or obstetrician. If the patient seems to be a good candidate, the surgeon or obstetrician can write for an APS consultation in the postoperative orders. (It should be noted that most third-party payors require a consultation from the primary physician in order to pay for postoperative pain management.) Thus, the preanesthetic interview is a more direct and useful venue for interfacing with the patient regarding postoperative analgesic management.

CONCLUSION

Whether one likes to admit it or not, APS care is a business to some extent. Associated with day-to-day patient care are the budgets, salaries, supplies, and pump procurement necessary to make the APS a viable functioning entity. Money matters have to be addressed. Bills have to be paid. This poses a dilemma, as management of an APS is not a business that can be reduced to mere credits and debits. APSs exist as a business in order to be about the business of providing good patient care. Unfortunately, many payors choose not to recognize postoperative pain management as a *new* legitimate service. Thus, many anesthesia departments and hospitals choose not to become involved with establishment of formal, organized APSs. Although management of an APS will never be lucrative, postoperative pain management by an organized service can be economically feasible and self-sustaining. As public awareness of the modalities provided by an APS grows, so too will demand and eventually payment. Unlike third-party payors, the public will view aggressive postoperative pain management not as a privilege but as a right.

ACKNOWLEDGMENTS

We wish to acknowledge the collaboration of Victor Vick, Vice President, Brigham and Women's Hospital, and Helen Gallahue, Administrator-Anesthesia, Brigham and Women's Hospital.

References
1. Guralnik DB, Friend JH: Webster's New World Dictionary of the American Language. The World Publishing Company, New York, 1966
2. Ready LB, Oden R, Chadwick HS et al: Development of an anesthesiology-based postoperative pain management service. Anesthesiology 68:100, 1988
3. Ramsey DH: Introducing patient-controlled analgesia into the hospital. p. 179. In Covino BG, Ferrante FM, Ostheimer GW (eds): Patient-Controlled Analgesia. Blackwell Scientific Publications, Boston, 1990
4. Acute Pain Management Guideline Panel: Acute Pain Management: Operative or Medical Procedures and Trauma. Guideline Report. AHCPR Pub. No. 92-0022. Agency for Health Care Policy and Research, Public Health Service, U.S. Department of Health and Human Services, Rockville, MD. 1992

29

Nursing Considerations for Acute Pain Management

Phyllis Hoopman

Nursing plays an essential role in postoperative pain management. Nurses have traditionally used effective pain management practices over the years. However, the experience in the development of a multidisciplinary pain treatment team has contributed to increased nursing satisfaction, increased consultation between and among professionals, and most importantly, improved patient satisfaction with high-quality health care delivery.

The need for the development of a multidisciplinary team grew out of the rapid increases in patient volume sustained by the Acute Pain Service at Brigham and Women's Hospital. A rapid growth in demand for analgesic services that far outstrips the ability to supply such services is a phenomenon not indigenous to our institution alone. This chapter, in part, focuses on our experience in development of a multidisciplinary team at Brigham and Women's Hospital. It is hoped that our experience may serve as a model for other such ventures, as formation of multidisciplinary acute pain management teams has now been promulgated by the Agency for Health Care Policy and Research of the federal government.[1]

THE FORMATION OF AN EFFECTIVE PAIN MANAGEMENT TEAM: BRIGHAM AND WOMEN'S HOSPITAL

A steering committee for pain management was organized in May 1989. This committee was and continues to be the base for carrying out the institution's initiative to offer high-quality and responsive pain management. The pain management steering committee includes members from a variety of disciplines:

Vice President for Surgical Services
Director of Pain Management Services (Department of Anesthesia)
Director of Surgical Nursing Services
Director of Operating Room/Recovery Room Nursing Services
Director of Pharmacy Services
Director for Cost-Effective Care
Administrator for Pain Management Services
Administrator for Anesthesia

Goals

The initiative began with a study of current epidural and patient-controlled analgesic (PCA) practices at our institution. The need to study these two methods of analgesia was due in part to the acute care patient population served and to the rapid increase in surgical patient volume being treated with epidural analgesia and PCA. Between fiscal year 1988 and the third quarter of 1989, use of epidural analgesia grew from 222 to 599 patients (a 169.8 percent increase) and use of PCA grew from 248 to 2,446 patients (a 886.3 percent increase). Meanwhile, limitation of physician time to respond to this growth and the desire of nursing to assume expansion in practice with PCA facilitated moving the steering committee's initiatives.

The steering committee was divided into three task forces. One was led by nursing for PCA, another was led by the Director of Pain Management Services for epidural analgesia, and the third was led by Pharmacy to assess distribution and storage of opioids for both PCA and epidural analgesia. Priority was placed on PCA because of the highest patient volume. We agreed that many practices could be shifted to registered nurses. The distribution and storage of opioids were part of the PCA program changes and, therefore, were addressed in parallel with the PCA program.

PCA Task Force

The PCA Task Force met every 2 weeks for 1 hour. Initially, activities were reported to the steering committee on a monthly basis and eventually on a quarterly basis. The PCA Task Force agreed to initially consider acute pain management for postoperative surgical, obstetric, and gynecologic patients. The introduction and/or expansion of PCA to the medical subspecialties would be considered at a later date.

When the PCA Task Force began to meet, nursing representatives from all surgical, obstetric/gynecologic (OB/Gyn), and recovery room areas met with Pharmacy, physicians and administrators of the Acute Pain Service, and at intervals, Equipment Pool representatives. A representative from Nursing Staff

Education was integral to the PCA Task Force in planning education and using her expertise as a Nursing Policy and Procedure Committee member. Education on pain and its relief was and continues to be a focus of all the task forces.

We decided to build a resource guide for PCA. The guide contained the following information:

1. information on the rationale for use of PCA in lieu of intramuscular opioids,
2. our revised nursing protocols for use of PCA in general care areas and OB/Gyn,
3. patient selection criteria for PCA,
4. a glossary of terms,
5. a nursing algorithm for inadequate analgesia, including titration of dose and administration of rescue doses,
6. a physician order sheet for PCA,
7. nursing procedure for use of the Abbott LifeCare PCA-PLUS II (the PCA infuser used at our institution),
8. fast load procedure for use in recovery room areas (to establish analgesia),
9. nursing guidelines for administration of naloxone, and
10. examples of infrequently used opioids for PCA administration.

Several of these protocols are included in the Appendix at the end of the chapter.

While the resource guide was being developed, educational efforts were intensified. Pain management literature was sent to each nursing care area. In-services were regularly given by the Acute Pain Service on individual nursing units. Pain Service physicians were assigned as liaisons to individual patient care areas to foster education and collaboration and to establish professional consultations between nurses and physicians. We began to see increasing informal consults between nurses, physicians, and pharmacists. The trust engendered by these relationships was probably the most important factor in helping us to reach our goal of improved delivery of care for PCA. These liaisons were established before beginning our pilot implementation of new nursing guidelines for PCA.

Drug Dispensing

The dilemma of opioid distribution was also addressed. At the start of our program, nurses were being called away from the patient in the recovery room areas to retrieve opioids for PCA. The interruption in patient care and the increased nursing time involved in this activity was more than an aggravation. The anesthesiologist, in turn, often had to wait for the nurse and the opioid while the patient's pain management was left unmet.

Hospital administration supported the idea of purchasing an automated medication vending device. It was decided to distribute PCA opioid cartridges and other pain medications through this machine. One new full-time pharmacy staff member was allotted to help in stocking the automatic vendor. Accounting for opioids with this device is patient-specific as to type and amount of opioid dispensed, time, and date. The device automatically records the user's identification number. Anesthesiologists have their own access to the vendor without going through nursing or pharmacy directly, and nursing staff are freed to deliver care to patients with fewer interruptions. The pharmacy has improved records of the dispensing of controlled substances through printouts from the automated vending machine. The savings in nursing, pharmacy, and physician time far outweigh an additional cost imposed by purchase of the automated vendor.

Nursing Acceptance of Task Force Changes

An evaluation of the program was undertaken 12 weeks after the pilot nursing units had worked with the new guidelines and protocols. Because original PCA pumps were exchanged for updated technology, we were interested in ascertaining nurses' perceptions regarding the new PCA infusers and the PCA Task Force directives. The evaluation was given to approximately 350 registered nurses with 141 respondents. The results were very positive.

A sample evaluation form is shown in Figure 29-1. There were nine questions; seven asked for ratings on a one (very poor) to six (outstanding) scale, and two questions required a yes or no response.

Seventy-five percent of the respondents stated a range of good to outstanding for questions 1 to 4. Question six (rating the PCA protocol/procedure) had 102 responses in the good to very good category and 13 in the outstanding category. Such a response was very positive for such a short period of education and actual practice time. Areas of concern were nurses' understanding of "titration" (see Glossary of Terms in Appendix) and flow sheet documentation. All staff were re-educated on the necessity for titration of analgesic dosage by nursing. The expectation that patients would initially require more nursing interaction during adjustment to their nursing care area after recovery room transfer was reinforced.

The most disturbing mechanical problem highlighted by the evaluation was the PCA infuser's lack of long battery life when not connected to an electric outlet (e.g., during ambulation). New batteries, additional electric outlets, and education to keep the infusers plugged in when patients were not ambulatory has reduced the incidence of battery failure to practically nil.

Ongoing Task Force Objectives

The PCA Task Force continues to meet quarterly. Annual revisions are made to the resource guide with updates on protocols and practices. Two major pain management workshops have been integrated into the nursing educational curriculum. One of these has been sponsored by the Anesthesia Department in

```
                 BRIGHAM AND WOMEN'S HOSPITAL

                    NURSING DEPARTMENT

              EVALUATION OF THE PCA-PLUS PROGRAM


Please rate the following questions on a 1 to 6 scale

1=Very Poor    2=Poor    3=Average    4=Good    5=Very Good    6=Outstanding


1.  The ease of learning to operate the equipment        1  2  3  4  5  6

2.  The patient's ability to operate the equipment       1  2  3  4  5  6

3.  Overall, how effective was the patient's pain
    controlled with PCA-Plus.                            1  2  3  4  5  6

4.  Did you feel the patient was satisfied with
    PCA-Plus therapy.                                    1  2  3  4  5  6

5.  The ease of administering a titration dose          1  2  3  4  5  6

6.  Overall, how would you rate the PCA-Plus
    Protocol/Procedure                                  1  2  3  4  5  6

7.  How does PCA-Plus compare to traditional
    pain management with respect to your
    autonomy in pain management.                        1  2  3  4  5  6

8.  The patients chosen for the PCA-Plus
    therapy meet the suggested criteria      Yes _____  No _____

    If no, please explain _____

    _____

9.  Does the PCA flowsheet meet the documentation needs    Yes ___  No ___

    If no, please explain _____

    _____

6/19/90

#13pcaeval
```

Fig. 29-1. Evaluation of the PCA-Plus program. (From Brigham and Women's Hospital. Pain Treatment Service, Boston, MA 1991, with permission.)

their commitment to ongoing education for all professionals. In addition, a nurse practitioner and clinical nurse specialist have been added to the staff of the Acute Pain Service. The addition of nurses to the team has strengthened nursing support and patient care. The service is visible, accessible, and trusted to respond to patient needs.

Our priorities have now shifted to the Epidural Task Force and educational efforts for patients and professionals regarding this modality. The Epidural Task Force is accessing use of up-to-date infusion devices and ultimately changing nurse and physician interactions in the delivery of care. A separate task force with representative groups similar to the PCA Task Force is presently at work redesigning policies and procedures regarding epidural analgesia.

Although PCA and epidural pain management have been the focus, the concern for education has continued to be a priority. The institution has provided resources to develop and print a pamphlet on postoperative pain management for patients. The pamphlet describes the services provided at the Brigham and Women's Hospital for the management of pain. These pamphlets are used for preadmission education.

Pain management services, led by anesthesiologists at our institution, provide excellent care to patients. Since the development of a multidisciplinary team to study global issues, we are realizing the effects of shared knowledge. Consultation and collaboration among many diverse services is being fostered. Certainly this will translate into more widespread and efficient patient care. Through collaborative efforts, the ultimate goal of aggressive postoperative pain management (i.e., the eradication or near eradication of postoperative pain as a phenomenon) can perhaps be attained.

ALTERNATIVE METHODS OF PAIN CONTROL

Encouraging patients to take control over self-administration of opioids is often negatively perceived by patients, at least initially, as it is inconsistent with more traditional values and beliefs regarding the administration of analgesics. The creation of an atmosphere conducive to effective PCA as well as epidural analgesia is accomplished when nurses use a combination of pharmacologic agents, psychoemotional knowledge and skills, and alternative methods of pain control.[2,3]

Posture/Position

Nonpharmacologic maneuvers can sometimes be used as singular methods to control or prevent pain. Patient positioning in bed or assisted sitting through use of specific supports to joints or noninjured areas can effectively reduce pain. Attention to corrective, therapeutic mattresses is also beneficial.

Sleep/Relaxation

The benefits of normal sleep-rest patterns during the postoperative period can help the individual to restore body needs. Attention to relaxation—whether by music, videos, silence, or privacy—have had positive effects in both intensive care units and general care areas.

Nausea/Vomiting

The concomitant use of medication and/or nutrition has been beneficial in the reduction of signs and symptoms that would otherwise potentially lead to increased pain. Nausea and vomiting could produce increased pain in the postoperative patient. Therefore, attention to the prevention of nausea and vomiting will alert the skilled practitioner to attend to patient needs and thereby avoid undue pain.

Mobilization

Inactivity can promote muscle wasting and joint stiffness. If the patient is nurse-dependent, arranging a regular activity schedule must be part of the nursing care plan. If the patient is independent, teaching them to incorporate activity is equally important for recovery.

Psychological State

All health care providers must be alert to the patient's psychological state. If the patient is depressed or anxious, pharmacologic management alone may not be addressing a causative factor for the patient's perception of pain. Therapy, with or without antidepressants, may improve mood, sleep, rest, and appetite.

Adjunctive Medications

The use of anti-inflammatory medications can produce potent analgesia in some patients. Used alone or in conjunction with hot or cold compresses, such treatments supplement the use of opioids.

CONCLUSION

Nurses have a vital role in pain management. As the caregivers spending the greatest amount of time in actual patient contact, nurses collect information, deliver pain management therapies, and make judgments in conjunction with the patient as to the overall efficacy of pain management. Nurses have a significant impact on the success of PCA and epidural analgesia. Nurses do so not only through their abilities to develop new policies and procedures for these modalities, but also by virtue of their role as providers of effective, beneficial, and therapeutic comfort measures.

References

1. Acute Pain Management Guideline Panel. Acute Pain Management Operative or Medical Procedures and Trauma. Guideline Report. AHCPR Pub. No 92-0022. Agency for Health Care Policy and Research, Public Health Service, U.S. Department of Health and Human Services, Rockville, MD, 1992

2. Muller RA, Pelczynski L: You can control cancer pain with drugs but the proper way may surprise you. Nursing 12:50, 1982
3. Paice JA: The phenomenon of analgesic tolerance in cancer pain management. Oncol Nurs Forum 15:455, 1986

Appendix 29-1*

BRIGHAM AND WOMEN'S HOSPITAL

PAIN MANAGEMENT

RESOURCE GUIDE

FOR

PATIENT CONTROLLED ANALGESIA

Developed By:

Marjorie Bowe, BSN, RN
Ellen Deering, MPA/H, RN
Frances Diggins, RN
Margaret Doyle, MS, RN
Michael Ferrante, MD
Phyllis Hoopman, MS, RN
Jeanne Lanchester, RN
Rosemary McErlane, RN
Evangeline McNeil, RN

Ruth Muller, MS, RN
Steve Powell, Pharm. D
Elisabeth Ollis, RN
Peggy Raeke, BSN, RN
Paul Souney, R.Ph, MS
Ellen Sullivan, BSN, RN
Tim VadeBoncouer, MD
Mary T. Walsh, BSN, RN

---

* From Brigham and Women's Hospital Pain Treatment Service, Boston, MA, 1991, with permission.

Brigham and Women's Hospital

The contents of the Pain Management Resource Guide as listed below have been developed and approved.

- Margaret Doyle, MS, RN
  Director OR/RR Nursing   _____

- Michael Ferrante, MD
  Pain Treatment Service   _____

- Phyllis Hoopman, MS, RN
  Director Surgical Nursing   _____

- Victor Yick
  Vice-President, Surgical Services   _____

Protocol for Patient-Controlled Analgesia (PCA-Plus) General Units
Protocol for Patient-Controlled Analgesia for Recovery Room and OB RR
Criteria for Patient-Controlled Analgesia
Patient-Controlled Analgesia Glossary of Terms
Considerations if Analgesia Inadequate
Patient-Controlled Analgesia Titration and Rescue
Physician Order Sheet for PCA-Plus
Patient-Controlled Analgesia Flow Sheet
Procedure for the Use of Patient Controlled Analgesia (PCA-Plus)
  Infuser Pump (Model 4100) - General Units
Fast Load for PCA-Plus - RR areas
PCA Narcan Guidelines
Incompatabilities
Additional Narcotics for PCA Administration

BRIGHAM AND WOMEN'S HOSPITAL
DEPARTMENT OF NURSING

PROTOCOL FOR PATIENT-CONTROLLED ANALGESIA (PCA)

Patient-controlled analgesia is an innovative and effective approach to pain relief. It allows the patient to self-administer a predetermined dose of intravenous narcotic. The interval between possible dosages is also predetermined, as well as the total possible dose in a four hour period.

The benefits of patient-controlled analgesia are multiple. The patient administers the narcotic when he feels that his discomfort is no longer tolerable (ie. when it increases above the minimal level). As the drug is administered intravenously at the time of patient need, comfort is achieved more rapidly and effectively than with the traditional IM/SC route of narcotic administration. Serum drug concentration remains relatively stable within the therapeutic range, obliterating the pain/ sedation cycle that accompanies fluctuation in serum drug concentration following IM/SC narcotic administration. Patient-controlled analgesia has proven successful in relieving acute pain associated with surgery, trauma (assuming that the patient's neurological status is normal) and burn debridement. It may also be utilized to relieve chronic, severe pain associated with malignancy.

General Information: Patient Controlled Analgesia

1. The goal of patient-controlled analgesia is to make the patient
   as comfortable as possible without excessive sedation.   A
   continuous 100% pain free state may not be realistic, as even
   with PCA the patient may experience some discomfort with ie.
   deep breathing/coughing and initial postop ambulation. Comfort
   level is assessed frequently after initiation of PCA using the
   0-10 pain scale.

2. Literature reports no significant increase in respiratory
   depression, hypotension or sedation with PCA over IM/SC
   narcotic administration. It is important to realize
   that these problems may be due to other causes than
   PCA, but their presence requires a reduction or
   cessation of PCA dosage and further patient evaluation.
   Nausea/vomiting and urinary retention may occur with narcotics
   in general. Gastric distress may also occur due to general
   anesthesia, paralytic ileus or nasogastric tube malfunction.

3. The venous access is to be assessed at a minimum of every two
   hours. In the event that this access can not be restarted,
   the physician (Pain Service) should be notified so
   that IM/SC "rescue" doses can be given to maintain comfort
   during the interval before PCA can be restarted or replaced by
   an alternative pain management plan. PCA administrative tubing
   is changed every 72 hours. Incremental doses of narcotics are
   recorded every two hours. Although narcotics are compatible
   with many medications, a second venous access may be necessary
   in the event of an incompatible product or blood therapy.

4. As narcotics are controlled substances, safety measures must be
   comprehensive to satisfy federal regulations. A key is used to
   lock the syringe cartridge into the pump and to lock the pump
   onto the pole. The key is maintained on the unit's narcotic key
   chain. Partially used syringe cartridges are to be disposed
   according to hospital policy. Two people (RN/MD or RN) are to
   witness the wasting of unused narcotic.

5. At any time, the patient may choose to terminate PCA therapy and
   switch to the traditional IM/SC narcotic method. Notify the
   M.D. (Pain Treatment Service Beeper #1842).

Patient Statement

   Patient-controlled analgesia may be initiated, monitored,
   adjusted and discontinued by a Registered Nurse upon a physician
   order. The nurse will assess and reinforce patient education
   prior to initiating PCA and throughout the patient pain
   management course.

PCA narcotic must be reordered every 72 hours, while maintenance IV solutions are ordered every 24 hours. The simultaneous use of <u>any</u> other narcotic analgesic is contraindicated without the approval of the Pain Service MD. IV tubing is to be changed every 72 hours. IV Peripheral access is preferred, but Central Line access may be used with a specific physician order.

<u>Criteria for Patient-Controlled Analgesia</u>

<u>SUGGESTED **CRITERIA FOR P.C.A. PLUS THERAPY**</u>:

Patient will be:

- alert and oriented

- able to communicate response to treatment

- physically able to push the demand button

<u>SPECIAL **CONSIDERATIONS**</u>:

Patients with a history of:

- narcotic addiction/substance abuse

- psychiatric disorder

- respiratory disorder

will be individually assessed for inclusion in the program.

<u>CONTRAINDICATIONS</u>

- language barrier

- inability to physically activate the demand button

- inability to cognitively activate the demand button

Patient Controlled Analgesia (PCA)

Glossary of Terms

Bolus (Loading Dose and Rescue Dose)

The goal of the bolus and rescue dose is to establish a therapeutic serum drug concentration. The initial dose of medication administered prior to initiation of PCA therapy or as additional doses to supplement PCA therapy.

Intermittent PCA dose (PCA dose)

The amount of drug administered when the patient activates the demand button.

Continuous Dose Rate

The rate, in ml/hr. of drug administered by continuous infusion.

Lockout Interval

(Time Delay)

The period of time following an administered dose during which the patient cannot receive additional narcotic, despite activation of the demand button.

Four Hour Limit

The maximum amount of medication the patient can receive over a four-hour period through the PCA.

Titration (Sliding Scale)

The incremental amount of narcotic which may be administered based on the patient's pain level.

Pain Scale

The patient's perception of the level or pain they are experiencing using the 0-10 measure.

0 = no pain   10 = excruciating
                          pain

0 1 2 3 4 5 6 7 8 9 10

Emetic Score

Degree of nausea experienced by the patient.

0 = nausea
1 = nausea present
2 = nausea with retching
3 = nausea with vomiting

0   1   2   3

General Guidelines:

PATIENT/FAMILY EDUCATION

Patient education is to take place prior to surgery. Instruction is
to be reinforced at the time of PCA initiation and throughout pain
management evaluation.

Topics include:

* Need for venous access
* Safety mechanisms of the pump and nursing practice
* Patient activation of the demand button
* Report to the nurse any pain despite activation of the demand
  button, pain/swelling/leakage at the IV site, respiratory
  difficulty, nausea/vomiting, urinary retention, or pruritus
  (itching).
* Option to discontinue PCA therapy for an alternative pain management
  program
* Activation of the pain control demand is to be done by the patient/
  nurse with emphasis to the family/visitors not to activate the PCA
  demand button.

NURSING GUIDELINES

1. All registered nurses must have documented attendance at
    the inservice on the PCA INFUSER and demonstrate competency.
    Under no circumstances can any staff nurse who has not attended
    the inservice manage a PCA infuser.

2. PCA is administered only upon the written order of the pain
    service physician or anesthesiologist.

3. It is the responsibility of the registered nurse to change
    the I.V. tubing every 72 hours. This includes PCA line and
    mainline infusion tubing.

4. It is the responsibility of the registered nurse to assess
    and document status on the PCA flow sheet:

    a. Date and time PCA was initiated and dosing parameters.

    b. Baseline vital signs as per protocol.

    c. Amount of milligrams of medication used and total doses.

    d. Patient's pain level, respiration rate, emetic score and
        IV access status at a minimum of every two hours.

    e. Blood pressure and pulse as indicated in physician order.

    f. MD/RN initial and validating signature.

Brigham and Women's Hospital
Department of Nursing
Protocol for Patient-Controlled Analgesia (PCA)
Recovery Room

Any post-op patient on whom a PCA pump is ordered will have the pump attached and programmed according to the physicians' orders by the Recovery Room nurse. It is within the clinical judgement of the nurse whether to administer the loading doses via the pump or the traditional I.V. push method. If the loading dose option is utilized, it should be recorded on the R.R. flow sheet and the pump's history should be cleared prior to calibration for patient use.

Those patients judged by the nurse to be capable of self pain control will be able to utilize the pump in the recovery room and during transfer to the patient unit. Whether or not the patient has begun self pain control is to be noted on the recovery room flow sheet and communicated during the nursing report to the patient unit.

Fast Load PCA Method for RR
    (40) Seconds)

Press On Button, read info screen.
Press Yes/Enter to clear history.
Press No to purge.
Press Yes/Enter for drug.
Press No to loading dose.
Press Yes for PCA mode.
Enter bolus dose, press Enter.
Press Enter for 5 minute bolus interval.
Press No for 4-hour limit. Press Enter.
Close and Lock door.
Press Button on blue pendant to give bolus.
Continue to press button PRN. (1 second)

To bolus before 5 minutes protocol; open door, press LOADING DOSE, press Yes, enter dose, press enter, press LOADING DOSE, close and lock door. (10 seconds)

Brigham and Women's Hospital
Nursing Department
Considerations If Analgesia Inadequate

Reminders   Points of Emphasis

If analgesia is inadequate, a
checklist evalution should be
performed to correct the problem.

A. Is I.V. patent?   A. Patient may be using PCA but
                                           not receiving drug secondary
                                           to nonpatent I.V.

B. Is patient using the demand PCA?   B. Patient may have
                                           misunderstood
                                           PCA instructions. Patient
                                           needs reinforcement of
                                           teaching and
                                           reassurance.

C. Is patient using demand PCA   C. If patient is only demanding
    maximally?   a PCA dose once or twice per
                                           hour, he/she needs to be
                                           reminded that
                                           button can be pressed
                                           whenever patient feels
                                           pain. Needs
                                           reinforcement/reassurance
                                           that addiction will not
                                           occur.

D. If answers to A, B, and C are
    Yes, the patient probably
    requires a titration dose of
    narcotic to obtain analgesia.
    Refer to PCA orders for
    titration dosing.

Brigham and Women's Hospital
Department of Nursing
Guidelines for
TITRATION AND RESCUE
FOR PCA-PLUS

Monitoring:
Record baseline: HR, BP, RR. Initiate PCA therapy and record HR,
BP, RR, q 15 min X 2 q 2° X 2 (i.e., for 4°), then HR, BP, q 4°,
thereafter. Record RR, response to narcotic and emetic score q 2°
on PCA flow sheet.

> **DRUG: Morphine Sulfate**
> **Concentration: 1 mg/1ml**

1. Initial Settings: as per
    anesthesiologist order.
    Customarily, PCA dose 2.0 mg (2 ml).
    Lockout interval time is 7 minutes
    Basal rate to be determined
    by MD, Pain Treatment Service.

2. IV
    Infuse D5W at KVO via Y-set
    if no maintenance IV solution
    ordered.

3. Rescue Loading Dose:
    Rescue Dose: if inadequate
    analgesia, RN may administer
    Morphine 1-3mg (1-3ml)
    I.V. q 5 minutes x 3 doses prn for
    pain via PCA pump. Thus, patient
    may receive 3 doses
    over 15 minutes to obtain
    analgesia. Maximum dose =
    9 mg (9ml). *Rescue may be
    exercised once every 8
    hours if necessary.

4. Titrated PCA Doses:
    If pain is still not controlled,
    increase initial PCA
    dose setting by 0.5mg (0.5ml)
    If analgesia not effective
    within one hour, then
    call the Pain Treatment Service.

5. If undue sedation, decrease PCA
    dose setting to: "Off position."
    Maintain IV. Call Pain Treatment
    Service.

6. Hold PCA and call Pain Treatment
    Service, beeper #1842 if these
    conditions occur

    (a) HR = 50
    (b) SBP ◄ 90
    (c) RR ◄ 8
    (d) 4-hour limit of drug is reached
        before 4 hours has elapsed

7. No systemic narcotics to be given
    except by order of Pain Treatment
    Service beeper #1842.

8. Notify Pain Treatment Service
    when PCA discontinued.

Brigham and Women's Hospital
Department of Nursing
Guidelines for
TITRATION AND RESCUE
FOR PCA-PLUS

Monitoring:
Record baseline: HR, BP, RR. Initiate PCA therapy and record
HR, BP, RR, q 15 min X 2 q 2° X 2 (i.e., for 4°), then HR, BP,
q 4 hr. thereafter. Record RR, response to narcotic and emetic
score q 2 hr PCA flow sheet.

> **Drug: Meperidine HCl (Demerol)**
> **Concentration: 10 mg/1ml**

1. Initial Setting: as per
   anesthesiologist order.
   PCA dose 13mg (1.3ml).
   Lockout interval time is 7 minutes.
   Continuous drip rate to be determined
   by MD, Pain Treatment Service.

2. IV:
   Infuse D5W at KVO via Y-set
   if no maintenance IV solution
   ordered.

3. Rescue Loading Doses:
   If inadequate analgesia,
   RN may administer
   Meperidine 10-30 mg.
   (1-3ml). I.V. q 5 minutes
   x 3 doses for pain. Thus,
   patient may receive 3 doses
   over 15 minutes to obtain
   analgesia. Maximum dose =
   90 mg (9ml). *Rescue dosing
   may be exercised once every
   8 hours if necessary.

4. Titrated PCA Doses:
   If pain is still not controlled,
   increase initial PCA dose
   setting by 5mg (0.5ml).
   If analgesia not effective
   within one hour, then
   call the Pain Treatment Service

5. If undue sedation, decrease PCA
   dose setting to: "Off position".
   Maintain IV. Call Pain
   Treatment Service.

6. Hold PCA and call Pain Treatment
   Service, beeper #1842 if these
   conditions occur

   (a) HR = 50
   (b) SBP ◄ 90
   (c) RR ◄ 8
   (d) 4-hour limit of drug is reached
       before 4 hours have elapsed

7. No systemic narcotics to be given
   except by order of Pain Treatment
   Service beeper #1842.

8. Notify Pain Treatment Service
   when PCA discontinued.

BRIGHAM AND WOMEN'S HOSPITAL

ADDITIONAL NARCOTICS FOR PCA ADMINISTRATION

Drug (concentration)	PCA Dose (mg)	Lockout Interval (min)
Dilaudid (0.2mg/ml)	0.05-0.25	5-10
Methadone (1mg/ml)	0.5-2.5	8-20
Oxymorphone (0.25 mg/ml)	0.2-0.4	8-10
Fentanyl (0.01 mg/ml)	0.01-0.02	3-10
Nalbuphine (1 mg/ml)	1-5	5-15

30

Management of a Postoperative Pain Service at a Teaching Hospital

Timothy R. VadeBoncouer
F. Michael Ferrante

Whenever the treatment of postoperative pain entails the concurrent management of several patients, a formally organized acute pain service (APS) is necessary. The APS should be physician-based, with anesthesiologists best suited to be the physicians-in-charge. Anesthesiologists possess knowledge and skills critical for the effective management of postoperative pain and the proper functioning of an APS: knowledge of local anesthetics and other analgesics, understanding of the effects of anesthesia on postoperative recovery, knowledge of nociceptive pathways and potential sites of pharmacologic modulation, and technical competence for performance of peripheral nerve, epidural, or subarachnoid anesthetic or analgesic techniques.

The formation of an APS allows for the prompt, efficient care of many patients in a hospital setting. It facilitates day-to-day analgesic management, provides a forum for resident teaching, and expands the visibility of the anesthesiologist as a caregiver *outside* the operating room.

As a gross generalization, the considerations underlying the organization of an APS are personnel- and equipment-oriented, and will be reviewed in the remainder of the chapter. The guidelines presented in this chapter are suggestions for the effective management of a university hospital-based service. They should be incorporated into a specific APS only within the constraints of a particular institution's standards of practice. Certainly, particular facets of this discussion will not be applicable to the private sector and should be ignored or adapted at the discretion of the individual practitioner.

PERSONNEL

The most important elements in the structure of an APS are the human elements. The APS should be viewed as a team composed of anesthesiologists, nurses, and pharmacists.

Anesthesiology

A staff anesthesiologist, interested and dedicated to pain management, should be the physician-in-charge of the APS. Responsibilities of the APS leader include consultation regarding pain-related problems, the teaching of residents and fellows, and assistance in the performance and teaching of procedures (e.g., nerve blocks, thoracic epidural techniques). Rounds should be made daily with the APS team leader in attendance to facilitate both patient care and teaching.

The simultaneous treatment of patients in widespread areas of a large hospital necessitates an adequately sized staff in order to respond promptly to the analgesic needs of individual patients. Residents (as part of a month-long rotation) and fellows (during 12 months of postgraduate training) make up the remainder of the anesthesiologists on the APS staff.

APS personnel—whether attending, resident, or fellow—must always be readily available to respond to the patient in pain, making adjustments in therapy and treating drug side effects. Physicians specifically dedicated to the APS should ideally be in-hospital 24 hours a day. (Under the most optimal circumstances, the responsibilities of the APS should **not** be divided between the operating room and the management of pain.) Where this is not practical, an in-hospital anesthesiologist covering for the operating room or recovery room should be responsible for overnight pain management. Staffing requirements should be tailored to the needs of a particular practice or institution. When many patients are being treated simultaneously, the expertise and dedication to pain management that will be provided by an in-hospital APS physician is invaluable and essential.

Nursing

Whether in the recovery room, on postsurgical wards, or in intensive care units, nurses are the primary moment-to-moment caregivers for patients managed by the APS. The frequent evaluation of the patient's level of pain and the observation of side effects of therapy are the task of the primary nurse. Critical information is then relayed to the APS. As such, nurses need to be extensively educated regarding all aspects of the various analgesic modalities used by the

APS. Most clinical aspects of patient-controlled analgesia (PCA) and epidural analgesia are new to the nurse. Thus, the level of education required for efficient APS operation is determined in the context of how day-to-day management will be carried out.

If epidural opioids and PCA are the only modalities in use, nurses can be taught to inject epidural catheters, to monitor side effects, to detect subarachnoid or intravenous catheter migration, and to change PCA drug cartridges. If this is not institutionally feasible, a more cursory education regarding basic aspects of the various analgesic techniques and the recognition of typical side effects will suffice. In all cases, extensive education regarding the technical aspects of equipment used by the APS (i.e., PCA and epidural infusion pumps) is mandatory.

If epidural local anesthetics are used, either alone or in combination with opioids, it is imperative that anesthesia personnel be available and responsive to any and all problems. The consequences of the untoward side effects of epidural local anesthetics are sufficiently severe to necessitate this degree of physician accountability. Nonetheless, nursing staff should be educated to recognize and anticipate hypotension, sensory and motor blockade, and inadvertent subarachnoid catheter migration in patients receiving epidural local anesthetics.

Familiarity with all aspects of PCA is also highly desirable when numerous patients use this modality on a widespread scale. Recognition of inadequate analgesia or the occurrence of side effects is crucial for the success of PCA. With appropriate training and education, adjustments in PCA therapy (including provision for rescue doses of opioid) can be performed by the nurse in accordance with physician orders. The routine use of a fixed-dose or a fixed-lockout interval for all patients is doomed to failure. Adjustment of these parameters by nursing in accordance with physician prescription enhances the efficacy and improves patient satisfaction with PCA.

Pharmacy

Hospital pharmacy services are essential for the day-to-day management of the APS. Pharmacy's most vital function is the preparation, storage, and dispensing of the solutions used for epidural analgesia and/or PCA. If continuous epidural infusions are used, they should be of a sufficient volume to permit renewal on at least a once-a-day basis. If solutions are of small volume and delivered at high rates, the necessity of frequent prescription renewal will become prohibitive. Since most epidural infusion rates do not exceed 15 ml/h, a 200–300-ml solution will usually last 24 hours.

In our practice, combinations of epidural local anesthetic and opioid are ordered daily, using preservative-free normal saline to bring the solution volume to 200 or 300 ml (Table 30-1). The use of a saline diluent permits easy preparation of a solution containing nearly any concentration of local anesthetic and/or opioid that is desired. Epidural solutions should be clearly marked in order to avoid inadvertent intravenous delivery or vice versa (see section on Equipment).

TABLE 30-1. Preparation of Selected Epidural Infusions

B 1/8 D2.5*		**D2.5**	
0.25% Bupivacaine	100 ml		
PF meperidine	10 ml (500 mg)	PF meperidine	10 ml (500 mg)
PFNS	90 ml	PFNS	190 ml
B 1/8 F5		**F5**	
0.25% Bupivacaine	100 ml		
Fentanyl	20 ml (1 mg)	Fentanyl	20 ml (1 mg)
PFNS	80 ml	PFNS	180 ml
B 1/8 M0.05		**M0.05**	
0.25% Bupivacaine	100 ml		
PF morphine	10 ml (10 mg)	PF morphine	10 ml (10 mg)
PFNS	90 ml	PFNS	190 ml

Abbreviations: PF, Preservative-free; PFNS, Preservative-free normal saline.
* Epidural solutions may be abbreviated by listing the local anesthetic and/or opioid followed by the respective concentration after each letter:
For example, B 1/8 D2.5 = 0.25% bupivacaine with 2.5 mg of demerol/ml
F5 = 5 µg of fentanyl/ml
M0.05 = 0.05 mg of morphine/ml.

Epidural solutions need to be stored and dispensed properly, as they usually contain opioid, a controlled substance. Anticipation of daily requirements can be made in advance by noting the number and type of surgical procedures to be performed on a particular day. In this way, several solutions can be prepared in advance so that epidural infusion therapy can begin promptly when patients arrive in the postanesthesia care unit.

Although a number of PCA infusers use prepackaged cartridges of opioid, it may be necessary with some systems for these cartridges or syringes to be prepared by the pharmacy. The issues of storage and dispensing of opioids for PCA are the same as those described for epidural solutions.

The input of pharmacy personnel is essential, especially when concerns of drug compatibility or side effects arise. In our practice, we are periodically joined by a member of the hospital pharmacy on APS rounds. Such collaboration provides a forum for understanding the peculiar pharmaceutic needs of the APS and facilitates the communication required to maintain a continuous working relationship between physician and pharmacist.

EQUIPMENT

Technical developments now allow the safe continuous epidural administration of local anesthetics or opioids via sophisticated infusion devices. Similarly, the technology of PCA infusers allows the administration of small doses of intravenous opioids at frequent intervals, ensuring continuous analgesic blood levels.

There are many commercially available PCA infusers, and these devices have been intensively reviewed in Chapter 10. Although experience with PCA infusers has been extensive (allowing determination of optimal pump characteris-

TABLE 30-2. Essential Design Features of Epidural Infusion Systems

Ease of operation
Rate-limited flow (not >25 ml/h)
Ease of identification as specific to epidural use (dedication)
Absence of accessory administration ports (Y-ports) on tubing
Security of drug (tamper protection)
Portability to allow ambulation
Extensive monitoring features (e.g., pulse oximetry, apnea monitors) are **not** essential or even desirable

tics), there is minimal to no literature guiding the optimal choice of features for epidural infusion devices. In the opinion of the authors, several key features are necessary for safe administration of epidural infusions via pumps. These pump characteristics are listed in Table 30-2. Infusion devices meeting most of these criteria are reviewed in Figures 30-1 to 30-3 and Table 30-3.

Ease of Operation

Although it may not seem obvious, ease of operation is the most important feature of pump design. If we can borrow from the experience with PCA devices, most problems associated with pump use occur at the machine-user interface.[1] Elimination of misprogramming and mishaps by simplification of operation will prevent serious untoward sequelae from accidental administration of large amounts of drug into the epidural space.

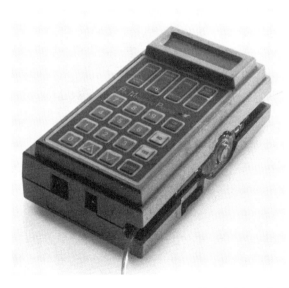

Fig. 30-1. Abbott Pain Management Provider (without lockbox).

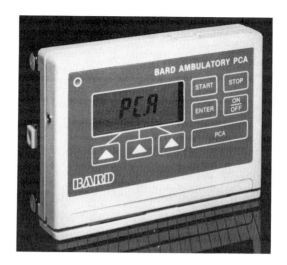

Fig. 30-2. Bard Ambulatory PCA.

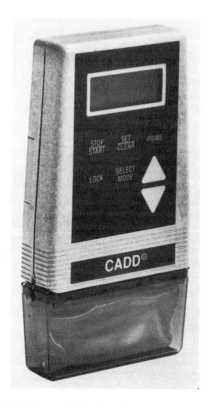

Fig. 30-3. Pharmacia Deltec CADD-PCA Model 5800.

TABLE 30-3. Epidural Infusion Devices

	Abbott Pain Management Provider	Bard Ambulatory PCA Pump	Pharmacia Deltec CADD-PCA Model 5800
Ease of operation	+ + + (adaptation of LifeCare PCA software)	+ + +	+ + (circular logic)
Rate-limited flow	<26 ml/h	<21 ml/h	<21 ml/h
Reservoir	100, 250, or 500 ml	100, 250, or 500 ml[a]	50 or 100 ml
Extension sets	No Y-ports (yellow stripe on tubing for ease of identification)	No Y-ports	No Y-ports
Security	Lockbox Keypad lockout	Access code	3 programmable lock levels
Portability	+ + +	+ + +	+ + +
Pump mechanism	Rotary peristaltic	Linear peristaltic	Linear peristaltic
Power requirements	AC or 9V battery	9V battery	9V battery
Printer	External	External	None

[a] At time of writing, 510K approval from the Food and Drug Administration is pending for the 500-ml reservoir.

Rate-limited Flow

A *mandatory* feature of epidural infusion devices is rate limitation of flow. Rate limitation can prevent the potentially catastrophic, accidental administration of massive amounts of drug into the epidural space. An optimal upper limit for speed of administration appears to be 20–25 ml/h.

Dedication

It is wise to specifically dedicate a particular infusion device to epidural use only. Practitioners will be immediately alerted to the presence of an epidural infusion by the physical appearance of the machine. Such distinctiveness in the mind of practitioners will prevent misprogramming and accidental administration of drugs into the epidural space.

At first glance, dedication of a device to epidural use only would not seem to be cost-effective. Furthermore, it would seem to add an increased layer of complexity to the administration of infusions within a hospital. However, the risk of a potential death from an accidental overdose of epidural drugs far outweighs any benefit from uniformity (use of one infusion device for all purposes).

It might be possible to design a single all-purpose infusion device suitable for epidural use. However, this device would be exceedingly complex and would need both hardware and software "fail-safes" for epidural use.

Besides dedication of epidural pumps, easily identifiable containers for epidural solutions should be used. Brightly colored labels or distinctive packaging designs are convenient ways to clearly mark solutions as dedicated for epidural use only.

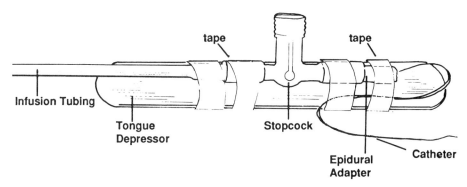

Fig. 30-4. Epidural injection port system.

Injection Ports

The plastic tubing connecting the solution to the epidural catheter should have *no* infusion (Y) ports, completely obviating the accidental administration of intravenous agents into the epidural space.

Since patients receiving epidural analgesia will periodically require epidural injections for "breakthrough" pain, it is necessary to have an easily accessible injection site. A three-way stopcock placed between the plastic tubing and the epidural adapter is a simple method of ensuring easy access to the injection port (Fig. 30-4). This assembly can be taped to a wooden tongue depressor along with a small loop of epidural catheter. The whole assembly may then be affixed to the patient's hospital gown by a safety pin. This assembly significantly reduces the incidence of accidental catheter disconnection associated with patient movement.

Security

No system is tamperproof, although manufacturers do their best to provide security. Devices use keypad lockout sequences, numeric codes, and different levels of lockout to prevent inappropriate access to the infuser. Unfortunately, resourceful patients can memorize sequences and codes to obtain access to the drug by reprogramming the infuser and increasing their dose or by administering an injection.

The containers for epidural solutions should preferably be situated within the infuser itself. This will minimize accidental administration of drugs not designated for epidural use. Some manufacturers encase both the infusion device and solution within a Plexiglass compartment (lockbox). Such systems are acceptable, if at times a bit awkward. A "spiked-vial" system with tubing and bottle external to the pump mechanism or lockbox should not be used as such a system increases the possibility of tampering and drug administration error.

Portability

Portability of the infusion device is not absolutely essential. However, epidural analgesia can promote earlier ambulation and shortened convalescence. Therefore, an infusion device promoting portability seems appropriate.

Monitors

The role of respiratory monitors has been extensively reviewed in Chapter 11. The reader is referred to that source for a lengthy discussion of this issue.

Clinical experience suggests that opioid-induced respiratory depression can be readily detected by frequent assessment of respiratory rate and wakefulness.[2] The use of respiratory monitors (e.g., pulse oximetry, apnea monitors) may offer no advantage over this approach and may actually provide a false sense of security. Bedside assessment of respiratory rate and level of arousal would seem to offer many advantages over a cumbersome respiratory monitor. Mandatory monitors or intensive care unit observation for all patients receiving epidural opioids could make management of a large service both financially and logistically prohibitive. Recently, a large prospective study has demonstrated the safety of epidural opioid administration to patients monitored on nursing floors with respiratory rates alone.[3] The incidence of respiratory depression was 0.2 percent. All cases of respiratory depression were discovered without the use of expensive monitors and were treated appropriately.

OPERATION OF AN ACUTE PAIN SERVICE

Figure 30-5 indicates the manner in which patients are admitted to the APS. An initial order must be written by the primary physician requesting a consult from the APS to evaluate the nature and severity of the pain and to institute the most appropriate analgesic regimen. Differences exist among various analgesic modalities in terms of the efficacy. In general, PCA is not as efficacious as epidural analgesia. However, side effects are more frequently associated with use of epidural analgesia.[4] If an APS is allowed to become only a PCA service, a number of patients will have inadequate analgesia because of the severity of pain attendant on their type of surgery (e.g., thoracotomy, total knee replacement). Similarly, an APS should not be allowed to become a purely epidural analgesia service because of the inadequate reimbursement for PCA in many states. Many patients do quite well with PCA and should not be subjected to invasive procedures because of unenlightened third-party payors.

From a practical point of view, the evaluation of the postsurgical patient and the institution of analgesic therapy is most conveniently initiated in the postanesthesia care unit (PACU). If PCA is to be used, nursing staff should institute PCA in the PACU. The analgesic agent, incremental dose, lockout interval, background infusion (if applicable) and 1- and 4-hour limits (if applica-

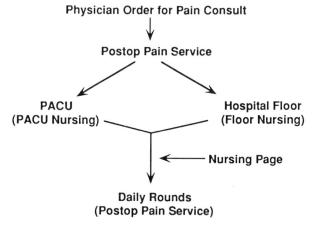

PATIENT-CONTROLLED ANALGESIA

Physician Order for Pain Consult

Postop Pain Service

PACU
(PACU Nursing)

Hospital Floor
(Floor Nursing)

Nursing Page

Daily Rounds
(Postop Pain Service)

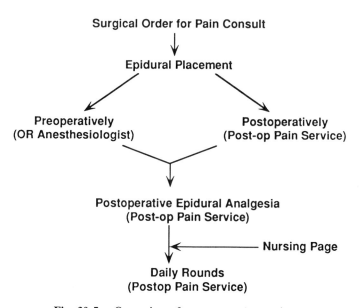

POSTOPERATIVE EPIDURAL ANALGESIA

Surgical Order for Pain Consult

Epidural Placement

Preoperatively
(OR Anesthesiologist)

Postoperatively
(Post-op Pain Service)

Postoperative Epidural Analgesia
(Post-op Pain Service)

Nursing Page

Daily Rounds
(Postop Pain Service)

Fig. 30-5. Operation of an acute pain service.

ble) are determined by the anesthesiologist. As PCA allows flexibility in analgesic regimen, nursing staff should be capable of increasing or decreasing dosage to provide an individualized analgesic regimen. An anesthesiologist must always be available for consultation if inadequate analgesia persists or serious side effects occur.

If epidural analgesia is used, the epidural catheter may be placed preoperatively by the anesthesiologist assigned to the anesthetic care of the surgical patient or postoperatively by the postoperative pain team. After placement of the epidural catheter, the appropriate local anesthetic, opioid, or combination may be administered either on an intermittent basis or as a continuous infusion.

Nursing staff on wards must be conversant with the potential side effects of epidural local anesthetics and/or opioids. A vigilant and well-educated nursing staff is the *best* monitor for anticipation of potential side effects related to analgesic therapy.

Documentation

Bedside rounds should be conducted each day by the APS for all patients receiving analgesic care. This contact accomplishes two goals. One, rounds permit a ready determination of patient satisfaction with analgesic treatment. A numeric pain score can be obtained from each patient, providing a raw objective measurement of the effectiveness of analgesia. The presence of side effects can also be determined at the bedside and appropriate measures instituted. Secondly, bedside rounds allow the anesthesiologist to be seen as a caregiver *outside* the operating room, helping to dispel the myth of the "anesthesiologist-as-technician." This image can only foster an improved relationship between the anesthesiologist and other health care providers.

A note summarizing the patients' analgesic course is written in the chart as a part of daily rounds. Any necessary change in therapy (e.g., a change in epidural solution rate or concentration, a change in PCA dose or lockout interval) are also prescribed and documented at this time.

At Brigham and Women's Hospital, a computer-generated worksheet is used to follow patients receiving APS care (Fig. 30-6). The patient's name and location, the surgical procedure, date of surgery, type of therapy, drugs used, location of epidural catheter (when appropriate), rate of infusion (for epidural analgesia), global pain score over the last 24 hours, and presence of side effects are noted for all patients followed by the APS. This worksheet is updated and distributed to all the members of the APS team before morning and afternoon rounds. Additional space for billing data and for other pertinent clinical information is also provided on the worksheet. (A worksheet specific for the needs of a particular institution can be easily developed through the use of commercially available computer "spreadsheet" programs.)

At the time epidural analgesia or PCA is instituted, a standard order sheet is completed (Figs. 30-7 and 30-8). These preprinted sheets include standing orders for treatment of common side effects, observation algorithms, procedures

PAIN TREATMENT SERVICE

BWH DEPT OF ANESTHESIA

5-Apr-92

BILL	LOC	NAME	NUMBER	A/S	PROCEDURE	DATE	Type	INFUSION	RATE	VNS	N	S	P	R	MB	OTHER
	15A	Doe, Jane	10485967	63F	Rt Total Knee Replacemen	3-Apr	L3-4	B1/8D2.5	6	1			X			mild pruritis (Rx with benadryl)
	11B	Jefferson, Tom	10097654	43M	Rt Thoracotomy	1-Apr	T6-7	B1/8F5	4	2						
	6A	Public, Jane	10574980	43F	Abd. Hysterectomy	4-Apr		PCA	Morphine	2/7/30	1	X					mild nausea, Rx with compazine
	5C	Calamity, Jane	10098345	32F	Ovarian cystectomy	1-Apr		PCA	Morphine	1/9/C1	1						

Fig. 30-6. Acute pain treatment service worksheet. This sheet is updated prior to morning and afternoon rounds. *Type* is usually PCA or epidural catheter location. *Infusion* is epidural solution or PCA drug. *Rate* is milliliter per hour for epidurals and demand dose per lockout interval (min) per 4-h limit or continuous infusion (C) (mg/h) for PCA. *VNS* is verbal numeric pain score from 0 (no pain) to 10 scale (worst pain). *N*, *S*, *P*, *R*, and *MB* refer to nausea, sedation, pruritus, respiratory depression, and motor block, respectively. *Other* allows room for communication about management problems among pain treatment staff. The worksheet is only a model.

BRIGHAM AND WOMEN'S HOSPITAL
A Teaching Affiliate of Harvard Medical School

PHYSICIAN'S ORDERS

Drug Allergies: _____

DATE	TIME	PHYSICIAN S ORDERS	POSTED
		PATIENT—CONTROLLED ANALGESIA ORDERS	
		1 While using PCA, patient is to receive no other	
		narcotics unless approved by the Pain Treatment Service.	
		2 Mode of operation will be PCA only, unless specified below.	
		3 Morphine: (1 mg/ml — 30 ml cartridge) Check: _____	
		Meperidine: (10 mg/ml — 30 ml cartridge) Check: _____	
		Other: ( ) Check: _____	
		4 Initial intermittent PCA dose: _____ (mg)	
		5 Initial lockout interval: _____ (min)	
		6 Initial 4 hr limit: _____ (mg/4 hr)	
		7 Rescue loading doses: Morphine: 1 — 3 mg q 5 min x3 prn	
		Meperidine: 10 — 30 mg q 5 min x3 prn	
		8 If pain not controlled after rescue doses x3, titrate PCA dose upward	
		by 0.5 mg if Morphine or 5mg if Meperidine.	
		9 If pain still not controlled 1 hour after titration, call Beeper 1842.	
		10 Tape ampule of Narcan (Naloxone - 1 ml - 0.4 mg/ml) to PCA device.	
		11 Benadryl 25 mg po or IM q4-6h prn pruritis	
		12 Compazine 10 mg IM q4h prn nausea (unless antiemetic ordered by primary care MD)	
		13 On patient units, RN will record venous access check, respiratory rate,	
		response to narcotic (0—10 scale), and emetic score (0—3 scale) q2h on PCA flowsheet.	
		Other vital signs as per nursing protocol or primary care MD orders.	
		14 Call Pain Treatment Service (Beeper 1842) for:	
		a) Pulse below: _____ ; b) Systolic B/P below: _____ ; c) RR below 8/min	
		d) 4 hour limit of drug is reached before 4 hours elapse.	
		M.D. SIGNATURE _____	

MEDICATIONS MAY BE GENERICALLY AND/OR THERAPEUTICALLY INTERCHANGED AS APPROVED BY THE PHARMACY AND THERAPEUTICS COMMITTEE.

IMPORTANT - BE SURE TO IMPRINT PATIENT IDENTIFICATION. DETACH ONE UNDERNEATH COPY
        EACH TIME MEDICATION ORDER IS WRITTEN AND FORWARD TO PHARMACY.
    IF NO YELLOW COPY SHOWS THROUGH HOLE AT RIGHT, START A NEW FORM   ⟶   PP-0067

Fig. 30-7. A typical standard order sheet for patients receiving PCA. (Courtesy of Brigham and Women's Hospital, Boston.)

BRIGHAM AND WOMEN'S HOSPITAL
A Teaching Affiliate of Harvard Medical School

PHYSICIAN'S ORDERS

Drug Allergies: _____

DATE	TIME	PHYSICIAN'S ORDERS	POSTED
		Orders for Epidural/Intrathecal Opiate and/or Local Anesthetic Infusion	
	1	Medication:	
	2	No parenteral or oral narcotics without notification of the anesthesiologist	
	3	Tylenol 325 mg tabs, 1-2 tabs q 3-4 h P.O. prn	
	4	Heplock or IV at all times	
	5	Heel pads	
	6	Apnea monitor or pulse oximeter	
	7	RR q _____ hour	
	8	Narcan 0.4 mg ampule at bedside	
	9	Page Beeper 1623 for:	
		a Inadequate analgesia	
		b RR _____ Systolic BP	
		c Pruritis, nausea, vomiting	
		d Somnolence or confusion	
		e Dressing problems - blood and/or saturation of dressing	
		f catheter problems - (Don't discontinue infusion because of seperation of catheter from hub)	
		g Increasing motor or sensory block	
		h Problems with apnea monitor	
	10	Call a code green anesthesia for an emergent problem	
	11	Straight cath q6° PRN	
	12	Please check BP q5 min X5 after each bolus	

MEDICATIONS MAY BE GENERICALLY AND/OR THERAPEUTICALLY INTERCHANGED AS APPROVED BY THE PHARMACY AND THERAPEUTICS COMMITTEE.

IMPORTANT . BE SURE TO IMPRINT PATIENT IDENTIFICATION. DETACH ONE UNDERNEATH COPY EACH TIME MEDICATION ORDER IS WRITTEN AND FORWARD TO PHARMACY.
IF NO YELLOW COPY SHOWS THROUGH HOLE AT RIGHT, START A NEW FORM ——➤

20-12
0515775
Rev 10/84

Fig. 30-8. A typical standard order sheet for patients receiving epidural analgesia. (Please note that use of apnea monitoring or pulse oximetry is *not* standard and must be ordered individually.) (Courtesy of Brigham and Women's Hospital, Boston.)

TABLE 30-4. Problems Associated with Management of an APS

Increasing demand for services
Lack of trained or interested anesthesia personnel
Inappropriate reimbursement
Nursing–anesthesia interactions
Surgical–anesthesia interactions

for notifying the APS when complications occur, and algorithms for nursing administration of opioid via the PCA infuser for breakthrough pain. Subsequent orders are written daily (e.g., renewal of epidural solutions) on standard physician's order forms.

PROBLEMS ASSOCIATED WITH AN ACUTE PAIN SERVICE

The management of acute pain, and specifically postoperative pain, is one of the most rapidly expanding areas of service for the hospital-based anesthesiologist. A number of problems still exist regarding the role of anesthesia in the organization and supervision of an APS (Table 30-4). There is clearly an ever-increasing demand for these analgesic services. Unfortunately, demand often outstrips supply, as there is still a lack of anesthesia personnel who are properly trained or even interested in the management of patients outside the operating room. In many areas, reimbursement for these services is clearly inappropriate, despite the obvious benefits to patients. The successful management of an APS requires close interaction between nursing, surgical, and anesthesia personnel. At times this may prove difficult but should not be impossible, provided that all recognize that the primary concern is to provide superior analgesia for all patients.

At the present time, the knowledge, equipment, and agents are available to essentially render most patients pain-free during and after surgery. Unfortunately, a number of practical problems must still be resolved before all patients can benefit from the knowledge and techniques that currently exist.

References
1. Callan CM: An analysis of complaints and complications with patient-controlled analgesia. p. 139. In Ferrante FM, Ostheimer GW, Covino BG (eds): Patient-Controlled Analgesia. Blackwell Scientific Publications, Boston, 1990
2. Ready LB, Oden R, Chadwick HS et al: Development of an anesthesiology-based postoperative pain management service. Anesthesiology 68:100, 1988
3. Ready LB, Loper KA, Nessly M, Wild L: Postoperative epidural morphine is safe on surgical wards. Anesthesiology 75:452, 1991
4. Eisenach JC, Grice SC, Dewan DM: Patient-controlled analgesia following cesarean section: a comparison with epidural and intramuscular narcotics. Anesthesiology 68:444, 1988

31

α_2-Agonists

F. Michael Ferrante

The α_2-adrenergic agonists are just beginning to be introduced into clinical practice. Although release of an α_2-agonist by industry for clinical use is several years away, there is accumulating clinical experience with these agents. Thus, a brief discussion of the molecular pharmacology, physiologic effects, and clinical experience with α_2-agonists is warranted. An introduction to the pharmacology of α_2-receptors[1] (and the autonomic nervous system in general) may be found in Chapter 3.

MOLECULAR PHARMACOLOGY

The α_2-adrenergic agonists may be grouped into three classes: (1) *phenylethylamines* (α-methylnorepinephrine), (2) *imidazolines* (clonidine, dexmedetomidine), and (3) *oxaloazepines* (azepexole). Clonidine (Fig. 31-1) is a *selective α_2-agonist* with an affinity ratio of 200:1 (α_2/α_1). In models of α_2-agonist action, clonidine has been identified as a partial agonist. Dexmedetomidine (another imidazoline) is an order of magnitude more selective than clonidine and is a full agonist at the α_2-receptor (termed *superselective*).[2]

The α_2-receptor itself is a glycoprotein with a single polypeptide chain. The polypeptide weaves back and forth through the cell membrane and folds back on itself to form the site for ligand binding. The cytoplasmic side of the receptor protein forms contact points for its coupling molecule, the guanine nucleotide binding protein (G protein). The G protein promotes transmembrane signaling to a discrete effector mechanism, which may be a transmembrane ion channel or an intracellular second-messenger cascade (Fig. 31-2).[3]

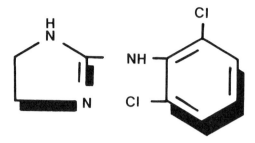

Fig. 31-1. Clonidine.

PHYSIOLOGIC RESPONSES MEDIATED BY α_2-RECEPTOR ACTIVATION

Neuroendocrine System

The α_2-agonists potently inhibit sympathoadrenal outflow. Decreased levels of circulating norepinephrine and diminished levels of catecholamine metabolites are found in the urine after clonidine administration.[4] In healthy human volunteers this sympathoinhibitory effect has been shown to result from decreased release of neurotransmitter at the synaptic junction.[5,6] Whether this results from a central effect on sympathetic outflow or presynaptic inhibition at the neuroeffector junction is unknown in humans. A central site of action is present in rats.[7]

Release of growth hormone is enhanced by α_2-agonists, although the underlying mechanism is unknown.[8] However, α_2-agonists inhibit the release of insulin by a direct effect on the islets of Langerhans.[9] This effect is short-lived and does not appear to present any clinical problems.[10]

As a class of drugs, all imidazolines can inhibit steroidogenesis in the adrenal gland as a result of their chemical structure rather than α_2-agonism per se.[11] Also, adrenocorticotropic hormone (ACTH) release from the pituitary gland is inhibited.[12]

Cardiovascular System

Postsynaptic α_1- and α_2-adrenoreceptors coexist on both arterial and venous smooth muscle. They mediate vasoconstriction independent of the nerve supply to the vasculature.[13]

The effects of α_2-agonists on the coronary circulation are controversial and may be species-specific. There is great interspecies variation in the presence and distribution of α_2-adrenoreceptors in the coronary circulation of different species. Poststenotic myocardial ischemia induced by stimulation of sympathetic nerves can be ameliorated by clonidine through centrally mediated reduction in sympathetic outflow.[14] It has been suggested that α_2-agonists mediate release of an endothelium-derived relaxation factor, as it is difficult to demon-

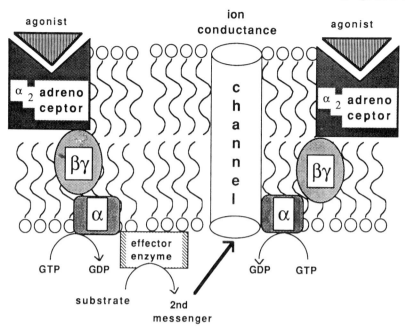

Fig. 31-2. Proposed molecular mechanism for analgesic action of α₂-agonists. After an α₂-agonist binds to the α₂-adrenoreceptor, guanosine diphosphate (GDP) is replaced by guanosine triphosphate (GTP) on the α subunit of the pertussis toxin-sensitive guanine nucleotide binding protein (G protein). This activated subunit can change the gating of an ion conductance channel by (1) a membrane-delimited process, or (2) alteration of the activity of an effector enzyme. The effector enzyme changes the rate of generation of a second messenger and, ultimately, modulation of the ion channel. (From Maze and Tranquilli,[3] with permission.)

strate α₂-adrenoreceptor mediated coronary vasoconstriction in vivo.[15,16] The effects of α₂-agonists on the regional blood flow in other vascular beds are even less well-studied.

The hypotension caused by administration of α₂-agonists is believed to be caused by central vasomotor effects.[17–19] The site of action within the brain remains obscure. The bradycardia induced by α₂-agonists is probably mediated by enhanced baroreflex sensitivity[20] and/or presynaptic inhibition of norepinephrine release at the synaptic junction[21] and/or vagomimetic effects.[22]

Respiratory System

Clonidine is the best studied of the α₂-agonists with respect to respiratory effects. Ventilatory and occlusion pressure response to carbon dioxide were shifted to the right by oral clonidine in healthy volunteers.[23] However, the effects of clonidine were minor in comparison with those of opioids.[23] Furthermore, synergism did not exist between the respiratory depressant effects of opioids and clonidine.[23]

Renal System

The α_2-agonists induce a diuresis in all animal models, although the mechanism(s) involved are species-dependent.[24–30]

Gastrointestinal System

Salivary gland secretion is reduced by α_2-agonists and is probably due to a direct effect.[21,31] Activation of prejunctional α_2-adrenoreceptors produces inhibition of vagally mediated release of gastric acid from parietal cells.[32] In humans, however, there does not appear to be any change in gastric pH.[33] The α_2-agonists also decrease vagally mediated gastric and small bowel motility.[34]

Central Nervous System

The α_2-agonists produce sedation.[35–37] The issue concerning the presynaptic[38] versus postsynaptic[39] mechanism underlying the sedative effects of α-agonists remains controversial.

The α_2-agonists (and particularly those with particularly high α_2 affinity, such as dexmedetomidine) exert anxiolytic effects similar to benzodiazepines.[2,40] Clonidine is biphasic in its effect. Clonidine exhibits anxiolytic characteristics at low α_2 concentrations but anxiogenic effects at higher doses, through an α_1 mechanism.[41] Other selective α_2-agonists (e.g., guanabenz, azepexole) exhibit such a paradoxical response at high doses.[42] In humans, clonidine has been administered acutely to patients with panic disorder.[43] Although effective for acute administration, the anxiolytic effect is lost with chronic administration.[43] The mechanism underlying this loss of effectiveness with chronic administration is unknown.

A summary of the physiologic effects of α_2-agonists is found in Table 31–1.

MECHANISM OF ANALGESIA

Schmitt et al[44] were the first to demonstrate profound analgesia associated with neuraxial (intracerebroventricular) administration of α-sympathomimetic compounds. The further investigation of neuraxial administration of α-adrenergic agonists has been fostered by the search for alternative and/or adjunctive agents to neuraxial opioids and their attendant side effects.

There is evidence suggesting that the analgesia attendant to administration of α_2-agonists may be partially mediated through opioid-dependent and opioid-independent mechanisms and pathways of the descending modulating system (see Ch. 2). Evidence supporting at least partial involvement of endogenous opioids include (1) the ability of naloxone to antagonize α_2-mediated analgesia,[45,46] (2) the existence of cross-tolerance between α_2 and opioid antinociceptive effects,[47–49] and (3) the release of endogenous opioids on stimulation of α_2-receptors.[50,51] However, the lack of *universal* cross-tolerance[52] and the inability of naloxone to reverse α_2-mediated analgesia in certain situations[53,54] support the presence of opioid-independent analgesic systems.

TABLE 31-1. Physiologic Responses Mediated by α_2-Agonists

Response	Mechanism
Neuroendocrine	
↓ adrenal medullary function	↓ neurotransmitter release
↑ growth hormone secretion	Postsynaptic hypophyseal effect
↓ insulin secretion	Direct effect on β cells
↓ adrenal cortical function	↓ ACTH secretion
	↓ steroidogenesis (imidazoline moiety)
Cardiovascular	
Vasoconstriction	Postsynaptic smooth muscle
Coronary vasodilation	Endothelium-derived releasing factor
Hypotension	Central vasomotor effect
Bradycardia	↓ baroreflex sensitivity, presynaptic inhibition of NE release, vagomimetic effect
Respiratory	
Shift of the CO_2 response curve	Direct effect on brain stem respiratory centers
Renal	
Diuresis	Inhibition of ADH release, blockade of ADH action, ↑ GFR, inhibition of renin secretion
Gastrointestinal	
↓ salivation	Inhibition of ACH release
↓ bowel motility	Inhibition of ACH release
Central Nervous System	
Sedation	↑ stage I and II sleep
Anxiolysis	↓ NE neurotransmission

Abbreviations: ACh, acetylcholine; ACTH, adrenocorticotropic hormone; ADH, antidiuretic hormone; GFR, glomerular filtration rate; NE, norepinephrine.

The greatest evidence in support of opioid-independent analgesia relates to the presence of noradrenergic descending modulating pathways (see Ch. 2).[55] There is clear evidence of α_2-adrenergic receptors in the dorsal horn.[56] Axons of noradrenergic cell bodies located in the rostroventral medulla and dorsolateral pons terminate in the dorsal horn of the spinal cord and are implicated in the modulation of nociception[57] (see Ch. 2).

Irrespective of the controversy surrounding opioid-dependent and opioid-independent mechanisms of α_2-induced analgesia, there is much data suggesting synergism between α_2-agonists and opioids at the level of the spinal cord. Omote et al[58] demonstrated a synergistic interaction between δ-receptor-mediated opioid analgesia and clonidine on the wide dynamic range neuron. Two studies using a rat model have demonstrated heightened analgesic responses from subanalgesic doses of subarachnoid clonidine and subarachnoid or systemic morphine.[49,59]

CLINICAL ANALGESIC STUDIES

Systemic Administration

Systemically administered dexmedetomidine,[60] as well as subarachnoid clonidine,[61] have been shown to relieve tourniquet-induced ischemic pain.

Patients recovering from spinal fusion have been administered clonidine by continuous intravenous infusion for postoperative analgesia. Patients received either saline or 5 mg/kg of clonidine over 1 hour as a loading dose followed by 0.3 mg/kg/h for an additional 12 hours. Significantly less morphine supplementation was required within the clonidine-treated patients. There was little hemodynamic instability if preload was maintained.[62]

Transdermal administration of clonidine has also been shown to reduce postoperative morphine requirements after abdominal surgery.[63]

Epidural Administration

The use of epidural clonidine was first reported in two patients with neuropathic pain.[64] Since that initial report of its effectiveness, a number of studies have examined the use of epidural clonidine for postoperative,[35,65–67] oncologic,[36] and obstetric[37,68] pain management. (The use of clonidine for postcesarean pain management[37,68] was previously discussed in Ch. 23.)

Eisenach et al[35] reported on the use of 100–900 μg of epidural clonidine for postoperative analgesia in an open-dose escalation study in total knee replacement and abdominal surgery patients. The highest dose produced greater than 5 hours of analgesia without sensory or motor blockade. Transient sedation was achieved with higher doses and was attributed to significant systemic blood levels (up to 3.3 ng/ml). Although respiratory function was not tested with provocative examinations (CO_2 response), epidural clonidine had no significant effect on arterial blood gases at any dosage.

Gordh[65] studied epidural clonidine as compared with placebo for post-thoracotomy pain. Administration of 3 mg/kg of epidural clonidine did not reduce supplemental meperidine requirements.

Addition of clonidine (1 mg/kg) to epidural sufentanil has been shown to prolong the duration of analgesia.[66]

In a comparison of epidural and intramuscular clonidine (2 mg/kg) for postoperative pain of orthopedic or perineal surgery, no difference in pain scores was reported between the two groups. Interestingly, plasma clonidine levels and the incidence of hypotension, bradycardia, and sedation were similar between the two routes of administration.[67]

Subarachnoid Administration

Coombs et al[69] were the first to administer subarachnoid clonidine. Administration of 300 μg of clonidine produced greater than 18 hours of analgesia in a patient with terminal cancer.

Little work has been performed with subarachnoid administration of α_2-agonists. A group of French investigators has used clonidine to supplement spinal anesthesia with isobaric bupivacaine.[70] Time to two-segment regression was considerably prolonged with coadministration of clonidine (150 μg) as compared with epinephrine (200 μg) or saline.[70] Using hyperbaric bupivacaine in a subsequent study, coadministration of 400 μg of epinephrine and 150 μg of clonidine produced similar times for two-segment regression.[71]

CONCLUSION

It is clear from the preceding review of extant clinical analgesic studies that much more research is necessary before the proper role for systemic, epidural, or subarachnoid administration of α_2-agonists is determined. Certainly, the search for alternative neuraxial analgesics to the opioids will continue to foment investigation of the α_2-agonists. Their exact role as analgesics is as yet undetermined, but it will surely be as part of a combination of analgesics in a "balanced" technique.

References

1. Nichols AJ, Hieble JP, Ruffolo RR Jr: The pharmacology of peripheral α_1- and α_2-adrenoreceptors. Rev Clin Basic Pharm 7:129, 1988
2. Scheinin H, Virtanen R, MacDonald E et al: Medetomidine—a novel α_2-adrenoreceptor agonist: a review of its pharmacodynamic effects. Prog Neuropsychopharmacol Biol Psychiatry 13:635, 1989
3. Maze M, Tranquilli W: Alpha-2 adrenoreceptor agonists: defining the role in clinical anesthesia. Anesthesiology 74:581, 1991
4. Hokfelt B, Hedeland H, Hansson BG: The effect of clonidine and penbutolol, respectively on cateholamines in blood and urine, plasma renin activity and urinary aldosterone in hypertensive patients. Arch Int Pharmacodyn Ther 213:307, 1975
5. Veith RC, Best JD, Halter JB: Dose-dependent suppression of norepinephrine appearance rate in plasma by clonidine in man. J Clin Endocrinol Metab 59:151, 1984
6. Conway EL, Brown MJ, Dollery CT: No evidence for involvement of endogenous opioid peptides in effects of clonidine on blood pressure, heart rate and plasma norepinephrine in anesthetized rats. J Pharmacol Exp Ther 299:803, 1984
7. Svenson TH, Bunney BS, Aghajanian GK: Inhibition of both noradrenergic and serotonergic neurons in brain by the α-adrenergic agonist clonidine. Brain Res 92:291, 1975
8. Grossman A, Weerasuriya K, Al-Damluji S et al: α_2-Adrenoreceptor agonists stimulate growth hormone secretion but have no acute effects on plasma cortisol under basal conditions. Horm Res 25:65, 1987
9. Angel I, Langer SZ: Adrenergic-induced hyperglyccmia in anaesthetized rats: involvement of peripheral α_2-adrenoreceptors. Eur J Pharmacol 154:191, 1988
10. Massara F, Limone P, Cagliero E et al: Effects of naloxone on the insulin and growth hormone responses to α-adrenergic stimulation with clonidine. Acta Endocrinol (Copenh) 103:371, 1983
11. Maze M, Banks S, Daunt D et al: Effect of dexmedetomidine, an imidazoline α-2 adrenergic agonist on steroidogenesis. In vivo and in vitro studies. Eur J Pharmacol 183:2343, 1990
12. Lanes R, Herrera A, Palacios A, Moncada G: Decreased secretion of cortisol and ACTH after clonidine administration in normal adults. Metabolism 32:568, 1983
13. Ruffolo RR Jr: Distribution and function of peripheral α-adrenoreceptors in the cardiovascular system. Pharmacol Biochem Behav 22:827, 1985
14. Heusch G, Schipke J, Thamer V: Clonidine prevents sympathetic initiation and aggravation of poststenotic myocardial ischemia. J Cardiovasc Pharmacol, suppl. 8: S33, 1986
15. Thom S, Hayes R, Calvete J, Sever PS: In vivo and in vitro studies of α_2-adrenoreceptor responses in human vascular smooth muscle. J Cardiovasc Pharmacol, suppl. 7:S137, 1985

16. Furchgott RF, Vanhoutte PM: Endothelium-derived relaxing and contracting factors. FASEB J 3:2007, 1989
17. Bousquet P, Schwartz J: α-Adrenergic drugs. Pharmacological tools for the study of the central vasomotor control. Biochem Pharmacol 32:1459, 1983
18. Bousquet P, Feldman J, Bloch R, Schwartz J: The nucleus reticularis lateralis: a region highly sensitive to clonidine. Eur J Pharmacol 69:389, 1981
19. Kubo T, Misu Y: Pharmacologic characterization of the α-adrenoreceptors responsible for a decrease of blood pressure in the nucleus tractus solitarii of the rat. Naunyn Schmiedebergs Arch Pharmacol 317:120, 1981
20. Harron DW, Riddell JG, Shanks RG: Effects of azepexole and clonidine on baroreceptor mediated reflex bradycardia and physiological tremor in man. Br J Clin Pharmacol 20:431, 1985
21. Reid JL, Wing LM, Mathias CJ et al: The central hypotensive effects of clonidine, Studies in tetraplegic subjects. Clin Pharmacol Ther 21:375, 1977
22. de Jonge A, Timmermans PB, van Zwieten PA: Participation of cardiac presynaptic $α_2$ adrenoreceptors in the bradycardic effects of clonidine and analogues. Naunyn Schmiedebergs Arch Pharmacol 317:8, 1981
23. Bailey PL, Sperry RJ, Johnson GK et al: Respiratory effects of clonidine alone and combined with morphine, in humans. Anesthesiology 74:43, 1991
24. Humphreys MH, Reid IA, Chou LY: Suppression of antidiuretic hormone secretion by clonidine in the anaesthetized dog. Kidney Int 7:405, 1975
25. Kimura T, Share L, Wang BC, Crofton JT: The role of central adrenoreceptors in the control of vasopressin release and blood pressure. Endocrinology 108:1829, 1981
26. Peskind ER, Raskind MA, Leake RD et al: Clonidine decreases plasma and cerebrospinal fluid arginine vasopressin but not oxytocin in humans. Neuroendocrinology 46:395, 1987
27. Smyth DD, Umemura S, Pettinger WA: $α_2$-Adrenoreceptor antagonism of vasopressin-induced changes in sodium excretion. Am J Physiol 248:F767, 1985
28. Stanton B, Puglisi E, Gellai M: Localization of $α_2$-adrenoreceptor-mediated increase in renal Na^+, K^+, and water excretion. Am J Physiol 252:F1016, 1987
29. Strandhoy JW: Role of α-2 receptors in the regulation of renal function. J Cardiovasc Pharmacol, suppl 8:S28, 1985
30. Smyth DD, Umemura S, Yang E, Pettinger W: Inhibition of renin release by α-adrenoreceptor stimulation in the isolated perfused rat kidney. Eur J Pharmacol 140:33, 1987
31. Watkins J, Fitzgerald G, Zamboulis C et al: Absence of opiate and histamine H_2 receptor-mediated effects of clonidine. Clin Pharmacol Ther 28:605, 1980
32. Cheng HC, Gleason EM, Nathan BA et al: Effects of clonidine on gastric secretion in the rat. J Pharmacol Exp Ther 217:121, 1987
33. Orko R, Poutto J, Ghignone E, Rosenberg PH: Effects of clonidine on haemodynamic responses to endotracheal intubation and on gastric acidity. Acta Anaesthesiol Scand 31:325, 1987
34. Wikberg J: Localization of adrenergic receptors in guinea pig ileum and rabbit jejunum to cholinergic neurons and to smooth muscle cells. Acta Physiol Scand 99:190, 1977
35. Eisenach JC, Lyzak SZ, Viscomi CM: Epidural clonidine analgesia following surgery: phase I. Anesthesiology 71:640, 1989
36. Eisenach JC, Rauck RL, Buzzanelli C, Lysak SZ: Epidural clonidine analgesia for intractable cancer pain: phase I. Anesthesiology 71:647, 1989
37. Mendez R, Eisenach JC, Kashtan K: Epidural clonidine analgesia after cesarean section. Anesthesiology 73:848, 1990

38. Zebrowska-Lupina I, Przegalinski E, Sloniec M, Kleinrok Z: Clonidine-induced locomotor hyperactivity in rats. The role of central postsynaptic receptors. Naunyn Schmiedebergs Arch Pharmacol 297:227, 1977

39. Maze M, Doze VA, Chen BX: Functional antagonism of α_2 mediated hypnotic action by α_1 adrenergic mechanisms in rats, abstracted. FASEB J 2:A1559, 1988

40. Ferrari F, Tartoni PL, Marginfico V: B-HT 920 antagonizes rat neophobia in the X-Maze test: a comparative study with other drugs active as adrenergic and dopaminergic receptors. Arch Int Pharmacodyn Ther 298:7, 1989

41. Soderpalm B, Engel JA: Biphasic effects of clonidine on conflict behavior: involvement of different α-adrenoreceptors. Pharmacol Biochem Behav 30:471, 1988

42. Handley SL, Mithani S: Effects of α-adrenoreceptor agonists and antagonists in a maze-exploration model of "fear"-motivated behavior. Naunyn Schmiedebergs Arch Pharmacol 327:1, 1984

43. Uhde TW, Stein MB, Vittone BJ et al: Behavioral and physiologic effects of short-term and long-term administration of clonidine in panic disorder. Arch Gen Psychiatry 46:170, 1989

44. Schmitt H, Le Douraec JC, Petillot N: Antinociceptive effects of some alpha-sympathomimetic agents. Neuropharmacology 13:289, 1974

45. Loomis CW, Jhamandas K, Milne B, Cervenko F: Monoamine and opioid interactions in spinal analgesia and tolerance. Pharmacol Biochem Behav 26:445, 1987

46. Mastrianni JA, Abbott FV, Kunos G: Activation of central mu-opioid receptors is involved in clonidine analgesia in rats. Brain Res 479:283, 1989

47. Paalzow G: Development of tolerance to the analgesic effect of clonidine in rats. Cross-tolerance to morphine. Naunyn Schmiedebergs Arch Pharmacol 304:1, 1978

48. Post C, Archer T, Minor BG: Evidence for cross-tolerance to the analgesic effects between morphine and selective α_2-adrenoreceptor agonists. J Neural Transm 72:1, 1988

49. Ossipov MH, Suarez LJ, Spaulding TC: Antinociceptive interactions between alpha-2 adrenergic and opiate agonists at the spinal level in rodents. Anesth Analg 68:194, 1989

50. Farsang C, Varga K, Vajda L et al: β-Endorphin contributes to the antihypertensive effect of clonidine in a subset of patients with essential hypertension. Neuropeptides 4:293, 1984

51. Xie CW, Tang J, Hans JS: Clonidine stimulated the release of dynorphin in the spinal cord of the rat: a possible mechanism for its depressor effects. Neurosci Lett 65:244, 1986

52. Yaksh TL, Reddy SV: Studies in the primate on the analgetic effects associated with intrathecal actions of opiates, alpha-adrenergic agonists and baclofen. Anesthesiology 54:451, 1981

53. Sullivan AF, Dashwood MR, Dickenson AH: α_2-Adrenoreceptor modulation of nociception in rat spinal cord: location, effects and interaction with morphine. Eur J Pharmacol 138:169, 1987

54. Curtis AL, Marwah J: Evidence for α adrenoreceptor modulation of the nociceptive jaw opening reflex in rats and rabbits. J Pharmacol Exp Ther 238:576, 1986

55. Fitzgerald M: Momoamines and descending control of nociception. Trends Neurosci 9:51, 1986

56. Fleetwood-Walker SM, Mitchell R, Hope PJ et al: An α_2 receptor mediates the selective inhibition by noradrenaline of nociceptive responses of identified dorsal horn neurones. Brain Res 334:243, 1985

57. Westlund KN, Bowker RM, Ziegler MG, Coulter JD: Origins and terminations of

descending noradrenergic projections to the spinal cord of monkey. Brain Res 292: 1, 1984

58. Omote K, Kitahata CM, Collins JG et al: Interactions between opiate subtype and alpha-2 adrenergic agonists in suppression of noxiously evoked activity of WDR neurons in the spinal dorsal horn. Anesthesiology 74:737, 1991

59. Drasner K, Fields HL: Synergy between the antinociceptive effects of intrathecal clonidine and systemic morphine in rats. Pain 32:309, 1988

60. Kauppila T, Kemppainen P, Tanila H, Pertovaara A: Effects of medetomidine, an α_2-adrenoreceptor agonist, on experimental pain in humans. Anesthesiology 74:3, 1991

61. Bonnet F, Diallo A, Saada M et al: Prevention of tourniquet pain by spinal isobaric bupivacaine with clonidine. Br J Anaesth 63:93, 1989

62. Bernard JM, Lechevalier T, Pinaud M, Passut N: Postoperative analgesia by IV clonidine, abstracted. Anesthesiology 71:A154, 1989

63. Segal IS, Jarvis DJ, Duncan SR et al: Clinical efficacy of transdermal clonidine during the perioperative period. Anesthesiology 74:220, 1991

64. Tamsen A, Gordh T: Epidural clonidine produces analgesia (letter). Lancet ii:231, 1984

65. Gordh T Jr: Epidural clonidine for treatment of postoperative pain after thoracotomy. A double-blind placebo-controlled study. Acta Anaesthesiol Scand 32:702, 1988

66. Vercauteren M, Lauwers E, Meert T et al: Comparison of epidural sufentanil plus clonidine with sufentanil alone for postoperative pain relief. Anaesthesia 45:531, 1990

67. Bonnet F, Boico O, Rostaing S et al: Clonidine-induced analgesia in postoperative patients: epidural versus intramuscular administration. Anesthesiology 72:423, 1990

68. Huntoon M, Eisenach JC, Boese P: Epidural clonidine after cesarean section. Appropriate dose and effect of prior local anesthetic. Anesthesiology 76:187, 1992

69. Coombs DW, Saunders RL, Lachance D et al: Intrathecal morphine tolerance: use of intrathecal clonidine, DEDLE, and intraventricular morphine. Anesthesiology 62:358, 1985

70. Racle JP, Benkhadra A, Pog JY, Gleizal B: Prolongation of isobaric bupivacaine spinal anesthesia with epinephrine and clonidine for hip surgery in the elderly. Anesth Analg 66:442, 1987

71. Racle JP, Poy JY, Benkhadra A et al: Prolongation of spinal anesthesia with hyperbaric bupivacaine by adrenaline and clonidine in the elderly. Ann Fr Anesth Reanim 7:139, 1988

Index

Page numbers followed by *f* indicate figures; those followed by *t* indicate tables.

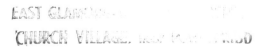